Textbook of
Orthopaedics,
Trauma and
Rheumatology

For Elsevier:
Commissioning Editor: Andrew Miller, Alison Taylor
Development Editor: Kim Benson
Production Manager: Elouise Ball
Design: Sarah Russell
Illustration Manager: Gillian Richards
Illustrator: Oxford Illustrations

Textbook of **Orthopaedics, Trauma** and **Rheumatology**

Edited by

Raashid Luqmani DM, FRCP, FRCPEdin
Consultant Rheumatologist/Senior Lecturer,
Nuffield Orthopaedic Centre and Oxford University, Oxford, UK

James Robb BSc(Hons), MD, FRCSEd, FRCSGlasg, FRCPEdin
Consultant Orthopaedic Surgeon, Royal Hospital for Sick Children, Edinburgh;
Honorary Senior Lecturer, University of Edinburgh, Edinburgh;
Senior Lecturer in Surgery, University of St Andrews, St Andrews, UK

Daniel Porter BSc(Hons), MD, FRCS(Tr & Orth)
Consultant Orthopaedic Surgeon and Senior Lecturer, University of Edinburgh, UK

John F. Keating MB, BCh, FRCSI, FRCSEd, FRCSEdOrth, MPhil
Consultant Orthopaedic Surgeon and Honorary Senior Lecturer, University of Edinburgh, UK

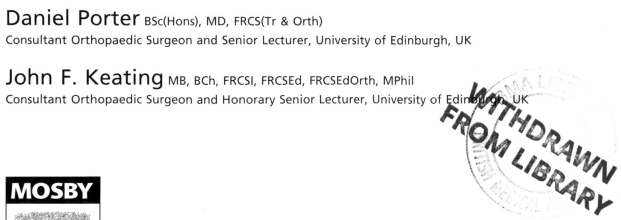
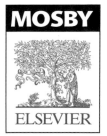

MOSBY

ELSEVIER

EDINBURGH LONDON NEW YORK OXFORD PHILADELPHIA ST LOUIS SYDNEY TORONTO 2008

MOSBY
ELSEVIER

ISBN: 978-0-7234-3389-7

British Library Cataloguing in Publication Data
A catalogue record for this book is available from the British Library.

Library of Congress Cataloging in Publication Data
A catalog record for this book is available from the Library of Congress.

Note
Knowledge and best practice in this field are constantly changing. As new research and experience broaden our knowledge, changes in practice, treatment and drug therapy may become necessary or appropriate. Readers are advised to check the most current information provided (i) on procedures featured or (ii) by the manufacturer of each product to be administered, to verify the recommended dose or formula, the method and duration of administration, and contraindications. It is the responsibility of the practitioner, relying on their own experience and knowledge of the patient, to make diagnoses, to determine dosages and the best treatment for each individual patient, and to take all appropriate safety precautions. To the fullest extent of the law, neither the Publisher nor the Editors assume any liability for any injury and/or damage to persons or property arising out or related to any use of the material contained in this book.

The Publisher

Printed in China

▌Contents

PAEDIATRICS   303

DEVELOPING WORLD   355

Problem-orientated section

CASES   365

ANSWERS   411

List of contributors

E. Nicole Amft MD, PhD, FRCP(Edin)
Consultant Rheumatologist, Rheumatic
Diseases Unit, Western General Hospital,
Edinburgh; Honorary Senior Lecturer,
University of Edinburgh, Edinburgh, UK

Ian Beggs FRCR
Consultant Musculoskeletal Radiologist, Royal
Infirmary of Edinburgh, Edinburgh, UK

Matthew A. Brown MD, FRACP
Professor of Immunogenetics, University of
Queensland, Queensland, Australia

Ian N. Bruce MD, FRCP
Reader and Honorary Consultant in
Rheumatology, arc Epidemiology Unit, School
of Translational Medicine, University of
Manchester, and The Kellgren Centre for
Rheumatology, Manchester Royal Infirmary,
Manchester, UK

Christopher D. Buckley MBBS, DPhil, FRCP
ARC Professor of Rheumatology, MRC Centre
of Immune Regulation, University of
Birmingham, Birmingham, UK

Anthony K. Clarke MD, FRCP
Honorary Consultant in Rheumatology &
Rehabilitation, Royal National Hospital for
Rheumatic Diseases, Bath, UK

Sally E. Edmonds MD, FRCP
Consultant Rheumatologist, Stoke Mandeville
Hospital; Consultant Paediatric Rheu-
matologist, The Nuffield Orthopaedic Centre,
Oxford, UK

Paul Eunson MB, ChB, FRCPCH
Consultant Paediatric Neurologist, Royal
Hospital for Sick Children, Edinburgh, UK

Hill Gaston MA, PhD, FRCP, FMedSci
Professor of Rheumatology, University of
Cambridge, Cambridge, UK

Sheena Hennell RGN, MSc
Nurse Consultant Rheumatology, Wirral
University Teaching Hospital NHS Foundation
Trust, Wirral, UK

Geoff Hooper MB, ChB, MMSc, FRCS,
FRCSEd(Orth)
Formerly Consultant Orthopaedic and Hand
Surgeon, St John's Hospital, Livingston, and
Honorary Senior Lecturer, University of
Edinburgh, Edinburgh, UK

Benjamin Joseph MS(Orth), MCh(Orth)
Professor of Orthopaedics, Kasturba Medical
College, Manipal, Karnataka, India

John F. Keating MB, BCh, FRCSI, FRCSEd,
FRCSEdOrth, MPhil
Consultant Orthopaedic Surgeon and Senior
Lecturer, University of Edinburgh, UK

Gabrielle H. Kingsley BSc, PhD, FRCP
Reader in Rheumatology, Department of
Rheumatology, King's College London School
of Medicine, London, UK

Mark Lillicrap MA, PhD, BM, BCh, MRCP, ILT(M),
PGCMedEd
Consultant Rheumatologist, Hinchingbrooke
Hospital, Huntingdon; Associate Clinical
Dean, University of Cambridge, Cambridge,
UK

Raashid Luqmani DM, FRCP, FRCP(Edin)
Consultant Rheumatologist, Rheumatology
Department, Nuffield Orthopaedic Centre,
Oxford, UK

Malcolm F. Macnicol MB, ChB, BSc(Hons), MCh,
FRCS, FRCSEd(Orth), FRCP(Edin), DipSportsMed
Consultant Orthopaedic Surgeon, Royal
Hospital for Sick Children and Royal
Infirmary; Part-time Senior Lecturer,
University of Edinburgh, Edinburgh, UK

Robert W. Marshall MB, BCh, FRCS(Eng)
Consultant Orthopaedic Surgeon, Royal
Berkshire Hospital, Reading, UK

Jacqueline Y. Q. Mok MD, FRCP(Edin), FRCPCH
DCH(Glas), MB, ChB
Consultant Paediatrician, NHS Lothian
University Hospitals Division; Part-time Senior
Lecturer, Section on Child Life and Health,
University of Edinburgh, Edinburgh, UK

Julia L. Newton DPhil, MRCP
Consultant Rheumatologist, Nuffield
Orthopaedic Centre, Oxford, UK

George Nuki MB, FRCP, FRCP(Edin)
Emeritus Professor of Rheumatology,
University of Edinburgh, and Honorary
Consultant Rheumatologist, Rheumatic
Diseases Unit, Western General Hospital,
Edinburgh, UK

Mark Paterson MB, BS, FRCS(Eng)
Consultant Paediatric Orthopaedic Surgeon, St
Bartholomew's and the Royal London
Hospitals, London, UK

Daniel Porter BSc(Hons), MD, FRCS(Tr & Orth)
Consultant Orthopaedic Surgeon and Senior
Lecturer, University of Edinburgh, UK

Stuart H. Ralston MB, ChB, MD, FRCP(Glas,
Edin) FMedSci
ARC Professor of Rheumatology; Head of the
School of Molecular and Clinical Medicine,
University of Edinburgh, Edinburgh, UK

James Robb BSc(Hons), MD, FRCSEd, FRCSGlasg,
FRCPEdin
Consultant Orthopaedic Surgeon, Royal
Hospital for Sick Children, Edinburgh;
Honorary Senior Lecturer, University of
Edinburgh, Edinburgh; Senior Lecturer in
Surgery, University of St Andrews, St
Andrews, UK

David L. Scott BSc, MD, FRCP
Professor of Clinical Rheumatology,
Department of Rheumatology, King's College
London School of Medicine, London, UK

David A. Sherlock DPhil, FRCS
Consultant Surgeon in Orthopaedics and
Trauma, The Royal Hospital for Sick
Children and Southern General Hospital,
Glasgow, UK

Zoe Stableford SRCh, BSc
Senior Podiatrist, Department of Podiatry and
Foot Health, Hope Hospital, Salford, UK

Athanasios I. Tsirikos MD, FRCS, PhD
Consultant Orthopaedic and Spine Surgeon,
Scottish National Spine Deformity Centre,
Royal Hospital for Sick Children, Edinburgh;
Honorary Clinical Senior Lecturer, University
of Edinburgh, Edinburgh, UK

Nick Wilkinson DM, MRCP, MRCPCH
Consultant Paediatrician and Paediatric
Rheumatologist, Rheumatology Department,
Nuffield Orthopaedic Centre, Oxford, UK

Acknowledgements

Moral support:	Our wives
Secretarial support:	Kathryn Cook and Michelle Cook
Illustrations:	Paul Cooper, Medical Illustration Department, Nuffield Orthopaedic Centre, Oxford
	Dr Colin Smith, Consultant Pathologist, Western General Hospital, Edinburgh
	Hinchingbrooke Healthcare NHS Trust
	Many colleagues in Oxford and Edinburgh
Chapter 2:	Mr Maurice Adkins, Dr Vaiyapuri Palaniappan Sumathi MD FRCPath and Mr Andrew Thomas FRCS

List of abbreviations

18FDG	[^{18}F]fluorodeoxyglucose
^{99m}Tc	Technetium-99m
ABCDE	Airway maintenance with cervical spine protection, Breathing and ventilation, Circulation with haemorrhage control, Disability (neurological status), Exposure/Environmental control – undress the patient, but prevent hypothermia
AC	Adhesive capsulitis
ACE	Angiotensin converting enzyme
ACL	Anterior cruciate ligament
ADAM-TS	A disintegrin and metalloproteinase with thrombospondin motifs
ADL	Activities of daily living
AFO	Ankle–foot orthosis
AIDS	Acquired immunodeficiency syndrome
AIS	Adolescent idiopathic scoliosis
AKA	Anti-keratin antibody
ALARA	As low as reasonably achievable
ALP	Alkaline phosphatase
ALPS	Autoimmune lymphoproliferative syndrome
AMPLE	Allergies, medications, past illnesses/pregnancy, last meal, events/environment of injury
ANA	Anti-nuclear antibody
ANCA	Anti-neutrophil cytoplasm antibody
Anti-Sm	Antibodies to Smith antigen
AP	Anteroposterior
APF	Anti-perinuclear factor
APL	Antiphospholipid
APS	Antiphospholipid syndrome
APTT	Activated partial thromboplastin time
ARDS	Acute respiratory distress syndrome
AS	Ankylosing spondylitis
ASA	American Society of Anesthesiologists
ASOT	Antistreptolysin O titre
ATLS	Advanced trauma life support
AVN	Avascular necrosis (also known as aseptic necrosis)
AZT	Azithromycin
BCP	Basic calcium phosphate
BMC	Bone mineral content
BMD	Becker muscular dystrophy
BMD	Bone mineral density
BMP	Bone morphogenetic protein
C1	Complement protein 1
C2	Complement protein 2
C3	Complement protein 3
C4	Complement protein 4
Ca(PO$_4$)OH$_2$	Calcium hydroxyapatite
CaH	Carbonic anhydrase
C-ANCA	Cytoplasmic anti-neutrophil cytoplasm antibody
CBFα1	Core binding factor α1
CCP	Cyclic citrullinated peptide
CD	Cluster of differentiation
CFS	Chronic fatigue syndrome
CINCA	Chronic infantile neurological cutaneous and articular syndrome
CK	Creatine kinase
CLCN7	Chloride channel 7
CMC	Carpometacarpal
CMV	Cytomegalovirus
CNS	Central nervous system
COL1α1	α1 chain of Type 1 collagen
COL1α2	α2 chain of Type 1 collagen
COX	Cyclo-oxygenase
CPPD	Calcium pyrophosphate dihydrate
CREST	Calcinosis, Raynaud's, (o)esophageal dysmotility, sclerodactyly, telangiectasia
CRP	C-reactive protein
CRPS	Complex regional pain syndrome
CS	Cushing's syndrome
Csk	C-terminal Rous sarcoma oncogene kinase
CT	Computed tomography
CTLA-4	Cytotoxic T-lymphocyte antigen-4
CTS	Carpal tunnel syndrome
DAS	Disease Activity Score
DC	Dupuytren's contracture
DEXA	Dual-energy X-ray absorptiometry
DIP(J)	Distal interphalangeal (joint)

DISH	Diffuse idiopathic skeletal hyperostosis
DM	Dermatomyositis
DM	Diabetes mellitus
DMARD	Disease-modifying anti-rheumatic drug
DMD	Duchenne muscular dystrophy
DNA	Deoxyribonucleic acid
DPL	Diagnostic peritoneal lavage
dsDNA	Double-stranded DNA
DVT	Deep vein thrombosis
DXA	Dual-energy X-ray absorptiometry
EBV	Epstein–Barr virus
ECG	Electrocardiograph
ECHO	Echocardiography
ECM	Extracellular matrix
ELISA	Enzyme-linked immunosorbent assay
EMG	Electromyography
ENA	Extractable nuclear antigen
ENPP1	Ectonucleotide pyrophosphatase/phosphodiesterase 1
ESR	Erythrocyte sedimentation rate
Fas	TNF receptor superfamily, member 6
Fc	Constant region of immunoglobulin protein
FCAS	Familial cold autoinflammatory syndrome
FCU	Familial cold urticaria
FES	Fat embolism syndrome
FGF	Fibroblast growth factor
FMF	Familial Mediterranean fever
FRZB	Frizzled-related protein
FSNGN	Focal segmental necrotizing glomerulonephritis
GALS	Gait, arms, legs, spine
GCS	Glasgow Coma Scale
GH	Growth hormone
GI	Gastrointestinal
GM-CSF	Granulocyte–macrophage colony-stimulating factor
GP	General practitioner
GSD	Glycogen storage disease
H2	Histamine receptor type 2
HA	Hydroxyapatite
HAD	Hospital Anxiety and Depression Scale
HAQ	Health Assessment Questionnaire
HIDS	Hyperimmunoglobulinaemia D and periodic fever syndrome

HIV	Human immunodeficiency virus
HKAFO	Hip–knee–ankle–foot orthosis
HLA	Human leucocyte antigen
HMSN	Hereditary motor and sensory neuropathy
HPRT	Hypoxanthine–guanine phosphoribosyl transferase
HRT	Hormone replacement therapy
HVR3	3rd hypervariable region
IBD	Inflammatory bowel disease
IBS	Irritable bowel syndrome
IGF-1	Insulin-like growth factor 1
IgG	Immunoglobulin G
IgM	Immunoglobulin M
IL-1	Interleukin 1
INR	International normalized ratio
IPJ	Interphalangeal joint
IVIG	Intravenous immunoglobulin
JDM	Juvenile dermatomyositis
JIA	Juvenile idiopathic arthritis
KAFO	Knee–ankle–foot orthosis
kD	Kilodalton
LAC	lupus anticoagulant
LCR	Locus control region
LFT	Liver function test
LJM	Limited joint mobility
LRP5	Lipoprotein receptor related protein 5
MCL	Medial collateral ligament
MCP(J)	Metacarpophalangeal (joint)
M-CSF	Macrophage colony-stimulating factor
MDP	Methylene diphosphonate
ME	Myalgic encephalomyelitis
MHC	Major histocompatibility complex
MHz	Megahertz
MICA	Major histocompatibility complex class I chain-related molecule A
mmHg	Millimetres of mercury
MMP	Metalloproteinase
MNC	Mononuclear cell
MR	Magnetic resonance
MRA	Magnetic resonance angiography
MRI	Magnetic resonance imaging
MRSA	Methicillin-resistant *Staphylococcus aureus*
MSUM	monosodium urate monohydrate
MTP(J)	Metatarsophalangeal (joint)
MVK	Mevalonate kinase
NAI	Non-accidental injury
NF	Neurofibromatosis

NICE	National Institute for Health and Clinical Excellence		RF	Rheumatic fever
NK	Natural killer		RF	Rheumatoid factor
NO	Nitric oxide		Rh	Rhesus
NSAID	Non-steroidal anti-inflammatory drug		RhF	Rheumatoid factor
			RNP	Ribonucleoprotein
NTPPH	Nucleoside triphosphate pyrophosphohydrolase		RSD	Reflex sympathetic dystrophy
			Scl-70	Scleroderma 70
OA	Osteoarthritis		SE	Shared epitope
OBPP	Obstetric brachial plexus palsy		SERM	Selective (o)estrogen receptor modulator
OE	Oestrogen			
OFC	Osteitis fibrosa cystica		SF	Synovial fluid
OI	Osteogenesis imperfecta		SF12	Short Form 12
ON	Osteonecrosis		SF36	Short Form 36
OPG	Osteoprotegerin		SI	Sacroiliac
OPLL	Ossification of posterior longitudinal ligament		SLE	Systemic lupus erythematosus
			SMA	Spinal muscular atrophy
P1NP	Procollagen type I nitrogenous propeptide		SpA	Spondyloarthritis (also known as spondyloarthropathy)
PAI	Plasminogen activator inhibitor		SPECT	Single-photon emission computed tomography
PAN	Polyarteritis nodosa			
P-ANCA	Perinuclear anti-neutrophil cytoplasm antibody		SSA	Sjögren's syndrome A antigen
			SSB	Sjögren's syndrome B antigen
PCL	Posterior cruciate ligament		STIR	Short T1 inversion recovery
pCO$_2$	Partial pressure of carbon dioxide		SUA	Serum uric acid
PCR	Polymerase chain reaction		TAR	Thrombocytopenia, absent radius
PD	Paget's disease		TB	Tuberculosis
PE	Pulmonary embolus		TCIRG1	T cell immune regulator 1
PET	Positron emission tomography		TENS	Transcutaneous electrical nerve stimulation
PFA	Persistent femoral anteversion			
PFAPA	Periodic fever, aphthous ulcer, pharyngitis, adenitis		TGF	Transforming growth factor
			TIMP	Tissue inhibitor of metalloproteinases
PG	Prostaglandin			
PIP(J)	Proximal interphalangeal (joint)		TLSO	Thoraco-lumbo-sacral orthosis
PIPJ	Proximal interphalangeal joint		TNF	Tumour necrosis factor
PM	Polymyositis		TRAPS	TNF receptor-associated periodic syndrome
PMN	Polymorphonuclear cell			
pO2	Partial pressure of oxygen		US	Ultrasound
PPi	Inorganic pyrophosphate		USS	Ultrasound scan
PSA	Prostate-specific antigen		UV	Ultraviolet
PsA	Psoriatic arthritis		VACTERL	(Abnormalities of) vertebrae, anus, cardiovascular tree, trachea, (O)esophagus, renal system and limb buds (syndrome)
PT	Prothrombin time			
PTH	Parathyroid hormone			
RA	Rheumatoid arthritis			
RANK	Receptor activator of nuclear factor kappa B		VRE	Vancomycin-resistant enterococcus
			Wnt	A family of highly conserved, signalling proteins that regulate cell–cell interactions during embryogenesis and carcinogenesis
RANKL	Receptor activator of nuclear factor kappa B ligand			
RCT	Randomized controlled trial			
ReA	Reactive arthritis		X-ANCA	Atypical anti-neutrophil cytoplasm antibody
REM	Rapid eye movement			

◼ Introduction

Welcome to this undergraduate textbook of orthopaedics, trauma and rheumatology. The book was designed with particular emphasis on undergraduate medical students who are about to undertake a training programme in musculoskeletal disease. Many medical schools in the UK have, for some time, been combining these three topics into one area for students, since there is considerable overlap. From the student's point of view it makes sense to learn one main way of assessing musculoskeletal problems, whilst acknowledging the variation in individual diseases. The common approach to history taking and physical examination is emphasized throughout the book. Where there are significant differences in practice between specialties, we have highlighted the reasons for the different approaches. Often it is a matter of perspective. The aim is to provide students with a comprehensive guide to the practical management of musculoskeletal conditions.

The book is divided into two sections:

1. Overview chapters on important musculoskeletal topics and a list of reference material for further reading
2. A series of problem cases that illustrate the diagnosis and management of common, as well as less common, musculoskeletal conditions; with answers to the problem cases and references back to the topic section.

In addition we have produced a series of MCQs available via the StudentConsult website. These self-assessment MCQs are based on the problems and topics.

The topic section of core knowledge contains text and illustrations, as well as tables designed to summarize the main points of each condition including aetiology, pathology, epidemiology, clinical features, investigations, management and prognosis. The style for these chapters is similar throughout so that students can easily scan through for the information they require.

The problem-orientated section consists of 100 cases. The section has short clinical vignettes, often with illustrations, followed by three or four pertinent questions about the problems related to diagnosis or management. The cases illustrate the clinical problems faced in everyday practice. The case answers are provided and highlight the clinical approach and thought processes that are necessary to deal with each problem. The cases are taken from our common clinical practice, and the emphasis is on conditions that students are likely to encounter during a musculoskeletal attachment. The case questions are linked to an answer section, which provides short paragraphs as answers for each vignette and is cross-referenced back to the topic section.

The answer section is in a separate part of the book from the question section, to allow students to practise their skills before being given the answers. We hope this will stimulate students to take a practical approach to diagnosis and management of musculoskeletal problems and to use the topic section to reinforce relevant learning points.

Inevitably, some rare conditions are not discussed in detail, but we have made some recommendations for further reading for those interested in knowing more. The book would also be of value to primary care physicians, nurse specialists and other members of the multidisciplinary team dealing with musculoskeletal problems. We hope you find the book of help to you in your everyday practice of orthopaedics, trauma or rheumatology.

MUSCULOSKELETAL DISORDERS

Musculoskeletal problems affect the health of all of us. Most general practitioners will spend around 20% of their working lives helping patients with these physical problems. For example, osteoarthritis is one of the top three causes of disability in Europe and poses a significant burden on health services, which is likely to increase as the population ages. Two important concepts applicable to all musculoskeletal disorders are, firstly, the definition of impairment, disability and handicap; and, secondly, the approach to evidence-based management. These will be considered in turn.

IMPAIRMENT, DISABILITY AND HANDICAP

It is important to be aware of the distinctions between impairment, disability and handicap. The World Health Organization has defined these as follows:

Impairment	Disability	Handicap
Any loss or abnormality of psychological, physiological, or anatomical structure or function	Restriction or lack, resulting from an impairment, of ability to perform an activity in the manner or within the range considered normal for a human being	Disadvantage for a given individual, resulting from an impairment or disability, that limits or prevents the fulfilment of a role that is normal (depending on age, sex and social and cultural factors) for that individual

WHO has also illustrated these definitions as follows:

'Impairments are disturbances at the level of the organ which include defects in or loss of a limb, organ or other body structure, as well as defects in or loss of a mental function. Examples of impairments include blindness, deafness, loss of sight in an eye, paralysis of a limb, amputation of a limb; mental retardation, partial sight, loss of speech, mutism.

Disabilities are descriptions of disturbances in function at the level of the person. Examples of disabilities include difficulty seeing, speaking or hearing; difficulty moving or climbing stairs; difficulty grasping, reaching, bathing, eating, toileting.

Handicap describes the social and economic roles of impaired or disabled persons that place them at a disadvantage compared to other persons. These disadvantages are brought about through the interaction of the person with specific environments and cultures. Examples of handicaps include being bedridden or confined to home; being unable to use public transport; being socially isolated.'

As a corollary to these, the WHO has also provided definitions for prevention, rehabilitation and equalization of opportunities as follows:

Prevention	Rehabilitation	Equalization of opportunities
Measures aimed at preventing the onset of mental, physical and sensory impairments (primary prevention) or at preventing impairment, when it has occurred, from having negative physical, psychological and social consequences (secondary prevention)	Goal-oriented and time-limited process aimed at enabling an impaired person to reach the optimum mental, physical and/or social functional level, thus providing the individual with the tools to change her or his own life. It can involve measures intended to compensate for a loss of function or a functional limitation (for example, by technical aids) and other measures intended to facilitate social adjustment or readjustment	The process through which the general system of society, such as the physical and cultural environment, housing and transportation, social and health services, educational and work opportunities, cultural and social life, including sports and recreational facilities, are made accessible to all

These concepts are applicable to many patients with longstanding musculoskeletal conditions.

PRINCIPLES OF EVIDENCE-BASED PRACTICE

Many currently accepted treatments in orthopaedics, trauma and rheumatology do have an evidence base, based on the 'gold standard' of the randomized controlled trial (RCT). The RCT is based on a systematic review of evidence and assignment of two groups of patients to separate treatment in an unbiased fashion. Although therapeutics lends itself to RCT analysis, the outcomes in many musculoskeletal conditions cannot simply be measured in the same way as an improvement in survival (chemotherapy) or blood pressure reduction (anti-hypertensives). Osteoarthritis, for example, results in disability that can be measured subjectively by the patient or objectively by the doctor. Patient-based assessment tools include the SF12 (Short Form 12), from which 12 questions can be derived to quantify the ease with which activities of daily living are performed. Pain scores are recorded on visual analogue scales. Improvement in power and range of movement can be recorded by health professionals using strength-testing machines. Normalization of locomotion and its increased efficiency can be measured using gait analysis laboratories.

Surgical procedures result in both minor and major complications. These should be recorded in the analysis together with patients 'lost to follow-up'. If many patients are lost this may invalidate the conclusions because those individuals may have died or had further treatment elsewhere but unknown. Joint replacement surgery results in an implant with a finite life. Revision rates can be measured in the same way as survival analysis from a fatal disease; the only difference is that the end-point is implant failure or revision rather than relapse or death.

Commonly used outcome tools include the Disease Activity Score (DAS) in rheumatoid arthritis, SF36 (Short Form 36), the Oxford joint scores, the Western Ontario and McMaster Osteoarthritis Index (WOMAC) scores, and the Charnley and Harris hip scores. These systems can be used to help individual hospitals and surgeons measure their own success rates against others. In the UK political considerations make publication of outcome data for organizations and individuals increasingly common. However, this information needs to be disseminated carefully, since raw data may reveal differences in outcome that mask a different patient-mix; for example, total hip replacement in primary hip arthritis is generally better than after hip fracture, and outcome data should reflect this through sub-stratification (including patient age, ASA status and pre-morbid factors, such as malignancy). Anonymized outcome data in orthopaedic practice include the *National Joint Register* reports in England and Wales, and the *Scottish Hip Audit* in Scotland. The latter does disseminate individual surgeon complication rates for internal hospital discussion with the aim of improving surgical practice. General post-surgical mortality data are collected by the *Confidential Enquiry into Perioperative Deaths (CEPOD)* in England and Wales, and the *Scottish Audit into Surgical Mortality (SASM)* in Scotland.

Nevertheless, even if outcome data are not placed in the public domain, their assessment remains a powerful tool for internal 'audit'. Here, audit allows outcome to be measured against a 'gold standard'. If current practice fails to achieve that standard, then the 'audit loop' should include the introduction of modifications in the treatment pathway. Finally, a further 'audit' will assess whether an improvement has occurred.

Common interventions allow 'care pathways' to be developed. These are usually produced as a booklet of tick-charts and free-field paragraphs in which the many professionals involved in the care of a patient can record pre-, peri- and post-operative events. These act as a checklist so that agreed protocols are carried out (for example perioperative thrombo-prophylaxis) and post-operative goals are set for the patient. The pathway is devised for an 'average' patient, and so needs to be supplemented by old-fashioned medical note-keeping when a patient develops complications requiring extra treatment.

In the UK, several bodies produce information to help doctors undertake best practice. Individual hospitals may develop protocols. In England and Wales the *National Institute for Clinical Excellence (NICE)* has produced guidelines on the use of metal on metal hip replacements and on the use of radio-frequency ablation of benign bone lesions. The equivalent Scottish body is *Quality Assurance*

Scotland (QIS). Also in Scotland the *Scottish Intercollegiate Guidance Network (SIGN)* publishes expert consensus reports on medical topics of concern. The Cochrane Collaboration has allowed assessment of all evidence for management of many musculoskeletal conditions. Consensus is gained based on studies representing several levels of evidence. These include literature reviews, case reports, retrospective series reviews, cohort studies, prospective non-randomized outcome studies and RCTs.

MUSCULOSKELETAL SYSTEM

1

CLINICAL HISTORY AND EXAMINATION

James Robb, Daniel Porter, John Keating and Raashid Luqmani

Cases relevant to this chapter

6, 11, 13, 16–21, 24, 28–31, 33, 34, 38, 39, 49–51, 55–57, 61, 66, 68, 69, 71, 73–76, 79, 82–85, 87, 88, 91, 93, 96, 97

●Essential facts

1. A diagnosis can usually be made from a good history and inspection of joints.

2. Careful inspection of joints is often more informative than palpation or movement.

3. Proximal joint and adjacent joints need to be included in the examination, because pain in one joint may be referred from pathology in other joints.

4. A systematic approach to examination is recommended.

5. Red flag symptoms include: pain preventing sleep; loss of appetite; loss of weight; visual loss; temporal headache and blurred vision; loss of bladder/bowel control; and rapidly progressive symptoms.

6. Red flag signs include: 'drawn' facial appearance; saddle anaesthesia; bilateral limb neurology; upper motor neurone signs; painful swelling; fever >38°C; inability to weight-bear; or a red, hot joint.

7. Malignant tumours of bone and soft tissues are typically rapidly growing, over 5 cm in size, painful, and deep to the deep fascia.

GENERAL CONSIDERATIONS

HISTORY

A diagnosis can often be made from a good history and inspection of joints. Many patients present with pain in a limb; this has a very wide differential diagnosis. It is always important to ask about precipitating factors, to find out if this is the first episode of the problem or a recurrence of a previous problem. The onset of the problem should be described, such as whether it occurred gradually and increased in severity or whether it came on very suddenly. It is useful to know if it started in one area of the body and spread to other areas, and, in particular, which joints were affected. Rheumatoid arthritis typically starts in the feet in the metatarsophalangeal joints (MTPJ) and the medium-sized joints, such as the ankle and wrist, and involves the metacarpophalangeal joints (MCPJ) and proximal interphalangeal joints (PIPJ) of the hand. By contrast, osteoarthritis in the hands typically involves the distal interphalangeal joints (DIPJ) and to some extent the PIPJ. Some conditions will move from one joint area to another and typically this occurs in infection-related arthritis. It is helpful to know how the problem varies during the course of the day. Is it worse first thing in the morning and associated with stiffness in the joints (which is typical in inflammatory joint disease) or does it tend to get worse with effort and use of the limb (which is more typical of a mechanical problem in the joints or soft tissue)? Are there associated systemic features such as weight loss or fever, rashes or other organ-specific problems? This would suggest that this joint problem might be part of an underlying multi-system condition, whether it is inflammatory or metabolic. For example, patients with diabetes commonly complain of stiff shoulders and sore fingers, and these may be the first manifestations of their condition. Patients have often tried some sort of remedy themselves using medications bought over the counter or prescribed by their general practitioner (GP). It is important to document what has been tried to determine what is unlikely to work and also what might have caused problems, such as side effects. Response to medication may help in deciding the type of problem. Patients may have sleep disturbance as a result of their musculoskeletal problem. Pain that wakes patients up from sleep may be an indication of more serious pathology, but some conditions that have no clear pathology, e.g. fibromyalgia, are associated with poor sleep quality. It is useful to know whether the activities of daily living or work have been affected by the condition. Can the patient still perform normal tasks, such as getting dressed, washed, getting up and down stairs, going to the toilet, cooking food, doing the household chores, driving a car or doing the shopping? When the patient comes to see you they may have already had some tests performed and it helps to know the results. The patients will have some expectation of the consultation and it is important to establish what they think so that you can give them appropriate information about their condition. Family history is particularly important in children, but also in some adults, and social history may be very relevant in terms of what support is available for patients. A history of alcohol consumption should be documented as some conditions, e.g. gout, are related to alcohol, smoking history and significant medical conditions such as diabetes.

For red flag symptoms see page 35.

GENERAL PHYSICAL EXAMINATION

A general physical examination will be necessary as well as a musculoskeletal assessment if the patient complains of pain that is not explained by the musculoskeletal findings. For example, you must check the peripheral pulses in a leg if you suspect ischaemic claudication as a cause of leg pain. Patients who appear to have systemic rheumatic disease will require a comprehensive medical examination as there may be extra-articular consequences of the condition. Examination of the elbows looking for subcutaneous nodules may be a clue to indicate rheumatoid arthritis; in patients with a history suggesting recurrent or chronic gout, search for hard subcutaneous lumps (tophi), which are full of uric acid and typically occur over extensor surfaces or at the pinna (ear). Skin lesions of vasculitis may be trivial findings such as nail-edge or nail-fold infarcts; in some cases there is much more severe skin involvement with full-thickness ulceration. Patients with connective tissue diseases often have skin involvement, such as the butterfly rash of systemic lupus erythematosus or the tight skin of patients with scleroderma. Involvement of internal organs, such as the lungs, heart or gut, may occur in connective tissue diseases and vasculitis. Medications used to treat systemic rheumatic disease may also have side effects in other areas or systems; for example, methotrexate is used widely for treating rheumatoid arthritis and may induce a higher risk of infection. It can cause a form of pneumonitis, which is rare, but if left untreated is fatal in over half of cases. Liver function can be affected by methotrexate and other drugs, but this is rarely a cause of symptoms or signs. Non-steroidal anti-inflammatory drugs (NSAIDs) commonly cause gastrointestinal toxicity, including peptic ulcers and haemorrhage, especially in the elderly. NSAIDs interfere with a number of other medications and may cause kidney and heart problems. Corticosteroids have well known effects including weight gain, moon face, osteoporosis, diabetes, risk of infection and risk of cataract. Similarly, medications used for other conditions may be responsible for, or contribute to, rheumatic problems. Thiazide diuretics used for a long time may increase levels of uric acid and lead to a form of chronic gout. A number of drugs can induce a lupus-like syndrome, e.g. anti-thyroid drugs can induce a vasculitis and many drugs can cause a skin vasculitis as part of an allergic reaction.

It is essential to remember that pain in a joint may be referred from other joints. The joint above and adjacent joints need to be included in the examination. Pain may also be referred from other areas, for example nerve root pain or shoulder tip pain arising from diaphragmatic irritation.

For red flag signs see page 35.

EVALUATION OF GAIT

Before examining the joints of the lower limbs ask the patient to walk and observe their gait. You should observe if the speed is normal, whether or not the patient has a limp and if there is asymmetry of the gait pattern. Do they use a walking aid? Look at the wear pattern of their shoes – is it symmetrical or is one part more worn than another?

The gait cycle consists of two phases: stance and swing, when the foot is on and off the ground respectively (Fig. 1.1). One gait cycle begins when one foot strikes the ground and ends when the same foot strikes the ground again, and a cycle is described as 0–100%. Stance lasts for 60% and swing for 40% of the cycle in normal gait. The stance phase can be subdivided into one period of single support when only one foot is in contact with the ground and two periods of double support when both feet are on the ground, which occurs at the beginning and end of stance. Step length is the distance from the point of contact of one foot to the same point contact of the other foot. Stride length is the distance from initial contact of one foot to the next initial contact of the same foot. Thus two steps equal one stride. Cadence is the number of steps per minute.

Prerequisites of normal gait are:

- stance phase stability
- swing phase clearance
- adequate foot pre-positioning
- adequate step length
- energy conservation.

In normal gait the hip has a total arc of about 45° of motion and the knee 60°. When considering abnormalities of gait it is useful to think of symmetry or asymmetry of stance time and step length, and whether or not a joint has a normal, reduced or excessive range of motion in gait. For example, arthritis of the hip will produce a stiff joint, which may result in loss of the normal range of hip motion in gait, diminished stance time on the affected side due to pain, increased stance time on the non-affected side and an increased upper body tilt over the affected side in stance to unload the hip. A patient who has had a traumatic division of the common peroneal nerve will have a drop foot in swing, difficulty in clearing obstructions with the affected foot, abnormal foot pre-positioning in late swing and will make initial contact with the ground through the forefoot. They may compensate for swing phase foot clearance difficulties by increasing lateral movement of the trunk away from the affected limb when it is in swing. A patient who has a paraplegia (traumatic or as a result of spinal cord pathology) or an above-the-knee amputation, for example, will have much higher energy costs than normal when walking. Stance phase instability might result, for example, from post-traumatic lateral ankle ligament instability resulting in a tendency for the foot to invert excessively.

EXAMINATION OF JOINTS

Too often, inspection of joints is neglected in the rush to feel and move them. It may be apparent from inspection that a deformity in a joint or in a bone may be a result of arthritis or a fracture. If you can see the abnormality, you can avoid causing the patient unnecessary discomfort and yet still achieve an accurate diagnosis. Table 1.1 summarizes the main points of examination.

The principles of examining joints are similar to those for examination of other body systems. It is best to adopt a systematic approach using 'Look, Feel, Move and Special Tests' or the GALS (gait, arms, legs and spine) method (Macleod). With the latter, ask the patient the following three questions:

1. Do you have any pain or stiffness in your muscles, joints or back?
2. Can you dress yourself without difficulty?
3. Can you walk up and down stairs without difficulty?

If all three replies are negative the patient is unlikely to have a significant musculoskeletal

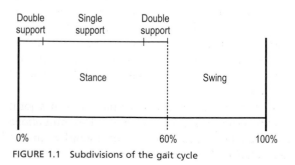

FIGURE 1.1 Subdivisions of the gait cycle

Table 1.1 Important points to observe in joints during clinical examination

Look	Scars, sinuses, swelling, deformity and erythema
Feel	Skin, soft tissues and joint
Move	Active and passive; normal range, reduced or increased range of movement; and stress tests
Special imaging (see Chapter 4 on Imaging)	Plain X-rays are the mainstay CT gives better bony definition MRI gives good definition of non-osseous structures Ultrasound is useful for joint effusions and rotator cuff tears of the shoulder Arthrography is used to confirm reduction of a hip in a child

problem. If not, examine their gait, arms, legs and spine.

The GALS and Look, Feel, Move and Special Tests approaches are complementary. For example, if you find as a result of your GALS screen there is a problem in the patient's knee, use the Look, Feel, Move and Special Tests approach to evaluate the knee further.

Look

Inspection of the joints will require adequate exposure. Look for swelling, deformity, redness and rheumatoid nodules to see if there is any asymmetry, but remember that some rheumatic diseases are symmetrical. You should look for associated features, such as rashes, psoriasis or muscle wasting around a joint that has not been used for some time. There may be scars from previous surgery or injury. The patient may look emaciated if there is an underlying malignancy or significant systemic disease (patients with severe rheumatoid arthritis may have lost a lot of weight). You may observe redness around a joint or limb, or swelling away from a joint. A ruptured Baker's cyst will cause swelling in the calf with redness and erythema of the overlying skin. Baker's cysts are common in patients with rheumatoid arthritis and there may also be an associated knee effusion.

Feel

Gently palpate the joints and limbs, to ascertain a difference in temperature in and around the joint and bony tenderness. Use the back of your hand to assess temperature; feel proximal and distal to the potentially abnormal area. There is usually a temperature gradient away from the heart so that the thigh is normally warmer than the knee, which is warmer than the shin. The back of your hand is very sensitive to these graded temperature changes and you should apply this evaluation routinely when examining large joints such as the knees. Feel the joints for evidence of swelling, which you will have detected on inspection. Feeling for swelling at this stage would confirm what you have seen, but also determines the nature of the swelling. You want to know whether it is fluid, soft tissue or bone. Massaging a joint may be a good way of detecting fluid within a joint, but remember that very swollen joints will fail this test because there is nowhere for the fluid to go. You should feel for tenderness, so you need to look at the patient's face during palpation. You should feel the structures around the joints, such as ligaments and tendons, as these could be the source of discomfort. You may observe a deformity; valgus is a deviation of a part away from the midline and varus the opposite.

Move

Finally, you want to move the joint. Active movement, i.e. that performed by the patient, should be observed first followed by passive movement performed by the examiner. Range of movement may be normal, reduced or excessive. If the patient has an excessive range of movement, this could suggest that they are hypermobile (Fig. 1.2).

If range of movement is restricted this may be due to pain, weakness, loss of neurological function, tissue stiffness, contracture or bony changes, such as ankylosis (fusion of a joint). After observing active movement, check passive movement, but stop if the patient complains of discomfort. The main benefit of checking passive movement is that, if weakness or stiffness is a limiting factor,

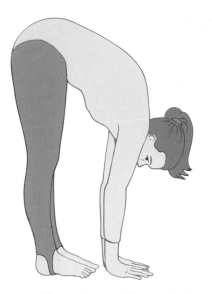

Score one point if you can bend and place your hands flat on the floor without bending your knees.

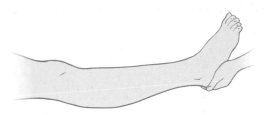

Score one point for each knee that will bend backwards.

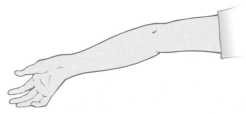

Score one point for each elbow that will bend backwards.

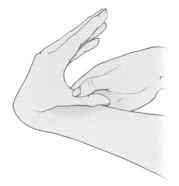

Score one point for each thumb that will bend backwards to touch the forearm.

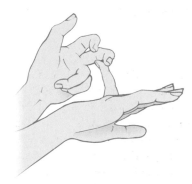

Score one point for each hand when you can bend the little finger back beyond 90°.

If you are able to perform all of the above manoeuvres then you have a maximum score of 9 points.

FIGURE 1.2　Five tests for hypermobility

you can assess the full range of joint movement with assistance.

All peripheral joints can be examined in this way, except for the hips, where there is no area to palpate, apart from a painful trochanteric bursa, and where inspection is unlikely to show a swelling; however, a deformity, for example a fixed flexion contracture, may be visible. Normal range of movements is shown in Figures 1.3 and 1.4.

The following is a regional guide to the major joints.

SHOULDER
ANATOMY OVERVIEW

Movement at the shoulder occurs at the glenohumeral and scapulo-thoracic articulations. The glenohumeral (shoulder) joint is multiaxial and has a strong capsule, which permits this very wide range of movement. Scapulo-thoracic movement is described as protraction (forward rotation over the thorax) and retraction (backward rotation over

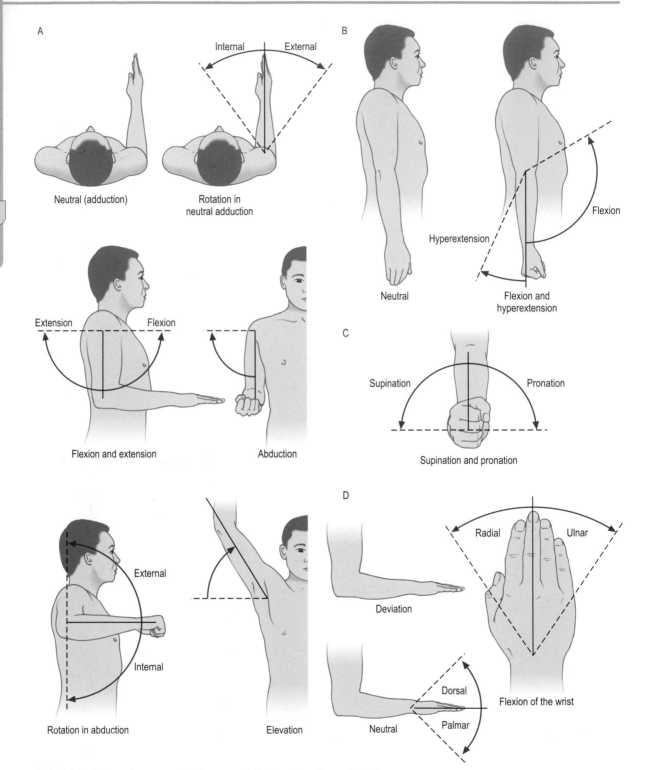

FIGURE 1.3   Range of movement in the upper limb (from Douglas et al 2005)

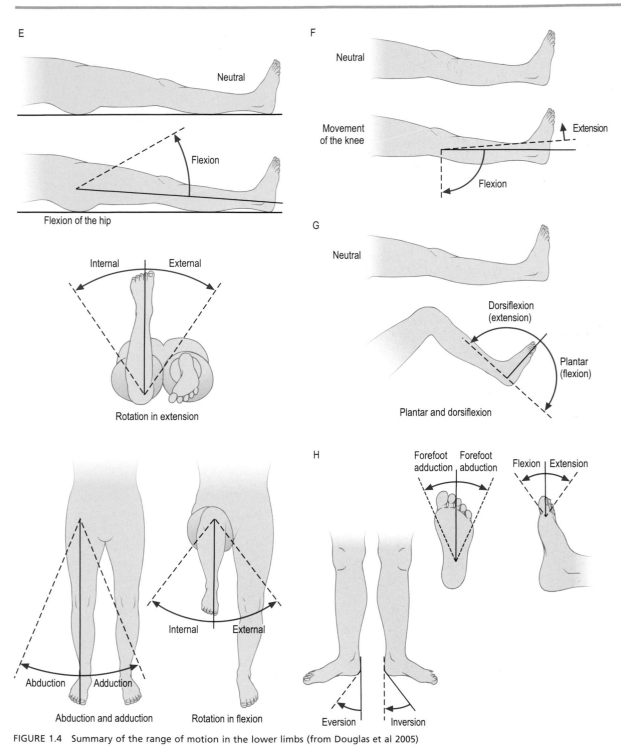

FIGURE 1.4 Summary of the range of motion in the lower limbs (from Douglas et al 2005)

the thorax), elevation (upward movement) and depression (downward movement). Most shoulder movements are composite and involve scapulothoracic and gleno-humeral movement. The rotator cuff muscles, supraspinatus, infraspinatus, teres minor and subscapularis, attach to the proximal humerus. Supraspinatus, infraspinatus and teres minor insert on to the greater tuberosity, and subscapularis to the lesser tuberosity. These muscles are important dynamic stabilizers of the shoulder joint as well as having a role in specific joint motions.

Subscapularis is a medial rotator of the shoulder, and teres minor and infraspinatus are lateral rotators of the shoulder. Glenohumeral abduction is initiated by supraspinatus and the deltoid abducts the arm beyond the initial 15°. The upper fibres of trapezius elevate the scapula, its middle fibres retract the scapula and the lower fibres depress the scapula. Teres major is also a medial rotator of the shoulder, but also extends the arm at the shoulder joint. Pectoralis major flexes, adducts and medially rotates the arm at the shoulder joint. Pectoralis minor pulls the tip of the shoulder inferiorly and protracts the scapula. Serratus anterior protracts the scapula and maintains close apposition of the inferior angle of the scapula against the thoracic wall. Latissimus dorsi adducts, medially rotates and extends the arm at the shoulder.

The muscles of the arm comprise biceps, coracobrachialis and brachialis anteriorly, and triceps posteriorly. Coracobrachialis flexes the arm at the shoulder joint; biceps flexes the elbow and supinates the forearm, and also contributes to flexion of the arm at the shoulder joint. Brachialis is a powerful flexor of the forearm at the elbow. Figures 1.5 and 1.6 show the details of muscle attachments of the arm.

The surface anatomy of the shoulder is important clinically, as patients with shoulder pathology may receive intra-articular injections of local anaesthetic, for example as a diagnostic test of impingement, and an injection of local anaesthetic with steroid in the management of inflammatory joint disease. The shoulder may be injected anteriorly by inserting the needle just lateral to the coracoid process, subacromially in the interval between the acromion and humeral head, and posteriorly just infero-medial to the most lateral prominence of the spine of the scapula.

Look

Look for asymmetry compared to the opposite side, swelling, muscle wasting, winging of the scapula (due to paralysis of serratus anterior), elevation of the scapula (due to Sprengel's deformity or Klippel–Feil syndrome). Wasting of the deltoid or supraspinatus and infraspinatus is commonly present in a wide range of shoulder disorders and can be detected by comparison with the normal side.

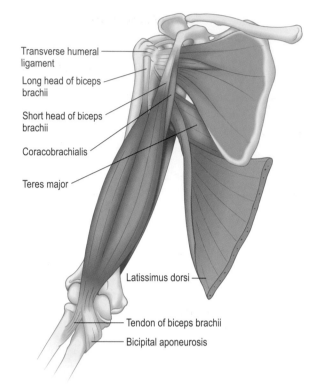

Transverse humeral ligament

Long head of biceps brachii

Short head of biceps brachii

Coracobrachialis

Teres major

Latissimus dorsi

Tendon of biceps brachii

Bicipital aponeurosis

FIGURE 1.5   Anterior muscles of the shoulder and arm (from Drake et al 2004)

Feel

Feel along the clavicle from sternoclavicular to acromioclavicular joints for a malunion, across the acromion for arthritis and along the spine of the scapula. Feel along the blade of the scapula both medially and laterally down to the angle. Feel trapezius and deltoid. Feel the anterior triangle of the neck to assess goitre and lymphadenopathy. Palpate the bicipital groove for bicipital tendonitis.

Move

The movements at the shoulder are forward flexion, extension, abduction/adduction, internal and external rotation. Movement occurs at both the scapulo-thoracic and glenohumeral joints and it may be necessary to distinguish between the two components. For example, during abduction the tip of the scapula is identified and palpated as the patient is asked to abduct the shoulder. The tip of the scapula will start to rotate away from the midline in the latter stages of abduction. For this reason the total arc of abduction may referred to as 'combined abduction'. You can use a quick screen-

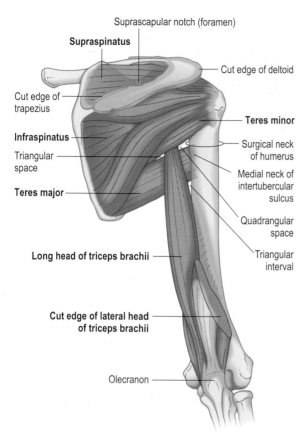

FIGURE 1.6   Posterior muscles of the shoulder and arm (from Drake et al 2004)

remove the abductor action of deltoid. Infraspinatus and teres minor, both of which act as external rotators, can be tested by asking the patient to hold their arm at 30° of flexion and then externally rotate the shoulder against resistance. This position removes the contribution of deltoid as an external rotator. Pain rather than weakness during these manoeuvres would suggest that the patient may have a rotator cuff tendonitis rather than a tear. A painful arc of movement of the glenohumeral joint may help to distinguish between inflammation and a tear (see Chapter 21).

A patient may have a positive apprehension test after a recurrent dislocation of the glenohumeral joint. To test this, the shoulder is abducted to 90° and externally rotated in this position. Pressure on the proximal humerus from behind causes discomfort and a sensation of shoulder instability when the test is positive.

ELBOW

ANATOMY OVERVIEW

Although there are three joints (humero-ulnar, humero-radial and radio-ulnar) in the elbow sharing a common synovial cavity, the elbow should be considered as a hinge joint producing extension and flexion. Figure 1.7 shows the anatomy of the elbow.

Look

Look specifically for swelling, effusion, deformity and the carrying angle, which is the angle subtended by the forearm in relation to the long axis of the arm. It is normally a valgus angle of 10–15° in the coronal plane when the elbow is extended. The carrying angle is generally greater in females than males. The carrying angle may be abnormal after an injury to the elbow.

Feel

Palpate the medial and lateral condyles and olecranon; these should form an equilateral triangle. If not, this may suggest a previous elbow injury. Tenderness over the common flexor and extensor muscle origins may indicate an epicondylitis, 'golfer's' and 'tennis' elbow respectively. The ulnar nerve can be palpated in its groove on the medial

ing test by asking the patient to put their hand behind their head and then to the small of their back. Both are composite movements and the first requires abduction, external rotation and extension of the shoulder, and the second abduction, internal rotation, extension and adduction.

A painful arc exists if the patient experiences pain when abducting the shoulder between 90° and 120°. Loss of active glenohumeral abduction may indicate a tear of the rotator cuff. The muscles of the rotator cuff can be tested individually. For subscapularis, ask the patient to put their hand behind their back and to internally rotate the shoulder against resistance. This may not be possible if the shoulder is stiff and, alternatively, the muscle can be tested by internal rotation of the forearm against resistance, keeping the elbow flexed at 90° and the shoulder in a neutral position. For supraspinatus, test abduction of the shoulder against resistance beginning with the arm by the patient's side to

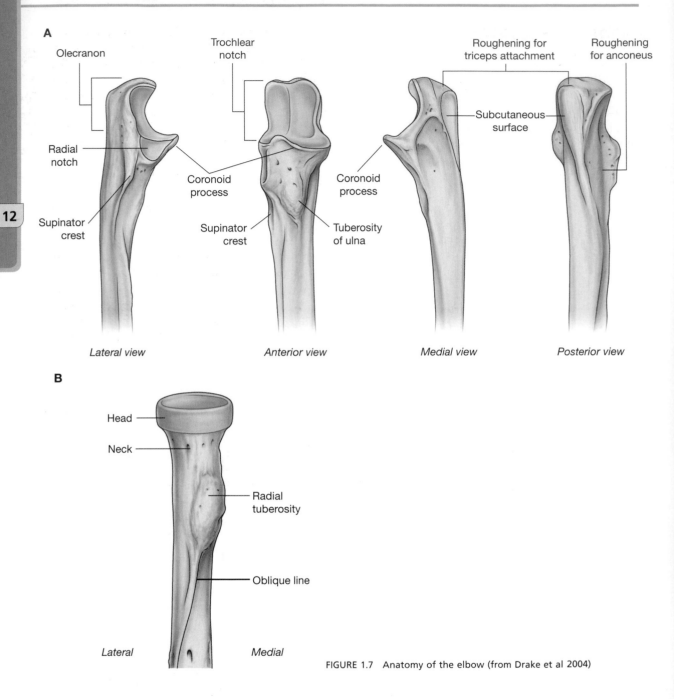

A

Olecranon

Trochlear notch

Roughening for triceps attachment

Roughening for anconeus

Radial notch

Coronoid process

Coronoid process

Subcutaneous surface

Supinator crest

Supinator crest

Tuberosity of ulna

Lateral view

Anterior view

Medial view

Posterior view

B

Head

Neck

Radial tuberosity

Oblique line

Lateral

Medial

FIGURE 1.7   Anatomy of the elbow (from Drake et al 2004)

side of the humerus where it can be compressed producing an ulnar nerve palsy.

Move

Many normal individuals have physiological hyperextension of the elbow and so this normal range of movement may be described as, for example, 10° of extension through neutral to 130° of flexion or 10–0–130° if using the Debrunner notation.

Epicondylitis may affect the extensor origin (tennis elbow and associated pain on resisted dorsiflexion of the wrist) or the flexor origin (golfer's elbow and associated pain on resisted palmar flexion of the wrist).

FOREARM, WRIST AND HAND

ANATOMY OVERVIEW

Figures 1.8 and 1.9 summarize the muscles of the forearm and Figure 1.10 shows the radiological appearance of the normal wrist. The radius and ulna have a proximal and distal radio-ulnar articulation. Pronation and supination of the hand occurs as a result of the radius rotating about the ulna and at the radio-capitellar joint. The hand is supinated when the palm faces anteriorly and is pronated when it faces posteriorly. Supination is produced by the action of biceps and supinator. Pronation is produced by pronator teres and pronator quadratus located at the proximal and distal ends of the forearm respectively.

The anterior compartment of the forearm contains the flexor muscles (Box 1.1). In the superficial layer flexor carpi ulnaris flexes and adducts the wrist joint, palmaris longus flexes the wrist joint, and flexor carpi radialis flexes and abducts the wrist joint. These muscles arise from the common flexor origin on the medial side of the distal end of the humerus. Flexor digitorum superficialis lies in the intermediate layer and acts principally as a flexor of the PIPJ of the fingers, but not the thumb, and can also flex the MCPJ of the fingers and flex the wrist. In the deep compartment the flexor digitorum profundus and flexor pollicis longus flex the DIPJ of the fingers and interphalangeal joint (IPJ) of the thumb respectively.

The superficial compartment of the posterior aspect of the forearm contains the extensor muscles and brachioradialis and these arise from the lateral aspect of the distal end of the humerus (Box 1.2). The brachioradialis inserts into the lateral aspect of the distal end of the radius and act as a flexor of the elbow when the arm is mid-pronated. Extensor

13

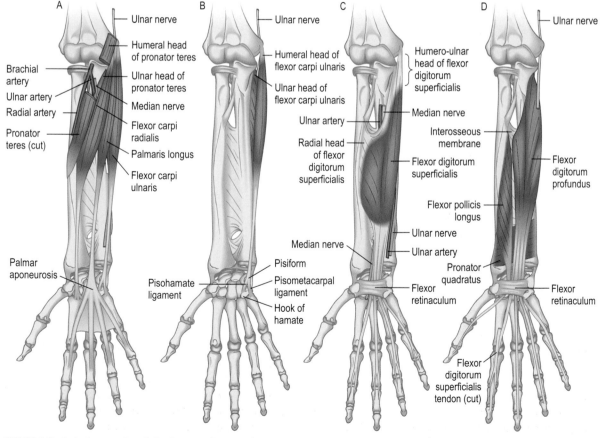

FIGURE 1.8　Anterior muscles of the forearm (from Drake et al 2004)

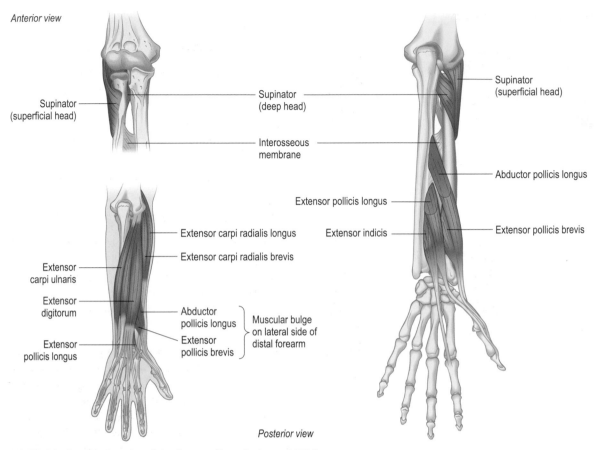

Anterior view

Supinator
(superficial head)

Supinator
(deep head)

Interosseous
membrane

Supinator
(superficial head)

Abductor pollicis longus

Extensor pollicis longus

Extensor indicis

Extensor pollicis brevis

Extensor carpi radialis longus

Extensor carpi radialis brevis

Extensor
carpi ulnaris

Extensor
digitorum

Abductor
pollicis longus

Extensor
pollicis brevis

Muscular bulge
on lateral side of
distal forearm

Extensor
pollicis longus

Posterior view

FIGURE 1.9   Posterior muscles of the forearm (from Drake et al 2004)

carpi radialis longus and brevis extend and abduct the wrist, extensor digitorum extends the fingers and also the wrist, extensor digiti minimi extends the little finger, and extensor carpi ulnaris extends and adducts the wrist. In the deep extensor compartment the abductor pollicis abducts the carpometacarpal (CMC) joint of the thumb mainly, but can also act to extend the thumb; extensor pollicis brevis extends the MCPJ of the thumb mainly, but can also extend the CMC joint; extensor pollicis longus extends the IPJ of the thumb mainly, but can also extend the CMC and MCP joints; and extensor indicis extends the index finger.

The flexion/extension axis of the thumb lies at 90° with respect to the fingers. Abduction, adduction and opposition also occur at the thumb. The muscles of the hypothenar eminence are supplied by the ulnar nerve and the muscles of the thenar eminence by the median nerve with the exception of adductor pollicis, which is supplied by the ulnar nerve. This is important to bear in mind when considering a peripheral nerve lesion affecting the hand. The interossei are supplied by the ulnar nerve and may be wasted in an ulnar nerve lesion.

Look

Look at the nails and nail-bed areas for signs of psoriasis or cutaneous vasculitis. Look specifically for swellings, such as synovitis of the extensor tendons, ganglia of the wrist, nodules or tophi, Dupuytren's contractures, rheumatoid deformities of the wrist and digits. In patients with inflammatory joint disease, the pattern of involvement may be characteristic; typically in rheumatoid arthritis, the metacarpophalangeal and proximal interphalangeal joints are swollen with sparing of the distal interphalangeal joints. By contrast, in osteoarthritis DIPJ and PIPJ involvement, with squaring of the carpometacarpal joint of the thumb, is most likely. Muscle wasting and sensory loss may accompany median or ulnar nerve compression.

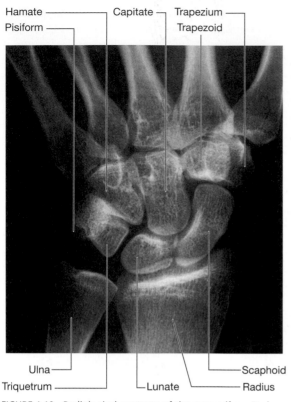

Hamate — Capitate — Trapezium — Trapezoid
Pisiform —

Ulna — Scaphoid
Triquetrum — Lunate — Radius

FIGURE 1.10   Radiological anatomy of the carpus (from Drake et al 2004)

> **Box 1.1**
> ## Anterior muscles of the forearm
>
> - Flexor carpi ulnaris and flexor carpi radialis
> - Flexor digitorum superficialis and profundus
> - Palmaris longus
> - Flexor pollicis longus

> **Box 1.2**
> ## Posterior muscles of the forearm
>
> - Extensor carpi radialis longus and brevis, and extensor carpi ulnaris
> - Extensor digitorum and extensor digiti minimi
> - Abductor pollicis longus

Feel

Feel for tenderness of abductor pollicis longus and extensor pollicis longus tendons at the base of the thumb, which may indicate de Quervain's tenosynovitis. Tenderness in the anatomical snuffbox and distal radius may suggest trauma to the scaphoid or distal radius. If swelling is present, it is helpful to determine whether it is soft tissue or bony, and also whether or not the swelling is painful; so remember to look at the patient's face and ask if the joints are tender.

Move

Forearm rotation is evaluated observing pronation and supination at the distal forearm. It may help for the patient to hold a pencil in both fists as they rotate the arm. This gives the observer a landmark to follow. Remember to have the patient's elbows tucked into their sides when doing this; otherwise shoulder abduction/adduction may mimic pronation/supination.

Wrist flexion and extension are tested by asking the patient to put their hands into the prayer (exten-sion) and reverse prayer (flexion) positions. Radial and ulnar deviations are then tested. Test the wrist extensor and flexor muscles by asking the patient to extend and flex the wrist against resistance.

Active extension of the fingers is then tested while the patient holds their wrist in the neutral position. The flexor digitorum superficialis flexes the PIPJ of the fingers, but so will the flexor digitorum profundus. To distinguish between the two ask the patient to flex the finger while you hold the PIPJ extended (profundus test) and then ask the patient to flex the PIPJ (superficialis test) while you hold the remaining fingers in extension. Flexion and extension at the IPJ of the thumb are tested as you hold the patient's thumb and then test abduction/adduction of the thumb.

Finally, compare grip strength between sides and evaluate the hand neurologically if indicated.

NEUROLOGICAL ASSESSMENT OF THE UPPER LIMB
GENERAL

A *dermatome* is an area of skin supplied by a single spinal cord level and a *myotome* is a portion of skeletal muscle innervated by a single spinal cord level. Myotomes will also generate movement at a joint and this information can be used as well in clinical examination to check if a particular spinal cord level is working or not. Myotomal innervation is subject to much less variation than dermatomal innervation.

Examination of the peripheral nervous system should follow these steps:

1. Observation of the limb
2. Passive movement of the joints in the area to be examined to detect any fixed deformity that will affect motor testing. This also allows evaluation of muscle tone
3. Manual motor testing of the muscles innervated by the nerve(s), beginning proximally and proceeding sequentially to the most distal muscles
4. Testing of the sensory branches/dermatomes supplied by the nerve(s)
5. Reflexes.

Look at muscles for evidence of wasting and fasciculation. Muscle tone will be increased in an upper motor neurone lesion and decreased or absent in a lower motor neurone lesion. Muscle strength can be tested by comparing one side with another or by using the MRC scale of 0–5 (Table 1.2).

Sensory testing involves vibration, position sense, subjective light touch and pain. Light touch is most commonly assessed. The sensory territories of the major peripheral nerves, dermatomes and myotomes of the upper limbs are shown in Figures 1.11 to 1.13.

Table 1.2 Medical Research Council scale for muscle power

Grade	Description
0	No muscle movement
1	Visible muscle movement, but no movement at the joint
2	Movement at the joint, but not against gravity
3	Movement against gravity, but not against added resistance
4	Movement against resistance, but less than normal
5	Normal strength

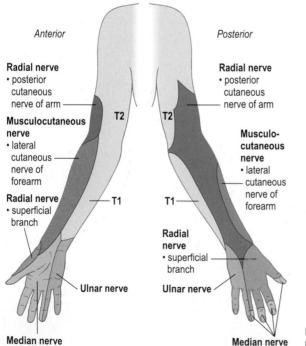

FIGURE 1.11 Sensory territories of the major upper limb peripheral nerves (from Drake et al 2004)

If you want to do a screening test of the motor components of the major nerve roots in the upper limb you should ask the patient to abduct the arm at the shoulder (C5), flex the elbow (C5, C6), flex the fingers (C8) and abduct/adduct the fingers (T1) (Table 1.3).

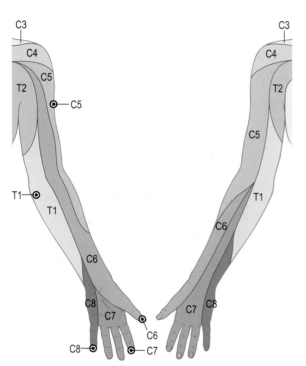

FIGURE 1.12   Dermatomes in the upper limb (from Drake et al 2004)

ASSESSMENT OF MOTOR FUNCTION OF PERIPHERAL NERVES

Radial nerve

A high radial nerve palsy will produce loss of extension at the wrist, fingers and thumb, whereas a lesion of the posterior interosseous nerve will produce loss of extension of the fingers and thumb, and loss of thumb abduction, but the wrist is spared. To test the nerve, begin proximally by testing triceps, brachioradialis and the radial supinator. Then proceed to the distal muscles innervated by the posterior interosseous nerve.

Ask the patient to extend the fingers and then the wrist while you support their wrist, which should be pronated and the elbow flexed to 90°. Extensor pollicis longus and abductor pollicis

Table 1.3 Motor innervation of upper limb

Movement	Innervation
Shoulder abduction	C5
Elbow flexion	C5 C6
Elbow extension	C7 C8
Flexion of fingers	C8
Finger ab/adduction	T1

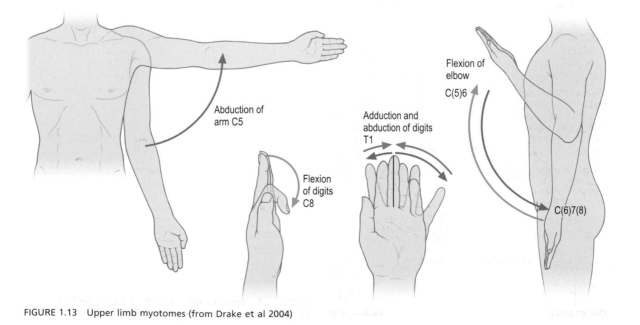

FIGURE 1.13   Upper limb myotomes (from Drake et al 2004)

longus can be tested by asking the patient to extend and abduct the thumb against resistance.

Median nerve

Begin by testing the forearm muscles supplied by the nerve (flexor pollicis longus, flexor digitorum profundus and the radial half of the flexor digitorum superficialis) as described above. In the hand it supplies the thenar muscles apart from adductor pollicis (ulnar nerve). The thenar muscles abduct and oppose the thumb. To test these, ask the patient to move their thumb upwards away from the palm (abduction) and to touch the little finger with the thumb (opposition).

Ulnar nerve

In the hand this nerve supplies the interossei and adductor pollicis muscles. To test adductor pollicis ask the patient to grip a piece of paper or card between the thumb and the palm. If there is an ulnar nerve palsy, the IPJ and MCPJs of the thumb will flex as the patient tries to grip the paper (Froment's sign). The same piece of paper or card can be used to test the interossei. Ask the patient to grip it between the little and ring fingers whilst holding the fingers extended. The first dorsal interosseus muscle can be tested by asking the patient to abduct the extended index finger against resistance.

Figure 1.14 demonstrates the complex movements of the thumb.

SPINE

ANATOMY OVERVIEW

The spinal column comprises seven cervical, twelve thoracic, five lumbar vertebrae, the sacrum and coccyx (Fig. 1.15). Correspondingly there are five lumbar and twelve thoracic rami, but paradoxically eight cervical rami, as the first cervical ramus exits between C1 and the occiput and the second between the atlas and axis (C1 and C2). The eighth cervical ramus exits between C7 and T1. The basic structure of a vertebra comprises a body, pedicle, lamina, facet joints, transverse and spinous processes.

There are modifications of the vertebrae in the thoracic and cervical spine. The bodies are separated by an intervertebral disc that consists of an outer annulus fibrosus and an inner nucleus pulpo-sus. The superior and inferior facet joints are synovial joints. In the thoracic spine there is an additional synovial demifacet for the articulation with the ribs as each rib articulates with two vertebral bodies. In the cervical spine the spinous processes are bifid and there is a foramen in the transverse processes to accommodate the vertebral arteries. The atlas (C1) and axis (C2) are modified further for their articulation with the occiput (atlas), and between the atlas and axis for the odontoid peg that arises from the axis. These are also synovial joints. At the other end of the spine the sacrum and coccyx have also been modified from the basic structure. The sacro-iliac joint is also a synovial joint.

Spinal ligaments (Fig. 1.16) constitute a longitudinal supporting system that permits movement. There are anterior and posterior longitudinal ligaments that link the vertebral bodies, and a supraspinous ligament that is modified in the cervical region to form the ligamentum nuchae. These three ligament systems run the entire length of the spine. In addition, the ligamentum flavum and interspinous ligaments link the pedicles and spinous processes at each level. A strong system of ligaments stabilizes the sacroiliac joints. At the cranio–cervical junction the transverse ligament spans the lateral masses and stabilizes the odontoid peg, and the alar ligaments connect the dens to the occiput and restrict excessive rotation of the head and atlas on the axis. The clinical importance of these synovial joints and ligaments is that they may be affected by inflammatory joint diseases and disrupted by severe trauma. A prolapsed intervertebral disc may produce irritation or compression of the lumbar or sacral nerve roots.

A powerful system of muscles helps to maintain spinal alignment and stability. The spinal extensor system runs from the occiput to the sacrum. Forward and lateral flexion are provided by a combination of spinal and abdominal muscle function, whereas rotation is more dependent on the spinal muscles themselves. Common spinal deformities are shown in Figure 1.17.

Look

The patient should be suitably undressed, usually down to their underwear, and chaperoned. Ask the patient to walk, observe their gait and then ask them to stand. Look at the spine from the side for an exaggerated thoracic kyphosis (curvature of the spine in the sagittal plane) and loss or exaggeration

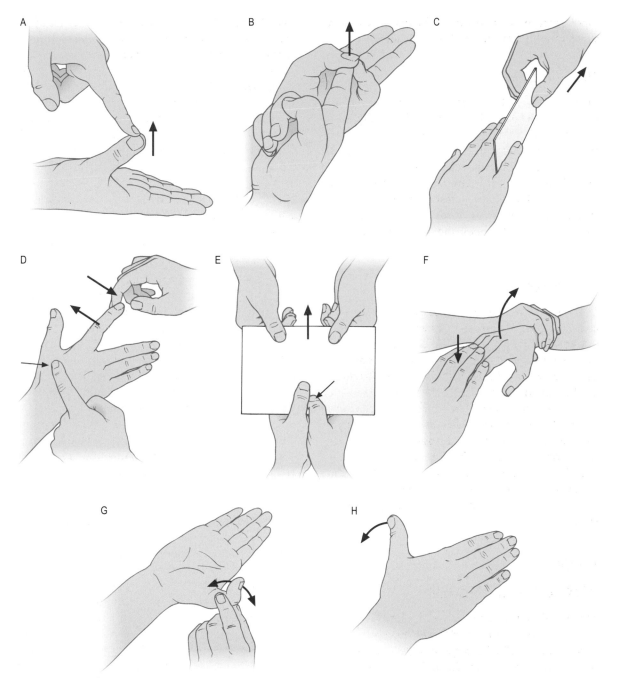

FIGURE 1.14 Thumb flexion, extension, abduction, opposition (median), interossei, first dorsal interosseus, adductor pollicis (ulnar) and wrist and finger extensors (radial) (from Douglas et al 2005)

of the cervical and lumbar lordoses (curvature of the spine in the sagittal plane). A gibbus is a marked increase in forward flexion of the spine due to anterior wedging at one or more vertebral levels. Look at the spine from behind, specifically for swellings; spasm of the erector spinae and an associated lumbar tilt that might suggest a disc prolapse; café au lait spots or nodules that might indicate neurofibromatosis; a hairy patch suggesting spinal dysraphism; asymmetry of shoulder height; trunk and pelvic alignment; rib hump and a lateral spinal curvature suggesting scoliosis; and leg length discrepancy, by observing pelvic orientation with respect to the horizontal.

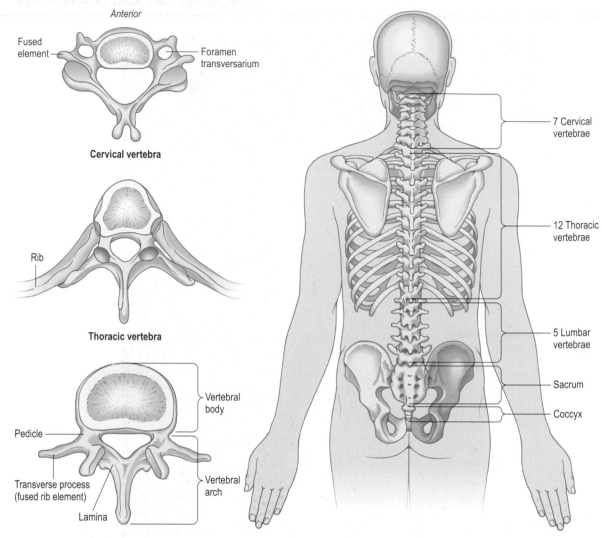

FIGURE 1.15   Cervical, thoracic and lumbar vertebrae (from Drake et al 2004)

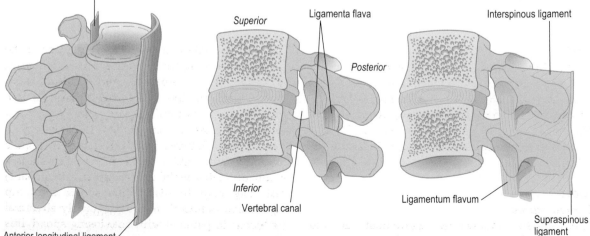

FIGURE 1.16   Ligaments of the spine (from Drake et al 2004)

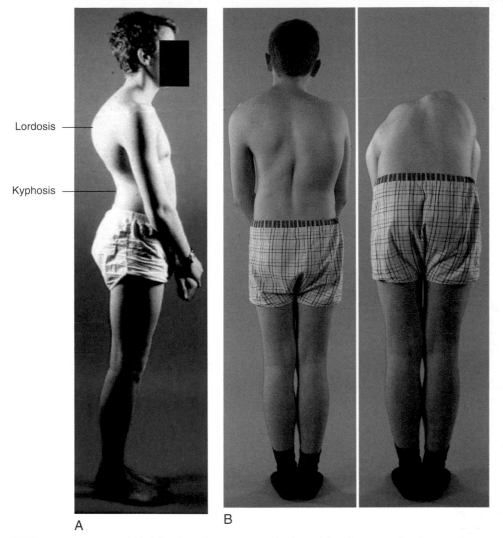

Lordosis

Kyphosis

A

B

FIGURE 1.17 Common spinal deformities. (A) Lordosis and kyphosis; (B) scoliosis: note that the curve is more prominent on Adam's (forward bend) test. Photographs by courtesy of Mr A. Tsirikos

Feel

Palpate the spinous processes to elicit tenderness. Note any paraspinal muscle tenderness.

In the neck check the thyroid gland, and the supraclavicular fossae for enlarged lymph nodes. Note any tenderness in the trapezius.

In the lumbar spine also palpate the sacroiliac joints.

Move

Lumbar spine

Figure 1.18 summarizes movement at the lumbar and thoracic spine. Flexion can be assessed by making a mark in the midline at the level of the 'dimples of Venus'. A second mark is made 10 cm proximal and a third mark 5 cm distal to the first mark, again in the midline. On forward flexion the uppermost and lowermost marks should separate by a further 5 cm. Patients who have a very stiff spine may appear to exhibit good forward flexion as a result of having mobile hips and this (Schober's) test may help to distinguish spinal from hip movement. Schober's test is commonly abnormal (reduced) in patients with ankylosing spondylitis (Fig. 1.19).

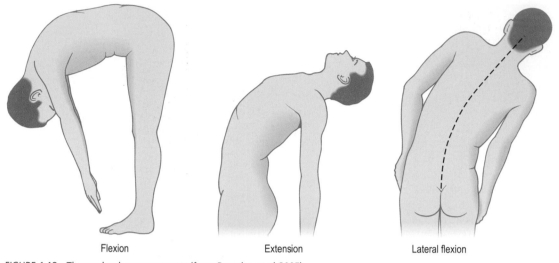

Flexion   Extension   Lateral flexion

FIGURE 1.18   Thoracolumbar movements (from Douglas et al 2005)

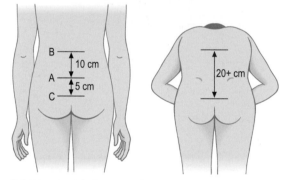

FIGURE 1.19   Schober's test (from Douglas et al 2005)

Thoracic spine

Most spinal rotation occurs through the thoracic spine. To test this, the patient's pelvis is stabilized by the examiner and the patient is asked to rotate their shoulders from side to side.

Chest expansion should differ by about 7 cm between full inspiration and full expiration. Typically in patients with ankylosing spondylitis, chest expansion is reduced significantly to 4 cm or below (use a measuring tape around the chest and ask patients to breathe deeply out, and then in).

There is no flexion in the thoracic spine, because it is splinted by the ribcage.

A 'forward bend' test may highlight a structural scoliosis, which will be more prominent on forward flexion by causing the rib hump on the convexity of the curve to be more noticeable. A postural scoliosis may disappear.

The patient is asked to arch backwards to test extension, but it is important that the knees are extended whilst doing so to minimize posterior pelvic tilt during the manoeuvre.

Lateral flexion is tested by asking the patient to slide their hand down the lateral aspect of the thigh towards the knee on the same side.

There is no rotation in the lumbar spine because the facet joints are vertical.

Cervical spine

There is a wide range of movement in the cervical spine, which diminishes as age increases (Fig. 1.20). Flexion and extension occur throughout the cervical spine. Extension is tested by asking the patient to look up towards the ceiling as far as they can. For flexion ask the patient to put their chin on their chest or to look down at the floor as far as they can. Rotation occurs throughout the cervical spine, but mainly at the atlanto-axial joint (C1/C2) and is tested by asking the patient to look over their shoulders. For lateral flexion ask the patient to attempt to put their ear on the ipsilateral shoulder.

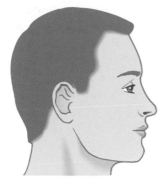

Neutral

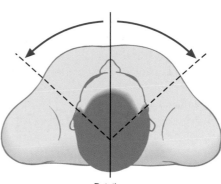

Rotation

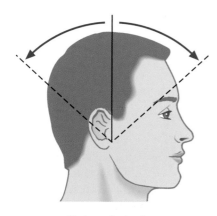

Flexion and extension

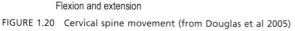

Lateral flexion

FIGURE 1.20   Cervical spine movement (from Douglas et al 2005)

Other features relevant to the spine

Ask the patient to lie prone. Sensation in the posterior aspect of the lower limbs and power in the hamstrings, quadriceps and plantarflexors can be tested in this position.

The *femoral nerve stretch* test is tested as follows: the knee is flexed to 90°, the pelvis stabilized by one of the examiner's hands and with the other hand the hip is extended whilst the knee is held flexed (Fig. 1.21). Pain in the anterior thigh indicates a positive test and suggests nerve root irritation of the femoral nerve or one of its component roots. It is often positive in upper lumbar disc prolapse involving the L2/3 or L3/4 discs. The Achilles' tendon reflexes (ankle jerks) can also be tested while the patient is prone.

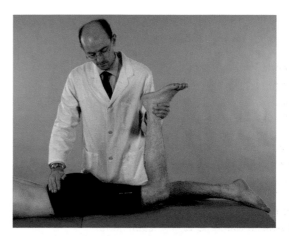

FIGURE 1.21   Femoral nerve stretch test

The patient is then asked to lie supine and again sensation in the lower limbs is tested as well as the pedal pulses. Muscle power of the hip flexors, knee extensors, knee flexors, ankle plantar, and dorsi-flexors, evertors and invertors are tested along with the patellar tendon reflexes. Hip, knee and ankle ranges of movement may also be tested.

The *straight leg raising* test is performed by keeping the knee extended and at the same time passively flexing the hip. The test is positive if there is a restriction of straight leg raising by pain radiating from the back down the posterior aspect of the thigh and calf. Tension on the sciatic nerve (sciatic nerve stretch test) can be increased by dorsi-flexion of the ankle which, if positive, increases the leg pain (Fig. 1.22).

The *tibial nerve stretch test* is also performed while the patient remains supine. The hip is flexed to 90° and the knee is extended. Press on the tibial nerve, which is located in the midline of the popliteal fossa. The test is positive if the patient complains of pain in the posterior calf or thigh. In this position the tibial nerve 'bowstrings' across the popliteal fossa. Hamstring shortening will also limit knee extension when the hip is flexed and the knee is being extended.

It is important to distinguish between nerve root irritation and nerve root compression. An example of the former is a positive straight leg raise test without any other neurological disturbances, and of the latter, loss of a reflex and muscle weakness. The two may coexist, however.

Loss of the ankle reflex may indicate a L5/S1 disc prolapse and weakness of extensor hallucis longus may be associated with a L4/5 disc prolapse.

It is also possible to test straight leg raising whilst distracting the patient. One way is to ask the patient to sit up straight when sitting on the bed or couch to see if they are able to keep their knees extended whilst having their hips flexed to 90°. If they are able to do so it would indicate the equivalent of a straight leg raise to 90°. The *flip test* is an alternative method. Ask the patient to sit on the edge of the bed whilst holding their hips and knees at 90° of flexion. Attempt to extend the knee of the leg under consideration; if they are able to tolerate full knee extension whilst maintaining hip flexion to 90°, this would suggest an equivalent of a straight leg raise of 90°. If the patient has sciatic nerve irritation or compression they may resist having their knee extended. Alternatively, they will arch their

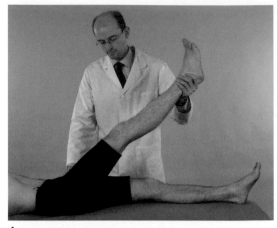

A

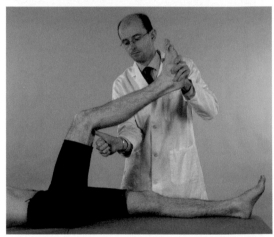

B

C

FIGURE 1.22 Stretch tests – sciatic nerve roots. In neutral position, the nerve roots are slack. (A) Straight leg raising may be limited by tension of root over prolapsed disc. (B) Root tension relieved by flexion at the knee. (C) Pressure over centre of popliteal fossa bears on posterior tibial nerve, which is 'bowstringing' across the fossa causing pain locally and radiation into the back

spine posteriorly, which will relieve tension on the sciatic nerve (flip).

During these manoeuvres the patient's demeanour and ability to carry out these tasks can also be observed.

HIP

ANATOMY OVERVIEW

The hip is a ball and socket joint and as a result is inherently more stable and less mobile than the shoulder joint. The muscles that act on the hip are shown in Table 1.4. In addition, the tensor fascia latae stabilizes the pelvis and rotates the tibia laterally on the femur.

The anatomy of hip and thigh muscles is shown in Figures 1.23 to 1.28. The vastus medialis, lateralis and intermedius extend the knee, as does rectus femoris, which also flexes the hip. The hamstrings (biceps femoris, semimembranosus and semitendinosus) extend the hip and flex the knee (Box 1.3).

The adductors are supplied by the obturator nerve (with the exception of magnus, which also receives a supply from the tibial division of the sciatic nerve), the vasti by the femoral nerve and the hamstrings by the sciatic nerve.

Look

The patient should be suitably undressed down to their underwear and chaperoned where appropriate. The presence of a hip deformity, for example a flexion contracture, muscle wasting, the

spine and a limb length discrepancy can be observed. Ask the patient to walk with and without walking aids if possible. The normal arc of motion at the hip in gait is about 45°. Does the hip have a normal, reduced or excessive range of motion in gait? Is there a limp and if so does it appear to be antalgic, i.e. painful (in which case there may be a reduced stance time on the affected side)? Does the patient have a 'waddling gait' suggestive of abductor insufficiency or a longstanding hip dislocation?

Perform Trendelenburg's test by asking the patient to stand on one leg for 30 s and then on the other (Fig. 1.29). You may help the patient by supporting their weight through their outstretched hands. The test is positive if the unsupported side of the pelvis drops, and is normal if the unsupported side of the pelvis rises. Factors producing a positive sign are weak hip abductors, hip disloca-

Table 1.4 Muscles acting on the hip

Muscle type	Example
Flexors	Psoas, rectus and sartorius
Extensors	Gluteus maximus and hamstrings
Abductors	Gluteus medius and minimus
Adductors	Adductor magnus, longus, brevis and gracilis
Internal rotation	Anterior half of gluteus medius
External rotation	Gemelli, obturator internus and quadratus femoris

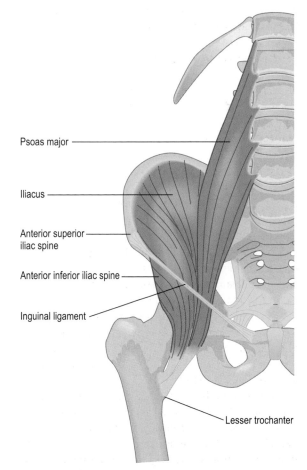

Psoas major

Iliacus

Anterior superior iliac spine

Anterior inferior iliac spine

Inguinal ligament

Lesser trochanter

FIGURE 1.23 Iliopsoas (from Drake et al 2004)

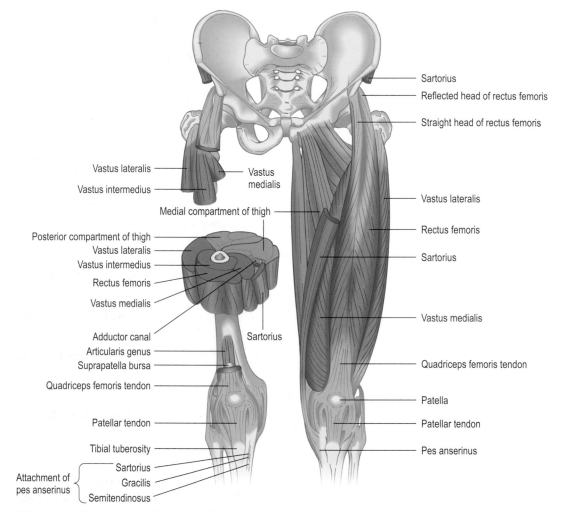

Sartorius
Reflected head of rectus femoris
Straight head of rectus femoris

Vastus lateralis
Vastus intermedius

Vastus medialis

Medial compartment of thigh

Vastus lateralis

Rectus femoris

Posterior compartment of thigh
Vastus lateralis
Vastus intermedius
Rectus femoris
Vastus medialis

Sartorius

Adductor canal
Articularis genus
Suprapatella bursa
Quadriceps femoris tendon

Sartorius

Vastus medialis

Quadriceps femoris tendon

Patellar tendon

Patella
Patellar tendon

Tibial tuberosity

Pes anserinus

Attachment of pes anserinus { Sartorius / Gracilis / Semitendinosus

FIGURE 1.24   Anterior aspect of the thigh (from Drake et al 2004)

tion or a longstanding fracture of the neck of femur and pain. Each condition results in gluteal insufficiency through either hip abductor weakness or an underlying muscle lever arm problem due to a skeletal or joint abnormality.

Feel
Since the hip is a deep-seated joint, palpation can be limited to the trochanteric region to elicit tenderness in the trochanteric bursa.

Move
Have the patient lie supine. When assessing the passive range of hip movement remember to be aware of the position of the patient's pelvis and

movement that occurs at the pelvis rather than at the hip itself. This may give a false indication of 'hip' movement.

Estimate true and apparent limb lengths (Fig. 1.30). True limb length is measured with a tape measure by using the anterior superior iliac spine, the tibial tubercle and the medial malleolus to measure indirectly femoral and tibial length or the overall limb length. These measurements are subject to errors from placement of the tape measure, from movement of the skin and subcutaneous tissues overlying the bony landmarks, and a natural difference between leg lengths within the population as a whole. The limbs should be placed symmetrically when taking these measurements. Apparent limb length is assessed by measuring the

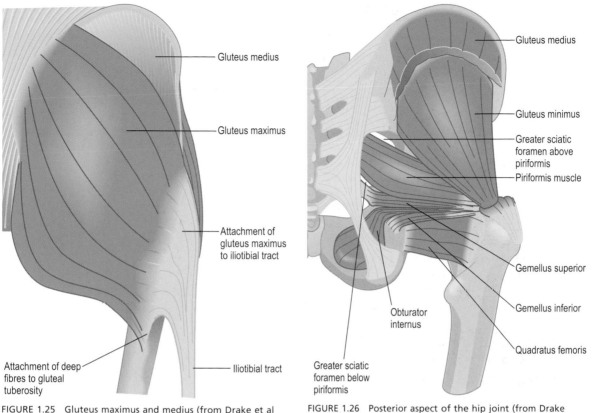

FIGURE 1.25   Gluteus maximus and medius (from Drake et al 2004)

FIGURE 1.26   Posterior aspect of the hip joint (from Drake et al 2004)

distance from the umbilicus or xiphisternum to the medial malleolus.

Hip stability in a baby or toddler is assessed by Ortolani's and Barlow's tests (see Chapter 26). The former is an assessment of hip reducibility. For Ortolani's test, the child's hip and knee are flexed and the examiner places their middle finger over the greater trochanter and thumb over the proximal thigh medially. The middle finger is used to pull the greater trochanter forward to attempt to reduce the hip. Barlow's test is the reverse of the Ortolani test where stability of the reduced hip is assessed by gently flexing the hip and knee and using the thumb to push the thigh backwards whilst adducting the hip. The test is positive if there is an exit clunk of the femoral head.

Hip flexion, internal/external rotation and adduction/abduction are assessed when the patient is supine. The femur may lie externally rotated after a fracture of the neck of femur or if the patient has a slipped upper femoral epiphysis. Thomas's test is used to detect a fixed flexion deformity of the hip. Flatten the lumbar lordosis by flexing the opposite hip as far as possible. You can check that the lumbar lordosis has been obliterated by placing your hand between the patient's lumbar segment and the bed. If there is a fixed flexion deformity (or loss of extension) of the hip under consideration, the thigh will lift up off the bed. Repeat the test for the other hip. A fixed flexion deformity of the hip will result in the patient not being able to lay the knee on the affected side flat on the examining couch. Remember that this may have nothing to do with hip pathology and be a result of a problem within the knee. It is important under these circumstances to examine both the hip and knee to determine where the pathology lies when a patient is unable to lay their knee flat on the examining couch. The patient's hip and knee can be examined whilst they lie on their side.

A child's *rotational profile* (femoral anteversion, tibial torsion and foot adductus) is assessed by

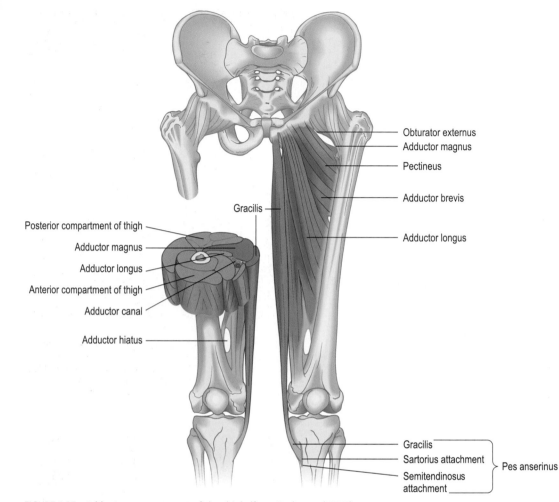

FIGURE 1.27 Adductor compartment of the thigh (from Drake et al 2004)

having them lie prone flexing the knee to 90° and rotating the hip whilst palpating the greater trochanter to determine its most prominent position. Once you have found this, estimate the angle of the tibial shaft to the vertical; this gives the value of anteversion and is usually about 10° and 15° in the skeletally mature male and female respectively. In young children the values may be much higher and can be nearer 40° in the neonate. Tibial torsion is assessed indirectly by bending the knee to 90° and visually superimposing the foot over the proximal thigh, thus giving the 'foot–thigh angle', an indirect estimate of tibial torsion, which in the skeletally mature individual is about 15–20° external. It is important that the mid-axis of the calcaneus is aligned with the mid-axis of the posterior part of the shank, i.e. the hind foot should be in neutral

varus/valgus alignment. Lastly, the shape of the foot can be evaluated with the patient in this position.

KNEE
ANATOMY OVERVIEW

The knee can be considered mainly as a hinge joint between the femur and tibia, but includes the patello-femoral joint within the same synovial cavity. Knee flexors are hamstrings and gastrocnemius. Knee extensors are the quadriceps muscles. There is also some rotation within the knee joint; when the foot is on the ground the last 30° of knee extension is associated with internal rotation of the femur on the tibia, and when the foot is off

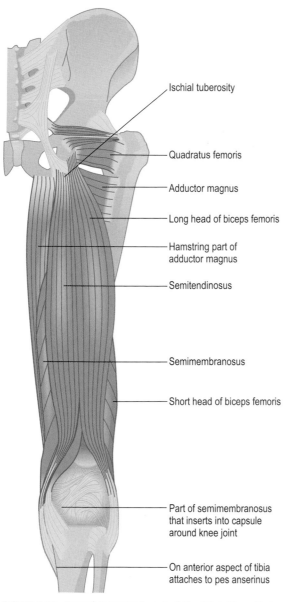

FIGURE 1.28 Posterior compartment of the thigh (from Drake et al 2004)

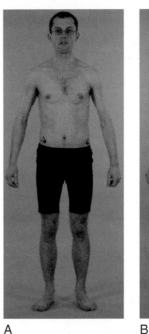
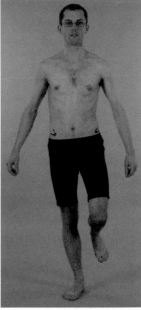

A   B

FIGURE 1.29 Trendelenburg's test. (A) In the neutral position, the patient stands on both legs; the iliac crests are level. (B) The patient then puts all his or her weight on the affected leg and raises the good leg. In a patient with a weak set of hip muscles, the buttock of the elevated leg will drop

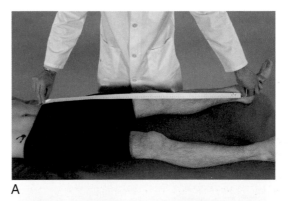

A

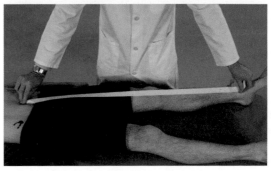

B

FIGURE 1.30 Measuring (A) true and (B) apparent limb length

Labels on Figure 1.28:

- Ischial tuberosity
- Quadratus femoris
- Adductor magnus
- Long head of biceps femoris
- Hamstring part of adductor magnus
- Semitendinosus
- Semimembranosus
- Short head of biceps femoris
- Part of semimembranosus that inserts into capsule around knee joint
- On anterior aspect of tibia attaches to pes anserinus

Box 1.3
Muscle compartments of the thigh

- Anterior: rectus, sartorius and vasti
- Posterior: biceps, semimembranosus and semitendinosus
- Medial: adductor magnus, longus and brevis, and gracilis

the ground extension is associated with lateral rotation of the tibia on the femur. The medial and lateral menisci act as 'shock absorbers' between the two major joint surfaces. The collateral ligaments originate from the corresponding epicondyle of the femur (Fig. 1.31). The lateral collateral ligament inserts onto the fibular head and the medial collateral onto the medial condyle of the tibia. The collateral ligaments impart coronal plane stability of the knee. The cruciate ligaments resist fore/aft

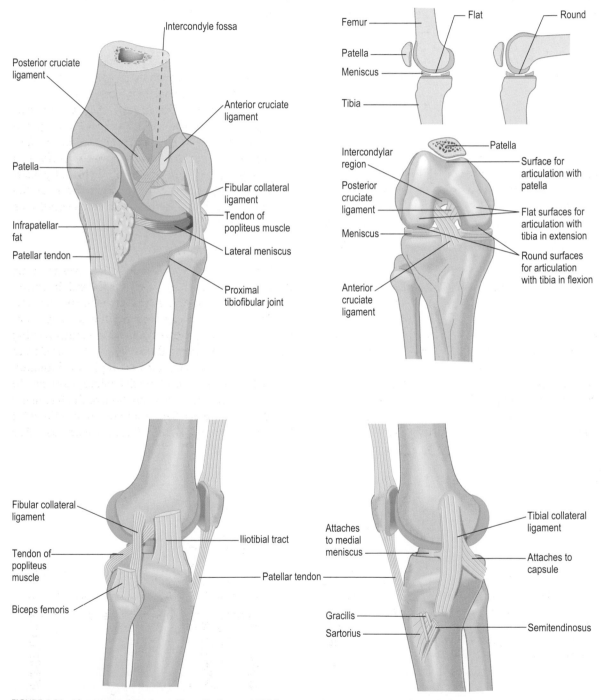

FIGURE 1.31   Ligaments of the knee (from Drake et al 2004)

forces in the knee. The anterior cruciate arises from the anterior intercondylar area of the tibia, and passes upwards and backwards to be inserted on the posterior part of the medial surface of the lateral femoral condyle. The posterior cruciate arises from the posterior intercondylar area of the tibia, and passes upwards, forwards and medially to be attached to the lateral aspect of the medial femoral condyle. The knee has about a dozen bursae associated with the joint. Clinically important ones are: anteriorly, the large supra-patellar bursa and the smaller pre-patellar bursa; posteriorly, in the midline of the popliteal fossa; and medially, those associated with the semimembranosus tendon.

Look

Observe the patient walking. The normal arc of movement of the knee in gait is 45° – is it normal, reduced or excessive, for example by hyperextending?

Look for an effusion, thigh muscle wasting, loss of full extension, varus/valgus malalignment and the popliteal fossa. Assess the shape of the knee when the patient stands; for example, does the varus/valgus worsen with load bearing?

Feel

Ask the patient to lie supine. Feel for warmth (using the back of your hand), synovial thickening, or an effusion. For small effusions, fluid can be milked out of the medial parapatellar 'dimple' into the suprapatellar pouch and then milked back into the dimple to produce a bulge of fluid – the 'cross-fluctuation test'. For larger effusions, fluid can be milked down from the suprapatellar pouch into the retro-patellar area and the patella 'balotted' down onto the femoral condyles in a bath of fluid – the 'patellar tap' test. Feel for tenderness along the medial and lateral joint line, and tenderness over the origin and insertions of the collateral ligaments, tibial tuberosity, inferior and superior poles of the patella and patellar facets.

Move

Assess the active and passive range of flexion and extension. The knee may hyperextend, which could be due to normal joint laxity or following posterior cruciate instability. Assess crepitus during passive flexion and extension. Check patellar tracking. If there is a history of patellar instability, a patellar apprehension test can be performed by attempting to displace the patella (usually laterally). Compare your findings with those of the opposite knee, but remember that some conditions cause bilateral abnormalities.

Ligament laxity tests

Abduction (valgus) and adduction (varus) tests (Fig. 1.32) are used to assess collateral integrity. Stand on the side of the knee to be examined. Lift the lower limb up and support the patient's foot and ankle in the crook of your elbow, thus leaving your hands free. Place the knee in 10° of flexion to relax the posterior capsule and apply an abduction stress to the knee joint whilst taking care not to rotate the hip when doing so. Repeat the test using an adduction stress. The test is positive if the joint 'opens up'. Compare your findings with the other

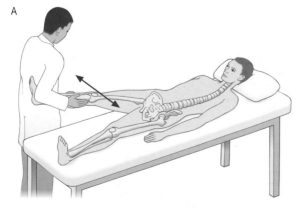
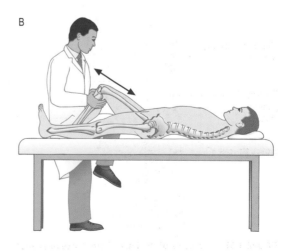

FIGURE 1.32 Ligament tests of the knee (from Douglas et al 2005)

knee. To test the cruciates, flex the knee to 90° and place the patient's foot on the examining couch. Observe the relationship of the femoral condyles to the tibial plateau – is the plateau displaced posteriorly (posterior sag test)? This would be consistent with a posterior cruciate injury. Stabilize the foot by sitting on it. Grasp the medial and lateral aspects of the upper tibia with both hands and attempt to draw the tibia forward over the femoral condyles. If there is excessive translation there may be an anterior cruciate injury (anterior drawer test), but remember to compare your findings with the opposite side. If you suspect a posterior cruciate injury, try translating the tibial plateau posteriorly over the femoral condyles (posterior drawer test). For both these tests it is important to verify that the starting point of the tibial condyles is in the normal anatomical position, otherwise you may have a false-positive test. Anterior cruciate integrity can also be tested by Lachman's test. Flex the knee to 10–15°, grasp the distal thigh with one hand and the proximal shin with the other, check that the tibial plateau is in its normal anatomical position and then attempt to translate the tibia forward in relation to the femur. Excessive forward translation would suggest an anterior cruciate injury. Again, compare the findings with the opposite knee.

Meniscal tests

The most common signs associated with a meniscal tear are the presence of a small effusion, reproduction of joint margin pain when squatting down and joint margin tenderness. To detect joint margin tenderness, ask the patient to flex the knee to 90°. The lateral joint margin is located just proximal to Gerdy's tubercle. The medial joint margin is at the same level on the other side. Meniscal tears are most common in the middle and posterior third of the meniscus, so tenderness is frequently maximal posteriorly.

FOOT AND ANKLE
ANATOMY OVERVIEW

The ankle joint comprises the tibia, fibula and talus, or talo-crural joint, and acts as a hinge joint; thus allowing plantarflexion (flexion) and dorsiflexion (extension). Inversion and eversion are composite movements occurring at the subtalar

(talo-calcaneal) and midtarsal joints (calcaneocuboid and talo-navicular) (Fig. 1.33). The movement of the foot has also been likened to that of the hand and the terms 'supination' and 'pronation' of the foot are also used, often interchangeably, with inversion and eversion. This is not strictly correct, and supination can be considered a composite movement incorporating adduction, plantarflexion and inversion, whereas pronation incorporates abduction, eversion and dorsiflexion. Inversion is produced by tibialis anterior and posterior, and eversion by the peronei. The plantar flexors are the gastrocnemius and soleus, and there is also a contribution from tibialis posterior, flexor hallucis longus and flexor digitorum longus, all of which pass around the back of the ankle. Dorsiflexion of the ankle occurs from the action of the anterior tibial muscles, tibialis anterior, extensor hallucis longus and extensor digitorum longus (Box 1.4).

There are three arches of the foot: medial, lateral and transverse.

Look

Observe the patient's gait. Which part of their foot contacts the ground, is the heel in varus/valgus/neutral during stance and swing, does the foot clear the ground during swing? Is the wear on the soles of the patient's shoes symmetrical? Is there a symmetrical distribution of callosities in the feet?

Look for calf muscle wasting suggestive of a neurological condition, flattening of the medial arch (if so, does the arch correct on standing?), pes cavus, bunions, club foot, metatarsus adductus and bony prominences, particularly of the metatarsal heads.

Feel

Feel for an ankle effusion or warmth, and for the dorsalis pedis and posterior tibial pulses, which may be reduced and point to an ischaemic cause for the patient's pain, or be of relevance when considering the potential for wound healing if surgery is being contemplated. Feel for painful bunions or metatarsalgia (under the metatarsal heads).

Move

Assess active and passive dorsi- and plantarflexion, and inversion and eversion. To distinguish between the hind and mid-foot components of inversion and eversion passively, grasp the shin with one hand and the heel with the other and invert and

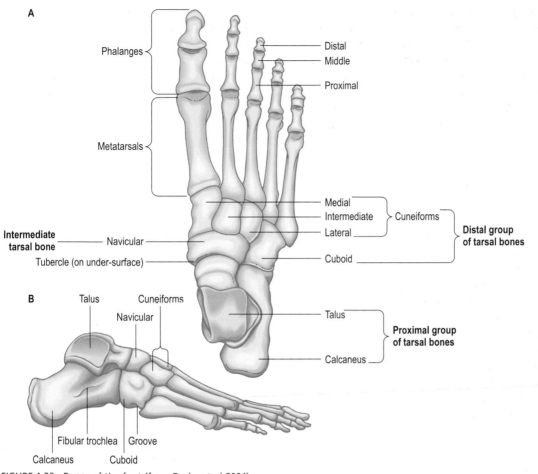

A

Phalanges
- Distal
- Middle
- Proximal

Metatarsals

Medial
Intermediate
Lateral
} Cuneiforms

Distal group of tarsal bones

Intermediate tarsal bone

Navicular

Cuboid

Tubercle (on under-surface)

B

Talus

Cuneiforms

Navicular

Talus

Proximal group of tarsal bones

Calcaneus

Fibular trochlea | Groove

Calcaneus | Cuboid

FIGURE 1.33 Bones of the foot (from Drake et al 2004)

evert the calcaneus (Fig. 1.34). This tests passive movement at the subtalar joint. To assess the midfoot component of inversion and eversion, grasp the heel in one hand and the midfoot in the other and repeat the manoeuvre. There is no active movement at the tarso-metatarsal joints. Mobility of the toes can be assessed actively and passively. Integrity of the Achilles tendon can be assessed by asking the patient to lie prone with their feet over the end of the couch. You can palpate the Achilles tendon to feel for a gap and then squeeze the patient's calf. The Achilles tendon is intact if the ankle plantar flexes on squeezing the calf (Simmonds or Thompson test).

NEUROLOGICAL ASSESSMENT OF THE LOWER LIMB

Dermatomes and myotomes in the lower limb can be used to check neurological function (Figs 1.35–1.37, Tables 1.5 & 1.6). Muscle wasting and fasciculation should be checked as well as abnormal tone

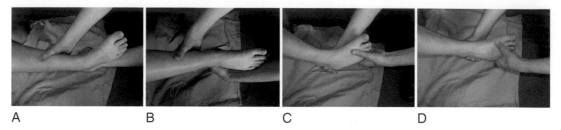

A   B   C   D

FIGURE 1.34 Subtalar and midtarsal movements

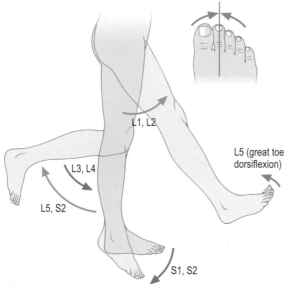

FIGURE 1.35 Movements generated by myotomes of the lower limb (from Drake et al 2004)

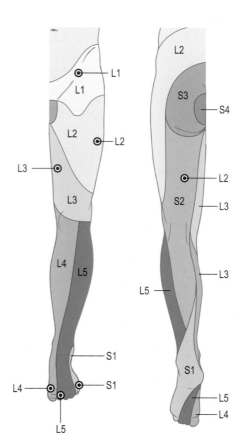

FIGURE 1.36 Dermatomes of the lower limb (from Drake et al 2004)

and strength. Of the other modalities, perception of light touch is commonly assessed. The dermatomes of the lower limbs and the sensory territories of the major peripheral nerves are shown in Figures 1.35–1.37.

In order to check the sensory components of the major nerve roots for the lower limb, you need to test sensation over the following areas: anterior part of the proximal thigh just distal to the inguinal ligament (L1), antero-lateral aspect of the mid thigh (L2), antero-medial aspect of the distal thigh (L3), the medial aspect of the shank (L4), lateral aspect of the shank (L5), the lateral aspect of the little toe (S1) and so on.

MOTOR FUNCTION

Muscles in the lower limb are supplied by the femoral, sciatic, obturator and gluteal nerves. The superior and inferior gluteal nerves supply the abductor muscles and the obturator nerve supplies the adductor muscles. The femoral nerve supplies the quadriceps muscle. All other muscles in the lower limb are supplied by the sciatic nerve and its branches. The two main branches are the common peroneal nerve and the tibial nerve. The peroneal nerve supplies the muscles of the anterior and peroneal compartment of the leg. The tibial nerve supplies the muscles of the deep and superficial posterior compartments.

34

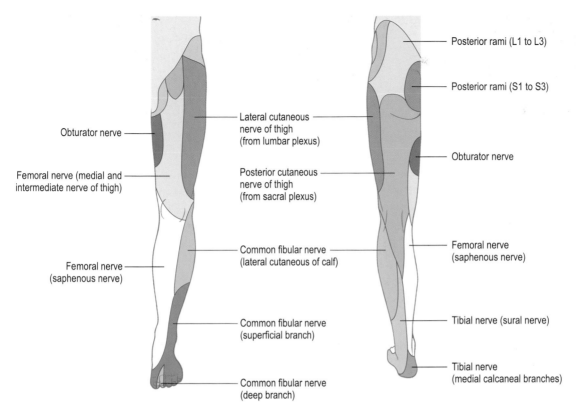

Obturator nerve

Femoral nerve (medial and intermediate nerve of thigh)

Femoral nerve (saphenous nerve)

Lateral cutaneous nerve of thigh (from lumbar plexus)

Posterior cutaneous nerve of thigh (from sacral plexus)

Common fibular nerve (lateral cutaneous of calf)

Common fibular nerve (superficial branch)

Common fibular nerve (deep branch)

Posterior rami (L1 to L3)

Posterior rami (S1 to S3)

Obturator nerve

Femoral nerve (saphenous nerve)

Tibial nerve (sural nerve)

Tibial nerve (medial calcaneal branches)

FIGURE 1.37   Sensory territories of the major lower limb peripheral nerves (from Drake et al 2004)

Table 1.5 Motor innervation of lower limb

Movement	Innervation
Hip flexion	L1 L2
Knee extension	L3 L4
Knee flexion	L5 S1 S2
Hindfoot inversion	L4
Great toe dorsiflexion	L5
Ankle plantarflexion	S1 S2

Table 1.6 Reflexes in the lower limb and trunk

Reflex	Innervation
Abdominal	T8 to T12
Knee	L2 L3 L4
Ankle	S1 S2

Emergency diagnoses in the locomotor system and the danger to which attention is drawn are listed in Table 1.8.

Clinicians frequently misdiagnose rare but dangerous conditions. In the early stages of such disorders, the clinical features may be similar to more common self-limiting conditions. Later, there is no excuse for missing an obvious swelling.

The absence of a traumatic cause for one or more of these clinical features should provoke suspicion, and stimulate further investigation. Patients who volunteer previous trauma, however, should not be ignored, even if the X-ray is normal. Parents of children with bone tumours, for example, frequently describe an earlier bruise or football injury, which 'went on to become a painful lump'. It is

'RED FLAGS' IN NON-TRAUMATIC DISORDERS

On the beach, never swim where a red flag is flying; a danger to life exists. In medicine, never ignore a 'red flag' symptom or sign; a danger to life or limb exists. These clinical features are shown in Table 1.7.

Table 1.7 Clinical 'red flag' features suggesting serious pathology

Symptom	Sign
Pain preventing sleep	'Drawn' facial appearance
Loss of appetite	Saddle anaesthesia
Loss of weight	Bilateral limb neurology
Visual loss	Upper motor neurone signs
Temporal headache and blurred vision	Painful swelling
Loss of bladder/bowel control	Fever >38°C
Rapidly progressive symptoms	Inability to weight-bear
	Red, hot joint

Table 1.8 Emergency diagnoses and dangers in musculoskeletal patients

Diagnosis	Danger
Tumour	Loss of life or limb
Infection	Bone or joint destruction
Central cord compression	Limb/bladder/bowel dysfunction
Cauda equina syndrome	Bladder/bowel dysfunction
Giant cell arteritis	Blindness
Slipped upper femoral epiphysis	Early hip arthritis

important for the alert clinician to believe his/her own examination findings, and act on them. This will often lead to an early diagnosis and a better patient outcome.

TUMOUR

Malignant tumours of bone and soft tissues are aggressive and, therefore, grow rapidly. Features indicative of malignant potential include lesions that are:

- rapidly growing
- over 5 cm size

- painful
- deep to deep fascia.

These lesions should be viewed as a potential malignant tumour until proven otherwise. Even one or two of these features should provoke early investigation. A delay of weeks will compromise treatment options and survival.

INFECTION

Features of bone and joint infection are those of local inflammation. These can be masked in the immunosuppressed; a high index of suspicion should exist in a patient with a musculoskeletal swelling who is unwell, on immunosuppressive therapy or suffering from an immunodeficiency disorder. In non-immunosuppressed children, clinical features predictive of osteomyelitis or septic arthritis include:

- inability to weight-bear
- temperature >38°C
- leukocyte count >12 000 cells/mm³
- erythrocyte sedimentation rate (ESR) >40 mm/h.

As in potentially malignant tumours, even one or two of these features should provoke early investigation. A delay of hours or days will lead to established infection, with bone or joint destruction and more extensive surgical reconstruction.

SPINAL DISORDERS

Symptoms predictive of potentially serious spinal pathology are as above; additional features identified by the Royal College of General Practitioners are:

- presentation under age 20 or over age 55
- non-mechanical pain
- thoracic pain
- past history of carcinoma, steroids, human immunodeficiency virus
- widespread neurological symptoms
- structural deformity.

Signs of an 'upper motor neurone' lesion indicating central cord compression include hypertonic weakness and rigidity, brisk reflexes and sustained clonus. Causes include spinal infection (pyogenic or tuberculosis), tumour, cervical vertebral subluxation secondary to trauma or rheumatoid arthritis or a cervical or thoracic central disc prolapse. Symptoms of sphincter and gait disturbance with saddle anaesthesia are highly suggestive of cauda equina syndrome, requiring an urgent magnetic resonance imaging scan for confirmation of central disc prolapse and appropriate urgent spinal decompression.

GIANT CELL ARTERITIS

When this vasculitic condition affects the temporal artery it is known as 'temporal arteritis' and can occasionally involve ciliary artery occlusion, leading to blindness. Symptoms of polymyalgia rheumatica should prompt questions about temporal pain and blurred vision, and examination for temporal tenderness. If these features are present then steroids should be commenced and an immediate rheumatological referral made to include temporal artery biopsy.

SLIPPED UPPER FEMORAL EPIPHYSIS

A mild form of this condition of late childhood and adolescence is important to identify early for the prevention of complete slip and a uniformly poor outcome. Acute groin, thigh or knee pain should suggest the possibility of hip pathology. An inability to weight-bear should result in an immediate orthopaedic referral. The classical description is of an older boy held between two parents with an externally rotated leg and non-weight-bearing. In an adolescent, a radiograph in the antero-posterior and (especially) lateral planes might reveal a slip of the proximal femoral physis. Long-term prognosis depends upon the degree of slip. Even in those able to walk, persistent limp or pain for longer than a week should be investigated promptly to avoid a progressive 'acute on chronic' slip.

SUMMARY

'Red flags' are key symptoms and signs that alert the clinician to the possibility of serious disease. To elicit them early is of vital importance to a satisfactory patient outcome.

FURTHER READING

Douglas G, Nicol F, Robertson C (eds) 2005 Macleod's clinical examination, 11th edn. Churchill Livingstone, Edinburgh.
Drake R, Vogl W, Mitchell A 2004 Gray's anatomy for students. Churchill Livingstone, Edinburgh.

APPENDIX

Figure 1.38 provides a structured proforma for use when assessing patients with rheumatic diseases.

38

New patient proforma for rheumatology patients

Name	New appointment	○
Address	Re-referral	○
Hospital no	Date	
Date of birth	Routine	○
Age	Urgent	○
Sex		

Main problem?

Joint pain	Muscle pain	Stiff	Swelling	Limp	Weak-ness	Other (specify)
○	○	○	○	○	○	○

Symptom onset month year	Precipitating event?

Current areas affected (if only one side affected, write R or L)

	Pain	Swelling	Stiffness	Weakness
Hand	○	○	○	○
Wrist	○	○	○	○
Forearm	○	○	○	○
Elbow	○	○	○	○
Upper arm	○	○	○	○
Shoulder	○	○	○	○
Hip	○	○	○	○
Thigh	○	○	○	○
Knee	○	○	○	○
Calf	○	○	○	○
Ankle	○	○	○	○
Feet	○	○	○	○
Neck	○	○	○	○
Back	○	○	○	○

	No spread	Symmetrical	Asymmetrical	Flitting
Spread?	○	○	○	○

Early morning stiffness duration (minutes)

Nil	<15	<30	<60	<120	>120	Specify
○	○	○	○	○	○	

What makes the problems worse/better?   nothing ○

	Drugs	Physio-therapy	Rest	Exercise	Other	Specify
Worse	○	○	○	○	○	
Better	○	○	○	○	○	

Variability of symptoms?   None ○

	Morning	Afternoon	Evening	Night
Worst time	○	○	○	○
Best time	○	○	○	○

Current job   Previous job if not working

Off sick from current job? ○   Medically retired? ○

Which activities are difficult to perform?	No problems	○
Dressing ○	Getting in/out of bath	○
Shopping ○		○
Walking ○		○
Walking up stairs ○		○
Walking down stairs ○		○
On and off toilet ○		

Family history	None	○
RA ○	OA	○
Psoriasis ○	SLE/CT	○
Psoriatic arthritis ○	Other	○
Back pain ○ Specify		

Current medications	nil ○	Drug name	Dose
Drug name	Dose		

Toxicity/allergy	nil	○

Other medical problems	None	○
Diabetes ○	Hypertension	○
Ischaemic heart disease ○	TB	○
Peripheral vascular disease ○	Rheumatic fever	○
Gastric/duodenal ulcer ○	Psoriasis	○
Hypothyroidism ○	Hyperthyroidism	○
Oesophageal reflux ○	Photosensitivity	○
COPD ○	Raynaud's	○
Asthma ○	Operations	○
Inflammatory bowel disease ○ Specify	Other	○

	Never	Ex	Current	No. per day
Smoker	○	○	○	○

Alcohol intake (units per week)	0	<10	10-20	21-30	31-40	>40	Binge
	○	○	○	○	○	○	○

Exercise/sports	Number of times per month					
	0	1-2	3-4	5-6	7-8	Other
	○	○	○	○	○	○

Sleep disturbance?	No	Yes	Due to pain
	○	○	○

FIGURE 1.38 A suggested history and examination proforma for rheumatology patients

Examination

Weight		Height		BMI
	Protein	RBC	Glucose	Normal
Urine				○

Skin/nails/hair	
Nail-edge infarcts	○
Nodules	○
CVS	
BP	
RS	
AS	
CNS	

Tests	Date	Ordered	Result
FBC		○	
ESR		○	
CRP		○	
ANA		○	
RF		○	
Other		○	
X-ray		○	
Ultrasound		○	
CT		○	
MRI		○	
Other		○	

Diagnosis

Management

Signature	
Print name	
Print designation	

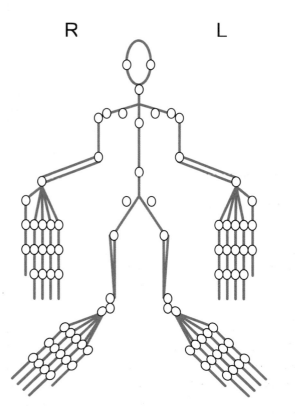

R   L

Joints – highlight on the mannekin any areas of Tenderness, Swelling, Restricted movement or Deformity

FIGURE 1.38 Continued

2

PHYSIOLOGY AND PATHOLOGY OF THE MUSCULOSKELETAL SYSTEM

E. Nicole Amft, Christopher D. Buckley and Stuart H. Ralston

Cases relevant to this chapter

66

●Essential facts

1. The function of the musculoskeletal system is to allow body movement and to protect and support vital organs.

2. The three main components of the musculoskeletal system are bone, joint and muscle.

3. Bone is a reservoir for calcium and phosphate in the preservation of calcium homeostasis.

4. Malfunction or failure of the skeletal system is the focus for rheumatology and orthopaedic practice.

5. Fractures are classified according to their pattern, causation or relation to surrounding tissues.

6. Fracture healing occurs in five stages: haematoma, organization, callus formation, modelling, and remodelling (completion).

7. Loss of hyaline articular cartilage by fragmentation or resorption is the commonest major joint problem.

8. Chronic synovitis leads to tissue hyperplasia, oedema and excess synovial fluid production resulting in joint stiffness, pain and loss of full joint function.

PHYSIOLOGY

In this section we review aspects of bone physiology beginning with an introduction to types of bones and bone composition, which is essential for an understanding of the different aspects of bone adaptation, including osteogenesis, modelling and remodelling. It will also provide the basis for understanding the mechanisms that lead to bone pathology. Finally, we discuss the functions of bone. Other skeletal components, such the cartilage and the synovial joints, are briefly addressed.

TYPES OF BONE

The skeleton contains two types of bone. These are cortical (or compact) bone, which makes up most of shafts (diaphysis) of the long bones, such as the femur and tibia, and trabecular (also known as medullary) bone, which makes up most of the vertebral bodies and the ends of the long bones (Fig. 2.1).

Trabecular bone has a greater surface area than cortical bone and because of this it is remodelled more rapidly. This means that conditions associated with increased bone turnover tend to affect

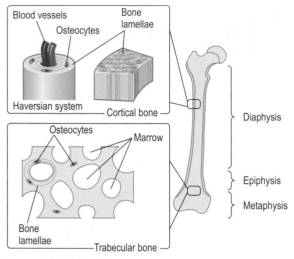

FIGURE 2.1   Types of bone

trabecular bone more quickly and more profoundly than cortical bone. Cortical bone is arranged in so-called Haversian systems, which consist of a series of concentric lamellae of collagen fibres surrounding a central canal that contains blood vessels. Nutrients reach the central parts of the bone by an interconnecting system of canaliculi that run between osteocytes buried deep within bone matrix and lining cells on the bone surface. Trabecular bone has a similar structure, but here the lamellae run parallel to the bone surface, rather than concentrically as in cortical bone.

BONE COMPOSITION

The organic component of bone matrix comprises mainly type I collagen: a fibrillar protein formed from three protein chains, wound together in a triple helix. Collagen type I is laid down by bone-forming cells (osteoblasts) in organized parallel sheets (lamellae) and, subsequently, the collagen chains become cross-linked by specialized covalent bonds, which help to give bone its tensile strength. When bone is formed rapidly (for example, in Paget's disease, or in bone metastases), the lamellae are laid down in a disorderly fashion giving rise to 'woven bone', which is mechanically weak and easily fractured. Bone matrix also contains small amounts of other collagens and several non-collagenous proteins and glycoproteins. Some of these, such as osteocalcin, are specific to bone, whereas others, such as osteopontin, fibronectin and various peptide growth factors, are also found

in other connective tissues. The function of non-collagenous bone proteins is unclear, but it is thought that they are involved in mediating the attachment of bone cells to bone matrix, and in regulating bone cell activity during the process of bone remodelling. The organic component of bone forms a framework, upon which mineralization occurs. During bone formation, osteoblasts lay down uncalcified bone matrix (osteoid), which contains the components described above, and small amounts of other proteins, which are adsorbed from extracellular fluid. After a lag phase of about 10 days, the matrix becomes mineralized, as hydroxyapatite $[Ca_{10}(PO_4)_6(OH)_2]$ crystals are deposited in the spaces between collagen fibrils. Mineralization confers upon bone the property of mechanical rigidity, which complements the tensile strength and elasticity derived from bone collagen.

BONE FORMATION, MODELLING AND REMODELLING

Bone is formed through the process of osteogenesis early during embryonic life and is *modelled* thereafter as the skeleton grows until early adulthood, when peak bone mass is attained. Thereafter, bone is constantly undergoing *remodelling*. The function of remodelling is to repair and renew damaged bone, but in later life the net amount of bone removed during remodelling exceeds that which is replaced, resulting in bone loss. In old age, subtle changes in bone shape occur with remodelling, particularly in the long bones, leading to a slight increase in cross-sectional area (cortical expansion) with cortical thinning.

Osteogenesis

Bone is formed in the embryo through the process of osteogenesis (or ossification), of which there are two main types. *Intramembranous ossification* refers to the process by which flat bones such as the skull, clavicle and mandible are formed. Accumulated mesodermal cells differentiate into osteoblasts at primary ossification centres. The osteoblasts synthesize bone matrix, which subsequently calcifies to form bone. Some osteoblasts become buried in lacunae within this tissue and these differentiate into osteocytes. The newly formed bone tissue is invaded by blood vessels and haemopoietic cells to form the bone marrow cavity. As bone formation advances, adjacent ossification centres fuse to form immature bone with a woven appearance. The long bones are formed by *endochondral ossification.* Here, the initial step is condensation of mesodermal cells to form a cartilaginous model (anlage) of the developing bone. The anlage undergoes vascular invasion, allowing haemopoietic cells access to form a marrow space in the developing bone. Osteoblast precursors, which will subsequently go on to form the new bone, are also derived from the invading vascular tissue. Following vascular invasion, the cartilage becomes calcified in centres of ossification, but the calcified cartilage is then removed by osteoclasts that form from haemopoietic precursors in the bone marrow. Mesenchymal cells present within the invading vascular tissue differentiate to form osteoblasts and these begin to form new bone to replace the calcified cartilage. In long bones, the primary ossification centre is situated in the middle of the diaphysis and this occurs pre-natally. By contrast, secondary ossification centres form at the metaphysis at different times after birth.

Endochondral bone growth and modelling

Skeletal growth occurs as the result of endochondral bone formation with subsequent modelling of the newly formed bone during childhood and adolescence. This results in longitudinal bone growth, changes in bone shape and an increase in cross-sectional area. Endochondral bone growth continues until fusion of the epiphysis occurs – mediated by an increase in circulating levels of sex hormones – at the end of puberty. Longitudinal bone growth primarily occurs as the result of proliferation of chondrocytes in the growth plate. These cells then undergo hypertrophy and the surrounding cartilage matrix becomes calcified. The calcified cartilage is then removed by osteoclast activity and replaced by new bone as a result of osteoblast activity, as in the developing bone.

Bone remodelling

The mechanical integrity of the skeleton is maintained by the process of bone remodelling, which

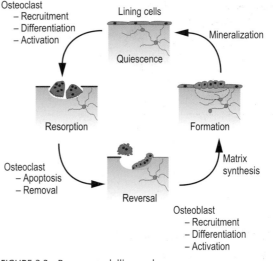

FIGURE 2.2   Bone remodelling cycle

occurs throughout life, in order that damaged bone can be replaced by new bone (Fig. 2.2). Remodelling of the bone occurs in response to alterations in type or amount of mechanical stresses (or to the lack of them). Remodelling can be divided into four phases: resorption, reversal, formation and quiescence. At any one time approximately 10% of bone surface in the adult skeleton is undergoing active remodelling, whereas the remaining 90% is quiescent.

OSTEOCLAST FORMATION AND DIFFERENTIATION

Remodelling commences with attraction of bone-resorbing cells (osteoclasts) to the site that is to be resorbed. These are multinucleated phagocytic cells, rich in the enzyme tartrate-resistant acid phosphatase, and are formed by fusion of precursors derived from the cells of monocyte/macrophage lineage. Osteoclast formation and activation is dependent on close contact between osteoclast precursors and bone marrow stromal cells. Stromal cells secrete the cytokine M-CSF (macrophage colony-stimulating factor), which is essential for differentiation of both osteoclasts and macrophages from a common precursor. Stromal cells also express a molecule called RANK ligand (RANKL) on the cell surface, which interacts with another cell surface receptor present on osteoclast precursors called RANK (*r*eceptor *a*ctivator of *n*uclear factor *k*appa B) to promote differentiation of osteoclast precursors into mature osteoclasts. The RANK–RANKL interaction is blocked by another molecule called osteoprotegerin (OPG), which is a 'decoy' ligand for RANK and is a potent inhibitor of osteoclast formation.

Mature osteoclasts form a tight seal over the bone surface and resorb bone by secreting hydrochloric acid and proteolytic enzymes through the 'ruffled border' into a space beneath the osteoclast (Howship's lacuna). The hydrochloric acid secreted by osteoclasts dissolves hydroxyapatite and allows proteolytic enzymes (mainly cathepsin K and matrix metalloproteinases) to degrade collagen and other matrix proteins (Fig. 2.3). Molecules that have been identified as being important in regulating osteoclast activity include carbonic anhydrase II (CA-II), which catalyses the formation of hydrogen ions within osteoclasts; *TCIRG1*, which encodes a subunit of the osteoclast proton pump, necessary to pump hydrogen ions into the space underneath the osteoclasts; *CLCN7*, which encodes a chloride channel necessary for transport of chloride ions into the space under the osteoclast; and cathepsin K, which degrades collagen and other non-collagenous proteins. Mutations in the genes that encode these proteins lead to *osteopetrosis,* which is a disease associated with increased bone density and osteoclast dysfunction. After resorption is completed osteoclasts undergo programmed cell death (apoptosis), in the so-called reversal phase, which heralds the start of bone formation. It has recently been discovered that many of the drugs that are used clinically to inhibit bone resorption, such as bisphosphonates and oestrogen, do so by promoting osteoclast apoptosis.

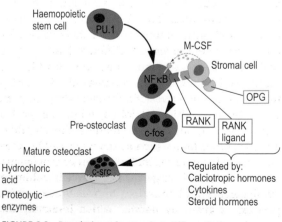

FIGURE 2.3 Regulation of osteoclast differentiation

OSTEOBLAST FORMATION AND DIFFERENTIATION

Bone formation begins with the attraction of osteoblast precursors, which are derived from mesenchymal stem cells in the bone marrow, to the bone surface. Although these cells have the potential to differentiate into many cell types, including adipocytes, myocytes and chondrocytes, it is now known that the key trigger for osteoblast differentiation is expression of a regulatory molecule called CBFA1 (core binding factor alpha1) in pre-osteoblasts. CBFA1 is a transcription factor that activates co-ordinated expression of genes characteristic of the osteoblast phenotype, such as osteocalcin, type I collagen and alkaline phosphatase. Recent studies have identified another molecule called 'osterix' that is equally important for the regulation of bone formation. Like CBFA1, osterix is a transcription factor, and is necessary for differentiation of mesenchymal cells into osteoblasts. The disease cleido-cranial dysplasia (absence of clavicles and cranial defects) is caused by haploinsufficiency of CBFA1 (complete deficiency is lethal). Haploinsufficiency means that the protein produced by a single copy of an otherwise normal gene is not enough for normal function. Another molecule called sclerostin also plays a role in bone formation. This is a secreted protein that binds a family of growth factors termed 'bone morphogenic proteins'. These are molecules that promote bone formation by stimulating growth and differentiation of osteoblast precursors.

Mature osteoblasts are plump cuboidal cells, which are responsible for the production of bone matrix. They are rich in the enzyme alkaline phosphatase and the protein osteocalcin, and circulating levels of these are used clinically as markers of osteoblast activity. Osteoblasts lay down bone matrix, which is initially unmineralized (osteoid), but which subsequently becomes calcified after about 10 days to form mature bone. During bone formation, some osteoblasts become trapped within the matrix and differentiate into osteocytes, whereas others differentiate into flattened 'lining cells', which cover the bone surface. Osteocytes connect with one another and with lining cells on the bone surface by an intricate network of cytoplasmic processes, running through canaliculi in bone matrix. Osteocytes are thought to act as sensors of mechanical strain in the skeleton, and release signalling molecules, such as prostaglandins and nitric oxide (NO), which modulate the function of neighbouring bone cells.

REGULATION OF BONE REMODELLING

Bone remodelling is a highly organized process, but the mechanisms that determine where and when remodelling occurs are poorly understood. Mechanical stimuli and areas of micro-damage are likely to be important in determining the sites at which remodelling occurs in the normal skeleton. Increased bone remodelling may result from local or systemic release of inflammatory cytokines like interleukin-1 and tumour necrosis factor in inflammatory diseases. Calciotropic hormones, such as parathyroid hormone (PTH) and 1,25-dihydroxyvitamin D, act together to increase bone remodelling, which allows skeletal calcium to be mobilized for maintenance of plasma calcium homeostasis. Bone remodelling is also increased by other hormones, such as thyroid hormone and growth hormone, but suppressed by oestrogen, androgens and calcitonin (Table 2.1).

BONE FUNCTIONS

The function of bone is to provide mechanical support for joints, tendons and ligaments, to protect

Table 2.1 Stimulators and inhibitors of bone remodeling

Stimulators	Inhibitors
Systemic hormones	
Parathyroid hormone	Sex hormones**
1,25-Dihydroxyvitamin D	Calcitonin
Parathyroid hormone-related protein	
Growth hormone	
Thyroid hormone	
Sex hormones**	
Locally acting factors	
Interleukin-1	Mechanical loading*
Parathyroid hormone-related protein	Interferon gamma
Tumour necrosis factor	OPG
Insulin-like growth factors	
RANKL	

*Mechanical loading inhibits bone resorption, but stimulates formation.
**Sex hormones stimulate bone turnover during skeletal growth, but inhibit turnover during adulthood.

vital organs from damage and to act as a reservoir for calcium and phosphate in the preservation of normal mineral homeostasis and haemopoiesis. Diseases of bone compromise these functions, leading to clinical problems, such as bone pain, bone deformity, fracture and abnormalities of calcium and phosphate homeostasis.

CARTILAGE AND ITS FUNCTIONS

Cartilage is a connective tissue consisting of cartilage cells (chondrocytes and chondroblasts) present in a matrix composed of type II collagen and proteoglycans. Four different types of cartilage are found in the body. They are elastic cartilage, fibrocartilage, hyaline (articular) cartilage and growth plate cartilage.

Elastic cartilage plays an important role in nasal septa, the ears, larynx and trachea, where it provides support and shape. Fibrocartilage is found in intervertebral discs and menisci. Hyaline cartilage covers articular surfaces, which provide a low friction surface allowing bones to slide over one another. It also acts as a shock absorber. Growth plate cartilage is found at the epiphyses of long bones. Since there are no blood vessels in cartilage, it does not heal readily when damaged. Metabolic needs of articular cartilage are obtained by nutrients diffusing through the synovial fluid. Removal of waste products occurs in the same way.

SYNOVIAL JOINTS

Joints are the sites at which two or more bones are united, regardless of whether there is movement between them. Synovial (diarthrodial) joints are especially important because they account for most of the body's articulations and are characterized by a wide range of movement. Different joints vary in their degree of movement and are classified as multi-axial, bi-axial and mono-axial, depending upon how many planes of movement they support. Examples of multi-axial joints, which support a wide range of movement, include the shoulder and hip; other joints such as the wrist, ankle, knee and elbow have more limited planes of movement. The stability and range of movement is achieved by ligaments and muscles. Information on joint position is given by nerves, which innervate the synovium.

46

Fully formed synovial joints are characterized by the presence of articular surfaces covered by a thin layer of hyaline cartilage, a joint cavity lined by a synovial membrane that contains synovial fluid and a fibrous capsule that surrounds the joint. The capsule is reinforced internally or externally (or both) by fibrous ligaments. Bursae are present in some joints, particularly large joints, such as the hip, knee, elbow and shoulder. Some joints, such as the knee, also contain menisci, which are made of fibrocartilage and play an important role as shock absorbers.

The synovial membrane (synovium) consists of two distinct layers known also as the intima (or synovial lining layer) and the subintima (or synovial sublining layer). The intima is in direct contact with the intra-articular cavity and normally comprises one to three cell layers without an underlying basement membrane. Synovial lining cells consist of macrophage-like (or type A) synoviocytes and fibroblast-like (type B) synoviocytes. The subintima is relatively acellular and contains scattered blood vessels, fat cells, fibroblasts and occasionally mononuclear cells. The synovial fluid is an ultrafiltrate of plasma, which also contains hyaluronic acid and glycoproteins secreted by the synovial cells. Its function is to lubricate the joint (to maintain low friction between cartilage and synovial surfaces) and to provide nutrients for the articular cartilage. The functions of synovium are to secrete synovial fluid and to provide a seal around the joint capsule so that the fluid does not escape.

INFLAMMATION AND HEALING

In this section, we review the basic aspects of inflammation and tissue healing and look at the pathological basis of diseases of the musculoskeletal system that compromise its supportive and mechanical functions.

PRINCIPLES OF INFLAMMATION

Inflammation is the primary process through which the body repairs tissue damage and defends itself against infection. It involves a complex interplay of cellular, humoral (fluid) and stromal (tissue) elements. Large numbers of leucocytes are recruited

from peripheral blood and expanded during the active phase of the inflammatory response. Most immune responses in healthy individuals are of limited duration and resolve completely, and normal tissue integrity is re-established. At this stage the immune response is commonly acute inflammation, dominated by granulocytes. Chronic inflammation is defined pathologically as a lesion dominated by mononuclear cells, principally lymphocytes and macrophages. We associate acute inflammation with resolution, whilst chronic inflammation tends to persist.

The hallmark signs of inflammation are tumour (swelling), rubor (redness), calor (heat), dolor (pain) and functio laesa (loss of function). In response to pathogen invasion, activated cells of the immune system release biologically active proteins, including plasma enzyme mediators, such as bradykinin and fibrinopeptides. Complement products act as opsonins (to bind foreign proteins) and chemotactic agents (to attract foreign proteins). Chemokines and cytokines are released, with upregulation of adhesion molecules on activated cells. Together, these chemical signals cause dilatation and increased permeability of blood vessels, which allows fluid and a large number of blood cells to enter the tissues. During an acute inflammatory response, neutrophil migration usually begins within 1 h of injury and is subsequently followed by an influx of monocytes and lymphocytes. Resolution of an inflammatory response requires the removal of the vast majority of immune cells that were recruited and expanded during this active phase of the response. The clearance of unwanted effector cells appears to be the result of the loss of survival signals from the interactions with stromal cells, leading to apoptosis and subsequent phagocytosis of dead cells.

In persistent inflammation, this resolution phase becomes disordered, and leads to the long-term survival of the inflammatory infiltrate, tissue hyperplasia and, ultimately, tissue destruction and scarring. Chronic persistent inflammation can develop during the persistence of an infectious agent (chronic infection). In addition, the failure to ignore self-antigens, as occurs in organ-specific autoimmune diseases (such as Graves' disease and myasthenia gravis), is a pathological process leading to tissue damage and disease. However, in many chronic inflammatory conditions, such as rheumatoid arthritis (RA) and arteriosclerosis, there is no convincing evidence that a specific antigen is involved in the persistence of the inflammatory response.

Fibroblasts, together with tissue macrophages, play a key role in the development of chronic persistent inflammation. The abnormal production of cytokines, chemokines and extracellular matrix (ECM) by fibroblasts leads to inappropriate survival and retention of leucocytes within inflamed tissues. Cytokines released by chronically activated macrophages stimulate fibroblast activation and collagen production, leading to tissue fibrosis. This type of scar tissue can interfere with normal tissue function.

IMMUNE SYSTEM

The immune system is a remarkable defence mechanism. It provides the means to make rapid, highly specific and often very protective responses against potentially pathogenic microorganisms including bacteria, viruses, fungi and parasites. Examples of immunodeficiency, as seen in both genetically determined diseases and the acquired immunodeficiency syndrome (AIDS), illustrate the central role of the immune response in protection against microbial infection. However, not only a deficient but also an excessive (overreacting) immune response, as seen in hypersensitivity reactions, can lead to tissue damage and fatal outcomes. A fundamental principle of the immune response is the differentiation of self from non-self. When this capacity fails, autoimmune diseases, such as RA and systemic lupus erythematosus (SLE), may develop.

The host defence system consists of two cooperative components: the innate immune system and the adaptive immune system. Their main distinction lies in the mechanisms and receptors used for immune recognition. They also differ in speed, defence specificity and involvement of effector cells.

Innate immune system or non-specific defence against infection

Innate (or natural) immunity acts as a first line of defence against infectious agents and other foreign components such as chemicals, drugs and pollen. These defences range from external physical and biochemical barriers to an internal defence involving the activity of phagocytes (neutrophils, monocytes and macrophages), cells that release inflammatory mediators (basophils, mast cells and eosinophils) and natural killer (NK) cells. The innate response has the advantage of speed, but lacks specificity. In addition, the magnitude of innate immune responses is identical, however many times the infectious agent is encountered.

Adaptive immune system

Adaptive or acquired immune responses involve the proliferation of antigen-specific B and T cells, which occurs when the surface receptors of these cells bind to specific antigens. B cells secrete immunoglobulins, the antigen-specific antibodies responsible for eliminating extracellular microorganisms. T cells help B cells to make antibody, but also eradicate intracellular pathogens by activating macrophages and by killing virally infected cells. Lymphocytes occupy a central stage because they are the cells that determine the specificity of immunity. Immune specificity is obtained by the distinct antigen receptor expression that arises by somatic gene rearrangement. However, lymphocyte function is absolutely dependent on signals that are provided by the innate recognition system.

The interaction between innate immunity and acquired immunity is a vulnerable position for the immune system. It should lead to the generation of immune memory and tissue repair. Specific defences against infection are distinct in primary and secondary immune responses. In the primary immune response (the body's first exposure to an antigen), lymphocytes proliferate and differentiate, and form a clone of short-lived effector cells, which ultimately give rise to long-lived memory cells. Secondary immune responses to the same antigen, which involve memory cells, are faster and often more protective. It is this characteristic that accounts for the designation 'acquired immunity'. In effect, this system compresses evolution into 2 weeks, allowing the selection of specific antigen receptors to keep pace with the selection of variant microorganisms, overcoming the deficiencies of innate immunity.

IMMUNE SURVEILLANCE AND HOMEOSTASIS

Immune tolerance

Tolerance is the process whereby immune responses to self-antigens are prevented. It occurs in three main ways: central tolerance, peripheral tolerance and inactivation (anergy or suppression). Central tolerance refers to the mechanisms that occur during lymphocyte development in the thymus (T cells) or bone marrow (B cells), and eliminates or inactivates lymphocytes that express receptors for self-antigens before they develop into functional cells (negative selection). Peripheral tolerance refers to the mechanisms acting on mature lymphocytes after they have left the primary lymphoid organs. This is necessary because not all self-antigens are expressed in the thymus; thus, not all T cells capable of recognizing self-antigens are deleted. Also, somatic hypermutation in B cells may generate antibody-forming cells specific for self-antigens. Peripheral deletion involves signalling pathways that induce apoptosis (programmed cell death) and are mediated by cell surface molecules, such as Fas and Fas ligand. Another molecule, cytotoxic lymphocyte antigen (CTLA)-4, is involved in making cells unresponsive in the presence of antigen (clonal anergy). Genetic deficiency of these molecules is associated with autoimmune diseases in mice and may contribute to autoimmunity in humans, as seen in the autoimmune lymphoproliferative syndrome (ALPS). Suppression is probably mediated by specific T cells, which secrete signalling molecules (cytokines) that suppress immune responses.

Apoptosis

Apoptosis is a physiological mechanism allowing the body to remove unwanted cells at various stages of development without the release of intracellular constituents that might cause breakdown of immunological tolerance or inflammation. It is a complex process by which an effector cell shuts down its normal function, including proliferation and deoxyribonucleic acid (DNA) repair mechanisms. Apoptotic cells package their constituents so that they can be safely phagocytosed by either a professional phagocyte or a neighbouring cell.

LEUCOCYTE HOMING AND TRAFFICKING

The circulatory and migratory properties of leucocytes allow efficient immune surveillance. Neutrophils and monocytes are rapidly recruited and accumulate at sites of injury and infection. These cells then die by apoptosis at the end of the inflammatory process. By contrast, lymphocytes recirculate through the body via the bloodstream to secondary lymphoid tissues, such as lymph nodes, or peripheral tissues where they search for their respective antigens, and then return to the bloodstream via efferent lymphatics to the thoracic duct. Lymphocytes acquire a predilection, based on the environment in which they first encounter antigen, to home or to recirculate through that same environment. Cell trafficking is not random, but rather targeted by active mechanisms of leucocyte–endothelial cell recognition, in which the endothelium selects from circulating immune cells. This has led to the current concept that all selectivity for leucocyte homing occurs at the point of entry (endothelial selection). Selection within tissues (stromal selection) has received little attention, despite well defined roles for stromal elements in the bone marrow and thymus during lymphocyte development.

BONES AND PATHOLOGY

Fracture and fracture healing

Definition
A fracture is defined as a break in the continuity of bone. Fractures are the most common abnormality of the bone. They are usually caused as a result of trauma.

Fracture types
Fractures can be classified according to their relation to surrounding tissues, according to pattern of fracture, or according to causation (Table 2.2).

Stages of fracture healing
Bone healing is unique because bone is the only tissue in the body that can replace itself without leaving a scar. The process of fracture healing occurs in five stages:

1. Haematoma
2. Organization

Table 2.2 Different types of fracture

Fracture type	Characteristics
Simple or closed	Clean break with intact overlying tissues
Compound or open	Direct communication between the broken bone and the skin surface
Transverse	Fracture line is at 90° to the longitudinal axis
Oblique	Fracture line is usually angled by 30° to 45° to the longitudinal axis
Spiral	Fracture line is oblique and encircles a portion of the shaft
Comminuted	Multiple bone fragments. Uncommon in infants and young children, but becomes more common in adolescence, particular in the tibia
Compression or crush	Often seen in vertebral bodies with compression of the trabecular bone
Greenstick or incomplete	The bone is incompletely fractured with a portion of cortex and periosteum remaining intact on the compression side. Common fracture in children
Trauma	As a result of a single violent injury
Stress	Small linear fragments as a result of repeated stress, commonly seen in athletes
Pathological or secondary	Fracture occurring in bones weakened generally or in a localized region by disease such in metabolic (e.g. osteoporosis, osteomalacia), infective, neoplastic processes or hereditary diseases (e.g. osteogenesis imperfecta, homocystinuria) of the bone

3. Callus formation
4. Modelling
5. Remodelling or completion.

After a fracture, bleeding from lacerated medullary blood vessels occurs between and around the fracture surfaces. This blood rapidly coagulates to form a clot (stage 1). Osteocytes near the fracture surface are deprived of their nutrition and the broken ends of the bone become necrotic. The necrotic material triggers a classical acute inflammatory response characterized by the invasion of neutrophils followed by macrophages in the clot with the production of granulation tissue and phagocytosis of dead and dying cells. Subsequently, capillaries and fibroblasts proliferate to form a fibrovascular granulation tissue. The capillary buds are of periosteal and medullary vessel origin. Osteoprogenitor cells (mesenchymal cells) differentiate into osteoblasts and migrate into the granulation tissue (stage 2). Within a few days, osteoblasts have synthesized a large amount of new bone (osteoid) that calcifies to form an osseous callus or woven bone around the fracture (stage 3) (Fig. 2.4).

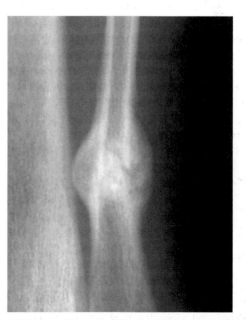

FIGURE 2.4 Plain radiograph showing advanced callus formation of a simple fracture of the fibula in a 60-year-old woman

Subsequently, modelling occurs due to the activity of osteoblasts and osteoclasts (stage 4). Eventually the woven bone is replaced by lamellar bone. Under load, the bone is gradually strengthened along the lines of stress (stage 5). If the alignment has been perfect, it may be impossible to see the fracture site.

The stages of haematoma and organization occur in the first 2 weeks of fracture. Between 3 and 6 weeks post fracture, a callus is well established and undergoes modelling and remodelling, which can take between 1 and 2 years. The timing is variable and is faster in children.

Conditions influencing and affecting fracture healing include local and systemic factors, which are discussed in Chapters 3 and 10.

Osteonecrosis

Definition
Osteonecrosis is the death of bone and marrow as a result of a poor blood supply to the region. Synonyms include avascular necrosis, aseptic necrosis, bone necrosis, ischaemic necrosis and bone infarction. Bones at high risk include the femoral and humeral heads, scaphoid and talus. Other areas frequently affected are the medial femoral condyle, proximal tibia, lunate, tarsal navicular, and metatarsal heads.

Pathogenesis
The principal mechanisms that lead to osteonecrosis comprise: vascular disruption owing to trauma; external vascular compression owing to marrow infiltration/hypertrophy; increased intraosseus pressure caused by drugs, such as corticosteroids; vascular occlusion owing to thrombo-embolism by fat/lipids, thrombi, sickle cells, nitrogen gas or caused by vasculitis; and impaired venous drainage that can occur in pregnancy owing to the gravid uterus. Chronic ingestion of alcohol is associated with osteonecrosis. Bone and marrow are undergoing medullary infarction, usually with cortical sparing. If the necrosis occurs next to a joint surface, further bone collapse is almost inevitable, which leads to joint deformity and secondary degenerative joint disease. Osteonecrosis is an irreversible process.

Clinical manifestations
These are discussed in Chapter 19.

CARTILAGE AND PATHOLOGY

Loss of hyaline articular cartilage is the commonest major joint problem. Loss may occur either by fragmentation or by resorption. The two processes often coexist. Cartilage fragmentation is characterized by formation of fissures and release of debris into the joint (Fig. 2.5). If a major cartilage fragment breaks, it may float like a loose body in the joint interfering with the normal joint motion. Cartilage fragmentation occurs as a result of a traumatic mechanical injury or progressive mechanical degeneration (wear and tear), leading to osteoarthritis. Cartilage wear occurs at points of load bearing.

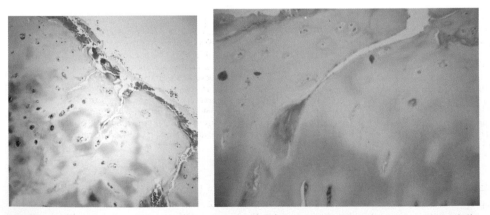

FIGURE 2.5 Histology of cartilage in osteoarthritis. Left: degenerative changes are present in this articular cartilage. Small tangential clefts and loose cartilage fragmentations are seen on the surface of the altered hyaline cartilage. A deeper vertical fissure has developed. Right: a vertical fragmentation at higher power. Haematoxylin–eosin staining method. Original magnification ×100 (left) and ×200 (right)

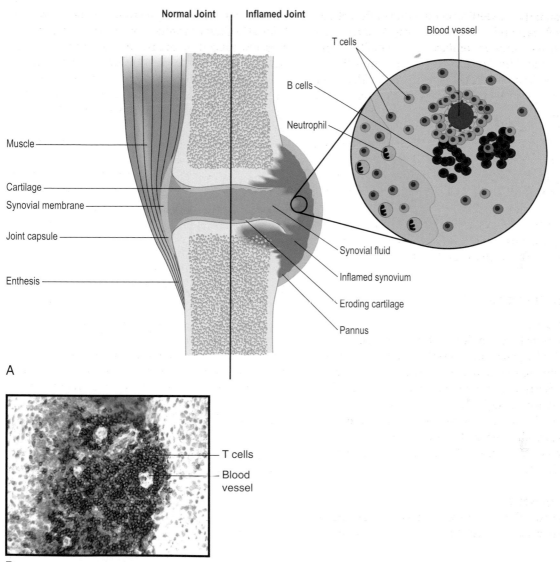

FIGURE 2.6 (A) Comparison between normal and inflamed joints. In the normal joint, the synovium is thin comprising only a few cell layers. In an inflammatory arthritis, such as rheumatoid (RA), the synovium is hyperplastic and oedematous, and villous projections of synovial tissue protrude into the joint cavity. Proliferating synovium is often referred as the pannus. The pannus has the capacity to migrate under the cartilage into the subchondral bone causing irreversible tissue damage with the characteristic marginal erosions observed on plain X-rays of joints in RA. Hyperplasia of the synovial lining results from a dramatic increase in the number of both type A and type B synoviocytes. An extensive network of new blood vessel formation, oedema and accumulation of mononuclear cells in the synovial sublining layer lead to a marked increase in synovial tissue volume. The cell infiltrate consists of T cells, B cells (some of which become plasma cells and secrete rheumatoid factor), macrophages, mast cells, natural killer cells (NK), dendritic cells and a few neutrophils. Paradoxically, neutrophils are the predominant cell within the synovial fluid. (B) Rheumatoid synovitis. Typical changes of blood vessel proliferation and increased cellularity are seen within the synovium. The predominant cell types are T cells, which are stained in a dark brown colour. Peroxidase staining method and counterstained with haematoxylin. Original magnification ×200

Resorption of cartilage occurs in inflammatory disease. Proliferating synovium, often referred to as pannus, has the capacity to migrate under the cartilage into the subchondral bone causing irreversible tissue damage. Since articular cartilage has no direct blood supply, it has little or no capacity to repair itself. When articular cartilage repairs, it initially heals as fibrocartilage and, if it survives, it can differentiate later on to hyaline cartilage, leaving no scarring.

SYNOVIAL JOINT AND PATHOLOGY

The synovium is of great clinical interest, since it is affected by many inflammatory conditions that lead to synovitis. Chronic synovitis leads to tissue hyperplasia, oedema and excess synovial fluid production resulting in joint stiffness, pain and loss of full joint motion (Fig. 2.6). For example, in rheumatoid arthritis, hyperplasia of the synovial lining results from a dramatic increase in the number of synoviocytes. An extensive network of new blood vessel formation, oedema and accumulation of mononuclear cells (MNCs) in the synovial sublining layer lead to a marked increase in synovial tissue volume. These cells secrete various cytokines as well as matrix metalloproteinases, which induce enzymatic degradation of cartilage and bone material and facilitate the local invasion of synovium at the synovial interface with cartilage and bone. Destruction of the bone matrix also leads to activation of bone osteoclasts and the further release of serine, aspartic and cysteine proteases, which degrade further the proteoglycan and collagen components of bone. This leads to bone demineralization and eventual fibrous fusion of the joint.

An excess production of synovial fluid leads to increased intra-articular pressures that can result in tamponade of the synovial vasculature, which can compromise its vasculature function, the formation of subchondral bony cysts and herniation of the synovium through weak points in the capsule. A Baker's cyst (popliteal cyst) is an example of synovial herniation into the popliteal region and this occurs frequently in rheumatoid arthritis and also osteoarthritis.

FURTHER READING

Allan D 1998 Structure and physiology of joints and their relationship to repetitive strain injuries. Clin Orthop 351: 32–38.

Buckley CD, Pilling D, Lord JM, Akbar AN, Scheel-Toellner D, Salmon M 2001 Fibroblasts regulate the switch from acute resolving to chronic persistent inflammation. Trends Immunol 22: 199–204.

Butcher EC, Williams M, Youngman K, Rott L, Briskin M 1999 Lymphocyte trafficking and regional immunity. Adv Immunol 72: 209–253.

Delves PJ, Roitt IM 2000 The immune system. N Engl J Med 343: 37–49, 108–117.

Firestein G 1998 Rheumatoid synovitis and pannus. In: Klippel JH, Dieppe PA (eds) Rheumatology, 2nd edn. Mosby, London.

Hughes DE, Boyce BF 1997 Apoptosis in bone physiology and disease. Mol Pathol 50: 132–137.

Kong YY, Yoshida H, Sarosi I et al 1999 OPGL is a key regulator of osteoclastogenesis, lymphocyte development and lymph-node organogenesis. Nature 397: 315–323.

Mundy GR 1996 Bone remodelling and its disorders, 2nd edn. Martin Dunitz, London.

Nakashima K, Zhou X, Kunkel G et al 2002 The novel zinc finger-containing transcription factor osterix is required for osteoblast differentiation and bone formation. Cell 108: 17–29.

Raisz LG 1988 Local and systemic factors in the pathogenesis of osteoporosis. N Engl J Med 318: 818–828.

Ralston SH 1997 Science, medicine and the future: osteoporosis. BMJ 315: 469–472.

Rodan GA, Harada S 1997 The missing bone. Cell 89: 677–680.

Tak PP 2000 Examination of the synovium and synovial fluid. In: Firestein GS, Panayi GS, Wollheim FA (eds) Rheumatoid arthritis, new frontiers in pathogenesis and treatment, 1st edn. Oxford University Press, New York, pp. 55–68.

Yasuda H, Shima N, Nakagawa N et al 1998 Identity of osteoclastogenesis inhibitory factor (OCIF) and osteoprotegerin (OPG): a mechanism by which OPG/OCIF inhibits osteoclastogenesis in vitro. Endocrinology 139: 1329–1337.

EPIDEMIOLOGY AND GENETICS OF RHEUMATIC DISEASES

Matthew A. Brown

Cases relevant to this chapter

25, 69, 74

•Essential facts

1. Musculoskeletal disorders are common, with osteoarthritis affecting 80% of the population over 75 years of age and 12.1% of the population between 25 and 74 years of age.

2. There is a genetic component to most musculoskeletal disorders.

3. The shared epitope hypothesis in rheumatoid arthritis (RA) suggests that the disease is associated with *DRB1* alleles encoding residues 70–74 in the third hypervariable region (HVR3) of the DRβ1 chain.

4. Ankylosing spondylitis has very high heritability and familiality, due to the presence of HLA-B27, but only 1–5% of HLA-B27 carriers actually develop disease.

5. Variation in a gene called *FRZB*, which is involved in the LRP5/wnt system controlling bone formation, contributes to the heritability of hip osteoarthritis in women.

6. Many genes have been implicated in osteoporosis, but the risk of fracture remains predominantly non-genetic.

All common rheumatic diseases have a substantial genetic component, which is not surprising given the importance of a functional musculoskeletal system in survival in times of hardship, and the inverse relationship between risk factors for auto-immunity and immunity. Genes do not, however, operate in isolation; they interact with one another and with environmental factors. Much is already known about environmental factors involved in rheumatic diseases, and the genes involved are steadily being identified.

HERITABILITY AND FAMILIALITY OF RHEUMATIC DISEASES

The relative magnitude of the genetic and environmental contributions to variation in the risk for developing a disease can be documented by measuring heritability in twins or families, or demonstrating familiality, which is the tendency of a condition to recur in families compared with the

Table 3.1 Demographic details of common rheumatic diseases

Disease	Incidence	Prevalence	Gender ratio (m:f)
Hip osteoarthritis	88/100 000	3.3–5.3% (>60 years age)	1:1 (<55 years of age). Female preponderance increases with age
Rheumatoid arthritis	10–40/100 000	0.5–1%	2:1
Ankylosing spondylitis	7/100 000	1.9%	2–3:1
Systemic lupus erythematosus	5.6/100 000	1.2/1000	9:1
Chondrocalcinosis		4.5%	1.3:1
Gout	1.2–1.8/100 000	1.4% (7% in men over 65 years of age)	2–4:1
Psoriatic arthritis	6.5–8/100 000	0.3%	1.3:1
Paget's disease	6/100 000	0.3% (age 55–59 years), 6–7% over 85 years	1:1 till later life, when male prevalence is greater

frequency in the general population. A weakness of both of these approaches is that they generally assume similar sharing of environmental risk factors for a disease, which is difficult to prove. Studies of concordance rates of twins or non-twin siblings raised either together or separately can at least partially address this question, although even such studies do not control for environmental sharing before the siblings are separated (e.g. in utero), and identifying sufficient numbers of families raised separately is very difficult unless the disease is common.

Heritability reflects the proportion of a population's risk of a disease or variance of a trait that is explained by genetic factors. Where everyone in the population is exposed to an environmental risk factor, then any variation in the trait influenced by that risk is not due to exposure to that environmental factor, but rather is genetic. For example, ankylosing spondylitis has a heritability of >90% in twins, but it is likely that an unknown environmental factor plays a significant role in its causation. A similar situation exists in osteoporosis, where the variation in bone density in the general population is high, but numerous environmental risk factors are known to be important. For example, poor dietary calcium intake causes low bone density, but in the range of intakes prevalent in the population there is little effect on bone density compared with the influence of genes, and thus the heritability is high.

The familiality of a condition compared with the general population, termed the 'recurrence risk ratio', is an important statistic in determining the difficulty of mapping genes, as it is related to the heritability, number of genes involved, their population frequencies and individual magnitudes of effect. The most frequently quoted statistic to assess familiality is the sibling recurrence risk ratio, λ_S, which is the recurrence rate in siblings of cases, compared with the population frequency of the disease. Demographic details for common rheumatic diseases are given in Table 3.1, and heritability and sibling recurrence risk ratios are given in Table 3.2.

Evidence for a role for genetic factors in a condition can also come from the finding of families with monogenic inheritance of the disease. Whilst in some conditions such as RA and ankylosing spondylitis no clearly monogenic causes have been established, other conditions, such as chondrocalcinosis, osteoporosis, osteoarthritis, systemic lupus erythematosus (SLE) and Paget's disease, can be caused by single gene diseases. Such monogenic traits tend to be rare, because natural selection prevents the disease-causing mutation from becoming common in the community.

RHEUMATOID ARTHRITIS

Despite case reports linking environmental exposure to infections, such as human parvovirus,

Table 3.2 Heritability, familiality (assessed by the sibling recurrence risk ratio) of common rheumatic diseases

Disease	Heritability (%)	Sibling recurrence risk ratio
Hip osteoarthritis		
Radiographic	58	
Requiring joint replacement	27	1.9
Osteoporosis		
Twins	80–90	
Families	40–80	5
Rheumatoid arthritis		
Systemic lupus erythematosus	60	14
Ankylosing spondylitis	66	24
Chondrocalcinosis	97	82

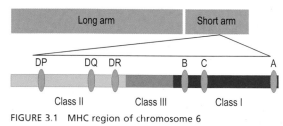

FIGURE 3.1   MHC region of chromosome 6

Epstein–Barr virus and hepatitis B, there is no convincing evidence of a relationship between any triggering environmental factor and RA. Genetic factors have an established role in severe disease, but genetic associations and heritability in less severe cases are much weaker. Nonetheless, strong established associations exist with MHC (major histocompatibility complex) and non-MHC genes (Figs 3.1 & 3.2 show some of the genetic sequences present on chromosome 6).

HLA-DRB1

The MHC is the major locus in all common inflammatory rheumatic diseases, and has even been implicated in a variety of non-inflammatory conditions as well, including osteoarthritis, osteoporosis and the common Japanese condition, ossification of the posterior longitudinal ligament. It is situated on chromosome 6 (6p21.3), extends over 3.6 million

base-pairs and is divided into three regions: class I, II and III. The class I region, at the telomeric end of the MHC, contains the HLA class I genes, HLA-A, -B and -C and extends over 2000 kilobases (kb). In the HLA class II region are the HLA-DR, -DP and -DQ loci, encoding the α and β chains of the various HLA class II molecules. The class III region lies between the class I and II regions and contains the tumour necrosis factor (TNF), complement and heat shock protein genes. The MHC is a highly gene-dense region containing about 224 genes, 40% of which are predicted to have immunoregulatory functions. Approximately 30% of the genetic risk for RA is encoded within the MHC.

Gregersen and colleagues first proposed the unifying 'shared epitope' (SE) hypothesis, demonstrating that RA is associated with specific HLA-DRB1 (*DRB1*) alleles that encode a conserved sequence of amino acids termed the SE, which comprise residues 70–74 in the third hypervariable region (HVR3) of the DRβ1 chain.

This hypothesis does not fully explain characteristics of the MHC associations of RA. In particular, it does not explain the differential strength of association of SE-carrying DRβ1 alleles. It is likely that further MHC genes are involved in RA susceptibility and that they either interact differently with or are carried on different haplotypes by various SE-carrying alleles, which are predisposed to presenting particular arthritogenic peptides.

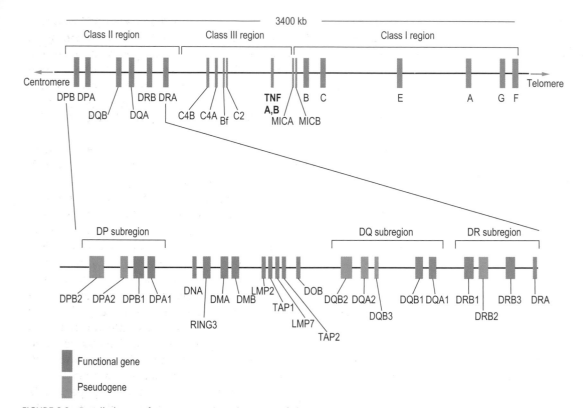

FIGURE 3.2 Detailed map of genes present on short arm of chromosome 6

PEPTIDYLARGININE DEIMINASE (*PADI4*)

PADI4 encodes the enzyme peptidylarginine deiminase, which is involved in post-translational conversion of arginine residues to citrulline. Identified as part of a genome-wide association study, association of a haplotype of single-nucleotide polymorphisms with RA has now been replicated in Japanese subjects, although replication of this finding in Caucasians has been inconsistent. The genetic findings are of particular interest because of the increasing evidence that anti-citrullinated peptide antibodies are highly specific and moderately sensitive for RA.

PROTEIN TYROSINE PHOSPHATASE 22 (*PTPN22*)

The gene *PTPN22* was found to be associated with RA having originally been identified as a susceptibility gene for type 1 diabetes mellitus. It encodes a 110-kD cytoplasmic protein, tyrosine phosphatase,

that is thought to function as a down-regulator of T cell-receptor-dependent responses through interaction with a negative regulatory kinase, Csk. Thus, the autoimmunity-associated allele is thought to have reduced binding affinity for Csk, in turn leading to reduced down-regulation of T-cell activation. The associated allele is found in 17% of white individuals compared with 28% of RA cases. This gene is also associated with a variety of other autoimmune diseases including systemic lupus erythematosus and Hashimoto's thyroiditis in addition to RA and type 1 diabetes mellitus, helping to explain the tendency for these conditions to segregate together.

SYSTEMIC LUPUS ERYTHEMATOSUS

SLE is both significantly heritable and highly familial. Some clear environmental factors known to play a role in SLE include oestrogen exposure, sunlight and some drugs (hydralazine, procainamide, quinidine, isoniazid and others). SLE occurs nine times as frequently in adult women compared with men, and flares are more common during pregnancy, thought to be due to high oestrogen levels. Oestrogen use in the oral contraceptive pill does not appear to pose a risk for SLE patients. Drug-induced lupus is an interesting example of gene–environment interaction, with 'slow metabolizers' of procainamide or hydralazine being at higher risk of disease. There are marked differences in the prevalence of SLE in different ethnic groups, with a high prevalence found in African Americans, Australian aboriginals and Asians compared with Caucasian individuals. To what extent this is genetic is uncertain, as, for example, SLE is rare in Africa, but common in African Americans.

Mutations in complement gene family members are rare, but significant, causes of SLE, as, quite apart from their significance to the individuals carrying them, they point to a pathogenic mechanism for disease. Complement deficiencies associated with SLE include deficiencies of C1q, C1r, C1s, C2, C3 and C1 esterase inhibitor. HLA-DRB1/DQB1 are also associated with SLE; the key genes involved are unknown.

A variety of other genetic associations with SLE have been reported, but on a population level these represent minor risk factors compared with the MHC.

ANKYLOSING SPONDYLITIS AND REACTIVE ARTHRITIS

Ankylosing spondylitis has very high heritability and familiality, the major gene responsible being HLA-B27. From 1% to 5% of HLA-B27 carriers develop ankylosing spondylitis, and in most populations worldwide, variation within B27 makes no difference to the likelihood of these individuals developing the condition (the exceptions are discussed below). As familial ankylosing spondylitis is in nearly all cases restricted to those carrying HLA-B27, it has been postulated that B27 is almost essential, but not adequate, to cause ankylosing spondylitis, and that other genes interact with B27 to cause the condition. There are now 22 subtypes of B27 known, but most are very rare. B*2706, which is found in South-East Asia, is paradoxically under-represented in ankylosing spondylitis cases, suggesting a protective effect. Ankylosing spondylitis is endemic in nearly all populations where

B27 occurs, the exception being west Africa, where in some ethnic groups B27 is as common as in Caucasians, but ankylosing spondylitis does not occur. HLA-B27 is rare in most African populations, where the development of seronegative arthritis, like ankylosing spondylitis, appears more closely related to HIV infection than genetic risk factors.

The strength of association of HLA-B27 with reactive arthritis is considerably lower than with primary ankylosing spondylitis, with most series reporting B27 carriage rates of 20–60%. Little more is known about the genetics of this condition. Environmental triggers for the disease are primarily either sexually acquired bacterial infections (chlamydia, ureoplasma) or enteric (salmonella, shigella, yersinia, campylobacter, clostridium and vibrio species). HIV carriers have a higher risk of developing the condition, though they also have greater exposure to triggering infections. Whilst there is a male gender bias in sexually acquired disease, enterically acquired disease occurs with equal frequency amongst men and women.

It is widely believed that ankylosing spondylitis is triggered by enteric infection similar to the aetiology of enteric reactive arthritis. However, the lack of epidemics of the condition, its worldwide distribution, and evidence from animal models that develop disease with exposure to normal enteric commensals, suggest that the infective trigger is likely to be ubiquitous. A variety of environmental factors are associated with greater severity of disease in ankylosing spondylitis, including cigarette smoking, socio-economic status and educational level. However, these factors account for a minority of the variation in severity of disease, which is also known to be highly heritable.

Whilst B27 is clearly the major gene in ankylosing spondylitis, twin and family studies indicate that other genes must be involved. There is strong evidence that genes of the interleukin-1 gene cluster are involved. This cluster of nine homologous genes is involved in controlling immune reactions, particularly to Gram-negative bacterial infection. Several studies have now demonstrated association of interleukin-1 variants with ankylosing spondylitis, with particularly strong association demonstrated with haplotypes involving interleukin-1β and another interleukin-1 gene cluster family member, IL-1F10. The key gene involved in this cluster is uncertain.

Seronegative arthropathies may also complicate inflammatory bowel disease and psoriasis (discussed below).

PSORIATIC ARTHRITIS

This complicates 5–7% of patients with cutaneous arthritis, and thus 0.3% of the general population. Whilst psoriasis itself shows moderate familiality (recurrence risk ratio in first-degree relatives 4–10), the figure for psoriatic arthritis has been reported to be as high as 55, similar to ankylosing spondylitis. A genetic role in psoriasis has been further demonstrated by the confirmed association with the gene HLA-Cw6. The extent of genetic correlation between psoriasis and psoriatic arthritis has not yet been established, nor has the consistency of segregation of the pattern of disease in psoriatic arthritis in families been reported. Psoriatic spondyloarthritis is also associated with HLA-B27 in up to 50% of cases, but the association is clearly much lower than in ankylosing spondylitis.

OSTEOARTHRITIS

This condition is extremely common, affecting 80% of the population over 75 years of age and 12.1% of the population between 25 and 74 years of age. The heritability of end-stage hip arthritis requiring hip replacement in female twins is 60%, and the recurrence risk of needing a hip replacement in siblings is 8.2%. Because the condition is so common in the community, despite the high heritability the recurrence risk ratios are quite low (see Table 3.2).

Whilst there are many monogenic forms of joint degeneration, the genes involved in skeletal dysplasias have not generally been demonstrated to have any significant role in osteoarthritis in the general community. Currently there are no genes that have been conclusively demonstrated to cause osteoarthritis, although there is strong evidence that variation in a gene involved in the LRP5/wnt system, *FRZB*, may contribute to the heritability of hip osteoarthritis in women particularly. This pathway is involved in controlling bone formation, and the genetic association may explain the known association of high hip-bone density and hip osteoarthritis.

Whilst the genetics of this condition remain to be fully elucidated, environmental factors involved have been well defined. Obesity and heavy physical labour are all known to be significant risk factors for primary osteoarthritis.

OSTEOPOROSIS

Osteoporosis is a heterogeneous condition characterized by increased fracture risk due to loss of bone quantity or impaired bone quality, and is not merely the state of reduced bone mineral density (BMD). However, because of the lack of easy methods of measuring bone quality, most information available about the epidemiology of the condition involves BMD.

Environmental factors that influence the later development of osteoporosis may be identified pre-natally. Maternal nutrition and cigarette smoking affect bone density measurements into late childhood and possibly beyond. Nutritional risk factors that are involved include vitamin D, calcium, and possibly also vitamin K and other factors. Physical activity is an important determinant of osteoporosis risk, with weight-bearing exercise increasing bone density during growth and physical inactivity/bed-rest leading to bone loss. Drug exposure, particularly to corticosteroid medications, but also anticonvulsants, heparin and excess thyroxine, predispose to osteoporosis. Extreme alcohol excess is also a potential cause of osteoporosis.

Heritability of BMD is high (60–90% measured in twins and families), and parent–child studies indicate that this in an important determinant of the inheritance of fracture risk. The heritability of fracture itself is uncertain (particularly of vertebral fracture), with estimates of heritability of Colles' fracture ranging from 20% to 54%. Other osteoporosis-related measures that have been shown to be heritable include hip geometry, bone turnover (resorption and synthesis) and growth.

There are many known monogenic conditions that can cause either high or low BMD. Monogenic low BMD most commonly is due to osteogenesis imperfecta. The four main types of osteogenesis imperfecta (OI) are inherited as autosomal dominant conditions, with occasional apparently recessive cases most likely occurring due to parental mosaicism. Types 1–4 osteogenesis imperfecta can be divided according to severity and presence of blue sclerae. Those with types 2 and 3 typically are born with fractures, with type 2 OI in particular being frequently embryonically lethal. Types 1 and 4 osteogenesis imperfecta are milder, with the blue sclerae of type 4 osteogenesis imperfecta resolving prior to adulthood. Other complications of these conditions include dentinogenesis imperfecta, aortic root dilatation leading to aortic regurgitation, hearing loss and joint hypermobility. These conditions are caused by mutations of the genes encoding the α1 and α2 chains of type 1 collagen (*COL1α1*, *COL1α2*).

Many genes have been implicated in the causation of osteoporosis, but few conclusively, and these explain at most a small proportion of the risk of osteoporosis.

CHONDROCALCINOSIS

Chondrocalcinosis is an extremely common condition affecting 25% of the population over 85 years of age, and found in the joints of 50% of patients undergoing total hip replacement. Although the genetics of chondrocalcinosis in the general community are not well defined, many families have been described with autosomal dominant inheritance of calcium pyrophosphate dihydrate (CPPD) chondrocalcinosis in which activating mutations of the *ankh* gene cause the condition. *Ankh* functions principally as a transmembrane transporter of inorganic pyrophosphate (PPi). PPi is known to inhibit hydroxyapatite formation, but when present in excess combines with calcium to form CPPD.

Other genetic disorders are also known to be associated with CPPD chondrocalcinosis, including haemochromatosis, hypophosphatasia, Wilson's disease, and rare disorders causing loss of function of ectonucleotide pyrophosphatase/phosphodiesterase 1 (ENPP1). All of these conditions are thought to act through influences on PPi levels to cause the CPPD deposition.

GOUT

The genetic epidemiology of gout has not been well characterized. Mutations in the *uromodulin* gene,

hypoxanthine-guanine phosphoribosyl transferase 1 deficiency and phosphoribosylpyrophosphate synthetase superactivity cause rare monogenic forms of the disease. These conditions cause uric acid overproduction, whereas the majority of cases with gout have low renal clearance of urate. Autosomal dominant medullary cystic kidney disease may also cause gout, though through underexcretion of uric acid. The heritability of the risk of developing gout has been estimated at 60–90%.

Environmental factors known to be involved in the disease include diet (purine-rich foods), alcohol intake and diuretic use. Lead poisoning, now a rare cause of the condition, has in the past been an important cause of gout, when lead-lined containers were used to store alcoholic beverages. There is some evidence to suggest that lower levels of lead exposure may have clinically relevant effects on uric acid excretion.

PAGET'S DISEASE

The risk of developing Paget's disease in first-degree relatives of patients is *seven* times greater than the risk in unrelated individuals, and is even greater if the condition is diagnosed early (under 55 years of age) and/or was more severe, as indicated by the presence of deformity. The heritability of the condition is unknown. Several families with monogenic segregation of the disease have been reported and mutations in two genes, *RANK* and *sequestosome*, have been demonstrated to cause the condition. *RANK* variation is not important in sporadic cases. One polymorphism of *sequestosome* gene has been found to be responsible for 8–16% of Paget's disease in the general population.

FURTHER READING

Klareskog L, Padyukov L, Lorentzen J, Alfredsson L 2006 Mechanisms of disease: genetic susceptibility and environmental triggers in the development of rheumatoid arthritis. Nat Clin Pract Rheumatol 8: 425–433.

Peach CA, Carr AJ, Loughlin J 2005 Recent advances in the genetic investigation of osteoarthritis. Trends Mol Med 4: 186–191.

4

INVESTIGATIONS

Raashid Luqmani and Ian Beggs

Cases relevant to this chapter

1–3, 12, 13, 18, 23–34, 68, 72, 74, 76, 77, 83, 87–90, 93, 94, 96, 97, 99

●Essential facts

1. Investigations are useful to support a diagnosis, but should not be performed in the absence of a clinical indication.

2. False-positive tests for autoantibodies are common, especially for rheumatoid factor and ANA.

3. A number of drugs can induce the development of autoantibodies, and only occasionally does this lead to clinical disease.

4. Anti-CCP antibody testing for rheumatoid arthritis is very specific in early disease, but lacks sensitivity.

5. Many rheumatic diseases and their treatments can result in systemic abnormalities including anaemia, low white cell count, thrombocytopenia and abnormal liver function.

6. The 'ALARA' principle ('as low as reasonably achievable') underpins the use of ionizing radiation.

7. Treat the patient, not the image.

8. Contraindications to MRI include electronic devices such cardiac pacemakers or cochlear implants, ferrous intracranial aneurysm clips and intraocular foreign bodies.

After a thorough history and clinical examination, further investigations can help to confirm or exclude a diagnosis. Important factors to consider are age, gender, family history of rheumatic disease, medication, pregnancy, infection, malignancy, and liver, pulmonary, haematological, endocrine or skin diseases. Laboratory or imaging investigations used in isolation will not usually provide a diagnosis and will depend on the pre-test probability of the diagnosis being present, which in turn is influenced significantly by the clinical findings. This principle is a very important one to follow. It can prevent unnecessary and sometimes costly tests being performed and potentially causing distress to patients. Laboratory tests are important in monitoring drug toxicity, especially for patients being treated with disease-modifying anti-rheumatic drug therapy, and can be used to monitor disease progress or to identify complications of disease.

HAEMATOLOGY

Most systemic rheumatic diseases are associated with normocytic normochromic anaemia and, occasionally, the anaemia may be the first clue to a diagnosis. Anaemia may be a result of drug therapy. Iron-deficient anaemia may result from non-steroidal anti-inflammatory drug (NSAID)-induced peptic ulceration and bleeding. Macrocytic anaemia can be due to methotrexate-induced folate deficiency, which can be avoided by providing routine folate supplements. Haemolysis may be a manifestation of systemic lupus erythematosus (SLE). Platelet counts are usually elevated in response to inflammation, but may be low as a direct result of disease such as SLE or, rarely, Felty's syndrome. More commonly, platelet counts are reduced as a result of drug toxicity. Neutropenia occurs in SLE, but can also be a sign of marrow toxicity from drug therapy. Raised neutrophil counts may warn of a possible infectious complication; however, it is important to remember that steroids reduce the ability of neutrophils to marginate in blood vessels, which results in an apparent rise in neutrophil counts, typically by one-third. Lymphopenia is common in SLE and may be induced by drugs. Very low lymphocyte counts predispose to fungal and viral infections. Abnormal clotting is typical of primary and secondary antiphospholipid syndrome, with delayed activated partial thromboplastin time (APTT) and prothrombin time (PT), together with the presence of a circulating lupus anticoagulant and, typically, anticardiolipin antibodies.

Most of the disease-modifying anti-rheumatic drugs have the potential to cause marrow toxicity. Regular monitoring of platelet counts and white cell counts, especially neutrophils, can anticipate and prevent serious illness, by withdrawing or reducing the dose of the drug before clinical problems arise.

ESR AND CRP

The erythrocyte sedimentation rate (ESR) is a very non-specific measure, which is usually increased in inflammatory states, but may also be increased in older people, or in individuals with high circulating levels of immunoglobulins or lipids. The C-reactive protein (CRP, an acute-phase protein) is a more direct measure of inflammation, since it is produced by the liver in response to systemic cytokine production. CRP is also increased in patients with infection. It is a useful investigation in bone and joint infection to monitor response to therapy.

MICROBIOLOGY

In all suspected cases of septic arthritis or osteomyelitis, attempts should be made to obtain a specimen of infected fluid or tissue prior to starting antibiotics. Blood and bone marrow culture may be helpful. Some infections can be inferred by using serial serological tests to demonstrate a change in the immune response to a specific antigen. For example, a transient rise in IgM antibodies directed against parvovirus B19, followed by a subsequent rise in IgG levels against the virus, is a good indicator of recent exposure to the virus, which is known to cause a self-limiting arthritis in adults.

BIOCHEMISTRY

All patients receiving methotrexate and sulfasalazine require regular monitoring of liver function. In patients with active inflammatory joint disease, it is common to observe a mild elevation of liver enzymes as part of the systemic inflammation, but this may cause confusion when starting disease-modifying anti-rheumatic drugs (DMARDs). In practice, it may be necessary to induce brief improvement in such patients with steroids, settling the inflammation, and normalizing liver function before starting a DMARD. Renal function should be tested regularly in patients with SLE and vasculitis. Patients receiving ciclosporin need to have regular creatinine monitoring for possible nephrotoxicity. Muscle enzyme levels are usually elevated in inflammatory muscle disease. Apart from creatine kinase, aldolase, lactate dehydrogenase, alanine aminotransferase and aspartate aminotransferase levels can also be increased.

Clues to a diagnosis of gout might include a good history, a normal physical examination, except during an acute attack, but supported by an elevated serum urate. Urate levels may be transiently normal following an acute attack, as a result of shedding of crystals into the joint, with a subsequent rise to above normal when the patient recovers.

Immunoglobulin levels may be elevated in many autoimmune diseases, especially if significant amounts of autoantibody are being produced. This will result in a polyclonal increase in immunoglobulins, typically of the IgG class. Monoclonal elevation of immunoglobulin suggests the presence of a myeloproliferative disease, such as myeloma, which may occasionally present with aches and pains and an elevated ESR, but typically a normal CRP level.

Muscle enzyme levels are usually elevated in inflammatory muscle disease and metabolic storage diseases, compartment syndrome and injuries associated with muscle necrosis. Estimation of creatine kinase (CK) levels may be helpful in patients who are suspected of having muscle necrosis, but who are unable to provide a reliable history. Apart from creatine kinase, aldolase, lactate dehydrogenase, alanine aminotransferase and aspartate aminotransferase levels can also be increased. Often the levels of CK are highest in cases of metabolic muscle disease (typically in the several thousands) compared to levels in inflammatory muscle disease (typically a few thousand or less).

Bone biochemistry includes serum calcium and phosphate levels, and the level of bone-derived alkaline phosphatase. It is now possible to measure parathyroid hormone levels in blood, as well as levels of vitamin D, so that a more precise diagnosis can be made. Markers of bone turnover, such as P1NP, can help in determining response to therapy in osteoporosis. Osteomalacia and rickets are typically associated with low calcium, high alkaline phosphatase and low vitamin D levels. High levels of alkaline phosphatase are typically found during active Paget's disease, but also occur in the presence of bony metastases, or in patients with liver disease. Alkaline phosphatase levels are higher than normal in pregnancy and during childhood and adolescence.

URINALYSIS

All patients with suspected connective tissue disease should have urine tested for blood and protein, since the presence of early renal involvement is often asymptomatic and untreated renal inflammation can lead to significant loss of function.

AUTOANTIBODY TESTING

Many healthy individuals make rheumatoid factor and anti-nuclear antibodies. Approximately 25% of healthy elderly people make rheumatoid factor (compared to around 4% of 20-year-olds); one-third of healthy individuals produce low-titre anti-nuclear antibody (ANA). At all ages, for unknown reasons, healthy females are more likely than healthy males to have circulating ANAs. Although up to one-third of first-degree relatives of patients with SLE have positive ANA tests, the majority never develop SLE.

In many pathological conditions involving tissue damage, immune activation may be directed against normal healthy tissue. The initial damaging events usually involve T cells, but released antigens may become targets for an antibody response. The detection and quantification of autoantibodies is an important aspect of diagnosis of autoimmune diseases, such as rheumatoid arthritis (RA), SLE, systemic sclerosis, and the systemic vasculitides. Many of these diseases are associated with a specific autoantibody or group of autoantibodies. They are usually detected by their reaction against tissue components using subjective methods such as indirect immunofluorescence. Positive samples should be further analysed using specific, quantitative methods. Autoantibodies are not 'gold standard' tests; they are markers of the disease, but with significant limitations. They should be used as part of a diagnostic workup, including the clinical history and examination findings, rather than as a marker indicating one particular disease.

Techniques are gradually improving, giving numerical results rather than titres, but a lack of standardization makes the results variable. Many of the antibodies show no correlation with disease activity, and should be regarded as indicators of the potential presence of disease. Their use should be restricted to the initial investigation and not repeated every time the patient is followed up (e.g. rheumatoid factor and ANA). Complement components levels in SLE and C-reactive protein in rheumatoid arthritis may provide useful information in the appropriate clinical context.

RHEUMATOID FACTOR AND ANTI-CYCLIC CITRULLINATED PEPTIDE ANTIBODIES

Rheumatoid factors are autoantibodies, usually of the IgM class, directed against the Fc portion of normal IgG molecules and are the commonest autoantibodies in humans. They are present in polyclonal form in a large number of autoimmune disorders as well as in some inflammatory states (Table 4.1). In monoclonal form, they are produced

Table 4.1 Conditions in which a positive rheumatoid factor test may be found

Normal health	Normal population, especially the elderly
Connective tissue disease	High prevalence in rheumatoid arthritis, but also seen in Sjögren's syndrome, systemic lupus erythematosus and hepatitis C-associated mixed cryoglobulinaemia; chronic inflammatory lung disease
Juvenile arthritis	Found in a small number of children with polyarticular juvenile idiopathic arthritis
Infectious diseases	Chronic bacterial infections, including sub-acute bacterial endocarditis, infective exacerbations of cystic fibrosis, tuberculosis, leprosy, trypanosomiasis, visceral larva migrans, infectious mononucleosis, influenza A, hepatitis A and cytomegalovirus infections
Endocrine diseases	Graves' disease and hypothyroidism
Liver disease	Chronic liver disease, autoimmune hepatitis
Malignancy	Some malignancies including B-cell proliferative diseases, adenocarcinoma of the bladder

by proliferating B cells (for example in Waldenström's macroglobulinaemia and chronic lymphoid leukaemia). In addition, rheumatoid factors are part of the normal antibody repertoire especially in the fetal and neonatal periods, suggesting that they may play a role in the development of the immune system. Healthy individuals are capable of making rheumatoid factor, but not usually in large amounts. Seventy per cent of patients with RA have elevated levels of rheumatoid factor. The presence of rheumatoid factor is associated with a worse prognosis and a higher incidence of systemic manifestations of the disease. Early in the course of RA, however, rheumatoid factor may not be detectable, and it is worth repeating the test some months later in patients who have clinical features of RA. Rheumatoid factor is also produced in other connective tissue diseases, chronic infection and vasculitis, resulting in low specificity for RA. Anti-filaggrin antibodies, anti-keratin antibody (AKA) and anti-perinuclear factor (APF) are more specific than rheumatoid factor and may be detected in early RA. However, the assays are not standardized. Cyclic citrullinated peptides (CCPs) of filaggrin are the target of those antibodies and a more specific enzyme-linked immunoassay (ELISA) has been developed. In established disease, anti-CCP antibodies have a specificity >90% and a sensitivity of 70%, and may replace rheumatoid factor testing in future. However, in patients with clinical evidence of early RA, although the specificity of rheumatoid factor and anti-CCP testing is very high (>95%), up to 45% of patients are negative for rheumatoid factor and anti-CCP.

ANA, DOUBLE-STRANDED DNA ANTIBODIES AND ENAS

Over 85% of patients with SLE will have a positive ANA, and in the correct clinical setting this is a very useful test in diagnosis. The ANA test is sensitive, but not specific (Table 4.2). Healthy people often have positive results. The test should not be used to evaluate vague symptoms, but to support a diagnosis of a connective tissue disease if a patient has appropriate symptom or signs. The final diagnosis is based on clinical findings, though test results may support the diagnosis, or prompt further specific investigation.

A number of drugs, including minocycline, penicillamine, hydralazine, procainamide, isoniazid, methyldopa and quinidine, can induce ANA production. Most patients have no rheumatic symptoms. A few, however, develop some clinical features of lupus. It is worth checking these patients for the presence of anti-histone antibodies, which are more specific for drug-induced lupus. Symptoms usually resolve when the drug is discontinued, but it may take 1 year or more for ANAs to disappear.

If the ANA test is positive in a patient with suspected connective tissue disease, it may be helpful to test for the presence of anti-double-stranded antibody, anti-extractable nuclear antigen (ENA), anti-ribonucleoprotein (RNP), anti-Smith (Sm), and antibodies seen in Sjögren's syndrome (SSA and SSB) tests. The finding of reduced complement levels (C3 and C4), indicating consumption, may help in determining disease activity in SLE.

Table 4.2 Conditions in which positive antinuclear antibody tests may be found

Normal health	Normal population, especially the elderly, transient during pregnancy
Connective tissue disease	High prevalence in systemic lupus erythematosus, but also seen in scleroderma, dermatomyositis, Sjögren's syndrome, mixed connective tissue disease and long-standing rheumatoid arthritis
Juvenile arthritis	Highest prevalence in girls with oligoarticular juvenile arthritis, but also seen in polyarticular and systemic disease
Infectious diseases	Malaria, bacterial infections, transient rise during many viral infections
Endocrine diseases	Type 1 diabetes, autoimmune thyroiditis
Liver disease	Chronic liver disease, autoimmune hepatitis
Malignancy	Breast cancer, squamous cell carcinoma of the lung and hepatocellular carcinoma
Haematological disease	Autoimmune thrombocytopenic purpura and haemolytic anaemia
Drugs	Many reported including minocycline, penicillamine, hydralazine, procainamide, isoniazid, methyldopa and quinidine

Anti-double-stranded DNA antibodies are found in 40% to 60% of patients with SLE during periods of disease activity, especially in active renal disease. Single-stranded DNA antibodies are of little clinical value. The anti-ENA, RNP, Sm, and SSA and SSB tests identify autoantibodies directed against nuclear antigens composed of non-histone proteins. Anti-RNP is typical of mixed connective tissue disease. The anti-Sm is more specific to SLE. In patients with suspected scleroderma, anti-scleroderma-70 (Scl-70) antibody and anti-centromere antibodies may be helpful, but anti-Scl-70 antibodies are seen in only 20% of patients with diffuse scleroderma. The anti-centromere antibody test is used to detect CREST syndrome, a variant of scleroderma characterized by calcinosis, Raynaud's phenomenon, oesophageal dysmotility, sclerodactyly (scleroderma of the digits) and telangiectasia (dilation of the capillaries and arterioles). The anti-centromere antibody is present in 90% of affected patients. ANA testing is important in children with juvenile arthritis; not only does it help in making the diagnosis if positive, but also its presence indicates a higher risk of chronic anterior uveitis, and may worsen the prognosis of the arthritis.

ANTI-NEUTROPHIL CYTOPLASM ANTIBODY

Anti-neutrophil cytoplasm antibodies (ANCAs) are autoantibodies directed against enzymes present in the primary granules of neutrophils and monocytes. Until the discovery of ANCAs, there was no specific laboratory method for the investigation of systemic vasculitis. The role of ANCAs in the pathogenesis of vasculitis is unclear. There is some controversy over the sensitivity, specificity, predictive value and antigen specificity of ANCAs, but they do represent a major advance in diagnosis of small vessel vasculitis. The diagnosis of vasculitis is often difficult because of the variable presentation. Wegener's granulomatosis, microscopic polyangiitis and Churg–Strauss syndrome are most often associated with ANCA. However, these diseases may occur in the absence of ANCA. The 'gold standard' for a diagnosis of vasculitis depends on clinical and pathological features. ANCA testing is supportive of clinical and pathological findings. The ANCA pattern, determined by indirect immunofluorescence, can be either cytoplasmic (C-ANCA), perinuclear (P-ANCA) or atypical perinuclear (X-ANCA). Proteinase-3 and myeloperoxidase are the most common autoantigens and are commonly associated with C-ANCA and P-ANCA, respectively.

HUMAN LEUCOCYTE ANTIGEN

Human leucocyte antigen (HLA) B27 is the tissue type most commonly associated with ankylosing spondylitis in adults. It may also help to define cases of juvenile arthritis with possible spinal involvement. It is likely that HLA-B27 is important in the pathogenesis of spondylitis, but the mechanisms remain unclear. Most population studies show that approximately 8% of normal healthy adults carry HLA-B27 compared to 90% of patients with ankylosing spondylitis. Most Native American and Eskimo populations studied have higher frequencies of HLA-B27 than the rest of the world, and some of the highest prevalence rates of spondyloarthritis occur in these patients, especially Reiter's syndrome and ankylosing spondylitis.

SYNOVIAL FLUID ANALYSIS

Aspiration of joint fluid for assessment of microbiology is an important diagnostic step in suspected septic arthritis (see Chapter 5). All such fluid should be examined with Gram staining and culture. Crystals may be seen in gout or pseudogout using polarized light microscopy. Electron microscopy is necessary for correct identification of hydroxyapatite crystals. Fluid can be tested for cell count, but is seldom of help in the diagnosis, since there is considerable overlap between numbers of neutrophils in inflammatory and infected fluid.

SYNOVIAL HISTOLOGY

Synovial histology seldom contributes to a diagnosis. In the case of suspected sepsis, especially tuberculosis, it is important to send tissue for culture as well as for histology. In patients with a persistent monoarthritis, the unusual condition of pigmented villonodular synovitis can be diagnosed by biopsy. It is a localized tumour of synovium, usually slow growing and rarely invasive. There is florid synovitis characterized by excess deposition of haemosiderin, giving rise to the pigmented appearance. Histology reveals macrophages laden with haemosiderin and lipid, and accompanying fibrotic changes.

MUSCLE BIOPSY

Histology of affected muscle tissue is important and can distinguish between predominantly immune myositis, found in dermatomyositis and polymyositis (with a combination of inflammatory cell infiltrates, muscle fibre necrosis and regeneration), and inclusion body myositis, which is less responsive to immunosuppression. Patients with weakness, pain and massively elevated muscle enzymes may have changes on muscle biopsy showing a metabolic myopathy due to a storage disease, with accumulation of excess precursors in muscle (e.g. McArdle's myopathy). Rhabdomyolysis due to muscle injury has a characteristic appearance of acute necrosis of muscle fibres. In children, some forms of hereditary muscular dystrophy can be diagnosed by genetic testing (see Chapter 27).

BONE BIOPSY

Biopsy of skeletal lesions can be performed using an open or closed technique. The usual indication is the suspicion of primary or secondary malignancy or infection. In the case of suspected malignancy, the bone biopsy should be done only after the affected part has been imaged. It is usually performed by the surgeon who will be responsible for the subsequent surgical care of the patient and done in a centre that deals with musculoskeletal malignancy (see Chapter 20). Bone biopsies may confirm a diagnosis of osteomalacia and can be performed using tetracycline labelling. The patient takes a course of tetracycline tablets before the biopsy is performed. Outpatient percutaneous biopsy of vertebral body lesions can be performed using a bone biopsy needle under imaging guidance. Aspiration biopsy of bone using a trephine needle is a simple and relatively safe procedure with a diagnostic accuracy of between 60% and 80%. Complication rates are under 1% in experienced hands.

IMAGING

The role of imaging is to complement clinical assessment and other investigations. Careful history-taking and physical examination are essential and cannot be replaced by imaging.

Guidance on appropriate use of imaging investigations is available from radiologists, radiology departments and radiological organizations such as *www.acr.org* or *www.rcr.ac.uk*. The indications for many examinations are straightforward. For more difficult or complex problems, it is best to consult a radiologist, who will advise on the most appropriate imaging strategy.

PRINCIPLES

- Imaging investigations should be obtained only if the result might alter patient management. For example, radiographs of the lumbar spine in adult patients with atraumatic low back pain and no 'red flag' clinical findings are of limited value.
- Conversely, radiographs are essential in patients with fractures that are clinically obvious because they will demonstrate the degree of deformity and help to guide appropriate treatment.
- The 'ALARA' principle ('as low as reasonably achievable') underpins all examinations that use ionizing radiation and aims to balance optimal images with low radiation doses. About 15% of the radiation experienced by the general population is human-made and, of this, 97% is due to medical radiation. Radiographs of the lumbar spine and computed tomography (CT) scans are radiation 'expensive'. Collectively, they account for 40–50% of the radiation dose of diagnostic imaging. Examinations that employ radiation should be used carefully. Particular care should be taken when irradiating children or the pelvis of women of child-bearing age. The lifetime risk of cancer due to a whole-body CT scan is 0.08% for middle-aged adults. The risk is significantly higher in children: abdominal CT in a 1-year-old has a 0.18% risk (Brenner et al 2001, Brenner & Elliston 2004, de González & Darby 2004).
- 'Treat the patient, not the image.' There are obvious exceptions, such as clinically occult malignancy that is demonstrated on imaging. However, modern imaging can show 'abnormalities' that may not be clinically significant. For example, radiographs and magnetic resonance imaging (MRI) of the lumbar spine often show 'abnormalities' that are asymptomatic. Radiographic 'abnormalities' are as common in asymptomatic patients as in those with low back pain.
- Trauma cases require radiographs in two planes to show adequately fractures and dislocations. Failure to obtain views in two planes may result in missing or under-estimating the extent of injuries and may significantly affect patient outcome. Additional views are occasionally required in some areas – notably the shoulder, hip, wrist and foot due to the complexity of the anatomy.
- Use the most appropriate examination for the clinical problem. In the shoulder, for example, radiographs may be sufficient. A vacuum phenomenon (Fig. 4.1) indicates with a high degree of probability that the rotator cuff is intact, whereas narrowing of the subacromial space (Fig. 4.2) shows that there is a complete thickness tear. Ultrasound (US) and MRI of the shoulder can be used to assess rotator cuff integrity. MRI provides additional information. Ultrasound is cheaper. Local preference and practice usually determine which will be used. MR arthrography is generally the best examination for the unstable shoulder, except for fractures, which are more clearly shown by CT.

RADIOGRAPHS

X-rays are produced by firing a stream of electrons at a tungsten anode. The resulting X-rays are absorbed or stopped to varying degrees by different tissues. The lungs consist mostly of air. They absorb very little radiation and appear translucent or radio-lucent. Bones contain calcium and produce considerable absorption of X-rays and appear dense or radio-opaque. Metal, calcium and most contrast

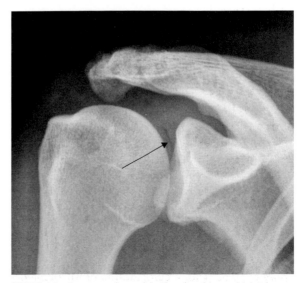

FIGURE 4.1 A vacuum (arrow) in the glenohumeral joint has a positive predictive value of 96% for an intact rotator cuff. From Beggs (2004)

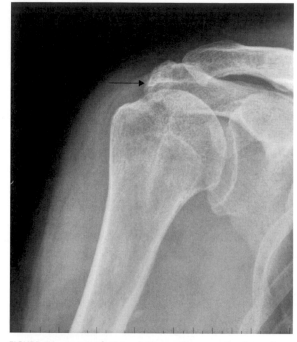

FIGURE 4.2 A gap of <7 mm between the acromion (arrow) and the humeral head indicates that there is a full-thickness tear of the rotator cuff. No further imaging is needed to confirm the diagnosis. The narrower the distance, the larger the tear. From Beggs (2004)

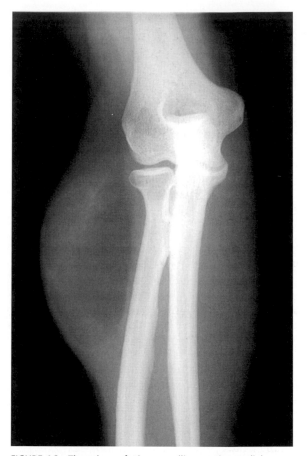

FIGURE 4.3 There is a soft-tissue swelling on the medial aspect of the forearm. It is radiolucent (less dense than the surrounding soft tissues). The appearances are typical of a lipoma, a benign tumour composed of fat. The other soft-tissue structures are indistinguishable

agents also appear radio-opaque. Soft tissues are intermediate and behave like water. Different soft-tissue structures are generally indistinguishable, with the exception of fat, which is radiolucent (Fig. 4.3). Lungs and bones are the tissues that are best demonstrated by X-rays (Fig. 4.4).

After passing through the patient, the X-rays are recorded directly onto X-ray film (conventional radiography), or onto a plate of re-usable photo-stimulable storage phosphors that are processed to give images (computed radiography) or onto a detector system that immediately converts the data into images (direct digital radiography). Images may be viewed on film (hard copy) or at the work-station (soft copy).

FLUOROSCOPY

Fluoroscopy uses an image intensifier to enhance the X-ray images, which can then be viewed in 'real time'. Simple image intensifiers are mobile. They can be used in operating theatres, e.g. to ensure that a fracture or dislocation has been reduced or to help with internal fixation. More powerful fluoroscopy equipment is available in radiology departments.

RADIONUCLIDE IMAGING

The isotope bone scan is the most frequently used radionuclide examination in musculoskeletal prac-tice. A radioactive isotope (technetium-99m) is attached to a phosphate compound (e.g. methylene diphosphonate; MDP) that accumulates on the surface of bone following intravenous injection. Accumulation of ^{99m}Tc-MDP is virtually uniform throughout the normal skeleton, but is higher in osteoblastic areas where there is increased bone formation. As ^{99m}Tc decays it emits gamma radia-tion that is detected by a gamma camera. Abnormal bone usually appears (Fig. 4.5) as a focus of

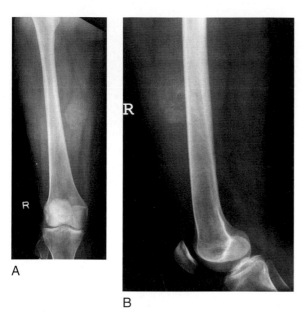

A

B

FIGURE 4.4 The radiograph of the thigh provides fine detail of the bone structure in the femur and an area of ectopic ossification (myositis ossificans) in the quadriceps muscle but there is poor soft-tissue detail

increased activity (a 'hot spot') on the bone scan. Myeloma or large lytic lesions that have little osteoblastic activity occasionally appear as photon-deficient areas (holes). Bone scans are sensitive but non-specific, and further imaging may be needed for a specific diagnosis.

SPECT (single-photon emission computed tomography) scans use the same basic technique, but produce tomographic and multiplanar images.

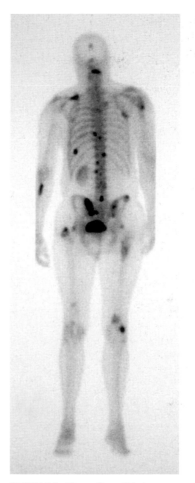

FIGURE 4.5 The radionuclide bone scan shows multiple 'hot spots' that are typical of bony metastases. Activity is uniform in the uninvolved skeleton. Isotope is usually excreted via the kidneys. This patient has a solitary kidney

POSITRON EMISSION SCANNING

Positron emission tomography (PET) uses isotopes such as ^{18}F that have short half-lives. The isotopes are attached to biologically active compounds, e.g. [^{18}F]fluorodeoxyglucose (18FDG), which mimics glucose and is taken up by many tumours. As the isotope decays it emits positrons, which collide with electrons giving off pairs of gamma rays that travel in opposite directions. PET scanners define the origin of the gamma rays and so identify areas of biological activity (Fig. 4.6). PET and CT images may be 'fused' to provide precise anatomical delineation of abnormal activity.

PET scanning is established in oncology, cardiology and neurology, but its role in musculoskeletal imaging has yet to be defined.

ULTRASOUND

Diagnostic ultrasound is generated by applying a pulse of electricity to a piezoelectric crystal, which vibrates and produces a sound wave. When sound is reflected it generates an electric potential in the piezoelectric crystal, which acts as both transmitter and receiver of sound waves. Sound is reflected at tissue interfaces and it is those echoes that allow images to be generated. Sound passes through fluid-filled structures without significant attenuation and is completely reflected by bone, calcification and metal. Ultrasound provides good soft-tissue, but not bony, detail, as it does not penetrate the surface of bone.

Frequencies >7 MHz are optimal in musculoskeletal ultrasound. There is a trade-off between

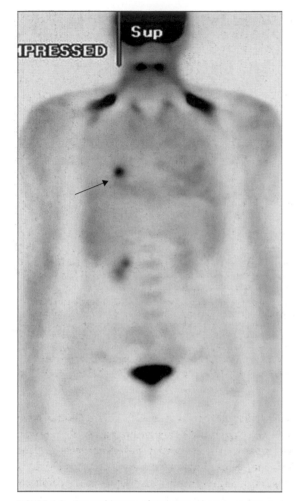

FIGURE 4.6 Coronal image of PET scan. There is a metastasis (arrow) in the right hemithorax from an osteosarcoma of the left femur. (Courtesy of Dr M Brooks)

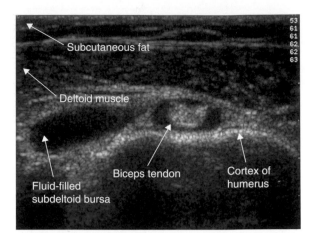

FIGURE 4.7 A transverse US scan of the shoulder shows the long head of biceps tendon in cross-section. The tendon is surrounded by fluid that lies within the tendon sheath. The fluid in the tendon sheath and bursa produce no echoes. In contrast the cortex of the humerus reflects all the sound waves and appears bright

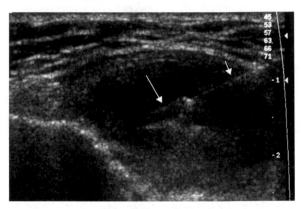

FIGURE 4.8 Ultrasound-guided biopsy of soft-tissue sarcoma. The tip of the needle (long arrow) lies in the centre of the mass. The shaft of the needle (short arrow) is also visible

spatial resolution and depth of penetration, i.e. spatial resolution is better for superficial than deep structures. Ultrasound is most useful in assessing superficial structures such as tendons, ligaments and muscles (Fig. 4.7). Ultrasound can also demonstrate masses, joint effusions and abscesses, and be used to guide interventional procedures such as aspiration, biopsy and steroid injection (Fig. 4.8).

Power and colour Doppler techniques allow assessment of vascularity.

COMPUTED TOMOGRAPHY

CT scanning was invented by Sir Godfrey Hounsfield. He subsequently received the Nobel Prize for Medicine. Hounsfield's original scanner had an X-ray tube that rotated round the patient and pro-

duced an axial image (Fig. 4.9). Current-generation CT scanners have multiple detectors; they produce high-quality images and have very fast scanning times: e.g. 10–12 s to scan the chest, abdomen and pelvis. Image reconstruction is also quick and the data can be manipulated to provide multiplanar and 3D views (Fig. 4.10). Intravenous and intra-articular contrast may be employed to provide more detailed images. CT provides exquisite bony detail.

MAGNETIC RESONANCE IMAGING

MRI scanners are effectively sophisticated magnets. As the patient lies in a scanner the body's protons

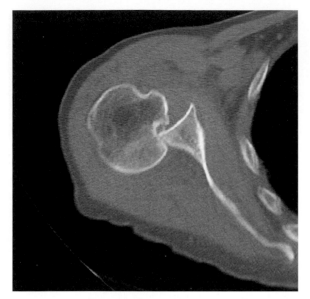

FIGURE 4.9 Axial CT scan of posterior dislocation of shoulder. The humeral head and glenoid are 'locked' and there is a depressed fracture (reverse Hill–Sachs defect) in the humeral head

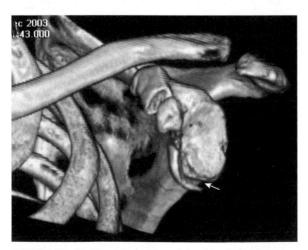

FIGURE 4.10 3D CT reconstruction of shoulder shows an undisplaced fracture fragment (arrow) on the antero-inferior margin of the glenoid. Soft-tissue structures and the humerus have been 'sculpted' to show the fracture

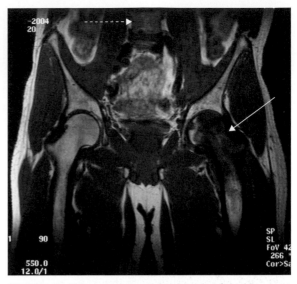

FIGURE 4.11 This coronal T1 weighted image of the hips provides good bone and soft-tissue detail. Subcutaneous fat is bright ('high signal intensity'). The medullary cavities of the pelvis and right femur are also bright because they contain yellow fatty marrow. The proximal left femur (solid arrow) is dark ('low signal intensity') because of marrow oedema. The marrow in the lumbar vertebra (dotted arrow) is also dark because it is red marrow and contains less fat than yellow marrow. Muscles are dark

are aligned along the long axis of the magnet. When an appropriate radiofrequency pulse is added, selected protons absorb energy and are deflected through 90°. The protons return to their previous state when the radiofrequency pulse is removed and this generates signals. T1 relaxation relates to the time required for the protons to line up in their original state after removal of the radiofrequency pulse, while T2 relaxation is the time for the deflected signal to disappear. Different tissues have different T1 and T2 relaxation times. By altering the times between initial radiofrequency pulses (TR) and subsequent refocusing pulses (TE) it is possible to manipulate the signals from different tissues to create images.

On T1-weighted images (Fig. 4.11) fat has high signal intensity (bright) and water is low signal (dark). T1 (and proton density)-weighted images provide excellent anatomical detail. On T2-weighted images (Fig. 4.12) water appears bright. Fat may be bright or dark depending on the technique used. T2-weighted images do not provide such crisp anatomical definition as T1-weighted images, but are sensitive for the detection of many abnormalities that are often associated with increased water content. The T2 effect can be enhanced by suppressing signal from fat. STIR (short T1 inversion recovery) sequences are also highly sensitive to the presence of increased water and possible pathology (Fig. 4.13).

MRI provides excellent detail of soft-tissue and bone marrow structures and pathology, and is used to look at joints, bone marrow and soft-tissue structures, such as muscles, tendons and ligaments. Intra-articular or intravenous contrast (Fig. 4.14)

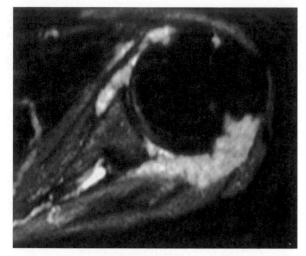

FIGURE 4.12   The axial fat-saturated T2-weighted image shows an extensive, bright synovial mass (due to synovial osteochondromatosis) that erodes the humeral head

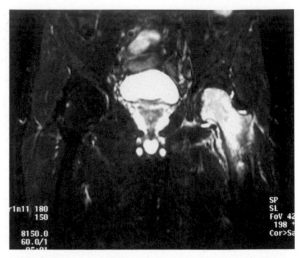

FIGURE 4.13   Coronal STIR image of hips (same patient as Fig. 4.11). Anatomical detail is poorer than on the corresponding T1-weighted image but the STIR sequence better shows the oedema in the proximal left femur

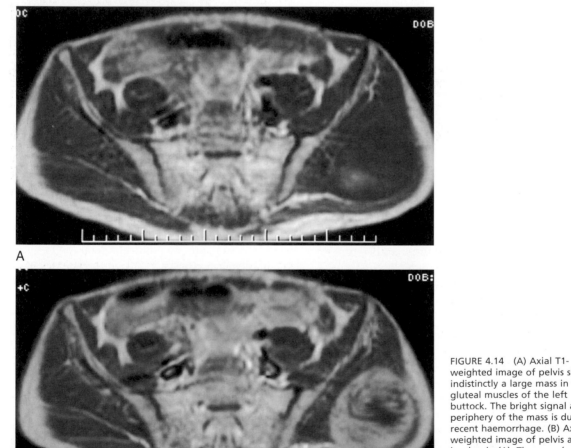

A

B

FIGURE 4.14   (A) Axial T1-weighted image of pelvis shows indistinctly a large mass in the gluteal muscles of the left buttock. The bright signal at the periphery of the mass is due to recent haemorrhage. (B) Axial T1-weighted image of pelvis at same level as in (A). The mass (recurrent sarcoma) enhances following an intravenous injection of gadolinium contrast agent. The dark central area is due to tumour necrosis

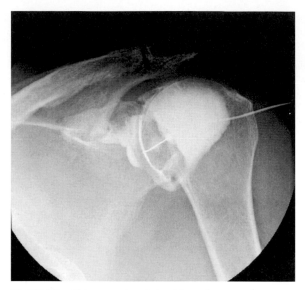

FIGURE 4.15 This conventional shoulder arthrogram shows no filling of the usually capacious joint recesses. The appearances are those of a 'frozen shoulder'

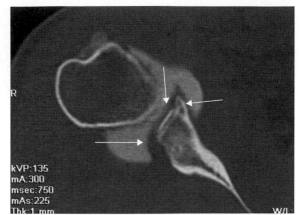

FIGURE 4.16 A CT arthrogram of the shoulder shows an old fracture (white arrow) of the anterior glenoid. Articular cartilage lies between the bone and the contrast

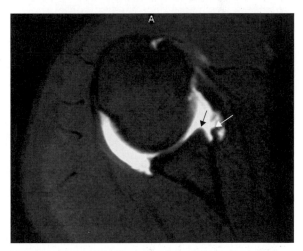

FIGURE 4.17 An MR arthrogram of the shoulder shows that the anterior glenoid labrum is deficient (black arrow) and has been displaced medially (white arrow)

may be needed to improve detail. Cortical bone, calcification and metal produce signal voids.

Contraindications to MRI include electronic devices such as cardiac pacemakers or cochlear implants, which will malfunction, and ferrous intracranial aneurysm clips and intra-ocular foreign bodies, which may move while the patient is in the magnetic field with catastrophic consequences. Patients are always carefully screened before being allowed in a scanner.

ARTHROGRAPHY

Imaging studies performed after injecting contrast into a joint are called arthrograms. Positive (iodinated) or negative (air) contrast or both (double contrast) are used in conventional (Fig. 4.15) or CT (Fig. 4.16) arthrography. Dilute gadolinium chelates are employed in MR arthrography (Fig. 4.17). Arthrograms are used to show or improve visualization of intra-articular structures that would otherwise not be seen or be seen poorly.

Conventional arthrograms can be used to assess loosening of joint prostheses or the integrity of ligaments and the triangular fibro-cartilage at the wrist or the rotator cuff at the shoulder. CT arthrograms of the knee show the menisci and cruciate ligaments in patients in whom MRI is contra-indicated. MR arthrography is the best way of assessing structures such as the glenoid labrum, glenohumeral

ligaments and capsular insertion in patients with shoulder instability, although CT provides better bony detail.

BONE DENSITOMETRY

Bone densitometry (Fig. 4.18) identifies osteoporosis (reduced bone mineral density), predicts fracture risk and indicates which patients require treatment in order to reduce morbidity and mortality. Different sites can be assessed. Cancellous bone changes more rapidly than cortical bone over time or with treatment and, therefore, the spine, calcaneum or distal radius are frequently used. Cortical sites such as the femoral neck and radial shaft are also used.

DEXA

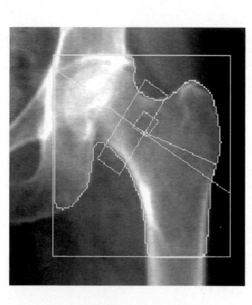

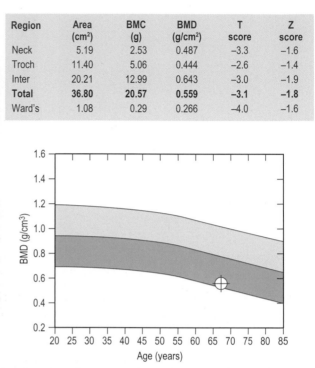

Region	Area (cm²)	BMC (g)	BMD (g/cm²)	T score	Z score
Neck	5.19	2.53	0.487	–3.3	–1.6
Troch	11.40	5.06	0.444	–2.6	–1.4
Inter	20.21	12.99	0.643	–3.0	–1.9
Total	**36.80**	**20.57**	**0.559**	**–3.1**	**–1.8**
Ward's	1.08	0.29	0.266	–4.0	–1.6

FIGURE 4.18   DEXA scan of hip in elderly osteoporotic female patient. The T score indicates the absolute fracture risk in standard deviations from normal; the Z score indicates the fracture risk adjusted for age in standard deviations from normal. Troch, trochanter; Inter, intertrochanteric region; Ward's, Ward's triangle. In the graph, the upper and lower shaded areas show the upper and lower ranges of the normal population, respectively

Several different techniques are available. Dual-energy X-ray absorptiometry (DXA or DEXA) scanning is the most popular as it can be used in multiple anatomical sites and has low precision error and radiation dose (less than a chest X-ray). DEXA scanning uses two different photon energies, either by altering peak voltage or by filtering the beam, to correct for soft-tissue attenuation. The spine and femoral neck are usually scanned. Osteoporosis is diagnosed when the patient's bone mineral density (BMD) or bone mineral content (BMC) is >2.5 standard deviations below a young adult reference mean.

REFERENCES

Beggs 2004 Alternative imaging techniques. Magn Reson Imaging Clin N Am 12: 75–96.

Brenner DJ, Elliston CD 2004 Estimated radiation risks potentially associated with full-body CT screening. Radiology 232: 735–738.

Brenner DJ, Elliston CD, Hall EJ, Berdon WE 2001 Estimated risks of radiation-induced fatal cancer from pediatric CT. AJR. Am J Roentgenol 176: 289–296.

de González AB, Darby S 2004 Risk of cancer from diagnostic X-rays: estimates for the UK and 14 other countries. Lancet 363: 345–351.

FURTHER READING

American College of Radiology. www.acr.org

Barland P, Lipstein E 1996 Selection and use of laboratory tests in the rheumatic diseases. Am J Med 100A: 2A16S–2A23S.

Bizzaro N, Wiik A 2004 Appropriateness in anti-nuclear antibody testing: from clinical request to strategic laboratory practice. Clin Exp Rheumatol 22: 349–355.

Lentle BC, Prior JC 2004 Osteoporosis: what a clinician expects to learn from a patient's bone density examination. Radiology 228: 620–628.

Radiation Protection Division, Health Protection Agency. www.hpa.org.uk/radiation

RadiologyInfo – radiology information resource for patients. www.radiologyinfo.org

Royal College of Radiologists. www.rcr.ac.uk

Sheldon J 2004 Laboratory testing in autoimmune rheumatic diseases. Best Pract Res Clin Rheumatol 18: 249–269.

Wiik AS, Gordon TP, Kavanaugh AF et al 2004 Cutting edge diagnostics in rheumatology: the role of patients, clinicians, and laboratory scientists in optimizing the use of autoimmune serology. Arthritis Care Res 51: 291–298.

74

MANAGEMENT OF MUSCULOSKELETAL PROBLEMS

5

MEDICAL MANAGEMENT OF ARTHRITIS

David L. Scott, Gabrielle H. Kingsley, Mark Paterson and Daniel Porter

Cases relevant to this chapter

12, 19, 20, 23, 26, 27, 32, 68, 70–77, 79–87, 90, 91, 93, 94, 96, 97

●Essential facts

1. Pain is an important feature of many musculoskeletal problems and adequate pain relief should be offered to patients.

2. Non-steroidal anti-inflammatory drugs (NSAIDs) control the symptoms of arthritis including pain, tenderness and stiffness, but they can induce gastrointestinal bleeding, erosion and ulceration in the elderly.

3. Disease-modifying anti-rheumatic drugs (DMARDs) are usually effective singly or in combination in the management of persistent inflammatory arthritis, and should be used as early as possible.

4. DMARDs are all capable of toxicity and their use must be carefully monitored.

5. Biologic therapy is an important advance in managing resistant cases of inflammatory joint disease.

6. Steroids have a short-term role in managing rheumatoid arthritis – as intra-articular injections, or by intramuscular injection

whilst waiting for a DMARD to become effective.

7. Musculoskeletal infections occur either by haematogenous spread, or by direct inoculation through open wounds or skin lesions.

8. Metaphyseal and epiphyseal regions of long bones are susceptible to infection where sharp loops of capillaries predispose to bacterial deposition.

9. The commonest organism involved in musculoskeletal infection is *Staphyloccocus aureus*, followed by *Streptococcus*.

10. Antibiotics should be given for 6 weeks; drainage is required if abscess formation has become established.

11. In chronic osteomyelitis, in addition to antibiotics, treatment involves radical surgical clearance of all non-viable material.

12. In the case of infected joint replacements, bacteria introduced at the time of surgery may produce a *biofilm* around the implant and are difficult to eradicate.

ANALGESICS
NEED FOR ANALGESIA

Pain is the dominant symptom in arthritis. It is present from the earliest stages of synovitis and persists throughout the course of the disease. In early inflammatory arthritis pain is predominantly related to the activity of the synovitis. In late disease it is influenced by the development of joint damage and failure. All forms of arthritis merit analgesia.

Pain can be controlled by analgesics or anti-inflammatory drugs, but equally important is the control of the underlying inflammatory disease process, replacing damaged joints and providing a range of other measures including exercise therapy, transcutaneous electrical nerve stimulation (TENS) and treatment of co-existent depression.

PRACTICAL USE OF ANALGESICS

Simple analgesics can be used in all patients with inflammatory arthritis to control pain (Table 5.1); they are an adjunct to other therapy. The available drugs include paracetamol, weak and strong opioids, tramadol and combinations of paracetamol and a weak opioid. There is some evidence from clinical trials that analgesics reduce pain in rheumatoid arthritis, but the amount of data is very limited. Most trials of these drugs were carried out more than 20 years ago and by current standards did not study enough patients and did not last long enough. However, almost all rheumatologists recommend using them. At the same time, only a very small proportion of patients with rheumatoid arthritis (RA) and other inflammatory arthropathies will have their symptoms relieved by analgesics alone.

HISTORICAL PERSPECTIVE

The development of paracetamol, the classic simple analgesic, stems from late nineteenth century searches for drugs to reduce fever in place of natural compounds like cinchona bark. Phenacetin was identified first, followed some years later by the drug we now call paracetamol (acetaminophen in the USA). In the 1940s paracetamol was shown to be the key, less toxic metabolite of phenacetin. It was introduced as a prescription drug in the 1950s, but paracetamol is now an over-the-counter analgesic.

PARACETAMOL

Paracetamol is the most widely used analgesic. A single dose of 1000 mg, paracetamol provides more than 50% pain relief over 4–6 h in moderate or severe pain compared with placebo. Its analgesic effects are comparable to those of conventional NSAIDs. There are virtually no groups of people who should not take it. Interactions with other treatments are not a problem. At the recommended dosage there are virtually no side effects and it is well tolerated by patients with peptic ulcers. Overdosage is a risk, as relatively small overdoses can cause hepatic failure.

Despite being used for many years its mechanism of action is not well understood. It may act centrally, producing analgesia through elevating the pain threshold by inhibiting prostaglandin synthetase in the hypothalamus. At therapeutic doses it does not inhibit prostaglandin synthetase in peripheral tissues, and consequently has no anti-inflammatory activity.

The drawback of paracetamol is that it is relatively ineffective; patients need to take 6–8 tablets daily to achieve any analgesic benefit. Consequently, patients rarely use it alone.

OPIOIDS: CODEINE AND DIHYDROCODEINE

Opioids bind to specific opioid receptors, which are principally found in the central nervous system and gastrointestinal tract. Endogenous opioid peptides are produced by the body and are essential in controlling responses to pain. There are several opioid drugs, including opium alkaloids (morphine and codeine), semi-synthetic opioids (heroin and oxycodone) and fully synthetic opioids (pethidine and methadone) that are structurally different.

The most widely used opioids in rheumatic diseases are codeine and dihydrocodeine. These weak opioids have centrally mediated effects. They are effective after 20–30 min and last for about 4 h. Dihyrocodeine has about twice the potency of codeine. They show a ceiling effect for analgesia

Table 5.1 An analgesic ladder for arthritis

Step	Pain level	Treatment
One	Mild	Paracetamol
Two	Moderate	Paracetamol plus mild opioid or opioid-like drug (e.g. codeine or tramadol)
Three	Severe	Paracetamol plus stronger opioid (e.g. dihydrocodeine or morphine)

and higher doses give progressively more adverse effects, particularly nausea and vomiting. These adverse effects outweigh any additional analgesic effect. One major drawback is that they are relatively constipating. They also cause central side effects, such as drowsiness.

TRAMADOL

Tramadol is effective in the relief of moderate to moderately severe pain. It is useful in some patients with inflammatory arthritis. It is a synthetic, centrally acting analgesic, with some opioid properties. Tramadol causes less constipation than opiates and dependence is not a clinically relevant problem. To be fully effective tramadol needs to be given at a dose of 50–100 mg every 4–6 h. A slow-release formulation can be useful if night pain is a particular problem. Common adverse effects of tramadol include headache, dizziness and somnolence, which often preclude its use in patients who need to be mentally alert in the day.

STRONG OPIATES

Analgesics such as oral morphine and oxycodone are virtually never used in treating inflammatory arthritis. The reason for not using strong opiates is the belief that their addictive nature is more disadvantageous than their therapeutic benefit. They can also have significant gastrointestinal side effects. However, such negative views reflect custom and practice rather than any rigorous scientific testing.

One new approach to pain relief is to give transdermal opioids such as fentanyl. This appears both effective and relatively free of gastrointestinal side effects and is advantageous in patients with otherwise uncontrolled pain. There are currently very limited data for arthritis.

COMPOUND ANALGESICS

Paracetamol is often combined with a weak opiate in a single tablet. Co-proxamol, the combination of paracetamol with dextropropoxyphene, was historically popular with clinicians, but is currently being withdrawn due its frequent use in suicide. Readily available alternative compound analgesics are paracetamol with codeine (co-codamol) and dihydrocodeine (co-dydramol). These compound drugs have the same effects and adverse reactions as the individual drugs.

OTHER DRUGS

Many other drugs are used to treat pain in arthritis. In particular tricyclic antidepressants, such as amitriptyline, can be used to control pain and improve sleep. The evidence base for this is incomplete and some clinicians use tricyclics extensively and others rarely. Their beneficial effects on pain must be weighed against their side effects and the drowsiness they can cause, which may be worsened by other concomitant therapy.

NON-STEROIDAL ANTI-INFLAMMATORY DRUGS

CLASSIFICATION

NSAIDs are a diverse group of drugs, so named to distinguish them from steroids and non-narcotic analgesics. Although they are one of the most frequently used groups of drugs, their benefits must be set against significant risks from gastrointestinal and other toxicity. Although they are usually given orally, they can also be used locally as creams or given parenterally.

INDICATIONS

NSAIDs are used to control the symptoms of arthritis including pain and inflammation; they also reduce tenderness and stiffness. Inflammatory synovitis due to rheumatoid arthritis or seronegative arthritis, inflammatory back pain due to ankylosing spondylitis, and degenerative arthritis due to osteoarthritis are all treated using NSAIDs.

MECHANISM OF ACTION AND COX1/COX2 EFFECTS

Inflammation involves many mediators, including prostaglandins. NSAIDs inhibit cyclo-oxygenase (COX), which has a key role in prostaglandin synthesis. COX has two isoforms. COX1 is responsible for 'housekeeping' prostaglandins involved in normal renal, gastric and vascular function. COX2 is induced at sites of inflammation. NSAIDs are classified by their effects on COX1 and COX2.

NSAIDs have other effects, including uncoupling oxidative phosphorylation, inhibiting lysosomal enzyme release and complement activation, antagonizing kinins and inhibiting free radicals. No single mechanism fully explains how NSAIDs work.

CONVENTIONAL NSAIDs

Although there are many NSAIDs, most specialists use only a few. Commonly used NSAIDs are shown in Table 5.2. NSAIDs reduce pain, joint tenderness and the duration of early morning stiffness. They have little impact on systemic effects of joint inflammation and do not reduce the elevated ESR of active rheumatoid arthritis.

Frequent dosing provides greater flexibility for individual patients, but also means taking more tablets at frequent intervals. Giving a NSAID once daily is more convenient, but risks greater toxicity. Side effects are minimized by giving the lowest dose compatible with symptom relief. Systematic

reviews have found no major differences in efficacy between the currently available NSAIDs, though there are differences in their adverse reactions. However, individual patients often show considerable variation in their responses to different NSAIDs.

ADVERSE REACTIONS TO NSAIDs

These are the main limiting factor to the use of NSAIDs. Overall NSAIDs are one of the commonest classes of drugs causing adverse events. Risks increase with age and NSAIDs must be used carefully in the elderly. Minor adverse effects such as dyspepsia and headache are commonplace, and rashes also occur. Renal, gastrointestinal and cardiac side effects cause more problems. Central nervous system side effects, such as drowsiness and confusion, are often underestimated. Haematological side effects are unusual. NSAIDs can exacerbate pre-existing asthma.

Renal adverse events are one area of concern. As prostaglandins regulate kidney function, NSAIDs can cause dose-dependent renal side effects, especially in patients with pre-existing renal disease. Common problems are peripheral

Table 5.2 Commonly used oral non-steroidal anti-inflammatory drugs

Drug	Suggested dose	Advantages	Limitations
Conventional NSAIDs			
Diclofenac	75 mg slow release bd	Rapid onset of action and relatively good efficacy	Risk of unusual toxicity, especially liver damage
Ibuprofen	600 mg tds	Well known and widely used with short half-life giving great flexibility of use	Requires frequent dosing
Naproxen	500 mg bd	Effective when used twice daily	Standard NSAID with no major benefits or drawbacks
Piroxicam	20 mg daily	Effective once daily	Increased side effects, especially gastro-intestinal ulceration
Indometacin	75 mg SR bd	Useful in acute gout or severe anklyosing spondylitis	Greater risk of side effects and frequent central nervous system adverse reactions
COX2-specific NSAIDs (coxibs)			
Celecoxib	200 mg daily	Effective, well tolerated and less gastrointestinal toxicity	Uncertain risk of cardiovascular side effects

oedema, hypertension, and reduced effects of diuretics and anti-hypertensive drugs. When renal blood flow is reduced, for example by cardiac failure or diuretic use, the added inhibition of prostaglandin synthesis by NSAIDs further impairs blood flow, and this can cause overt renal failure, particularly likely in the elderly. Other renal problems seen occasionally include acute renal failure, hyperkalaemia, and interstitial nephritis and papillary necrosis.

Gastrointestinal toxicity is the main problem with NSAIDs. The range of adverse effects includes dyspepsia, gastric erosions, peptic ulceration, bleeding, perforation, haematemesis or melaena, small bowel inflammation, occult blood loss and anaemia. The most serious problems are perforations, ulcers and bleeds. Many patients who have serious gastrointestinal complications do not have prior dyspepsia. In the absence of warning signs there is no way to ascertain if a patient is on the point of developing serious problems.

If NSAID use is unavoidable, some protective strategy is needed, particularly in those patients at greatest risk. There are several potential options. One choice is to co-prescribe proton pump inhibitors, such as omeprazole. This is effective and acceptable to patients. H2-receptor antagonists also help, but are less effective than proton pump inhibitors. A third choice is to co-prescribe prostaglandin analogues, such as misoprostol. This is also effective, but causes added side effects, such as diarrhoea, and is less well tolerated than proton pump inhibitors. The final option is to use a safer NSAID – one of the newer COX2 drugs.

COX2 DRUGS (COXIBS)

Identification of the COX2 isoenzyme provided a new therapeutic target. The hope was to achieve similar anti-inflammatory action and pain relief to conventional NSAIDs, but without the gastrointestinal toxicity associated with COX1 inhibition. Several new drugs in this class are now available including celecoxib and etoricoxib. Celecoxib was introduced several years ago and etoricoxib is relatively new. Rofecoxib, another member of this group, has been withdrawn due to cardiac adverse effects.

Coxibs are all equally effective as conventional NSAIDs. They undoubtedly have less gastrointestinal toxicity and decrease the risk of gastric ulcers. However, they may carry an increased risk of cardiac toxicity, particularly in patients with pre-existing cardiac disease and associated cardiac risk factors. Other side effects are similar to those of conventional NSAIDs.

Their use is likely to be restricted to patients most at risk of serious upper gastrointestinal side effects, who do not have cardiac risk factors. Patients at 'high risk' of developing serious gastrointestinal adverse events include those of 65 years of age and over, those using concomitant medications known to increase the likelihood of upper gastrointestinal adverse events, those with serious co-morbidity or those requiring the prolonged use of maximum recommended doses of standard NSAIDs. The risk of NSAID-induced complications is particularly increased in patients with a previous clinical history of gastroduodenal ulcer, gastrointestinal bleeding or gastroduodenal perforation. The use of even a COX2-selective agent should, therefore, be considered especially carefully in this situation.

TOPICAL NSAIDs

NSAIDs can be used topically as creams or gels, for example Voltarol Emulgel. These local NSAIDs are modestly effective and extremely safe. They are used mainly in osteoarthritis.

DISEASE-MODIFYING ANTI-RHEUMATIC DRUGS

This diverse group of drugs is considered collectively because they improve symptoms and also modify the course of the disease. This means they slow down or halt erosive joint damage and reduce disability.

INDICATIONS

DMARDs are used to reduce swollen joints, improve global health and decrease an elevated acute-phase response. They are used mainly in RA, but are also given to patients with seronegative arthritis, including psoriatic arthritis. Some patients achieve a major clinical response; a minority achieves sustained remission. Treatment also slows erosive damage and improves function.

HISTORICAL PERSPECTIVE

Injectable gold, the first DMARD, was first used in the 1920s. Early observational studies showed it helped two-thirds of patients. Between 1950 and 1980 several DMARDs were introduced, including antimalarials and sulfasalazine. They were all used after chance observations by individual clinical rheumatologists allowed existing pharmaceuticals to be adapted for RA.

COMMONLY USED DMARDs

Methotrexate is the dominant DMARD, given to over 80% of patients treated with DMARDs. Leflunomide and sulfasalazine are also used in a reasonable number of cases (Table 5.3). Most other DMARDs are only rarely used.

RESPONSES

Not all patients respond to methotrexate; over 30% show poor responses. There is no ideal way to predict who will respond; responses are better in early disease and worse in patients who have failed on other DMARDs. If there is no improvement after 3 months, success is unlikely and methotrexate should be stopped if there is no evidence of benefit by 6 months.

METHOTREXATE

Methotrexate is an anti-metabolite that inhibits folate metabolism. Low doses are used in arthri-

Table 5.3 Main disease-modifying anti-rheumatic drugs

Commonly used	Infrequently used	Rarely used
Methotrexate	Hydroxychloroquine/ chloroquine	Ciclosporin
Leflunomide	Injectable gold	Penicillamine
Sulfasalazine	Azathioprine	Auranofin (oral gold)
		Cyclophosphamide

tis and these may have other effects, such as changing adenosine metabolism and accumulation.

Low-dose methotrexate is given weekly. It is usually given orally, but can be given by subcutaneous or intramuscular injections. Methotrexate is strongly bound to plasma proteins, and free methotrexate could be displaced by drugs like NSAIDs; this is not a problem in clinical practice.

Methotrexate is usually started orally at a dose of 7.5 mg/week. This is gradually increased to a target dose of 15–25 mg/week. Lower doses are given if the drug is poorly tolerated. It is given with low-dose folic acid to reduce adverse reactions.

Methotrexate causes many side effects; most develop in the early months of treatment and are minor. Common gastrointestinal adverse effects often resolve with dose reduction or parenteral administration. Stomatitis is frequent. Alopecia causes concern in women. Methotrexate may cause accelerated nodulosis, with small nodules on the fingers or elbows. Infections, including opportunistic infections and herpes zoster, sometimes occur.

Serious side effects include cytopenias, most commonly leucopenia, which respond to methotrexate withdrawal. Mild transaminase elevations are common, but serious hepatotoxicity, which can lead to fibrosis or frank cirrhosis, is rare. Methotrexate should be avoided in patients with a risk of liver damage, such as a high alcohol intake or diabetes mellitus. A potentially fatal acute pneumonitis occurs rarely, and methotrexate should be stopped if patients develop respiratory symptoms, such as a persisting cough.

Patients should be monitored prior to and during treatment with methotrexate. Conventionally, full blood counts and liver function tests are undertaken monthly. A chest X-ray is usually recommended at the beginning of treatment, so subsequent lung problems can be evaluated from a known baseline.

LEFLUNOMIDE

This new DMARD was developed as an immunosuppressant. It is a pyrimidine synthesis inhibitor with anti-proliferative activity. Leflunomide is a prodrug, converted in the gastrointestinal tract and plasma to its active metabolite. The prodrug has a long half-life of 2 weeks.

The effective dose of leflunomide is 20 mg daily; some patients benefit from 10 mg daily. Loading doses (100 mg for 3 days) facilitate rapid steady-state levels of the active metabolite. Otherwise dose steady-state plasma concentrations need 2 months' treatment. The loading dose causes a more rapid response, but also results in more early side effects, especially gastrointestinal reactions.

Common adverse reactions include diarrhoea, nausea, reversible alopecia and rashes. Diarrhoea often leads to patients stopping treatment. Omitting the loading dose reduces the frequency and severity of diarrhoea. Hypertension is seen in some cases. There is also a small increase in the risk of infections, in common with other immunosuppressive drugs. Occasionally patients develop low white cell counts or low platelet counts and, in these, treatment should be stopped.

One particular concern is liver damage. Transient increases in liver enzymes are commonplace, and only need careful observation. If the levels rise by more than threefold, normal treatment should be stopped. A few patients have developed cirrhosis or liver failure. Patients receiving leflunomide need regular monitoring of liver function and also blood counts. These are undertaken every 2 weeks for the first 6 months and then less often.

A washout procedure, using cholestyramine or activated powdered charcoal for 1–2 weeks, can be considered with severe side effects or in younger patients who wish to conceive.

SULFASALAZINE

Sulfasalazine is given orally with a target dose of 2–3 g daily or up to 40 mg/kg/day, using the enteric-coated formulation. To minimize upper gastrointestinal side effects, such as nausea, treatment is initiated at 500 mg daily rising slowly to 2 or 3 g. Sulfasalazine causes a number of side effects in addition to gastrointestinal disturbances including rashes, reduced white cell counts and liver damage. It requires monitoring for blood and liver toxicity in the early stages. A particular concern is an allergic neutropenia that occurs in both early and late treatment and is unpredictable.

OTHER DMARDs

Gold injections are effective in a minority of cases, but cause many adverse reactions, which can be serious. The use of gold has, therefore, markedly reduced in recent years. Gold is given as weekly injections of 50 mg intramuscularly and after 20 injections is decreased to 50 mg monthly. It often causes proteinuria or rashes, which may persist long after treatment is stopped. It also causes marrow failure and blood counts need careful monitoring.

Hydroxychloroquine is modestly effective in RA, especially in early disease. It is usually given at a dose of 400 mg/day. It is less effective than other DMARDs, but is relatively safe. Common adverse effects include rash, abdominal cramps and diarrhoea. Its main toxicity is retinopathy and an annual visual screening is required to monitor visual acuity, using the standard Royal College of Ophthalmologists test types.

Ciclosporin is an immunosuppressive drug that improves symptoms and decreases erosive damage. Its adverse effects, particularly nephrotoxicity and hypertension, limit its long-term use.

Azathoprine is also used because of its immunosuppressive effects. It improves symptoms but has only a weak effect. It can result in serious haematological toxicity and this limits its value. It is not contra-indicated during pregnancy.

COMBINING DMARDs

Despite conventional therapy with DMARDs many patients have an aggressive course with progressive joint destruction and marked disability developing over 5–10 years or longer. There is evidence that early therapy with DMARDs improves outcome and that two or more DMARDs used together are more effective than single DMARDs used sequentially.

Effective combinations include methotrexate with sulfasalazine and hydroxychloroquine, methotrexate with ciclosporin, and methotrexate with leflunomide. Using two DMARDs increases the chance of toxicity, and some effective combinations need to be used with some caution, such as methotrexate and leflunomide.

CURRENT BEST PRACTICE WITH DMARDs

Early treatment

There is a growing consensus that DMARDs should be used as early as possible. Observational studies show that patients with active RA in whom DMARDs are started early have better functional and radiological outcomes after 5 years. Randomized trials support these observational findings. Trials of early treatment with sulfasalazine, or weaker drugs like auranofin and hydroxychloroquine, all show that early treatment reduces disease activity. With sulfasalazine there is also evidence that it reduces erosive damage.

Withdrawing DMARDs

When RA patients taking DMARDs are in remission, stopping therapy increases the risk of a flare-up. For this reason it is usually best to continue therapy.

Pregnancy

Many DMARDs, including methotrexate and leflunomide, are teratogenic and best avoided before and during pregnancy. Treatment should be stopped before attempting conception; the optimal gap differs between drugs (3–6 months for methotrexate and 2 years for leflunomide).

BEST APPROACH

There is no doubt that DMARDs are effective and safe in RA. The evidence from randomized clinical trials is inevitably incomplete and best practice reflects not only that available evidence, but also the overall current consensus amongst practising clinicians. The main points about using these drugs are:

- DMARDs are most effective in patients with active RA.
- They should be started early in the course of the disease.
- Methotrexate is the drug of first choice.
- Leflunomide or sulfasalazine is the best alternative.
- If patients have an adverse reaction to a DMARD they should move on to another.
- Those patients who have an incomplete response should have another DMARD added.
- Continue DMARDs in patients who have entered complete or partial remission.

BIOLOGICS

Biologics have changed the treatment of RA. They rapidly improve symptoms and modify disease progression. Conventional drugs inhibit small molecules. However, the cytokines are large peptides and can be inhibited only by large molecules. Biologics are proteins, usually based on immunoglobulins, produced using new biotechnological methods. The presently used biologics mainly focus on inhibiting one key cytokine: tumour necrosis factor α (TNFα).

INDICATIONS

TNFα inhibitors should be considered when patients continue to have active RA after an adequate trial of other effective DMARDs. Methotrexate is the best example. Within the UK current guidance is for two effective DMARDs to be given for 6 months; one must be methotrexate. TNFα inhibitors can be added to pre-existing treatment with DMARDs. In some cases they may replace previous DMARDs. Currently three TNFα inhibitors can be used (Table 5.4). Despite prompt and continued responses, drug-free remission remains rare. Many patients have increased disease activity when they discontinue therapy and the majority continue on long-term treatment. Biologics are also indicated in uncontrolled psoriatic arthritis and ankylosing spondylitis.

CLINICAL EFFECTS

TNFα inhibitors, when given in adequate doses, produce major improvements in symptoms, signs and laboratory measures. This improvement occurs within 12 weeks of starting treatment. Provided there is some evidence of benefit, treatment should be continued. In patients with an incomplete response, there is some evidence that increasing the dose or reducing dosing intervals may provide additional benefit, as may the addition or substitution of other DMARDs. If patients show no response, therapy should be stopped. There is no reason that any specific TNFα inhibitor should be used first. There is also no evidence that any TNFα inhibitor is more effective than any other. Switching from one TNFα inhibitor to another is well documented, though not supported by evidence from clinical trials.

Table 5.4 Currently available TNFα inhibitors

TNFα inhibitor		Site of action	Dosing schedule	Methotrexate
Infliximab	Chimeric IgG1 anti-TNFα	Binds soluble and transmembrane TNFα and inhibits binding of TNFα to TNF receptors	Intravenous administration every 4–8 weeks	Essential to co-prescribe
Etanercept	Soluble TNF-receptor fusion protein	Binds TNFα and lymphotoxin and competitive inhibitor of TNF receptor	Subcutaneous twice weekly	Optional to co-prescribe
Adalimumab	Recombinant human IgG1 monoclonal antibody	Binds soluble and transmembrane TNFα and inhibits binding of TNFα to TNF receptors	Subcutaneous fortnightly	Optional to co-prescribe

ADVERSE EFFECTS

Local reactions such as minor redness and itching at the injection site are common with etanercept and adalimumab. They last a few days. Minor symptoms, such as headache and nausea, are common in patients during infliximab infusions. Symptoms suggesting immediate hypersensitivity response with infliximab infusions, such as urticaria, are uncommon but well described; serious anaphylaxis is rare. Antihistamines, steroids and adrenaline (epinephrine) should be available while infusions are being given, though they are rarely needed.

Serious and opportunistic infections occur in patients receiving TNFα inhibitors. They should not be started or should be discontinued when serious infections occur. Examples include septic arthritis, infected prostheses, acute abscesses and osteomyelitis. TNFα inhibitors should be avoided in patients with viral infections, particularly hepatitis B and C. Tuberculosis is of particular concern. There is increased susceptibility to primary tuberculosis. More importantly, previous tuberculosis may be reactivated. The incidence of reactivation of latent tuberculosis by TNFα inhibitors is highest in the first 12 months of treatment and maximum vigilance is needed during this period. Screening patients for tuberculosis reduces the risk of activating the condition. All patients should be evaluated for the possibility of latent tuberculosis. This evaluation should include a detailed history and examination, together with screening tests, such as skin tests and chest radiography, depending on recom-

mendations. Treatment for the possibility of latent tuberculosis should be considered if patients might be at risk.

Demyelinating-like disorders and optic neuritis have been reported in patients receiving TNFα inhibitors. A few cases of pancytopenia and aplastic anaemia have been seen. Although heart failure is associated with high levels of TNFα, there is no evidence that TNFα inhibitors are clinically useful in this setting and they may even increase mortality. For this reason the biologics should be used with caution in patients with significant heart failure.

IMMUNE RESPONSES TO TNFα INHIBITORS

Patients develop antibodies to etanercept and adalimumab, but their clinical significance is unknown. Antibodies to infliximab are seen more often and may accelerate the clearance of infliximab, increase the risk of infusion reactions and reduce responses. These antibodies form less often when infliximab is given in combination with methotrexate, which is the standard way of using infliximab.

DMARDs AND BIOLOGICS DURING SURGERY AND MAJOR MEDICAL ILLNESS

Many clinicians advocate stopping DMARDs and biologics in patients who are undergoing elective surgical procedures or are admitted with serious medical disorders. There are circumstances, particularly the onset of a serious infection, in which these drugs are contra-indicated. However, this consideration does not apply to the average hospital admission. Custom and practice varies between units and some stop DMARDs at the time of surgery and others do not. There is insufficient evidence to assess whether this is beneficial or not and it is unlikely that units that stop these drugs will change practice in the immediate future. In any event they need to be restarted as soon as possible, otherwise the arthritis may flare up.

NEW BIOLOGICS

Treatment with biologics remains a rapidly evolving area. It is likely that new anti-TNF agents will soon become available with potential improvements in efficacy or reductions in cost. Other types of agent have been developed successfully. For example, rituximab, which inhibits B cells in arthritis and other conditions, has now been approved for use in arthritis. Abatacept, which prevents full T-cell activation in arthritis, is also available. Biologics still undergoing clinical trials and associated evaluations in arthritis include inhibitors of interleukin 6.

STEROIDS
BACKGROUND

Steroids have been used to treat inflammatory arthritis for over 50 years. They often show dramatic short-term effects on inflammation, but their clinical benefits diminish with time. Side effects limit their use. Steroids are usually given orally. Intravenous pulses and intramuscular, soft-tissue or intra-articular injections are also used, mainly to minimize or avoid side effects and to deal with acute or local problems. The choice of preparation depends on the required anti-inflammatory potency and duration of action. Cortisone and hydrocortisone are not recommended for long-term use in arthritis. Prednisolone has mainly glucocorticoid (anti-inflammatory) activity; it is the most commonly used oral corticosteroid for long-term treatment.

SYSTEMIC STEROIDS

Oral steroids have an immediate benefit through reducing inflammatory synovitis and also some of the extra-articular features seen in a minority of RA patients. They are used in a variety of specific situations. Examples include patients refractory to other treatments; to obtain symptomatic control; in defined combination regimens particularly in early RA; in elderly patients (in whom steroids may be better tolerated than anti-inflammatory drugs); and during pregnancy, when other drugs may be contra-indicated. In most of these circumstances, the dose should be low (in the region of 7.5 mg daily).

They are used to treat extra-articular features of RA, such as vasculitis, and for systemic connective tissue disorders, such as systemic lupus erythematosus. They are also specifically used to treat polymyalgia rheumatica and temporal arteritis. In most of these situations high doses may be needed, depending on the clinical situation. One notable exception is polymyalgia rheumatica, which usually responds to low doses, such as 10–15 mg per day, then progressively reducing to withdraw over the next 2–3 years.

Intramuscular steroid injections, such as 120 mg methylprednisolone, are often used to treat an arthritis flare or given when disease-modifying drugs, such as methotrexate, are being started. This approach is simple to administer and rarely causes significant side effects if continued for up to four injections only. Intravenous steroids are rarely used because, although rapidly effective, they often are followed by a severe rebound in symptoms after 2–3 months; there are also reports of fatalities due to arrhythmias.

SIDE EFFECTS

The disadvantages of systemic steroid use are almost entirely related to their side effects, which are frequent and often serious. Patients are typically concerned by general changes, such as weight gain and oedema. Other problems include the development of diabetes mellitus, gastrointestinal reactions including gastric ulcers, mood changes and depression, myopathy and cataracts. On balance, the cardiovascular risks, especially hypertension and accelerated atherosclerosis, are the main threat to health. Certain adverse events are preventable; this is particularly true for osteoporosis. Oral steroid treatment is associated with a significant increase in fracture risk at the hip and spine. Though the greatest increase in risk is seen with high-dose therapy, increased risk is also seen at doses of prednisolone under 7.5 mg daily. Fracture risk increases rapidly after the onset of steroid treatment and declines equally rapidly after cessation of therapy. Loss of bone mineral density associated with oral steroids is, therefore, greatest in the first few months of their use. Patients at high risk of fracture, particularly those aged 65 years or over and those with a prior fragility fracture, should commence bone-protective therapy at the time of starting steroids.

ASPIRATION/INJECTION OF JOINTS AND SOFT TISSUES

The purpose of joint aspiration is to yield diagnostic joint fluid for synovial analysis or to drain a joint for therapeutic relief (for example in acute knee joint haemarthrosis). From other structures, aspiration may also be diagnostic and therapeutic (for example aspiration of ganglion or bursal fluid). Injection of a joint with local anaesthetic will allow temporary pain relief, which may be diagnostic if there is debate on the origin of pain. Injection of locally acting steroid may give medium- or long-term relief in inflammatory arthropathy or early osteoarthritis.

As infection may be introduced by the needle, a careful aseptic technique is followed. The patient should be positioned in a clean environment. The doctor should at least have washed hands to elbows and sterile gloves should be worn. With an immunosuppressed patient this may have to be undertaken in a completely sterile environment, such as an operating theatre with antiseptic washing of hands beforehand. A trolley should be prepared with skin antiseptic for cleaning the patient's skin area. Sterile drapes should also be applied. Depending on the size of the needle for aspiration (large bore for ganglion aspiration), a small amount of local anaesthetic may be required for skin anaesthetization. Following skin preparation, the needle for aspiration/injection should then be introduced in an aseptic manner. The tip of the needle can often be felt to 'give' as it penetrates through the joint capsule into the synovial space.

The safe introduction of a needle into any structure relies upon a sound knowledge of anatomical structures. As a result, certain areas cannot safely be approached without the use of ultrasound or fluoroscopy (for example, the hip joint, vertebral joints). For these the services of a radiologist should be sought.

Steroid injections are used in individual joints to control local synovitis and patients usually show an improvement in symptoms that lasts for a few weeks to a few months. Other sites that can be injected include entheses – where tendons are inserted into bones – and areas of compression – such as the carpal tunnel when there is median nerve compression.

Adverse effects of local steroid injections are uncommon. Iatrogenic infection is the most serious, but least common, complication, occurring in less than 1 in 10 000 cases. More common, but less clinically important, complications include local irritation, atrophy of soft tissues at the sites of injection and post-injection flares. There have been isolated reports of weakening and even rupture of tendons after local steroid use. Some patients suffer a loss of pigmentation, which can be permanent; this can be a problem for dark-skinned individuals.

Common joints for aspiration and injection are described below:

- *Glenohumeral joint*
  A safe posterior window is identified 2 cm inferior to the tip of the acromion. The skin here has widely spaced sensory end-organs and frequently no pain is felt at all. The needle penetrates the posterior deltoid, rotator cuff tendon and capsule.
- *Subacromial bursa*
  Identical to above, except the needle is introduced 1 cm inferior to the acromion and is angled superiorly to enter the space for injection of steroid and local anaesthetic.
- *Elbow*
  The interval between the olecranon posteriorly and the radial head laterally is safe. The radial nerve runs anterior to the radial head here.
- *Common flexor and extensor origins of the distal humerus*
  These can be injected with steroid in intractable golfer's or tennis elbow. The injection is often extremely painful.
- *Wrist*
  There are several dorsal windows here. Introduction immediately ulnar to the extensor carpi radialis longus tendon is safe.

- *Digits*
  Dorsal injections just ulnar or radial to the extensor tendon are recommended.
- *Greater trochanteric bursa*
  In slim patients a long spinal needle may reach the bursa, which lies deep to the fascia lata over the trochanter. It can be painful, and a radiologist using ultrasound to guide the steroid to the area of inflammation may be more reliable.
- *Knee*
  A dorso-lateral approach into the suprapatellar pouch will penetrate quadriceps fascia and capsule. Alternatively an infero medial approach aimed towards the superolateral aspect of the patella is effective.
- *Ankle*
  A dorsal window just medial to tibialis anterior is safe.
- *Ganglia*
  Viscid material will be slow to enter even a large-bore needle. A 20-ml syringe will be needed to apply the necessary suction.

If infection or crystals are suspected then diagnostic material is sent for analysis to the microbiology laboratory. A large aspirate can be sent in a sterile universal container for both Gram stain and culture. Smaller volumes can be instilled into blood culture broth medium for culture. Synovial fluid that will allow 'stringing' of fluid between surfaces is unlikely to be infected since this phenomenon is due to the presence of chains of chondroitin sulphate. Most bacteria produce proteolytic enzymes that will prevent this phenomenon.

OTHER DRUGS
ALLOPURINOL

Allopurinol lowers blood uric acid levels, which are elevated in patients with gout. It achieves this by inhibiting the conversion of hypoxanthine to uric acid, the final step in purine metabolism. Allopurinol is used to prevent recurrent attacks of gout or when gout is likely to be induced by high uric acid levels, for example during cancer chemotherapy. Allopurinol is ineffective in acute gout.

When started, allopurinol can induce acute gout in some patients. It is, therefore, started with NSAID cover for the first few weeks of treatment. Colchicine is an alternative to NSAIDs in some cases.

Allopurinol is taken indefinitely when there have been recurrent attacks of gout. The initial dose is usually 100 mg daily and this may rise to 300 mg or more if uric acid levels remain high. Its main adverse reaction is rash.

COLCHICINE

Colchicine, an alkaloid from the crocus, has been used to treat and prevent gout for over 200 years. It is given at an initial dose of 0.5 mg in acute gout. Many experts recommend repeating this dose every 1–2 h until gastrointestinal symptoms ensue or pain resolves, ensuring no more than 4–5 mg is given in 24 h. Other experts prefer to use a lower dose and to combine this with steroid injections. Low-dose colchicine can also be used to prevent recurrent attacks of gout. Colchicine frequently causes gastrointestinal side effects, such as nausea, vomiting and diarrhoea. It rarely causes bone marrow toxicity.

BISPHOSPHONATES

These are used to prevent osteoporosis and treat Paget's disease of bone. They decrease bone turnover. Several drugs are available:

- *Disodium etidronate* is the oldest drug and is taken as a 14-day pulse of oral etidronate followed by 76 days of calcium supplementation. This cycle is repeated.
- *Alendronate* can be taken as a single tablet, once daily, continuously. It is more often taken as a single weekly tablet.
- *Risedronate* is similar and is usually taken weekly.
- *Oral bisphosphonates* require to be taken on an empty stomach, with water, with the additional need for alendronate and risedronate to be taken in an upright position to reduce the chance of upper gastrointestinal dyspepsia, including oesophagitis. Less frequent dosing is popular with patients and produces similar benefits on bone density.

MUSCULOSKELETAL INFECTION

Various musculoskeletal tissues can become infected, giving rise to a variety of clinical problems (Table 5.5). The underlying causes and the

Table 5.5 Spectrum of musculoskeletal infection

Tissue	Infection	Typical organism	Typical medical treatment	Typical surgical treatment
Bone	Osteomyelitis	*Staphylococcus aureus* *Streptococcus* sp.	Intravenous (IV) antibiotics	Periosteal incision, bone drainage
Joint	Septic arthritis	*Staphylococcus aureus* *Neisseria gonorrhoeae*	IV antibiotics	Joint aspiration and lavage
Muscle	Pyomyositis	*Staphylococcus aureus*	IV antibiotics	Incision and drainage

basic principles of management are similar, irrespective of the tissue concerned. Here we will look at why and how tissues become infected, consider the clinical presentation and describe the principles governing management of these conditions. Specific types of infection will then be considered in greater detail.

PATHOLOGY OF MUSCULOSKELETAL INFECTION

In this section we are concerned exclusively with bacterial infection. In some parts of the world, fungal infections are of importance, but, even so, these are relatively uncommon.

Musculoskeletal infections occur either by haematogenous spread (that is, via the bloodstream) or by direct inoculation through open wounds or skin lesions. Bacteria may come from an established infection elsewhere (for example, in the respiratory tract) or may simply be circulating in the bloodstream.

The presence of bacteria in the circulation (bacteraemia) does not usually lead to established infection either in the bloodstream (septicaemia) or in a local site, such as a joint. It is not uncommon for bacteria to circulate in the blood without being able to establish a focus of infection. Infection occurs when the infecting organism is present in sufficient numbers and with sufficient virulence to overcome the body's defence mechanisms. These latter include the non-specific inflammatory response as well as specific immunological responses. There is, thus, a balance between host resistance and infection. Organisms that are normally considered to be of low virulence can cause infections when the host's immune protection is compromised.

Certain tissues and regions are more susceptible to bacterial colonization than others. These include the metaphyseal and epiphyseal regions of the long bones. This is attributed to the vascular arrangement in these areas, where sharp loops of capillaries predispose to bacterial deposition. Other susceptible tissues include any bone or muscle that has been damaged or otherwise has an impaired blood supply.

The commonest organism involved in musculoskeletal infection is S*taphyloccocus aureus*, followed in frequency by species of S*treptococcus*. *Haemophilus influenzae* infections used to be common in children prior to the introduction of immunization against this organism. Other organisms are associated with the specific infections described below.

CLINICAL PRESENTATION OF MUSCULOSKELETAL INFECTION

In general terms, acute infection is accompanied by a systemic response, including fever, malaise and tachycardia. With increasing severity of infection and the presence of bacterial products in the bloodstream, there may be rigors and signs of shock (septic shock). The fever is classically a swinging fever, with peaks of high temperature corresponding to the release of bacterial toxins in the bloodstream. The site of the infection will show the classic signs of inflammation, with local warmth, redness, swelling and tenderness. These signs will be most obvious in infections of tissues near the surface and, conversely, will be difficult to elicit in deep sites, such as the hip joint. The patient will complain of pain and will be reluctant to move the affected part (so-called pseudo-paralysis).

Typically, the white cell count will be raised, with a neutrophilia in acute bacterial infection. Inflammatory markers, such as the erythrocyte sedimentation rate (ESR) and the acute-phase protein, C-reactive protein (CRP), will be raised. These markers may be useful in monitoring the progress of the treated infection.

The indications for diagnostic imaging vary according to the specific types of musculoskeletal infection and will be described below.

PRINCIPLES OF MANAGEMENT OF MUSCULOSKELETAL INFECTION

As far as possible the causative organism should be identified and its antibiotic sensitivities confirmed. Blood cultures may be positive during a bacteraemic phase, but ideally material from the infection site should be obtained for culture and sensitivity before any antibiotic therapy is started.

In the early stages of infection, antibiotics alone may be sufficient to control and eradicate the infection. Initially, these may need to be administered intravenously in order to obtain adequate levels of antibiotic in the tissues concerned.

The affected part should be rested and splinted if appropriate, and analgesia prescribed as necessary. Antibiotics alone will not cure musculoskeletal infection at any site once abscess formation has become established, or where pus is accumulating in significant volumes. Under these circumstances drainage is indicated. Simple aspiration and washout of an involved joint may be all that is necessary, but open surgery and more radical measures will be required for bone infection.

Following an appropriate period of rest and protection, mobilization, with the help of physiotherapy, will be necessary to restore range of joint movement and muscle power, and minimize osteoporosis in affected bones.

SPECIFIC INFECTIONS

Acute pyomyositis

Acute infection of the muscle is rare in Western countries, but common in tropical developing countries. The organism is usually *Staphyloccus aureus*. Abscess formation is common and surgical incision and drainage is necessary. Despite the large abscesses often encountered, these occur between the muscle bundles and long-term disability through contracture and scarring is not generally seen.

Immunocompromised patients are predisposed to infections, such as pyomyositis, and awareness of this form of infection is important when dealing with patients with compromised immune systems (see below).

Acute septic arthritis

Infection of a joint may occur by blood-borne infection, by direct penetrating injury (this may take the form of a surgical procedure on the joint), or by spread of infection from an osteomyelitic focus in an adjacent bone. Over all age groups the commonest organism is *Staphylococcus aureus*. In sexually active adults, the commonest cause is *Neisseria gonorrhoeae*, the causative organism of gonorrhoea. About half of all cases of septic arthritis are under the age of 3 years. Across all age groups, the commonest joint affected is the knee, but in infants and young children septic arthritis of the hip is more common.

The clinical presentation is of pain and loss of movement in a joint together with fever and malaise. Prompt diagnosis and treatment is necessary, as articular cartilage does not survive long in the presence of a tense effusion of pus. A high index of suspicion for infection is required in all cases of an acutely swollen and painful joint, particularly in a young child. Aspiration of the joint (Fig. 5.1) may not yield the causative organism, and diagnostic

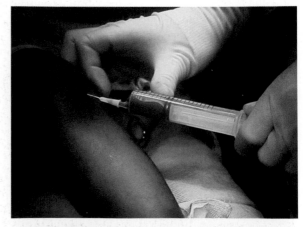

FIGURE 5.1 Aspiration of blood-stained pus from the knee of a child with septic arthritis

imaging modalities such as radiography and ultrasound will simply confirm the presence of a joint effusion. However, the clinical picture together with abnormally high values for the inflammatory markers should be enough to make the provisional diagnosis of infection. After blood cultures have been obtained, 'best guess' antibiotic treatment can be started and the joint drained. At the hip, this will require open surgery.

There is much controversy over the duration of antibiotic therapy required in septic arthritis, but most clinicians agree that intravenous therapy should continue at least until the temperature and CRP have returned to normal levels, with maintenance oral therapy for 4–6 weeks. The antibiotics used initially should include a cephalosporin to cover Gram-positive cocci, such as *Staphylococcus aureus*.

Complications include joint damage with subsequent osteoarthritis. In growing children, involvement of the nearby growth plates can give rise to progressive deformity and shortening of the affected limb segment.

Acute osteomyelitis

Acute osteomyelitis is an acute infection of the bone. It is usually caused by blood-borne organisms (haematogenous infection), but can spread from a severe soft-tissue infection into the adjacent bone, or from an open fracture or penetrating wound. The commonest organism is *Staphylococcus aureus*, followed by haemolytic *Streptococcus* sp. Haematogenous infections generally localize to the metaphysis of long bones because of the vascular arrangement described above.

This is mainly a disease of children. Clinically, the child presents with pain, malaise and a high fever. He or she will resent and resist movement of the affected limb, but generally not to the same extent as in a septic arthritis. The inflammatory markers will be raised above normal. In the first few days, there will be no changes in the bone on the plain radiograph, but soft-tissue swelling can be appreciated. Ultrasound may show the presence of pus developing in the subperiosteal region (Fig. 5.2). Isotope bone scan will show increased uptake in the infected part. MRI scan will show non-specific changes in the bone marrow, but will clearly show any periosteal abscess formation.

The initial management is directed at determining the causative organism as outlined above. Intravenous antibiotics may be all that is necessary in the early case. If these are unable to eliminate the infective focus, or in cases that present later, further action may be required. Pus accumulates under tension in the metaphysis, causing localized bone destruction and leaking through the cortex to elevate the periosteum (Fig. 5.3). Once this process starts, surgical drainage is necessary. The periosteum is incised and the underlying bone is drilled to release pus under tension.

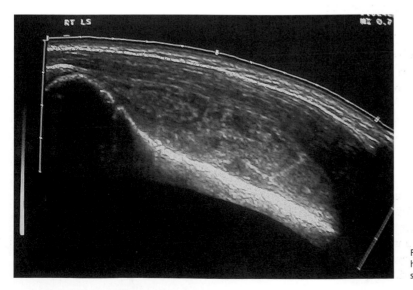

FIGURE 5.2 Osteomyelitis of proximal humerus; ultrasound scan showing subperiosteal collection of pus

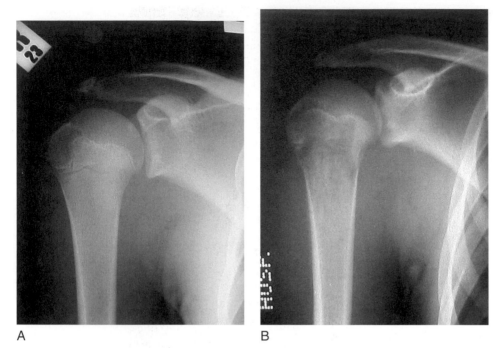

A   B

FIGURE 5.3 Radiographic appearance of acute osteomyelitis. (A) Proximal humerus at day 1 of infection – no visible changes. (B) Proximal humerus at day 12 of infection – bone destruction in the metaphysis

The duration of antibiotic therapy is a controversial issue, but commonly a course of 6 weeks of appropriate antibiotic is prescribed.

Complications of acute osteomyelitis include deformities due to damage to the growth plates of the bone in growing children (Fig. 5.4), and the persistence of infection to produce chronic osteomyelitis (see below).

Chronic osteomyelitis

Failure to eradicate infection of the bone in the acute stage results in persistence of the organism in the bone. It is characterized by continuing destruction of the bone by the infective process. Periosteal stripping results in parts of the bone becoming avascular and necrotic. These dead fragments are called *sequestra*. The surrounding periosteum lays down new bone, which surrounds the sequestrum. This is known as the *involucrum*. Necrotic material and pus continue to make their way out of the bone through tracks that may eventually traverse through the soft tissues to the skin, where they form *sinuses*. These are all characteristic features of chronic osteomyelitis (Fig. 5.5).

By this stage, antibiotics cannot be expected to exert anything other than a suppressive effect on the infection, which flourishes in a bed of avascular or poorly vascularized tissue. Treatment involves radical surgical clearance of all nonviable material. This will inevitably leave large defects in the affected bone, and extensive bone and soft-tissue grafting may be necessary. In a few cases these measures are insufficient to eliminate infection, and amputation has to be considered.

SPECIAL SITUATIONS

Tuberculosis of bones and joints

Tuberculosis (TB) is a chronic granulomatous infection caused by *Mycobacterium tuberculosis*. Osteomyelitis and septic arthritis generally occur by haematogenous spread from foci elsewhere, usually the lungs. After many years of decline in the prevalence of TB infections, these are now on the rise again in the UK. Worldwide, it remains a common and serious problem. In the musculoskeletal system, the spine is the commonest site of involvement, followed by the large joints of

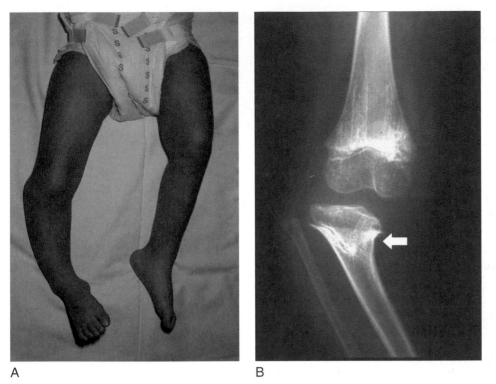

A

B

FIGURE 5.4 Partial growth arrest due to damage to the growth plate in the proximal tibia by a meningococcal infection. (A) Clinical appearance of deformity. (B) Radiographic appearance; arrow indicates area of growth arrest caused by damage and premature fusion of part of the growth plate or physis

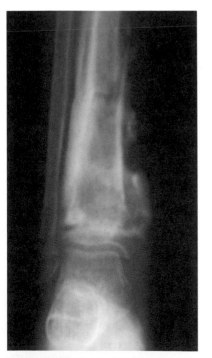

FIGURE 5.5 Radiograph of distal tibia affected by chronic osteomyelitis; pathological fracture and sequestrum formation

the lower limb. Involvement of the small bones of the hands and feet is known as tuberculous dactylitis.

Clinically, the presentation may be indistinguishable from that of septic arthritis or osteomyelitis caused by other organisms. An affected joint will develop chronic effusion and thickened synovium, and infection may spread into the adjacent bones. In the spine, paravertebral abscesses may form, and these can track down alongside the psoas muscle to present as swellings ('cold abscesses') in the groin. Bone involvement can lead to extensive destruction and subsequent deformity (Fig. 5.6).

In musculoskeletal TB the rise in white cell count may not be dramatic, but typically the ESR is quite markedly raised. Material from an infected bone or joint will usually show the acid-fast bacilli on Ziehl–Nielsen staining, and it is important to ask for this stain when requesting microbiological analysis in suspected cases. *Mycobacterium tuberculosis* is difficult to culture and it may take 6–8 weeks to obtain a positive result. However, there

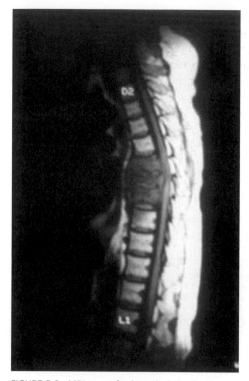

FIGURE 5.6   MRI scan of tuberculosis in the thoracic spine; note destruction of vertebral bodies, anterior abscess formation and acute angulation (kyphus or gibbus) of spine

are now immunoassays available that detect T cells specific for the mycobacterium antigens, and these provide a more rapid diagnosis. As in other tissues, tuberculous infections of the bone and joint are characterized histologically by the production of granulomata with Langhans' giant cells and central caseation.

Management principles are the same as for other forms of septic arthritis and osteomyelitis. In early disease, prompt diagnosis and institution of anti-TB chemotherapy may avoid the need for surgical intervention. Affected joints can be mobilized gently following a period of rest, and a good result can be expected. Abscess formation has to be dealt with by drainage. In advanced disease, bony destruction often leads to an ankylosis or fusion of the joint. Future joint replacement may be complicated by reactivation of infection even after many years.

Other mycobacteria may be responsible for bone and joint infections, particularly in immuno-compromised individuals such as HIV patients.

Sickle cell disease

In sickle cell disease, abnormal red blood cells result in sluggish blood flow and reduced oxygen tension in the bones, creating ideal conditions for bacterial colonization and the establishment of infection. Sickle cell disease sufferers are particularly prone to osteomyelitis caused by *Salmonella*. The possibility of osteomyelitis should always be considered in a sickle cell patient presenting with bone pain.

Implant-related infection

Infection can complicate the use of orthopaedic implants, such as total hip replacements or fracture fixation plates. Bacteria introduced at the time of surgery may flourish in the damaged tissue surrounding the implant. Such infections may be extremely difficult to eradicate, particularly if the bacteria produce a *biofilm*. This is a slimy layer of polysaccharide and protein that acts as a barrier to the body's defence mechanisms and to antibiotics. Organisms commonly implicated in joint replacement surgery are *Staphylococcus aureus* and *Staphylococcus epidermidis*.

Infection around an implant will ultimately destroy the surrounding bone and cause loosening of the implant (Fig. 5.7). Although such infections may be kept under control by the use of antibiotics, elimination of the infection can generally be secured only by removal of the implant and thorough clearance of the infected bone and soft tissues. In order to reduce the risks of catastrophic outcomes such as this, orthopaedic operating theatres often use laminar air-flow systems that reduce the risk of bacterial contamination of the operation site. In addition, prophylactic antibiotics are prescribed during the operating period. In this way, the risk of deep infection in a total hip replacement should be less than 2%.

Immunocompromised patients

Severe chronic disease such as HIV/AIDS results in reduced competence of the body's immune systems. Under these circumstances, bacteria that might not normally be regarded as pathogenic, together with fungi and yeasts, may cause musculoskeletal infections, such as chronic osteomyelitis. However, these patients are also at increased risk

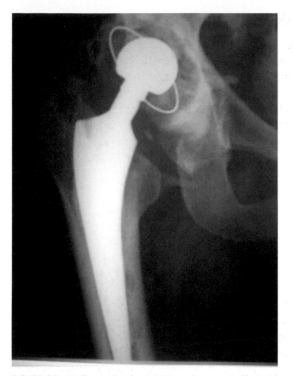

FIGURE 5.7 Radiograph of total hip replacement affected by deep infection; note scalloped appearance of the medial femoral cortex as a result of lysis from areas of infection

of the more usual infections, including tuberculosis of the bones and joints. The same applies to patients whose immune responses are being deliberately suppressed to reduce the risk of organ rejection, or who are on prolonged steroid or cytotoxic therapy regimens for rheumatoid disease or neoplastic disease.

FURTHER READING

Cole WG 1990 The management of chronic osteomyelitis. Clin Orthop Relat Res 264: 84–89.

Nade S 1983 Acute septic arthritis in infancy and childhood. J Bone Joint Surg 65-B: 234–241.

Scott RJ, Christofersen MR, Robertson WW et al 1990 Acute osteomyelitis in children: a review of 116 cases. J Pediatr Orthop 10: 649–652.

ROLE OF THE ALLIED HEALTH PROFESSIONAL

Sheena Hennell, Zoe Stableford and James Robb

Cases relevant to this chapter

2–4, 9, 10, 14–17, 19–21, 26, 27, 31, 50, 53, 63, 68, 74–76, 79, 80, 83, 91, 96, 97

> ## ●Essential facts
>
> 1. Nurse specialists provide key support for patients with rheumatic diseases.
>
> 2. Physiotherapists aim to reduce pain and restore or maintain physical function through education about exercise, pain relief, improving muscle strength, joint mobility and cardiovascular status.
>
> 3. Gait re-education is important after lower limb joint replacement or trauma.
>
> 4. Walking aids should be adjusted to the correct height to ensure maximum benefit.
>
> 5. Occupational therapists aim to enable patients to reach their full potential in self-care, productivity and leisure.
>
> 6. Occupational therapists can measure pre-operative functional status assessment, predict outcome and help patients to understand and cope with post-operative rehabilitation.
>
> 7. Joint protection reduces the load on individual joints, which in turn reduces pain and increases performance and independence.
>
> 8. Podiatry relieves pain, maintains mobility and function, minimizes deformity and protects vulnerable tissues from ulceration.
>
> 9. An orthosis may prevent unwanted motion, limit a normal range of motion, correct a mobile deformity, or accommodate fixed deformity.
>
> 10. The biomechanical principles of orthotic function involve long lever arms and large surface areas to minimize pressure to soft tissues.

Many musculoskeletal afflictions are longstanding and patients can benefit from a multi-disciplinary approach where time is devoted to education and clinics run by specialist allied health practitioners. This chapter will consider some of these roles.

NURSE SPECIALIST

The main function of the nurse specialist is to support patients through education, drug monitoring and management of their condition.

NURSE-LED CLINICS

Verbal communication and patient education leaflets provide information for patients. Leaflets may provide information on disease-modifying anti-rheumatic drugs (DMARDs), non-steroidal anti-inflammatory drugs (NSAIDs) (see Chapter 5), coping with a flare or early morning stiffness, for example. Some leaflets may be developed in individual hospital departments or provided by the Arthritis Research Campaign. Patients are given the opportunity to discuss any concerns and ask questions. The aim is to improve their understanding of their condition, awareness of drug therapy effects as well as their side effects, and to promote self-help of their condition.

Nurses undertake a formal review of disease activity in patients with rheumatoid arthritis (RA), including assessment for tender and swollen joints. The nurse examines the upper limb joints and knees, and records the patient's erythrocyte sedimentation rate (ESR) and a global health visual analogue score. The Disease Activity Score (DAS 28), based on an assessment of 28 joints, is in widespread use (Table 6.1) and is a reliable, valid and practical assessment tool. Locally agreed protocols based on the severity of the patient's DAS 28 score are used to determine changes in treatment; the higher the score, the more likely the need to increase or change treatment.

Assessment of functional status in RA may be undertaken using a standardized, structured, self-completed questionnaire, such as the Health Assessment Questionnaire (HAQ, Table 6.1), to assess physical activity. It may also be helpful to assess a patient's mood using the Hospital Anxiety and Depression Scale (HAD, Table 6.1). If direct interview or the use of these questionnaires reveals significant reduction in physical functioning, changes in medication, further advice and information, and referral to physiotherapy and occupational therapy may be necessary. Patients with decreased mood may benefit from psychological support provided by nurse/therapy specialists and sometimes also require antidepressants.

Education

Educational support and self-management techniques can be organized to suit, either individually or as group support. Computer-based initiatives, such as web-based packages and local websites, are also available. The aim is to provide patients with the necessary skills and knowledge to understand their disease and symptoms, as this can improve their ability to cope with chronic illness.

DMARDs and blood monitoring

All DMARDs require blood monitoring and, in addition, leflunomide and ciclosporin require blood-pressure monitoring. This is checked either at the hospital or as part of a shared-care agreement with local general practitioners (GPs) and practice nurses. If monitoring is carried out in a rheumatology department it is usually the responsibility of the specialist nurse to organize regular blood tests according to national guidelines and to check results. Patients with abnormal results attributed to their medication may have to stop their DMARD treatment or reduce the dose until stable, according

Table 6.1 Common assessments used in patients with rheumatoid arthritis

Type of assessment	Abbreviation	Description	Role/disease specific
Disease Activity Score	DAS 28	The number of tender and the number of swollen joints (28 joints including small joints of both hands, wrists, elbows, shoulders, knees) are entered into a calculation with the erythrocyte sedimentation rate (ESR) and global health visual analogue scale (VAS) determined using a 100-mm line	The overall score is a measure of disease activity in patients with rheumatoid arthritis (RA). The higher the score, the higher the disease activity
Health Assessment Questionnaire	HAQ	This is a questionnaire that is given to patients to assess functional status	The overall score is a measure of functional ability for those patients with RA. The higher the score, the greater the disability
Hospital Anxiety and Depression Scale	HAD	This questionnaire is used to assess mood. Patients with chronic illness can often display symptoms of depression	Using this scale in patients with chronic illness can help to direct treatment strategies

to agreed guidelines. Treatment is usually restarted when blood tests have returned to normal.

When DMARD monitoring is managed in primary care using local protocols, the specialist nurse is available to assist with decision-making. Patients are usually issued with a shared-care booklet in which blood test results are recorded and trends observed. If blood values fall outside protocol guidelines, careful consultation between primary and secondary care services is important and it may be appropriate for the specialist nurse to take over care temporarily. For example, a patient with RA and Felty's syndrome may be treated with methotrexate. These patients are often neutropenic as a result of their disease and the DMARD may help to control their disease and also help to correct the immune-mediated neutropenia. However, DMARDs may also induce a drug-related neutropenia and such patients require close monitoring.

Rheumatology helpline

Rheumatology specialist nurses in many rheumatology departments operate an advice/helpline for patients, GPs, practice nurses and other health-care professionals. Patients may contact the helpline if they require advice on coping with a flare-up, medication, general advice or information. Details of any treatment change are recorded in the patient's hospital notes and a letter is sent to the GP. Emergency appointments at the nurse-led clinic are available in most departments if a patient requires urgent review. Patients requiring urgent help from specialist occupational therapy and physiotherapy should be able to access this via the helpline, the whole multidisciplinary team liaising well with one another.

Specialist clinics

Specialist nurses are often responsible for pain management and monitoring of biological agents. Patients requiring the latter for rheumatological diseases require screening before TNF therapy and assessment of disease activity in line with nationally agreed guidelines. After starting TNF therapy, patients require regular review and collection of DAS 28 scores to assess response to treatment. These data may be collected and held in national registers, and specialist nurses are often responsible for the collation of these data.

Specialist nurses are often involved in pain management, which usually involves patient education as well as prescribing. Obtaining a balance between rest and exercise, using symptomatic measures, such as ice or heat, adapting to the condition and using self-help techniques to manage social and psychological issues are all important components of coping with a chronic condition. Counselling is complex and nurses are generally not trained counsellors, but it is important to recognize the need for additional support for the patient. Sometimes it is appropriate for patients to be seen in a combined session with a number of therapists, either at an outpatient appointment or at home.

Non-medical prescribing

Nurses with a prescribing qualification are now able to prescribe any medication, except some controlled drugs and unlicensed agents. For patients who have a chronic illness and where care is managed using a team approach, supplementary prescribing can be used. The consultant acts as the independent prescriber and the nurse specialist is a supplementary prescriber, who may prescribe using an agreed clinical management plan. The plan must be patient specific with supporting prescribing rationale, but may be generic to cover all rheumatological conditions.

SUMMARY

The role of the nurse specialist is evolving. Many have expanded their roles to include full examination and assessment, ordering of investigations and interpreting results, administering joint injections and prescribing to control disease activity and symptoms. However, education and teaching remain central to their role.

ROLE OF THE PHYSIOTHERAPIST

The primary function of the physiotherapist is to reduce pain, and to restore and maintain physical function. Educating the patient about exercise and management of their condition, helping with pain relief, preventing recurrence of symptoms, combined with physical therapies to improve muscle strength, mobility of joints and cardiovascular status is the major part of their role.

PHYSIOTHERAPY ASSESSMENT

The physical function of the patient as well as the range of movement and stability of joints is assessed. Patients' function can be affected by a flare-up of a rheumatological problem, as a result of a longer-standing problem, such as osteoarthritis of a major joint or in recovering from acute musculoskeletal trauma. Physiotherapists have a valuable role in assessing patients before joint replacement surgery, to advise about the recovery and what the patients may expect post-operatively and to ensure that equipment required as part of their rehabilitation is available for the patient on their return home. Many orthopaedic departments have leaflets that describe major joint replacement, the recovery, and risks and benefits of the procedure.

THERAPY

The main emphasis is education and exercise tailored to the individual's need and diagnosis. Exercises are necessary to help to restore muscle balance and strength, to increase joint movement and lubrication, to improve joint stability and to improve posture and circulation. Generally, it is important to maintain a general level of fitness to help patients to feel better and to improve function; this may also help to improve mood and psychological wellbeing. Patients with inflammatory arthritis, osteoarthritis and spondyloarthropathies require education about the benefits of exercise, which should become part of a daily routine. Patients with mechanical back pain may benefit from exercise programmes to improve abdominal muscle and spinal muscle strength.

Therapies include applications of ice and heat, electrical therapy and hydrotherapy to provide relief from pain and stiffness. Application of transcutaneous electrical nerve stimulation (TENS) may also provide effective pain relief. Exercise is more effective when pain is reduced, physical function is improved and patients can use exercise to condition themselves.

WALKING AIDS

Gait re-education is an important component after lower-limb joint replacement or trauma. Assessment before using a walking aid to ensure the correct height of a walking stick or crutches is essential to ensure maximum benefit. Patients whose upper limbs are affected by inflammatory joint disease often benefit from using an appropriate walking aid, where the handles have been modified to spread loads through the hand and wrist or forearm. Some patients require two walking sticks or crutches for bilateral joint problems. A four-poster frame may be required if a patient has to walk partially weight-bearing through one of their lower limbs or if they have problems with stability or balance.

POST-OPERATIVE REHABILITATION

The physiotherapist has a key role in helping patients with their rehabilitation after orthopaedic surgery for arthritis or following injury to optimize joint and muscle function, relief of pain and the ability to walk again if the surgery has been to the lower extremity. Patients are also helped with tasks such as climbing stairs and learning to get in and out of bed safely after surgery.

ROLE OF THE OCCUPATIONAL THERAPIST

The role of the occupational therapist is to enable the patient to reach their full potential in achieving and maintaining social/functional roles within the context of self-care, productivity and leisure. To achieve this, the therapist uses core skills to gain a good understanding of the patient's functional needs and priorities. Knowledge of relevant housing details, home circumstances and social support is needed. Assessment and treatment is based on occupation and encourages active participation of the individual in problem-solving. Psychological as well as practical support is given in coping with life-style changes. The approach is holistic and will take into account the impact upon family and other relevant personnel, such as work colleagues and carers. Psychological support will focus on enabling the patient to maintain their role and a sense of control especially where social situations or active disease, e.g. in rheumatoid arthritis, make the patient particularly vulnerable. Examples of the common roles played by occupational therapists are shown in Boxes 6.1 and 6.2.

Box 6.1
Examples of specialized assessment and treatments used by occupational therapists

- Seating assessments
- Work assessments
- Upper limb functional assessments
- Splinting

Box 6.2
Aims of occupational therapy treatment within the home

- To prepare ahead for post-operative rehabilitation
- To assist patients to cope with flare-up
- To meet patients with a diagnosis of rheumatoid arthritis during pregnancy and to plan for coping after childbirth and to help those with a new diagnosis following childbirth
- To facilitate application of joint protection and energy conservation
- To advise on equipment, housing alterations and adaptations
- To build confidence and facilitate discharge following surgery and recovery from illness

Box 6.3
Principles of joint protection

1. Distribute load over several joints.
2. Use each joint in its most stable anatomical and/or functional position.
3. Avoid positions of deformity and forces in their direction.
4. Use the strongest, largest joints available for the job.
5. Avoid staying in one position for too long.
6. Avoid gripping too tightly.
7. Avoid adopting poor body positioning, posture, and using poor moving and handling techniques.
8. Monitor pain levels and adjust activity accordingly (also referred to as 'respect for pain').
9. Maintain muscle strength and range of movement.

PRE-OPERATIVE ASSESSMENT

The occupational therapy pre-operative assessments are crucial to maintain quality of care, reduce stress for the patient and avoid unnecessary delays in discharge. Addressing post-operative rehabilitation problems by early problem-solving, sometimes requiring a home visit, is essential for some patients. An example would be patients with upper limb problems who are not allowed to weight-bear for a period of time after their surgery.

Pre-operative assessment is also fundamental to determining functional status and predicted outcomes, and in the ability of the patient to understand and cope with post-operative rehabilitation.

An example of this is the need for occupational therapy assessment of upper limb function in the patient with rheumatoid arthritis (RA) prior to hand surgery.

ENERGY CONSERVATION ADVICE

Fatigue is often under-appreciated. Indeed, it may be a greater problem than pain. Occupational therapists give education and support using task analysis and encouraging behaviour changes using appropriate prioritization and delegation to reduce fatigue, but still maintain function and roles.

JOINT PROTECTION

The aim of joint protection is to reduce load and effect on joints by evaluating activities to adopt working methods. The principles underlying joint protection advice are shown in Box 6.3.

These principles reduce pain and increase ease in activities of daily living, which in turn improve independence and self-efficacy. Occupational therapists will facilitate patients to apply these to relevant activities of daily living at an appropriate time and stage of their disease.

COGNITIVE BEHAVIOURAL APPROACHES

This problem-oriented approach aims to help patients to identify and modify dysfunctional thoughts, assumptions and patterns of behaviour. Patients and therapists work together to identify thinking patterns and behaviour that may contribute to the patient's disability. Therapy challenges those thinking patterns and works to implement behavioural change by goal-setting and activity timetabling, relaxation, role-playing and modelling coping behaviours.

This approach can be useful for the control of physical and behavioural aspects of pain if patients come to understand the interaction of emotion and cognitive behaviour in chronic rheumatic diseases.

ROLE OF THE PODIATRIST

The main emphasis of podiatry treatment is to relieve pain, maintain mobility and function, minimize deformity and protect vulnerable tissues from ulceration in the foot. Podiatrists manage foot, toe and nail pathologies, and are members of the multidisciplinary team.

PODIATRY EXAMINATION OF THE LOWER LIMB

This includes a biomechanical examination to ascertain the range of movement at the ankle, subtalar, mid-tarsal and toe joints, and an overall observation of the knee, hind foot, arch profile in weight-bearing and during the gait cycle. The use of force plates and in-shoe pressure systems provides a profile of high-pressure areas on the plantar surface of the foot and ground reaction forces. These are helpful when prescribing foot orthoses to unload areas of high pressure on the foot and to unload areas at risk of skin ulceration in inflammatory joint disease.

A general assessment of nail and skin pathologies is undertaken, paying particular attention to callus formation on prominent areas, such as metatarsal heads, retracted digits and bursae, and interdigital neuroma formation. Removal of a callus may not always provide relief, as it does not deal with the underlying problem.

TREATMENT

This includes:

- nail and skin management to maintain comfort
- nail surgery performed under local analgesia
- minor toe surgery under local analgesia
- ulcer care including the management of infections.

ROLE OF THE ORTHOTIST AND ORTHOSES

An orthosis is an externally applied device used to modify the structural and functional characteristics of the neuromuscular and skeletal systems. In doing so the orthosis may control body motion or alter, or prevent alteration in, the shape of body tissues. An orthotist is a professional who measures and fits orthoses.

An orthosis is manufactured by taking a cast from the patient's limb or trunk. Plaster of Paris is the usual material used for the trunk and limbs, but a negative image can also be taken of the foot by having the patient stand on a deformable material. This produces a negative cast of the patient and a positive cast of the area to be treated can then be manufactured from the negative cast. The orthoses are usually made from lightweight thermoplastic materials that can be moulded and vacuum-formed to the patient's positive cast. The thermoplastic material can then be trimmed, rectified and fitted to the patient.

ORTHOTIC TERMINOLOGY

The orthotic term describes the area encompassed by the orthosis (Table 6.2).

ORTHOTIC FUNCTION

In controlling joint motion an orthosis may prevent unwanted motion, limit a normal range of motion and correct a mobile deformity. If the deformity is fixed or not fully correctable, the orthosis can accommodate the deformity (Box 6.4).

BIOMECHANICAL PRINCIPLES OF ORTHOTIC FUNCTION

Orthoses are in direct contact with the patient and, since pressure = force/area, long lever arms can

Table 6.2 Orthotic terminology

Term	Area
Foot orthosis (FO)	Encompasses the whole or part of the foot
Ankle–foot orthosis (AFO) (see Fig. 6.1)	Encompasses the whole or part of the ankle and foot
Knee–ankle–foot orthosis (KAFO)	Encompasses the whole or part of the knee, ankle and foot
Thoraco-lumbo-sacral orthosis (TLSO) (see Fig. 6.2)	Encompasses the whole or a part of the thoracic, lumbar and sacroiliac regions of the trunk

Box 6.4
Orthotic Function

- Control joint alignment
- Control joint movement
- Alter load transmission
- Redistribute pressure
- Correct deformity

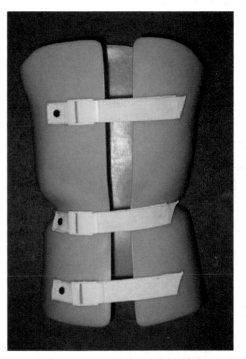

FIGURE 6.2 A thoraco-lumbo-sacral orthosis (TLSO)

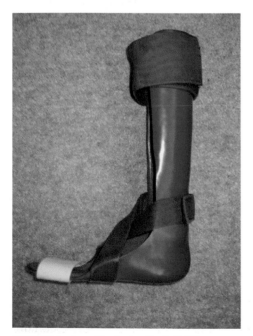

FIGURE 6.1 An ankle–foot orthosis (AFO)

help to reduce force and large contact areas reduce pressure.

The ankle–foot orthosis (AFO) will extend from the calf to the foot (Fig. 6.1).

AFOs are used to control movement and posture at the ankle, and help to control events in the gait cycle, for example dropping of the foot in swing phase or control of the progression of the ground reaction force along the foot in stance. Total contact foot orthoses are widely prescribed to unload forces acting across the foot (see above).

An example of the thoraco-lumbo-sacral orthosis (TLSO) is shown in Figure 6.2. This is most widely used in the non-operative management of adolescent idiopathic scoliosis (see Chapter 27). Here the application of the three-point force system (Box 6.5) to control the scoliosis will be firstly at the bony pelvis, secondly directed via the ribs to just under the apical vertebra, and thirdly above the apex in the region of the axilla (Fig. 6.3). Large contact areas optimize pressure distribution from

Box 6.5
Three-point force systems

- Long lever arms
- Large surface areas
- Minimize pressure to the soft tissues

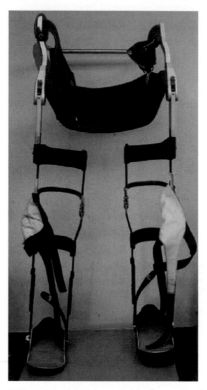

FIGURE 6.4   A hip–knee–ankle–foot orthosis

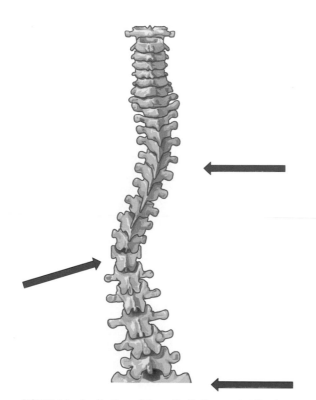

FIGURE 6.3   Application of the orthotic three-point fixation principle to a scoliosis

SUMMARY

We need a multidisciplinary approach to patients with longstanding musculoskeletal problems. The educational role of the allied health professionals is integral to the management of these patients.

FURTHER READING

Albert S, Rinoie C 1994 Effect of custom orthotics on plantar pressure distribution in the pronated diabetic foot. J Foot Ankle Surg 33: 598–604.

Enright SJ 1997 Cognitive behaviour therapy – clinical applications. BMJ 314: 1811–1816.

Hawley DJ 1995 Psycho-educational interventions in the treatment of arthritis. Baillieres Clin Rheumatol 9: 803–823.

Kitas G, Erb N 2003 Tackling ischaemic heart disease in rheumatoid arthritis. Rheumatology 42: 607–613.

Laughton C, McClay-Davis I, Williams DS 2002 A comparison of four methods of obtaining a negative impression of the foot. J Am Podiatr Med Assoc 92: 261–268.

the orthosis. There are two limitations to bracing for idiopathic scoliosis – curve magnitude and the position of the apical vertebra. A curve magnitude of more than 45° is usually an indication for surgery. If the apical vertebra is higher than the 7th thoracic vertebra, there is insufficient space above this before the axilla to give sufficient lever arm length for the orthosis to work effectively.

Figure 6.4 shows an example of a hip–knee–ankle–foot orthosis (HKAFO) that can be used to enable a patient who has spinal paraplegia to use a reciprocal walking pattern.

Philips JW 1995 The functional foot orthosis, 2nd edn. Churchill Livingstone, London.

Prevoo ML, van Riel PL, van't Hof MA et al 1993 Validity and reliability of joint indices. A longitudinal study in patients with recent onset rheumatoid arthritis. Br J Rheumatol 32: 589–594.

Root ML, Orien WP, Weed JN 1977 Normal and abnormal function of the foot. Clinical biomechanics, Vol. II. Clinical Biomechanics, Los Angeles.

Scott DL, Houssein DA 1996 Joint assessment in RA. Br J Rheumatol 35(Suppl. 2): 14–18.

Smolen JS, Breedveld FC, Eberl GL et al 1995 Validity and Reliability of the 28 count for the assessment of RA activity. Arthritis Rheum 38: 38–43.

Van Riel PLCM, van Gestel AM, Scott DL 2000 The EULAR handbook of clinical assessment in rheumatoid arthritis. Van Zuiden Communications, Alpen an den Rijn, The Netherlands.

Woodburn J, Barker S, Helliwell PS 2002 A randomized controlled trial of foot orthoses in rheumatoid arthritis. J Rheumatol 29: 1377–1383.

7

SURGICAL MANAGEMENT OF JOINT DISORDERS

John Keating

Cases relevant to this chapter

2, 16, 26, 27, 55, 56, 76, 82, 97

●Essential facts

1. Joint surgery is indicated when medical management has failed to adequately control pain or restore function.

2. Arthroscopic surgery is indicated for a number of joint disorders.

3. Surgical synovectomy is an effective, conservative approach to inflammatory arthritis, especially in younger patients.

4. Osteotomy is less commonly used due to an improvement in joint replacements, but is effective in younger male patients with medial compartment osteoarthritis of the knee.

5. Loosening is the most common mode of failure of total arthroplasties, especially in patients under the age of 60.

6. Hemiarthroplasty is commonly used following trauma involving only one side of the joint.

7. Excision arthroplasty is used as a last resort or as an interim treatment; it can be part of the treatment protocol of an infected total joint replacement.

8. Arthrodesis is most often used for small joints in the hands, wrists, feet and ankles.

INTRODUCTION

Surgery for arthritis is generally considered when medical management fails to control troublesome symptoms. The most common indication for surgery is to relieve pain. However, there may be other indications, including progressive deformity and disability resulting from the acquired stiffness that is a feature of most progressive arthritic conditions. More detailed information on these surgical procedures may be found within the chapters dealing with regional joint pathology.

ARTHROSCOPY

Arthroscopy is examination of a joint with a rigid endoscope. It was first used in the knee joint, but is now used for most major joints including the wrist, elbow, shoulder, hip, knee and ankle (Fig. 7.1). Arthroscopy was formerly commonly used for diagnostic purposes, but the use of computed tomography (CT) and magnetic resonance imaging (MRI) has largely supplanted this. In most situations arthroscopy is now used for operative treatment of joint disorders (Box 7.1). Although it can

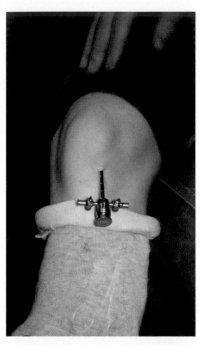

FIGURE 7.1   Photograph showing knee arthroscopy

Box 7.1
Indications for arthroscopy

- Excision or repair of meniscal tears (knee)
- Removal of loose bodies
- Joint debridement for osteoarthritis
- Repair of muscle tears (e.g. rotator cuff tear in the shoulder)
- Ligament repair (e.g. anterior cruciate ligament in knee)
- Fixation of osteochondral fractures
- Correction of joint instability (shoulder)
- Arthrodesis
- Synovectomy for inflammatory arthropathy
- Diagnosis (now less frequent)

---

be used in many joints, the majority of arthroscopies in clinical practice are performed on the knee or shoulder joint.

The scope of surgical procedures that can be carried out using arthroscopic surgery has greatly increased in the past two decades.

REPAIR OR EXCISION OF INTRA-ARTICULAR SOFT-TISSUE STRUCTURES

Many joints have intra-articular structures that can be injured during normal or sporting activity. These structures include the meniscus of the knee, the glenoid labrum in the shoulder and the acetabular labrum in the hip joint. When these structures tear they can cause mechanical symptoms. Surgical excision of the damaged structure by arthroscopy has largely supplanted open surgery to deal with these problems.

JOINT STABILIZATION

Recurrent joint instability usually requires open surgery to correct the problem. However, anterior shoulder instability is now amenable to arthroscopic stabilization and success rates approach those that can be achieved by open surgery. Similarly, patellar instability in selected cases can be treated by arthroscopic lateral release, which avoids more major open surgery.

LOOSE BODIES

Loose bodies may form in joints due to a variety of conditions, most commonly trauma, osteochondritis dissecans and synovial osteochondromatosis. Retrieval or replacement and fixation can be carried out arthroscopically.

LIGAMENT RECONSTRUCTION

Arthroscopic ligament reconstruction is most commonly used in the knee to deal with anterior and posterior cruciate ligament tears.

SYNOVECTOMY

Synovectomy is surgical removal of inflamed synovium. It is an operation that is now less commonly performed, but was formerly used quite regularly in the treatment of inflammatory arthropathies. The advantage of this procedure is that it represents a conservative approach with preservation of the joint, which is a particular advantage in younger patients. In modern practice it is usually performed arthroscopically. The main disadvantage is that the degree of symptomatic relief obtained is variable and is often temporary. It is usually indicated in younger patients with marked synovitis but well preserved joint spaces, and in some florid forms of synovitis that can be quite destructive of articular cartilage. These may result from frequent bleeding (haemoglobinopathies) or tumour-like synovial proliferations (pigmented villo-nodular synovitis).

OSTEOTOMY

An osteotomy is an operation that alters the alignment of a bone. It was formerly used quite commonly in the treatment of arthritis but is less frequently used now due to the wider availability of successful joint replacements. The rationale for using an osteotomy adjacent to a joint is to alter the distribution of forces across the joint. In the case of the knee, osteoarthritis most commonly involves the medial compartment with a varus deformity (Fig. 7.2). A high tibial osteotomy converting the alignment to valgus will alter the balance of forces across the joint with more weight being transferred to the lateral compartment, which is usually well preserved. This operation is still used particularly in younger male patients with medial compartment osteoarthritis of the knee. Total knee replacement

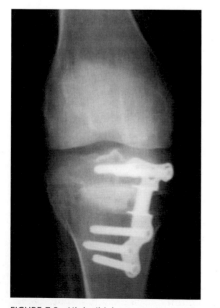

FIGURE 7.2 High tibial osteotomy to offload the medial compartment of the knee in a young patient with osteoarthritis

should be avoided in these patients if possible, particularly if they have a manual occupation. High tibial osteotomy provides good relief of pain for 7–10 years in 70% of patients and can usefully defer the requirement for a knee replacement until the patient is of a more suitable age.

Osteotomies were also commonly used around the hip, but are now seldom performed due to the success of total hip replacement. However, there is still a role for acetabular osteotomy in patients with acetabular dysplasia who present in early adult life with hip pain.

Another main indication for osteotomy is to correct acquired or congenital deformity of bone. Acquired deformities are most commonly the result of fractures and their complications. The development of a symptomatic malunion may need consideration of a corrective osteotomy to restore normal alignment and prevent the development of late osteoarthritis.

ARTHROPLASTY

Arthroplasty is replacement of a joint. There are three possibilities:

1. Total arthroplasty
2. Hemiarthroplasty
3. Excision arthroplasty.

TOTAL JOINT REPLACEMENT

Total arthroplasty implies that both articulating surfaces of the joint are replaced. The most common examples in clinical practice are total hip (Fig. 7.3) and knee replacement for osteoarthritis. Most modern joint designs comprise a metal replacement on one side and high-density polyethylene on the other side. In the case of the hip a common combination is a high-density polyethylene socket, and a metal femoral head and stem. However, other materials such as ceramic are now commonly used.

Successful replacement joints are now available for the shoulder, elbow, hip and knee. Replacements for the wrist and ankle have proved less successful. Specific complications of joint replacement include:

- infection
- dislocation
- stiffness
- loosening.

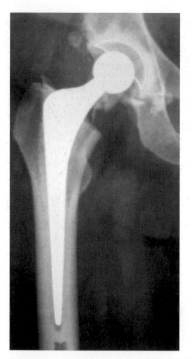

FIGURE 7.3 Total hip arthroplasty with femoral head and acetabular replacement

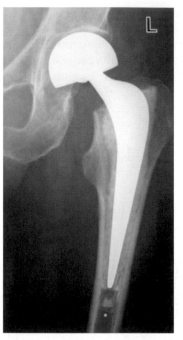

FIGURE 7.4 Hemiarthroplasty of the hip carried out for a subcapital fracture. Only the femoral head has been replaced

General complications include deep vein thrombosis, pulmonary embolus, myocardial infarction and stroke, although these usually occur in more elderly patients.

Infection is the most troublesome early complication. Although it is uncommon (usually no more than 1%) it often entails further surgery to remove the implant in order to control infection with later reimplantation. Loosening is the most common mode of failure in the longer term. The risk of this complication varies with the implant used, the indication for surgery and the age of the patient at the time of surgery. In the case of knee and hip replacements used for osteoarthritis in patients over 60 years, the incidence of loosening is low and 80–90% survivorship can be expected at 15 years after surgery.

However, less satisfactory results can be expected in younger more active patients, when loosening rates may be higher. Orthopaedic surgeons, therefore, prefer to avoid joint replacement in patients under the age of 60 years. However, there is no specific age limit and some patients with severe symptomatic arthritis may require joint replacement at a much younger age if there is no other surgical alternative.

HEMIARTHROPLASTY

This refers to a form of joint replacement in which only one side of the joint is resurfaced. This is commonly used following trauma in which one side of the joint is damaged but the other surface is involved. Examples include displaced subcapital hip fractures (Fig. 7.4), complex proximal humeral fractures and comminuted radial head fractures. All of these injuries can be treated with a hemiarthroplasty that replaces the articular surface involved by the fracture, but the other side of the joint is not replaced and articulates with the artificial component. The complications of hemiarthroplasty are the same as those associated with a total joint replacement.

EXCISION ARTHROPLASTY

In certain situations, a synovial joint is excised, but no implant is used to replace the joint surfaces. This is termed an excision arthroplasty. This treatment option was used in the past more frequently. In modern orthopaedic practice it is usually employed only as a last resort or as an interim treatment. It can be part of the treatment protocol of an infected total joint replacement. This may entail excision of the infected artificial joint, leaving the patient with an excision arthroplasty until clinical and haematological markers of infection return to normal, at which stage a revision joint replacement is undertaken. It can be utilized as a final option, for example where the functional expectation is low, such as to treat an arthritic 1st metatarsophalangeal (MTP) joint (Keller's hemiarthroplasty).

ARTHRODESIS

This term describes any operation to fuse a joint. Fusion of joints for arthritis is most often used for small joints in the hand or foot. It is generally avoided for major upper and lower limb joints, since there is considerable disability associated with fusion of these. A notable exception is the ankle joint (Fig. 7.5). Joint replacement of the ankle is not particularly successful. Fusion of the ankle is carried out for post-traumatic arthritis as this provides good relief of pain and functional disabil-

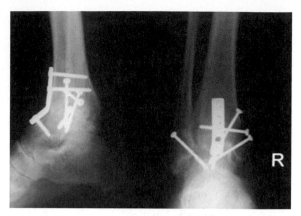

FIGURE 7.5   Fusion of the ankle joint for osteoarthritis in a 60-year-old man. The functional outcome and relief of pain were excellent

ity is not severe. This also applies to the wrist joint. Fusion of the shoulder, elbow, hip or knee is best avoided since these fusions are associated with major functional impairment and are not well tolerated by patients.

TRAUMA

8

PRINCIPLES OF FRACTURE MANAGEMENT

John Keating

Cases relevant to this chapter

35, 37, 38, 40–43, 45–48, 50, 51, 53, 54, 57–65, 67

●Essential facts

1. A fracture is any loss in the continuity of bone, most frequently due to trauma.

2. Most displaced fractures must be reduced and stabilized, followed by rehabilitation to restore function.

3. Many fractures are suitable for non-operative reduction (under anaesthesia).

4. External fixation is minimally invasive, but can be complicated by infection and malunion.

5. Lower-limb diaphyseal fractures are best managed using internal fixation with an intramedullary nail.

6. Upper-limb diaphyseal fractures in adults are usually treated by plating if surgery is required.

7. Periarticular fractures or intra-articular fractures that result in joint incongruity or malalignment are best treated with internal fixation.

8. Most paediatric fractures are amenable to non-operative treatment.

9. Fractures involving the growth plate are common in children and require accurate reduction and occasionally internal fixation.

10. Dislocations may be associated with neurovascular injury and require urgent reduction.

FRACTURE DEFINITION

A fracture is any loss in the continuity of bone and is most frequently the result of trauma. The term fracture encompasses all bony injuries from simple undisplaced cracks in bone, to major complex long-bone fractures with extensive soft-tissue injuries. Some additional terms in common use help describe the fracture. An open (compound) fracture is one in which there is a wound in communication with the fracture site. A comminuted fracture is one in which there are more than two main fragments. Inspection of radiographs allows description of the deformity. Angulation describes the relation of the long axis of the proximal and distal segments of bone. Displacement refers to the degree of separation between the bone ends (Fig. 8.1). Rotation is best judged on clinical examination and refers to the degree of rotational malalignment at the fracture site. Angulation, displacement and rotation are described in relation to the major proximal fragment (even if this is quite short).

PRINCIPLES OF TREATMENT

Despite the wide spectrum of injury, there are some basic principles of treatment underlying

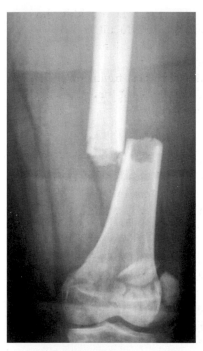

FIGURE 8.1 Completely displaced femoral diaphyseal fracture. Note associated patellar fracture

management that can be applied to most fractures. The fundamental aims are:

- Reduce the fracture under anaesthesia (if displaced)
- Maintain the reduction until the fracture heals
- Optimize the long-term functional outcome.

Reduction is usually desirable in displaced or angulated fractures, but is not always required (e.g. most clavicular fractures heal uneventfully with a satisfactory outcome despite some displacement). The fracture can be reduced by closed methods (e.g. manipulation or traction) or by direct surgical exposure – open reduction. Once the fracture is reduced, the surgeon then has to choose some method of treatment to maintain the reduction until union occurs. Non-operative or operative methods can be chosen. Each method has advantages and disadvantages, and several options can be considered in most situations. The decision is influenced by location and morphology of the fracture, the presence of associated injuries and the experience of the surgeon.

Fracture union is mainly dependent on the blood supply of the bone at the site of the injury. This is related to the intrinsic quality of the bone blood supply in a given location and the energy of the injury. In general, cancellous bone has a better blood supply than cortical bone and heals more rapidly and reliably. The nature of the injury also has a major influence. Higher-energy injuries do more damage to the blood supply and are, therefore, associated with more prolonged healing times.

NON-OPERATIVE TREATMENT

Fractures can be treated non-operatively by a variety of methods. The advantages of non-operative methods include the following:

- Non-invasive – no surgery required
- Cheap – no modern theatre facility and implants needed

The disadvantages include:

- Reduction not always precise
- Stability is often inadequate for major injuries
- Malunion rates are higher in adults
- More outpatient visits and radiographs are required to monitor treatment.

RELATIVE INDICATIONS FOR NON-OPERATIVE TREATMENT

- Low-energy undisplaced injuries
- Fractures in cancellous bone
- Phalangeal/metacarpal/metatarsal fractures
- Fractures that do not require anatomical reduction (e.g. clavicle, many humeral fractures)
- Some children's fractures.

TYPES OF NON-OPERATIVE TREATMENT

1. Bed rest: some fractures can be treated with rest and analgesia alone, e.g. isolated pubic ramus fractures.
2. Cast treatment: reduction and cast application is suitable for many common injuries in adults and children, particularly distal radial fractures.
3. Splints: there is a variety of modern splints available that can be introduced at the outset or during the course of treatment to assist in immobilizing the fracture.

4. Traction: this method of treatment confines the patient to bed, sometimes for long periods, and is seldom used now in adults.

OPERATIVE TREATMENT METHODS

EXTERNAL FIXATION

External fixation devices are attached to bone by pins or wires and consist of an external frame (Fig. 8.2). Devices vary in design from simple uniaxial frames to complex circular frames for more difficult problems. The main advantages are minimally invasive surgery and versatility of application. Disadvantages are problems with pin-track infection, poor patient acceptance and a higher rate of malunion. These devices are particularly suitable for use in situations where application of internal fixation would be difficult or risky. Examples include distal metaphyseal fractures, bone where there has been previous osteomyelitis, multiple fractures or extensive skin damage and swelling following high-energy trauma. External fixation may be used temporarily in these situations until internal fixation is deemed safe.

Indications for external fixation

- Closed fractures with extensive soft-tissue trauma
- Some open fractures

- Juxta-articular fractures where nailing and plating are technically difficult
- Temporary stabilization of long-bone fractures in multiple trauma
- Leg lengthening after post-traumatic shortening
- Correction of complex post-traumatic angular/rotational deformity.

INTERNAL FIXATION

Internal fixation devices fall into two main categories: intramedullary devices and plates. Other variations are used, such as screws or wiring techniques. Intramedullary nails are widely used in the treatment of lower-limb long-bone fractures in adults. They can be inserted with minimally invasive surgery and are excellent for restoring normal length, alignment and rotation. They are biomechanically very strong and are ideal for lower-limb diaphyseal fractures, where union times may be prolonged (Fig. 8.3). They are associated with a reliably high rate of union and very low rates of malunion. Other complications, such as infection, are also very low. They cannot be so easily applied to the bones in the upper limb. The narrow medullary canals in forearm bones make nailing difficult

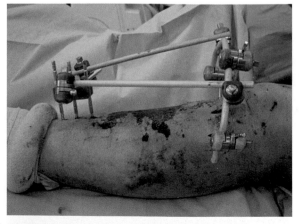

FIGURE 8.2 External fixator applied to proximal tibial shaft fracture. Note extensive skin swelling and soft-tissue contusions that would have been associated with a high risk of soft-tissue complications if internal fixation had been chosen

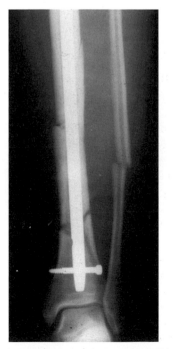

FIGURE 8.3 Complex segmental tibial shaft fracture fixed with interlocking intramedullary nail

to apply in the radius and ulna. The humerus can be more readily nailed, but the entry points at the elbow and shoulder are associated with complications. In children, flexible intramedullary nails can be used to stabilize long-bone fractures and the radius and ulna. Nails should not cross an open physis in a child.

Plating is most commonly used for metaphyseal fractures, displaced intra-articular fractures and diaphyseal fractures in the upper limb in the adult (Fig. 8.4). The main advantage is that a very precise reduction can be achieved, which is important when anatomical reduction is closely related to functional outcome (e.g. displaced intra-articular fractures). It is a more invasive technique and the complication rate associated with plating of diaphyseal fractures in the lower limb is higher than with intramedullary nailing.

Internal fixation is the treatment of choice for displaced unstable fractures where a poor reduction would compromise healing or functional outcome. It is often used in higher-energy open fractures and fractures with associated nerve or vascular injury to produce a stable wound environment.

Isolated screws are used in epiphyseal injuries (Salter–Harris types III and IV; see Chapter 12) to maintain continuity of the reduced articular surface and to stabilize a slipped upper femoral epiphysis

(see Chapter 26). Percutaneous pinning of unstable fractures that have been reduced by manipulation is a useful and widely used technique in children and is effective when combined with the application of a plaster cast. Examples include percutaneous pinning of a supracondylar humeral fracture and a bayoneted distal radial fracture.

Indications for internal fixation

- Displaced intra-articular fractures – plates, wiring techniques
- Periarticular fractures – plates
- Lower-limb long-bone fractures – intramedullary nails
- Fractures with vascular or nerve injury
- Salter–Harris III and IV physeal fractures in children.

DISLOCATIONS

A dislocation of a joint refers to complete loss of joint congruity (Fig. 8.5). A subluxation indicates a partial loss of joint congruity. Traumatic dislocations of the small joints of the hand, particularly interphalangeal joints, are common sports injuries. Dislocations of large joints are less frequent. Shoulder (glenohumeral) dislocation is the most common large joint dislocation in clinical practice. Dislocations may be associated with neurovascular injury (e.g. hip dislocation is associated with sciatic nerve palsy in 10–15% of cases). Diagnosis of dislocation is based on the history, the presence of character-

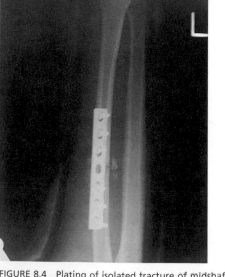

FIGURE 8.4 Plating of isolated fracture of midshaft radius forearm fracture

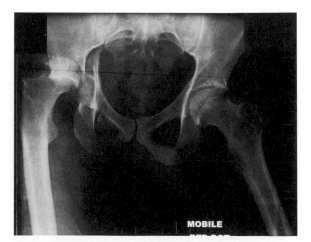

FIGURE 8.5 Traumatic posterior dislocation of right hip

istic deformity and radiographic confirmation. Most dislocations can be treated by a prompt closed reduction under sedation or local anaesthetic. Traumatic hip dislocations often require general anaesthesia to allow reduction. If a closed reduction cannot be achieved then a surgical open reduction is required.

ARTHROPLASTY

Joint replacement is not applicable to many fractures as the initial treatment. It is used, however, for displaced subcapital hip fractures in the elderly.

Since these are very common injuries, hip arthroplasty is a common operation in most trauma units. Joint replacement is also used in the elbow and shoulder, although these are less common indications.

FURTHER READING

Parker MJ, Gurusamy K 2006 Internal fixation versus arthroplasty for intracapsular proximal femoral fractures in adults. Cochrane Database Syst Rev 4: CD001708.

9

LOCAL COMPLICATIONS OF FRACTURES

John Keating

Cases relevant to this chapter

35–43, 45, 47, 48, 50, 51, 53, 54, 57–65, 67

●Essential facts

1. Trauma is the most common cause of compartment syndrome; muscle swells within a restrained fascial compartment and eventually occludes its blood supply, resulting in an infarction and a late ischaemic contracture (Volkmann's ischaemic contracture).

2. A clinical diagnosis of compartment syndrome is based on a high index of suspicion and the presence of increasing pain despite adequate analgesia and fracture immobilization.

3. Fractures and dislocations can be associated with nerve injury.

4. Dislocation of the hip or posterior wall acetabular fractures cause sciatic nerve injury in 15% of cases; most injuries are due to a traction neuropraxia, which will recover.

5. Vascular injuries are rare complications of fractures with the exception of high-energy open fractures.

6. Early infection typically occurs in open fractures; the risk is minimized by appropriate early management – wound excision and debridement, skeletal stabilization and early wound closure or coverage.

7. Non-union affects about 5% of fractures; it is more common in susceptible patients who sustain high-energy or open fractures with extensive damage to the bone blood supply.

8. Malunion is a relatively common after fracture, especially following non-operative treatment. Some degree of malunion is relatively well tolerated in some locations, such as the clavicle and humeral shaft.

9. Post-traumatic osteoarthritis is associated with displaced intra-articular fractures; the risk is proportional to the degree of residual joint incongruity.

10. Avascular necrosis is an occasional complication especially in displaced fractures, where the blood supply to one major fragment crosses the plane of the fracture and is disrupted. It is most commonly associated with talar neck, femoral neck and scaphoid fractures.

Complications after fracture may be considered to be local or general and subdivided into early or late. There is no accepted time for a complication to be considered 'early', but the term is usually applied to complications that occur during the acute phase of treatment.

EARLY

COMPARTMENT SYNDROME

Compartment syndrome occurs when muscle swells within a restrained fascial compartment and eventually occludes its blood supply, resulting in an infarction and a late ischaemic contracture (Volkmann's ischaemic contracture). Trauma is the most common cause, although the condition is often seen in patients with alcohol and drug abuse problems who lie for prolonged periods on a limb (Fig. 9.1). In clinical practice the condition occurs in the calf and forearm most frequently, although it can occur in the thigh and foot.

The pathophysiology is characterized by swelling of the muscle due to post-traumatic bleeding and oedema. As the compartment pressure rises, the muscles initially occlude the venous outflow, but not the arteriolar inflow, which hastens the development of the condition. Eventually the compartment pressure exceeds the arteriolar pressure and a muscle ischaemia results. The main arterial vessels running through the compartment have a higher pressure than the arterioles and are not occluded until very late in the sequence of events (if at all). Similarly, the nerves in relation to the compartment are less sensitive to ischaemia than the muscles.

The implication is that distal pulses and neurological function are normal until very late. The presence of reduced or absent pulses with or without neurological signs indicates the diagnosis has been made too late and there is a significant risk of irreversible ischaemic muscle necrosis.

Clinical diagnosis is based on a high index of suspicion, and the presence of increasing pain despite adequate analgesia and fracture immobili-zation. Young adults with tibial shaft fractures, forearm fractures or crush injuries to the foot are most at risk. Interestingly, the problem is seen less often in children who have equivalent fractures. The most useful physical sign is the presence of increased pain on passive flexion and extension of the fingers of toes of the affected limb. If there is any doubt then measurement of the compartment pressure is advisable. A pressure of less than 30 mmHg can be considered normal and a pressure of more than 40 mmHg is high, but the most useful guide is the pressure differential between the diastolic blood pressure and the compartment pressure. This should be above 30 mmHg to have adequate muscle perfusion. Compartment pressure monitoring is not routine practice after fractures in children.

The treatment of a compartment syndrome is a prompt fasciotomy of the muscle compartments involved. If there is any diagnostic doubt then fasciotomy is safer than procrastination, which may result in a disastrous outcome if the diagnosis is delayed.

NERVE INJURY

Certain fractures and dislocations are associated with nerve injury (Table 9.1). Anterior dislocation of the shoulder may result in an injury to the axillary nerve or even the brachial plexus. Diaphyseal

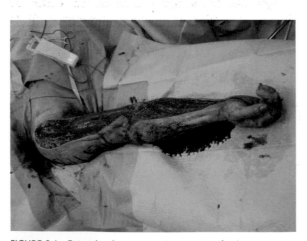

FIGURE 9.1 Extensive forearm and upper arm fasciotomy carried out in a patient with a history of drug abuse who lay unconscious on the arm for a period in excess of 24 h

Table 9.1 Fractures commonly associated with nerve injury

Fracture or dislocation	Associated nerve injury
Shoulder dislocation	Axillary nerve
Humeral shaft	Radial nerve
Supracondylar humeral fracture	Anterior interosseous or median nerve
Monteggia fracture dislocation	Posterior interosseous or radial nerve
Distal radial fracture	Median nerve
Posterior hip dislocation	Sciatic nerve
Knee dislocation	Common peroneal nerve

fractures of the humerus may be associated with radial nerve injury. Supracondylar fracture of the humerus in children is quite commonly associated with neuropraxia; the anterior interosseous nerve (see Chapter 1) is most commonly affected. Dislocation of the hip or posterior wall acetabular fractures cause sciatic nerve injury in 15% of cases. Although most nerve injuries are due to a traction neuropraxia, which will recover, documentation of the injury is important. A thorough evaluation of the neurological status of the limb is necessary. If the nerve injury is missed and surgery is subsequently undertaken, the nerve injury may be blamed on the operation. In general, the prognosis for some recovery is good, although it is often incomplete. Poor prognostic factors are more extensive nerve injuries, very dense palsies and older age groups.

Local pressure to the common peroneal nerve, particularly in thin individuals and after prolonged recumbency, is seen as a result of direct pressure on the nerve as it passes around the neck of the fibula (see Table 9.1).

VASCULAR INJURY

Vascular injuries are a well recognized but, fortunately, rare complication of fractures. They are most commonly associated with high-energy fractures, many of which are open. Some closed injuries, particularly complete knee dislocation and supracondylar fracture of the humerus in children, also carry the risk of this complication. The diagnosis is often obvious on clinical examination with the classic signs of acute ischaemia – pallor, pulselessness, paralysis, paraesthesia and a cold limb. The first step in management is a closed reduction of the fracture, which often improves circulation, particularly if the ischaemia is due to kinking or spasm of vessels. If there are signs of ischaemia then it must be assumed that there is arterial disruption until proven otherwise. Angiography is required to confirm the diagnosis, followed by surgery to revascularize the limb.

Plan of management for fracture with vascular injury

- Angiogram to confirm diagnosis
- Temporary vascular shunt to perfuse distal limb

- Skeletal stabilization – temporary external fixation often used
- Definitive vascular repair
- Staged definitive skeletal internal fixation if required.

INFECTION

Infection may occur as an early or late complication. Early infection is limited to open fractures. The risk is minimized by appropriate early management – wound excision and debridement, skeletal stabilization and early wound closure or coverage. Antibiotics are also given, but correct surgical management of the wound and fracture are the key to minimizing the risk of infection. If these principles are followed the incidence of infection will be low, even in open fractures. Infection following an open fracture or wound infection after internal fixation usually entails a further wound debridement and possible revision of soft-tissue cover. In general, some form of skeletal stabilization must be maintained, as infection is difficult to control in a wound with an unstable fracture.

LATE LOCAL COMPLICATIONS
NON-UNION

A non-union occurs when a fracture fails to heal. Delayed union is a less well defined term that implies that a fracture may unite, but is taking longer than the expected time for that particular injury. Non-union is uncommon, but overall affects about 5% of fractures. Most bones heal with a favourable biological and mechanical environment. Non-union may be affected by patient risk factors, the nature of the injury and the treatment selected. It is more common in high-energy or open fractures with extensive damage to the bone blood supply. It is very unusual in children. Some patient risk factors have also been shown to increase the risk of non-union.

Patient risk factors for delayed or non-union

- Smoking
- Alcohol abuse

- Increasing age
- Steroid use
- Diabetes mellitus
- Chronic renal failure.

Fracture risk factors for delayed or non-union

- High-energy fractures
- Open fractures
- Infection
- Bone loss.

The mode of treatment may also contribute to the development of a non-union. Treatment may be poorly selected for a particular fracture type or inexpertly carried out (Fig. 9.2). Surgery may increase the damage to the blood supply of the bone and, thus, increase the risk of non-union. Fixation failure or infection after internal fixation will also frequently result in non-union.

Non-union is often classified from radiographic appearances. Hypertrophic non-unions are those characterized by a hypertrophic appearance of the bone ends adjacent to the non-union. They are due to an unfavourable mechanical environment where there is excessive motion at the fracture site. Stabilization of the fracture results in union in most cases. Atrophic non-unions are typified by complete lack of radiographic evidence of any bone healing. This was considered to be due to poor blood supply, but is now thought to be a more general problem with healing, possibly due to lack of bone morphogenetic proteins to initiate the normal healing response. They require skeletal stabilization and stimulation of bone healing, most commonly by addition of autogenous bone graft.

MALUNION

Malunion is a relatively common problem after fracture. It is more common after non-operative treatment. In many locations, some degree of malunion is well tolerated. Fractures of the clavicle and humeral shaft heal reliably with non-operative treatment with some degree of malunion, but this seldom causes disability. Clavicular fractures remodel well and humeral malunion is compen-

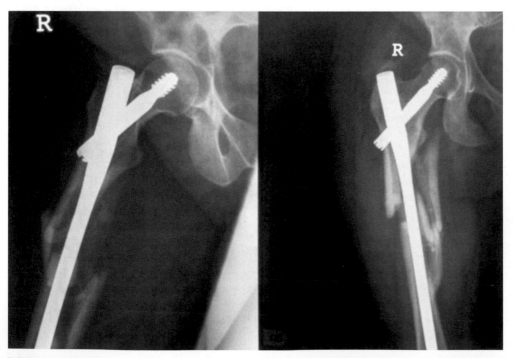

FIGURE 9.2 Complex proximal femur fracture treated with intramedullary nail. At 9 months after the injury, the fracture has failed to heal and there is shortening of the femur with malunion

sated for by the range of shoulder motion. In the lower limb, remodelling of femoral and tibial shaft fractures will occur if length and alignment are maintained. Angular and rotational malalignments will not remodel and are not well tolerated if in excess of 10°. For articular fractures, anatomical reductions are the goal in most cases. Incongruity at joint surfaces will result in a high risk of post-traumatic osteoarthritis. Favourable and unfavourable risk factors for remodelling in children are detailed in Chapter 12.

POST-TRAUMATIC OSTEOARTHRITIS

Post-traumatic osteoarthritis is associated with displaced intra-articular fractures. Most of these fractures are treated with reduction and internal fixation to minimize this risk. Occasionally a satisfactory reduction cannot be achieved due to extensive comminution. The risk of osteoarthritis developing is proportional to the degree of residual joint incongruity. Osteoarthritis may develop slowly over many years, but if there is sufficient damage to the joint surface the onset may be rapid (Fig. 9.3). In older patients the complication

is often treated by arthroplasty. In younger patients consideration may have to be given to arthrodesis.

AVASCULAR NECROSIS

Avascular necrosis is an occasional complication after fracture. It tends to occur in bones where the blood supply to one major fragment crosses the plane of the fracture and is disrupted, especially if the fracture is displaced. This complication affects displaced fractures of the femoral neck, scaphoid and talus in adults and after an intracapsular fracture of the neck of femur in a child. The blood supply of these bones enters at one location and crosses the fracture line. Significant displacement will almost invariably damage the blood supply and late avascular necrosis is, therefore, a risk after reduction. The clinical and radiological manifestations of avascular necrosis may develop slowly over 18–24 months, and the timing and duration of follow-up must take this into consideration.

COMPLEX REGIONAL PAIN SYNDROME

Complex regional pain syndrome is an occasional late local complication of an upper or lower limb fracture and is further described in Chapter 13.

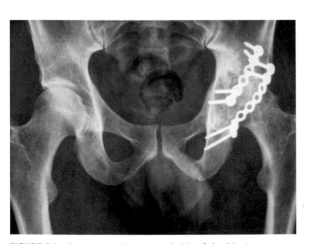

FIGURE 9.3 Post-traumatic osteoarthritis of the hip 4 years after fixation of complex acetabular fracture. Note almost complete loss of joint space on left side

FURTHER READING

Ashwood N, Challanor E 2003 Managing vascular impairment following orthopaedic injury. Hosp Med 64: 530–534.

LaStayo PC, Lee MJ 2006 The forearm complex: anatomy, biomechanics and clinical considerations. J Hand Ther 19: 137–144.

Marsh D 1998 Concepts of fracture union, delayed union, and non-union. Clin Orthop Relat Res 355(Suppl): S22–S30.

Olson SA, Rhorer AS 2005 Orthopaedic trauma for the general orthopaedist: avoiding problems and pitfalls in treatment. Clin Orthop Relat Res 433: 30–37.

GENERAL COMPLICATIONS OF FRACTURES

10

John Keating

Cases relevant to this chapter

50, 51, 54, 62, 64, 65

●Essential facts

1. Fat embolism is complication of long-bone fractures and results in symptoms similar to acute respiratory distress syndrome.

2. Lower-limb deep venous thrombosis (DVT) and pulmonary embolism (PE) occur in <1% of fractures; risk factors include older age, multiple trauma, lower limb trauma and concomitant head injury.

3. Low-molecular-weight heparin, unfractionated heparin and foot pumps prevent DVT in patients with fractures.

4. Immobility and recumbency associated with fractures increases the risk of respiratory and urinary infection.

5. Pressure sores occur after fractures, particularly in elderly immobile patients; the usual sites are the heel, the greater trochanter and the sacrum.

Complications after fracture may be considered to be local or general and subdivided into early or late. There is no accepted time for a complication to be considered 'early', but the term is usually applied to complications that occur during the acute phase of treatment.

FAT EMBOLISM

Fat embolism syndrome (FES) is a clinical syndrome that is an occasional complication of long-bone fractures. It is characterized principally by respiratory dysfunction, but is a generalized condition that is associated with organ dysfunction elsewhere. The respiratory picture is similar to acute respiratory distress syndrome (ARDS), but FES is a distinct condition, although the final physiological pathways mediating the two conditions are similar. FES has been a well recognized complication of fractures for over a century. The feature of fat embolism was noted in pathological specimens and it was assumed that marrow fat from fractured long bones was responsible for the condition. It is now known that this is not the sole explanation. There is a biochemical theory that supports the view that mediators and cellular debris released from the fracture site alter lipid solubility and contribute to the formation of micro-emboli that are also filtered out in the lung capillaries. Local complement activation occurs and an intense inflammatory response results in the lung parenchyma.

The net result of these processes is a decreased permeability of the alveolar membrane with poorer gas diffusion, resulting in hypoxia.

RISK FACTORS FOR DEVELOPMENT OF FES INCLUDE

- Lower-limb diaphyseal fractures, especially the femur
- Multiple fractures
- Closed fractures
- Young patients (<35 years).

If it occurs, FES usually develops within 72 h (and often sooner) in 90% of patients. Early recognition is the key to effective treatment. The characteristic clinical features are related to the underlying pathophysiology and include:

- Tachypnoea
- Dyspnoea
- Confusion/agitation
- Petechial rash (usually on the trunk, head and neck area)
- Tachycardia
- Other occasional features are fat in the urine (lipuria), retinal emboli on fundoscopy and fat in the sputum.

Investigation may demonstrate a low pO_2 and a low pCO_2, and thrombocytopenia. The pCO_2 is initially low due to the hyperventilation that is an early feature. More severe cases with progressive lung involvement eventually exhibit elevated pCO_2. The chest radiograph demonstrates diffuse bilateral infiltrates (Fig. 10.1). Deposition of emboli in the kidneys and liver may be associated with altered urea, electrolytes and liver enzymes.

Treatment of the condition is based on prevention and supportive measures in patients who develop the syndrome. The weight of evidence supports early fixation of long-bone fractures as an effective measure in reducing the incidence and severity of the condition. For lower-limb long-bone fractures the usual treatment method is intramedullary nailing. In multiple trauma patients who may not tolerate prolonged surgery, temporary external fixation followed by definitive fixation several days later is an option. FES is very unusual before skeletal maturity.

DEEP VENOUS THROMBOSIS AND PULMONARY EMBOLUS

Lower-limb deep venous thrombosis (DVT) and pulmonary embolism (PE) are occasional complica-

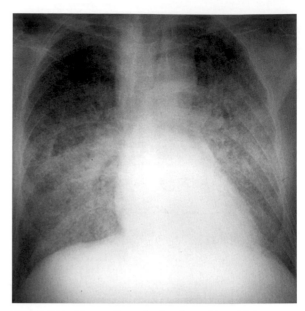

FIGURE 10.1 Chest radiograph of patient with multiple long-bone fractures with adult respiratory distress syndrome showing bilateral diffuse infiltrates throughout both lung fields

tions of fractures. The overall incidence of both complications in all fractures is low (<1%). However, the risk of DVT is considerably higher in patients with multiple trauma, lower-limb trauma, concomitant head injury and patients >40 years. Obesity, smoking and a previous history of DVT also increase the risk. In some studies of hip fractures, DVT rates have been between 20 and 50%. For this reason DVT prophylaxis is routinely used in patients with lower-limb trauma and any patient requiring inpatient hospital treatment. Randomized trials have confirmed the efficacy of low-molecular-weight heparin, unfractionated heparin and foot pumps for prevention of DVT. However, the studies have not conclusively proved that any of the methods currently used prevent PE. In multiple trauma patients there may be contraindications to the use of these methods due to coagulopathy, and in high-risk patients inferior vena cava filters may have to be used.

DVT and PE are very unusual after trauma in children

COMPLICATIONS OF IMMOBILITY

Most of the other general complications are associated with the enforced immobility and recumbency associated with fractures. Respiratory tract infec-

128

tion is a common occurrence in the early post-operative period in the elderly. Basal atelectasis contributes to development of this complication, which is also a higher risk in patients with pre-existing lung disease. Urinary-tract infection in the elderly is another consequence of immobility and poor bladder drainage. Use of catheters and pre-existing bladder drainage problems increase the risk.

Pressure sores are a significant risk after fractures, particularly in elderly patients. The incidence of this problem is related to the level of immobility, the fracture and the quality of nursing care. The usual sites are the heel, the greater trochanter and the sacrum. They are a source of considerable morbidity if they occur and are best prevented. Early identification of high-risk patients with institution of preventative methods is the pre-ferred strategy. Disuse osteoporosis and joint stiffness may occur in patients who have prolonged periods of immobility after fractures. These also occur in children. Patients who have deficient sensation, e.g. following spinal paraplegia, are particularly at risk.

FURTHER READING

Brogen J, Kelsberg G, Safranek S, Nadalo D, Janki P 2005 Clinical inquiries. Does anticoagulation prevent thrombosis for persons with fractures distal to the hip? J Fam Pract 54: 4376–4377.

Hedstrom M, Ljungqvist O, Cederholm T 2006 Metabolism and catabolism in hip fracture patients: nutritional and anabolic intervention – a review. Acta Orthop 77: 5741–5747.

Parisi DM, Koval K, Egol K 2002 Fat embolism syndrome. Am J Orthop 31: 9507–9512.

11

MANAGEMENT OF MULTIPLE TRAUMA

John Keating

Cases relevant to this chapter

54, 62

•Essential facts

1. Clinical evaluation, resuscitation, investigation and treatment have to be performed systematically in order to avoid errors leading to an adverse outcome for the patient.

2. The Advanced Trauma Life Support (ATLS) system guides clinicians in the early stages of management.

3. The history should focus on obtaining information about allergies, medications, past illnesses, pregnancy, the last meal consumed and the events and environment of the injury.

4. The primary survey identifies immediate life-threatening injuries; it includes maintaining the airway with cervical spine protection, establishing breathing with ventilation if required, restoring circulation and controlling haemorrhage, assessing disability and neurological status, determining exposure and controlling the environment around the injured patient.

5. The most useful radiographic investigations initially are: lateral cervical spine, chest X-ray, and a plain anteroposterior (AP) view of pelvis.

6. Haemorrhagic shock is common in multiple trauma; the key early signs are tachycardia and cutaneous vasoconstriction.

7. There are six causes of life-threatening respiratory compromise: upper airway obstruction, tension pneumothorax, open pneumothorax, flail chest, massive haemothorax and cardiac tamponade.

8. Abdominal distension, absent bowel sounds and guarding or rebound tenderness suggest an intra-abdominal injury; a rectal (and vaginal examination in females) should be performed, a gastric tube inserted and an urgent computed tomography (CT) scan should be requested.

9. For suspected head injury, a CT scan should be considered in all patients with a Glasgow Coma Scale score of less than 15, a loss of consciousness for more than 5 min or any patient with a focal neurological deficit; space-occupying lesions or a midline shift of greater than 5 mm are indications for craniotomy.

10. Early skeletal stabilization of major long-bone fractures reduces complications; for patients with severe extra-skeletal injuries or who are haemodynamically unstable, definitive internal fixation may not be feasible and temporary external fixation is necessary.

Patients with multiple injuries are a difficult challenge and require a multidisciplinary approach to evaluate and treat all injuries present. Clinical evaluation, resuscitation, investigation and treatment have to be carried out in a systematic fashion to avoid errors leading to an adverse outcome for the patient. The standard method of initial assessment and management is the Advanced Trauma Life Support (ATLS) system, which has been developed to guide clinicians in the early stages of management. The ATLS system recognizes that the usual model of a detailed history, followed by a systematic head-to-toe physical assessment is ideal for the multiply injured patient. The ATLS system is based on recognizing life-threatening conditions immediately, instituting treatment even if the exact diagnosis is not established, and limiting the history obtained in the acute setting to collecting facts relevant to the initial task of saving the patient's life. There are equivalent systems for the child, e.g. Paediatric Advanced Life Support (PALS) system.

HISTORY

The history obtained is defined by the mnemonic AMPLE:

- Allergies
- Medications
- Past illnesses/pregnancy
- Last meal
- Events/environment of injury.

This abbreviated history will collect the essential information needed about the patient in the acute situation.

INITIAL ASSESSMENT

The initial assessment after hospital admission is divided into the following phases:

1. Primary survey
2. Adjuncts to primary survey and resuscitation
3. Secondary survey (head-to-toe evaluation and history)
4. Adjuncts to the secondary survey
5. Continued post-resuscitation monitoring and re-evaluation
6. Definitive care.

PRIMARY SURVEY

The primary survey is aimed at detecting and simultaneously treating injuries that pose an immediate threat to survival. The sequence is identified by the mnemonic **ABCDE**:

Airway maintenance with cervical spine protection
Breathing and ventilation
Circulation with haemorrhage control
Disability: neurological status
Exposure/Environmental control – undress the patient but prevent hypothermia.

The *patency of the airway* must be established and intubation may be required. It has to be assumed that the *cervical spine* may be injured and it should be immobilized in a collar. Excess motion of the cervical spine must be avoided until injury has been excluded by radiography or other imaging. Once the airway is secure the chest must be examined particularly to detect a tension pneumothorax, flail chest or an open pneumothorax, which may compromise *ventilation*. The major cause of early death after multiple injury is *haemorrhage*. Disability refers in this situation to the *neurological status*, which may be impaired due to the presence of a head injury. The Glasgow Coma Scale is the simplest way of documenting this. The patient needs to be fully *exposed* to allow a thorough examination – this entails removal of clothing. Once this is done the patient's *environment* needs to be controlled by warm blankets and warm intravenous fluids to prevent hypothermia.

The most useful radiographic investigations initially are:

- Lateral cervical spine
- Chest X-ray
- Plain AP view of pelvis.

The CT scan is the most accurate investigation to detect head, chest and abdominal injury. It should ideally be obtained in all multiply injured patients, but occasionally patients with haemorrhagic shock may not be stabilized adequately until definitive control of the blood loss is achieved.

SHOCK

Haemorrhagic shock is the most common cause of shock in a multiple trauma patient, but other causes need to be considered.

- Cardiogenic shock
- Tension pneumothorax
- Neurogenic shock
- Septic shock.

The key early signs of haemorrhagic shock are tachycardia and cutaneous vasoconstriction. In healthy young adults hypotension occurs later and signifies a blood loss in excess of 1500–2000 ml. Patients who feel cool and are tachycardic should be assumed to be in shock until proven otherwise. The treatment of shock is aimed at control of the source of blood loss and rapid volume replacement. Two large-bore intravenous cannulas are inserted, usually into the antecubital fossa and warmed isotonic electrolyte solutions are given. The initial fluid bolus is 1–2 litres for an adult and 20 ml/kg for a child. This is followed by blood transfusion. Fully cross-matched blood is preferable, but in an urgent situation type specific (ABO- and Rh-matched blood) can be used. In life-threatening hypotension type O packed cells can be used. The return of blood pressure and pulse to normal is an encouraging sign. Restoration of urinary output to 0.5 ml/kg/h suggests that adequate renal perfusion has been restored.

THORACIC TRAUMA

The importance of establishing an airway and dealing with any upper airway obstruction has been mentioned. Causes or contributing factors to upper airway obstruction include aspiration, laryngeal injury, mandibular injury, penetrating tracheal injury and posterior sternoclavicular injury. More commonly hypoxia, hypercarbia and acidosis are due to thoracic trauma. Examination of the chest and the chest radiograph will identify most causes. There are six causes of life-threatening respiratory compromise that must be sought in the primary survey:

1. Upper airway obstruction
2. Tension pneumothorax
3. Open pneumothorax
4. Flail chest
5. Massive haemothorax
6. Cardiac tamponade.

ABDOMINAL TRAUMA

Abdominal trauma is not unusual in multiple injury and clinical examination alone rarely suggests the specific diagnosis. Abdominal distension, absent bowel sounds and guarding or rebound tenderness suggest an intra-abdominal injury. A rectal (and vaginal examination in females) should be performed. A gastric tube should be inserted. CT scanning is the most accurate investigation. Diagnostic peritoneal lavage (DPL) is sensitive but nonspecific. Abdominal ultrasound is more sensitive but is dependent on the skill of the user. Laparotomy is indicated for:

1. Blunt abdominal trauma with hypotension and evidence of intraperitoneal blood loss
2. Blunt abdominal trauma with blood-stained lavage, or a positive abdominal ultrasound or CT scan
3. Hypotension with penetrating intra-abdominal wound
4. Evisceration
5. Peritonitis
6. Free intra-abdominal air.

HEAD INJURY

Head injuries can be classified using the Glasgow Coma Scale:

Mild GCS score 14–15
Moderate GCS score 9–13
Severe GCS score 3–8.

The most useful additional investigation is the CT scan. This should be considered in all patients with a GCS score of less than 15, a loss of consciousness of more than 5 min or any patient with a focal neurological deficit. Space-occupying lesions or a midline shift of greater than 5 mm are indications for craniotomy.

MUSCULOSKELETAL INJURIES IN MULTIPLE TRAUMA

Most patients with multiple trauma have fractures. The present evidence strongly supports a policy of early skeletal stabilization of all major long-bone fractures. This has a number of benefits:

- Reduction in severity and incidence of pulmonary problems (acute respiratory distress syndrome and fat embolism syndrome)

- Reduction in blood loss
- Reduction in pain
- Earlier mobilization – reduced risk of deep vein thrombosis, pulmonary embolus and other complications associated with immobility.

In patients with severe extra-skeletal injuries and who are haemodynamically unstable, definitive internal fixation may not be feasible and temporary external fixation may have a role to play (Figs 11.1 & 11.2). Minor fractures or relatively stable metaphyseal or articular fractures can be splinted during the acute phase and undergo later reconstruction when the patient is stabilized. These more severely traumatized patients have a higher incidence of neurovascular injuries and compartment syndrome associated with the fractures sustained, and these complications should be carefully sought during the secondary survey.

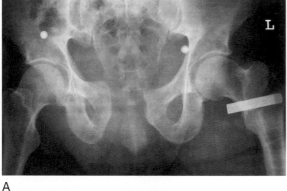

A

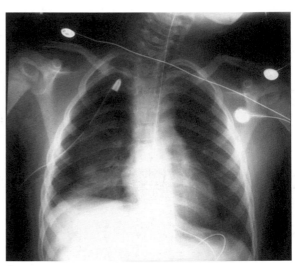

C

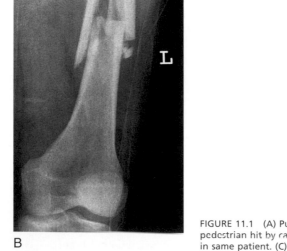

B

FIGURE 11.1 (A) Pubic symphysis disruption and left intertrochanteric hip fracture in pedestrian hit by car. (B) Left femoral shaft fracture below left intertrochanteric fracture in same patient. (C) The patient also had a pneumothorax treated with a chest drain

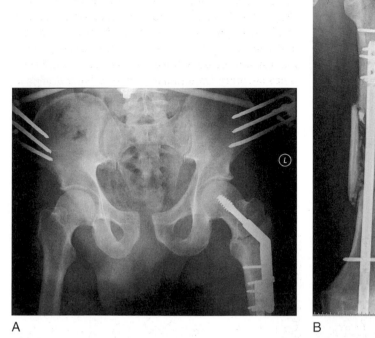

A   B

FIGURE 11.2   (A) Postoperative radiograph showing external fixation of pelvis and internal fixation of the intertrochanteric hip fracture. (B) The femoral fracture was fixed with a retrograde intramedullary nail

FURTHER READING

Bose D, Tejwani NC 2006 Evolving trends in the care of polytrauma patients. Injury 37: 20–28.

Harris MB, Sethi RK 2006 The initial assessment and management of the multiple-trauma patient with an associated spine injury. Spine 31(Suppl): S9–S15.

Renaldo N, Egol K 2006 Damage-control orthopedics: evolution and practical applications. Am J Orthop 35: 285–291.

CHILDREN'S FRACTURES 12

James Robb and Jacqueline Mok

Cases relevant to this chapter

39, 43, 44, 46, 52, 65

●Essential facts

1. Children's bones have a lower modulus of elasticity than adult bones and are more susceptible to bending forces.

2. Children's fractures are more likely to occur in the metaphysis, where there is less cortex than medulla, than in the diaphysis, which has an equal amount of cortex and medulla.

3. Fracture patterns in children are as follows: plastic deformation, buckle or torus fracture, greenstick fracture, complete fracture and physeal (growth plate) injury.

4. Fracture healing is the same as that for adults except that it is more rapid.

5. Children's fractures have the capacity to remodel and so some residual angulation or translation after reduction may be acceptable.

6. Physical abuse is the most common category of non-accidental injury and is characterized by bruises, lacerations, thermal injuries and fractures.

7. The prevalence of non-accidental fractures is between 11% and 55% of physically abused children.

8. The following features suggest non-accidental injury: a vague history; inconsistency with clinical findings or child's developmental stage; unexplained delays in seeking help; evasive or aggressive parents or carers; the presence of other injuries; and previous concerns regarding the child or sibling(s).

STRUCTURE OF A CHILD'S BONE

Children's bones have a lower modulus of elasticity than adult bones and thus are more susceptible to bending forces. Their bone is more porous and less dense than adult bone, but the periosteum is much thicker.

A cross-section of the diaphysis and metaphysis of a child's long bone will show that the diaphysis is approximately circular in cross-section and there is also approximately an equal amount of cortex and medulla. On the other hand the metaphyseal region is generally oval in cross-section and there

is relatively less cortex with respect to the medulla. Figure 12.1 illustrates this using the femur as an example. If forces are applied to the bone it is more likely to fail in the metaphyseal region and this accounts for the large number of metaphyseal injuries of long bones seen after low-velocity trauma in children. A greater amount of energy is required to fracture the diaphysis (Fig. 12.2).

TYPES OF FRACTURE

There are five distinct fracture patterns in children (Box 12.1). The first four will be considered here and physeal injuries in the section on growth plate

138

injuries. The fracture patterns result from the direction and amount of energy that has been applied to the bone (see Fig. 12.2). Initially the bone will bend, plastic deformation occurs as a result of micro-fractures of the cortex and the bone will not return to its original shape. This pattern is not usually seen in adults. It is seen most often in the forearm and leg where plastic bowing of the ulna or fibula may accompany a radial or tibial fracture. With an increasing amount of energy the bone will start to fail and buckle. Eventually the bone will fail on the tension side whilst the compression side will continue to bend thus producing the characteristic greenstick fracture (Fig. 12.3). More energy applied to the bone will cause a complete fracture of the compression side.

An axial or longitudinal force applied to a long bone in a child may produce buckling of the metaphysis. This type of fracture is also known as a torus fracture (Fig. 12.4). Torus is the name given to the band around the base of a Grecian column and in geometry represents the shape of a doughnut.

In a complete fracture three anatomical patterns are recognized (Box 12.2). These may also be comminuted (those containing more fragments of bone other than the proximal and distal components) or segmental (the same bone has been broken at two distinct sites).

Spiral fractures are produced as a result of rotational forces being applied to the bone; they are usually low-velocity injuries and may arise where one part of a limb is fixed relative to another. Oblique fractures are unstable and arise as a result of an increasing amount of force being applied to the bone. Transverse fractures tend to occur as a result of three-point bending. Comminuted and segmental fractures are a feature of high-velocity trauma (Fig. 12.5).

PHYSEAL (GROWTH PLATE) INJURIES

Children are unique in having growth plates, and the growth plate is thought to be an area of relative mechanical weakness when compared to the bone of the metaphysis and epiphysis. Physes are more susceptible to injury from rotational forces rather than angulation or traction. The commonly used classification of physeal injuries by Salter and Harris is illustrated in Figure 12.6. The type I injury is a fracture through the physis without involving the bone of the metaphysis or epiphysis. The type II injury is the commonest and carries the best prognosis. Here the fracture propagates through the

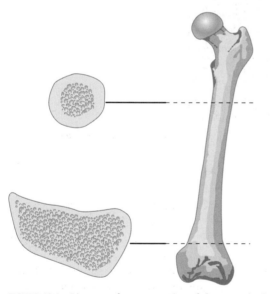

FIGURE 12.1   Diagram of a cross-section of the metaphysis and diaphysis of a child's femur

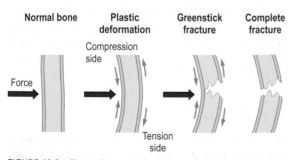

FIGURE 12.2   Shows how plastic deformation, greenstick and complete fractures occur

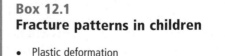

Box 12.1
Fracture patterns in children

- Plastic deformation
- Buckle or torus fracture
- Greenstick fracture
- Complete fracture
- Physeal injury

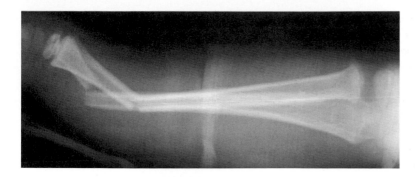

FIGURE 12.3 Greenstick fracture of the radius (there is one intact cortex) and complete fracture of the ulna

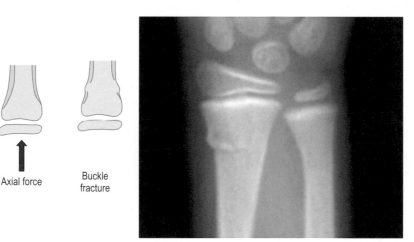

Axial force

Buckle fracture

FIGURE 12.4 Shows that an axial force can produce a buckle or torus fracture of the metaphysis. The radius is buckled on the lateral side

Box 12.2
Patterns of complete fractures

- Spiral
- Oblique
- Transverse

physis and includes a triangular portion of the metaphysis (always on the compression side of the fracture where periosteum is intact). The type III fracture passes through part of the physis and then across the epiphysis, whereas the type IV passes across the epiphysis, physis and metaphysis. Both type III and IV injuries involve the articular surface of the joint as well as the physeal plate and should be reduced anatomically, which often entails open reduction and internal fixation. The type III and IV injuries generally carry a worse prognosis because of the likelihood of physeal growth arrest from the disruption to the physis and the risk of post-traumatic arthritis of the joint if the articular surface is not reduced accurately. A growth arrest may cause an angular deformity because the uninjured part of the physeal plate continues to grow whilst the arrested side does not (Fig. 12.7). Type V is a compression injury to the physis and like type I does not involve the bone of the metaphysis or epiphysis. The injury may only be diagnosed in retrospect if a partial growth arrest of the plate becomes evident later.

PERIOSTEUM

This is much thicker in children than in adults. Part of the periosteum will be torn in a fracture, but the intact part can be used to ensure fracture stabil-

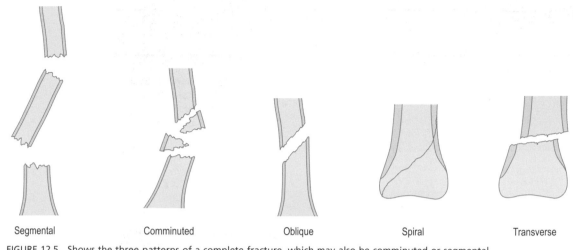

Segmental   Comminuted   Oblique   Spiral   Transverse

FIGURE 12.5 Shows the three patterns of a complete fracture, which may also be comminuted or segmental

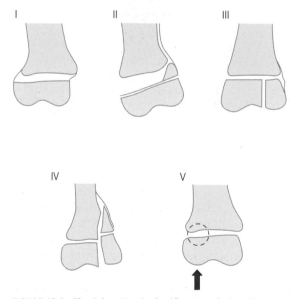

FIGURE 12.6 The Salter–Harris classification of physeal injuries

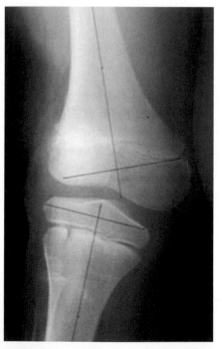

FIGURE 12.7 Growth arrest of the lateral side of the distal femoral epiphysis following an open Salter–Harris IV injury

ity after reduction. In Figures 12.8A and B there is a complete fracture of the distal end of the radius. The periosteum is intact posteriorly, whereas it has ruptured anteriorly. The diagram shows how the periosteum can be used as an intact tether on the dorsal side of the fracture to assist in reducing and maintaining the reduction.

Occasionally periosteum from the torn side may fold into the joint as illustrated in Figure 12.9. Here it is not possible to reduce the epiphyseal injury because the periosteum has folded into the fracture and this has to be retrieved from the fracture surgically.

FRACTURE HEALING

The mechanism is the same as that for adults (see Chapter 13) except that it occurs more rapidly. For

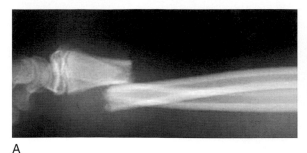

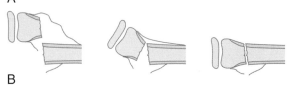

A

B

FIGURE 12.8 (A) Lateral X-ray of the forearm showing complete fractures of the radius and ulna. (B) Line drawing of the radial fracture showing that the periosteum is intact dorsally, but torn anteriorly due to dorsal displacement of the distal fragment. The middle and right-hand figures show how the periosteum can be used to help hinge the distal fragment back into position when it is reduced by manipulation

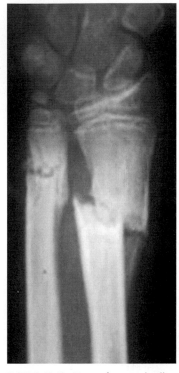

FIGURE 12.10 X-ray of external callus. There is radial translation of the distal radius in relation to the radial shaft. This fracture is stable; the alignment is acceptable in a child of this age and the fracture does not need surgical fixation

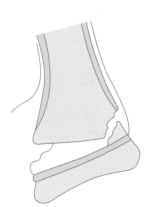

FIGURE 12.9 Shows incarcerated periosteum in a Salter–Harris II physeal fracture of the distal tibia

example, a femoral fracture in a 5-year-old will have united by about 5 weeks, yet for an adult may take 20 weeks. Fractures that have not been rigidly fixed heal by producing external callus (Fig. 12.10).

REMODELLING

Children's fractures have the capacity to remodel and so some residual angulation or translation after reduction (Fig. 12.11A) may become acceptable (Fig. 12.11B). Factors favourable and unfavourable for remodelling are shown in Table 12.1.

Bony remodelling in the plane of motion of the joint occurs at about 1° per month until the physis tends to lie at 90° to the axial forces on the limb. Physeal reorientation also occurs as a result of asymmetrical forces placed across the physis due to the residual angulation. Since malrotation does not remodel, it is essential that fractures, particularly of the forearm, femur and tibia, are correctly reduced. As a guideline, residual angulation of no more than 10° in the coronal and transverse planes is acceptable in the pre-adolescent child.

SUMMARY

- Some fracture patterns are unique to children.
- Healing of children's fractures is quicker than in adults, but will depend on the age of the child.

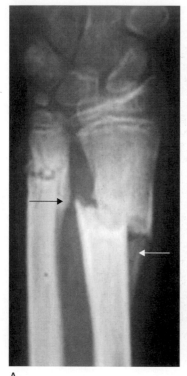

A

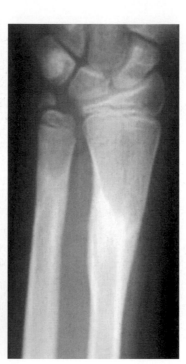

B

FIGURE 12.11 X-ray of remodelling of the same fracture as in Figure 12.10.
(A) Radiograph taken 6 weeks after the fracture; the arrow indicates callus.
(B) Radiograph taken 1 year later shows that the translation of the radial fracture is less noticeable

Table 12.1 Factors that have favourable and unfavourable effects on remodelling

Favourable	Unfavourable
Young child	Child approaching skeletal maturity
Fracture close to the physis	Fracture distant from the physis
Residual deformity in the plane of motion of the joint	Residual deformity out of the plane of motion of the joint
	Residual malrotation

- Physes are unique to children and the potential problems associated with physeal injury should be recognized and treated.
- Remodelling will occur in children's fractures, but factors influencing this should be recognized.

- Fractures affecting specific sites in children are discussed in Chapter 13.

NON-ACCIDENTAL INJURY

Physical abuse is the most common category of non-accidental injury, and the majority of children who have been physically abused present with bruises, lacerations, thermal injuries and fractures. The prevalence of non-accidental fractures is between 11% and 55% of physically abused children, depending on the age of the population studied. Distinguishing abusive from accidental fractures is crucial to the protection of children, but the evidence on which to base decisions is scanty. Eighty per cent of children with abusive fractures are <18 months old, whereas 85% of accidental fractures occur in children >5 years old. High-quality radiographs and interpretation by a skilled paediatric radiologist will increase the fracture detection rate. In one large study the distribution of affected sites were long-bone diaphyses (36%), ribs (26%), metaphyses (23%) and skull (15%). A

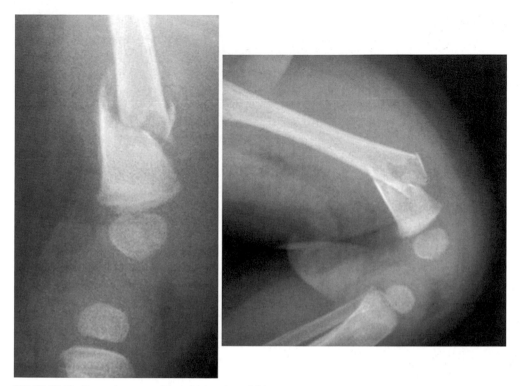

FIGURE 12.12 X-ray of a non-accidental injury in a child

recent systematic review of fractures in child abuse has shown that rib fractures in children without explicit explanation have the highest specificity of abuse. For other fractures, factors that should be taken into account are: the age and developmental stage of the child, the number of fractures present and the details of the reported mechanism of injury (Fig. 12.12).

Factors that should alert the clinician to suspect non-accidental injury are:

- History that is vague, inconsistent and discrepant with clinical findings or child's developmental stage.
- Significant delay between injury and seeking medical attention, without credible explanation.
- Evasive or aggressive responses from parent when details of injury are sought.
- Presence of other injuries.
- Previous concerns regarding child or sibling(s), e.g. lack of care; unusual injuries; repeated attendances at an accident & emergency department.

ASSESSMENT

The role of the doctor is to perform a comprehensive medical assessment, in the same systematic and rigorous manner as would be appropriate to the investigation and management of any other potentially fatal disease. Be aware of the referral pathways to senior colleagues with specialist skills to help you assess whether the child has been abused. Make sure your record keeping is contemporaneous, comprehensive and legible. Record negative as well as positive findings. Write down verbatim any statements from the child or parent.

A thorough medical history should be taken, as outlined in Table 12.2.

DIFFERENTIAL DIAGNOSIS

- Normal variant/physiological finding, e.g. periosteal new bone formation.
- Accidental injury.
- Birth injury, in a young infant. Most fractures sustained at birth heal within a few weeks. Check obstetric and neonatal records.

Table 12.2 Important aspects of history taking in children with suspected non-accidental injury

Pointer	Comment
Circumstances of injury	When the injury occurred; what happened; how did it occur; where did it occur; who witnessed the injury?
Growth and development	Recorded either in the parent-held Child Health record or from the health visitor. Examine weight chart for any evidence of failure to thrive
Birth history	Was the baby born pre-term? If so, check the neonatal records for details of gestation, delivery, any investigations and treatments given, e.g. intravenous nutrition, vitamin supplements, X-rays which might show rickets of prematurity
Child-care concerns	About the child or the sibling; from the health visitor or social worker
Past medical history	Of the child, sibling or parents; from the general practitioner

- Bone disease, e.g. osteogenesis imperfecta, osteopenia of prematurity, rickets, copper deficiency, osteomyelitis and metastatic lesions. Note that sometimes the autosomal dominant disorder hereditary multiple exostosis presents with rib exostosis, which can be misinterpreted as healed rib fractures.

INVESTIGATIONS

Blood must be taken to exclude metabolic bone disease (calcium, phosphate, alkaline phosphatase, copper and magnesium levels). Discuss with a radiologist about the necessity for further radiological investigations, e.g. special views and MRI scans. Where a non-accidental fracture is suspected in a child <2 years old, a full skeletal survey must be performed to exclude occult fractures (see Fig. 12.12). Repeat X-rays of doubtful areas should be obtained after 1–2 weeks, to identify callus (to assist with dating injury) and previously occult injuries.

INTER-AGENCY WORKING

When non-accidental injury is suspected, you must consider other explanations for the injuries, in addition to co-existing forms of abuse. The Child Protection Register should be checked by telephoning social services. Follow your local as well as national guidelines to ensure the safety of the child.

A multi-agency child protection enquiry should be commenced, by contacting the social services department who should in turn discuss the case with the police. Referrals should be followed up in writing within 24 hours. Social services have a statutory responsibility to make enquiries when concerns are expressed about a child, while police have a duty to investigate. A multi-agency meeting, attended by parents (case conference), is the forum where professionals decide, based on the available information, whether the child has suffered harm. If so, the child is placed on the Child Protection Register and a Child Protection Plan agreed to ensure the safety and wellbeing of the child.

FURTHER READING

Carty H, Pierce A 2002 Non-accidental injury: a retrospective analysis of a large cohort. Eur Radiol 12: 2919–2925.

Welsh Child Protection Systematic Review Group. A systematic review of fractures in child abuse. *www.core-info.cf.ac.uk/fractures/index.htm*

Worlock P, Stower M, Barbor P 1986 Patterns of fractures in accidental and non-accidental injury in children: a comparative study. BMJ 293: 100–102.

13

REGIONAL INJURIES

John Keating, Geoff Hooper and James Robb

Cases relevant to this chapter

35–49, 52–64, 66, 67, 73, 82, 95, 100

●Essential facts

1. Non-operative treatment is used for most clavicle, humeral, distal radial, metacarpal and phalangeal fractures.

2. Operative treatment is required for displaced fractures of the distal humeral fractures, olecranon or forearm fractures in adults and displaced intra-articular fractures of the distal radius and small hand joints.

3. Glenohumeral dislocation is the most common major joint dislocation and is associated with recurrence in younger patients and rotator cuff tears in older patients.

4. Displaced supracondylar humeral fractures in children are associated with a significant risk of vascular and neurological injury.

5. Distal radius fractures are very common; 30% are unstable in a cast.

6. Scaphoid fractures may not be obvious on initial radiographs and are associated with a risk of avascular necrosis.

7. Metacarpal and phalangeal hand fractures can be treated conservatively unless there is rotational or angular malalignment.

8. Most unstable pelvic fractures occur as a result of high-energy trauma and 70% are associated with other injuries.

9. Intracapsular hip fractures interfere with femoral head blood supply and are frequently complicated by non-union and avascular necrosis.

10. Extracapsular hip fractures heal with internal fixation.

11. The 1-year mortality rate after hip fracture is 30%.

12. Displaced intra-articular fractures of the knee usually require internal fixation.

13. Intramedullary nailing is the treatment of choice for most femoral and tibial diaphyseal fractures.

14. Compartment syndrome occurs in 2–5% of tibial shaft fractures.

15. Unstable ankle fractures should be treated by internal fixation.

16. Displaced intra-articular calcaneus fractures in young patients should be treated by internal fixation.

17. Talar neck fractures are associated with a high incidence of avascular necrosis.

18. Most metatarsal and foot phalangeal fractures can be treated non-operatively.

UPPER LIMB INJURIES

FRACTURES OF THE CLAVICLE AND SHOULDER GIRDLE

Clavicular fractures

These are common injuries in adults and children. The majority of cases follow a fall on the shoulder. Most fractures involve the middle third of the bone. Clinical diagnosis is not difficult in most cases – there is tenderness with visible and palpable deformity at the site of the fracture. A small percentage of these patients have high-energy trauma and in these cases there is an association with brachial plexus injuries and vascular injury. Clinical assessment should include an assessment of the neurovascular status of the upper limb.

Virtually all of these fractures can be diagnosed with plain radiographs. In the majority of cases, management is non-operative using a collar and cuff sling for 4–6 weeks, and analgesic medication. Patients should be advised to avoid overhead activity for the first 6 weeks and heavy manual work for 3 months. In adults radiographs should be obtained at 2 weeks, 6 weeks and 3 months to ensure the fracture progresses to union.

In children (Fig. 13.1), complications are unusual; very few require any additional treatment and the fracture heals rapidly. Full function can be expected but the child and parents will be aware of a swelling over the fracture for several months after healing. This is due to external callus formation, which usually remodels well.

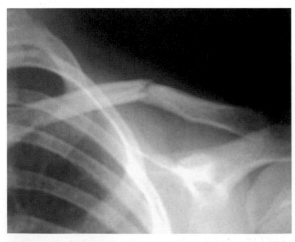

FIGURE 13.1 Angulated midshaft clavicular fracture in a child; this will heal uneventfully

Surgical treatment of clavicular fractures is occasionally indicated. Patients with a vascular injury or brachial plexus palsy will usually require plating of the clavicle. Non-union occurs in 10% of adult clavicular fractures and is more common in midshaft fractures with more than 1 cm of displacement or with comminution. Non-union of midshaft fractures can be successfully treated in most cases with plating. In lateral third fractures, delayed union or non-union is the norm if the coraco-clavicular ligaments are ruptured, which results in superior migration of the medial fragment. They can be treated non-operatively if asymptomatic. In patients with troublesome pain, internal fixation is indicated.

Scapular fractures

These are uncommon injuries but are associated with high-energy trauma. They have a well recognized association with rib fractures, clavicle fractures, brachial plexus injuries and intra-thoracic injury. The most important aspect of management is identification of the associated injuries. In general, most scapular fractures can be treated non-operatively in a sling for 4–6 weeks.

Although most scapular fractures can be treated non-operatively, fractures involving the glenoid fossa with significant displacement are best treated by internal fixation.

Shoulder injuries

Fractures and dislocations involving the proximal humerus and shoulder girdle are very common and affect all age groups. There are three common injuries: acromio-clavicular dislocation, glenohumeral dislocation and proximal humeral fractures.

Acromio-clavicular dislocations

These injuries result from a fall directly onto the shoulder. They are common in contact sports. The lateral aspect of the clavicle is attached to the scapula by strong coraco-clavicular ligaments. If these are disrupted, the weaker acromio-clavicular joint ligaments can be disrupted allowing superior displacement of the clavicle in relation to the acromion. There are three grades of injury:

- Grade I – The acromio-clavicular ligaments are damaged, but there is no superior displacement of the clavicle. Patients are tender on palpation of the joint, but there is no deformity.

- Grade II – The ligaments are damaged sufficiently to allow subluxation, but not complete dislocation of the joint.
- Grade III – There is complete dislocation with superior displacement of the joint. The coraco-clavicular and acromio-clavicular ligaments are torn. This injury is not usually seen in the younger child, but may be seen in adolescents.

Treatment of grade I and II injuries is non-operative with a sling for comfort until early mobilization is commenced 1–2 weeks after injury. Most grade III injuries can also be treated non-operatively. However, occasionally the clavicle is widely displaced and comes to lie in a subcutaneous position. These injuries are best treated surgically. The clavicle can be repositioned using a coraco-clavicular screw.

Glenohumeral dislocation

The glenohumeral joint is the most frequently dislocated major joint. The usual mechanism is a fall on the extended arm with the shoulder in extension. The humeral head dislocates in an anterior dislocation and comes to lie medial to the glenoid, just below the coracoid process. Posterior dislocation also occurs, but is uncommon, and accounts for less than 5% of shoulder dislocations. It is often associated with high-energy trauma, an epileptic fit or as a consequence of an electric shock. Glenohumeral dislocation is a very unusual injury in a child.

The diagnosis of anterior dislocation is obvious on clinical examination. There is swelling and deformity of the shoulder and the humeral head is palpable in the anterior subcoracoid position. Posterior dislocations are less obvious on physical and radiographic examination, but one key clinical feature is that the glenohumeral joint is fixed in internal rotation. If there is a history of unusual trauma, and the shoulder is in fixed internal rotation, it should be assumed there is a posterior dislocation. A plain anteroposterior (AP) radiograph shows anterior dislocations readily, but posterior dislocations are easily missed. Axillary or modified oblique views are better for diagnosis of posterior dislocation. Axillary nerve injury, brachial plexus palsy and rotator cuff tears are all well recognized complications of glenohumeral dislocation and should be looked for clinically.

Closed reduction of the dislocation under sedation is usually possible. Occasionally general anaesthesia is required and should always be used in a child. Posterior dislocations are often associated with an impaction fracture of the humeral head, which becomes locked on the edge of the glenoid, rendering closed reduction difficult. Open reduction is more frequently required. After closed reduction of a shoulder dislocation a period of 3–4 weeks of immobilization is recommended in younger patients to minimize the risk of recurrent dislocation. In patients over the age of 40 years this is less of a risk and early mobilization is encouraged.

In younger patients the main risk is recurrent dislocation and in those under 20 years of age the risk is 80%. In patients over the age of 40 years, rotator cuff tears and nerve injury are more frequent. Greater tuberosity fractures or rotator cuff tears are present in 10–30% of glenohumeral dislocations. They are more common in older patients. Nerve injuries (most commonly the axillary nerve) can be treated non-operatively as they recover spontaneously in 95% of cases. They are present in 30% of patients over the age of 50 with dislocation. Rotator cuff tears are easily missed since they are difficult to diagnose at presentation after reduction of the dislocation due to pain and limited motion. In patients who have not regained active abduction by 4–6 weeks after injury an urgent ultrasound or MRI scan is indicated to diagnose a rotator cuff tear and carry out surgical repair in suitable patients.

PROXIMAL HUMERAL FRACTURES

Fractures of the proximal humerus are most frequent in elderly female patients. Clinical examination reveals bruising and swelling of the shoulder. The bruising migrates down the arm in the first 10–14 days after injury and eventually may be more obvious at the elbow. Neurological injuries are present in 20–30% of older patients and tend to involve the axillary nerve or brachial plexus.

Most of these fractures are not markedly displaced and unite reliably with non-operative treatment in a sling in a few weeks. Wide displacement of the fragments or the presence of displaced tuberosity fragments warrants consideration of internal fixation or humeral head replacement (Fig. 13.2). Non-operative treatment is associated with a high rate of malunion and shoulder stiffness, but operative treatment in osteoporotic bone seldom produces superior functional results except in the most displaced fracture patterns.

In children the injury may involve the physeal plate (see section on physeal injuries) or the proximal metaphysis (Fig. 13.3). Most injuries can be treated non-operatively and, even if there is noticeable angulation at the fracture site, the proximal humerus has excellent potential for remodelling in the child.

HUMERAL SHAFT FRACTURES

Humeral shaft fractures occur as a result of direct or indirect trauma applied to the upper arm. Although they are often the result of high-energy trauma they are quite a frequent injury in elderly patients or alcohol abusers as a consequence of simple falls. The diagnosis is based on the history, physical examination and plain radiographs. The radial nerve has a close relationship to the humeral diaphysis and radial nerve palsy occurs in 12% of humeral fractures.

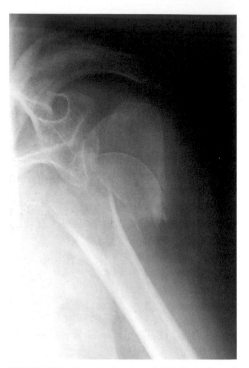

FIGURE 13.2　Complex fracture dislocation of proximal humerus

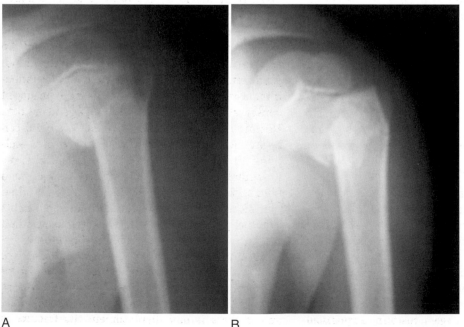

A　　　　　　　　　　B

FIGURE 13.3　(A) Anteroposterior and (B) lateral views of a fracture of the proximal humerus in a child; the angulation is acceptable and will remodel

The humerus has a good blood supply and the majority of these fractures will heal with non-operative treatment. Moderate degrees of malunion (angulation and/or rotation of up to 20° with shortening of up to 3 cm) can be accepted due to the range of motion of the shoulder, which allows compensation for the malunion. The usual treatment is immobilization in a plaster U-slab, which can be replaced after the first 2–4 weeks by a functional brace. Fractures usually unite between 8 and 12 weeks. The presence of a radial nerve palsy is not an indication for surgery since 95% of these can be expected to recover spontaneously. Humeral shaft fractures in children are managed in the same way as for the adult.

Not all humeral shaft fractures can be treated non-operatively. Indications for surgery include:

- Open fractures
- Fractures with a brachial plexus palsy
- Fractures associated with a vascular injury
- Bilateral humeral fractures
- Humeral fractures associated with an ipsilateral forearm fracture
- Multiple trauma patients
- Pathological humeral fractures
- Displaced transverse fractures – high risk of non-union with closed treatment.

If surgery is required, plating is the preferred fixation option for most fractures. Intramedullary nailing is possible, but has been associated with a high rate of non-union and other surgical complications. In children, rigid nails and any fixation device that crosses a physis are not used. Flexible intramedullary nails or plate fixation are appropriate.

FRACTURES AROUND THE ELBOW

Distal humeral fractures

Fractures involving the distal humerus are not common, but are difficult to treat in adults. They usually occur as a fall directly onto the elbow. They may be extra-articular, but more commonly the elbow joint surface is involved.

Non-operative treatment of these injuries is difficult, but an above-elbow cast is the usual method. Most injuries are treated by internal fixation. This treatment has the advantage of restoring anatomical reduction of the joint surface and is associated with the best long-term outcome. In older patients ana-tomical reconstruction may be difficult and use of total elbow arthroplasty is an alternative to internal fixation in this situation.

Complications of this injury include ulnar nerve injury, heterotopic ossification, post-traumatic arthritis and infection. However, the most common complication is stiffness. Stiffness may be associated with heterotopic ossification. It is usually treated by a soft-tissue release and excision of ectopic bone.

Fractures of the distal humerus and metaphysis in children are usually managed non-operatively.

Supracondylar fractures of the humerus are the commonest elbow injury in children aged 5–7 years and result from a fall onto the outstretched hand. The force is transmitted up the forearm and the humerus fails in the metaphysis, the area of least structural strength. Ninety-five per cent of supracondylar fractures are extension types and the remainder have a flexion pattern. The degree of displacement of the distal fragment may range from being undisplaced to some displacement, but with posterior cortical continuity or complete displacement (Fig. 13.4). Completely displaced fractures may be associated with loss of circulation to the forearm and hand as the brachial artery is trapped in the fracture site. Neurological damage may also occur as peripheral nerves at the elbow are contused or stretched by the injury and the anterior interosseous nerve is the most commonly affected (see Chapter 2). Loss of circulation to the hand is a surgical emergency and urgent reduction of the fracture under general anaesthesia is required. Displaced fractures are generally pinned after reduction. Neurological injury is usually managed conservatively and generally carries a good outlook. Healing of the fracture is rapid and the child can begin mobilizing the elbow after 3 weeks. Malunion of the fracture may occur and cubitus varus (a medial deviation of the forearm) may be seen (Fig. 13.5). This is a cosmetic deformity that does not affect function, but most children and parents eventually find the appearance unacceptable and it can be corrected by supracondylar osteotomy.

Fracture of the lateral condyle in children (Fig. 13.6) is the second commonest injury at the elbow in children aged 5–7 years. The injury passes through the elbow joint and across the growth plate and if there is any displacement the fracture is fixed to ensure anatomical reduction of the joint surface and growth plate. If a displaced lateral

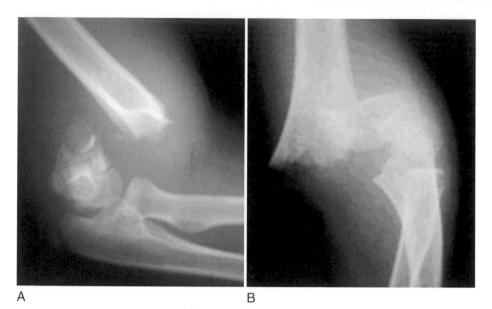

FIGURE 13.4 (A) Anteroposterior and (B) lateral view of supracondylar humeral fracture in a child. This is completely displaced and requires reduction and pinning

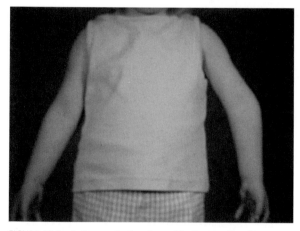

FIGURE 13.5 Anteroposterior view of both arms in a 6-year-old who had sustained a supracondylar humeral fracture 2 years earlier. There is a malunion and resulting cubitus varus

condyle is not fixed and a non-union ensues, there is a likelihood of the child developing a progressive lateral drift of the forearm and tardy ulnar nerve palsy as an adult.

Olecranon fractures

The olecranon process is commonly fractured in falls on the elbow. The triceps inserts onto the olecranon and this commonly results in distraction of the fracture. Non-operative treatment is, therefore, seldom feasible. Internal fixation using a tension-band wire system is the most common method of operative treatment (Fig. 13.7). Post-operatively a short period of immobilization is usual for 10–14 days after which cautious mobilization of the elbow out of a cast may begin. The main complication is failure of fixation with delayed or non-union of the fracture. In children the injury can be treated conservatively if the articular surface has not been disrupted or surgically if there is loss of continuity of the joint surface.

Radial head and neck injuries

Fractures of the radial head and neck are quite frequent and result as a consequence of a fall on the outstretched hand. Force transmitted up the radial shaft results in a compressive axial force on the radius with a fracture of the head itself, or the neck. Radial neck fractures are often minimally displaced and if the angle subtended by the radial articular surface is less than 30° no specific treatment is needed. Fractures with tilt of the head in excess of 30° usually need to be manipulated or have open reduction and fixation. Complete dislocation of the

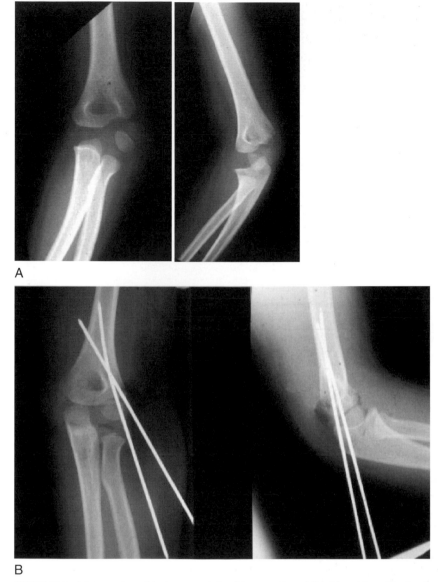

A

B

FIGURE 13.6   (A) Lateral condyle fracture of distal humerus in a child. (B) Position after fixation

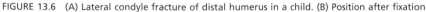

radial head may require radial head replacement. In children an angulation of up to 20° can be accepted, but a greater tilt is an indication for closed reduction, which can be achieved by manipulation or by using a percutaneous wire to reduce the fracture (Fig. 13.8).

Radial head fractures are treated according to the degree of comminution and displacement. Undisplaced fractures can be treated in a sling with early mobilization. Two-part or three-part fractures require internal fixation with screws if displaced. Very comminuted head fractures that cannot be

reconstructed are treated by radial head replacement. Radial head fractures are rare in children and the head should not be excised.

Elbow dislocations and fracture dislocations

The elbow may dislocate as a result of a fall on the outstretched hand with the elbow extended. The olecranon and radial head dislocate in a postero-lateral direction. Neuropraxia of the nerves round the elbow is an occasional complication. Closed

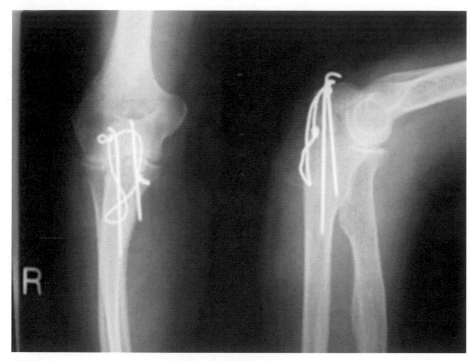

FIGURE 13.7   Post-operative view of tension-band wiring of olecranon fracture

reduction can be achieved in the majority of cases by application of manual traction with the elbow slightly flexed. Sedation is necessary, but general anaesthesia is not generally required. The elbow is usually stable after reduction. After 10–14 days of immobilization in a back-slab plaster, the elbow is mobilized. Some high-energy dislocations are associated with more extensive degrees of soft-tissue disruption and the joint may be unstable. In the majority of these adult cases exploration of the elbow with ligament repair is necessary. The same principles apply to children (Fig. 13.9) except that operative repair of disrupted ligaments is not usually indicated. The injury may also be associated with an avulsion of the medial epicondyle, which can then be incarcerated in the joint as a result of either the injury or the subsequent reduction. If this occurs the elbow should be opened, the fragment retrieved and pinned back in place (Fig. 13.10).

Fracture dislocations of the elbow are rare, but are more serious injuries often associated with poor outcomes in adults. The 'terrible triad' of the elbow refers to a dislocation in association with a coronoid process fracture and a radial head fracture in adults. There are several varieties of fracture dislo-

cation, but the principles of treatment are similar. Restoration of bony anatomy is essential to relocate the joint and restore stability. This usually requires internal fixation of the fractures involving the olecranon, coronoid process and ulnar shaft. The radial head may also need to be reconstructed, but in comminuted cases radial head replacement is needed. Careful early follow-up of these patients is needed to detect any loss of joint stability. The functional outcome is often compromised by stiffness and a soft-tissue release is frequently required to restore a functional range of motion.

FRACTURES OF THE FOREARM

Fractures of the forearm are very common injuries in children, but are much less common in adults. The peak age of fractures in children is between the age of 5 and 12 years, and fractures in this age group account for 50% of children's fractures. These injuries vary from plastic deformation (Fig. 13.11), to greenstick fractures, to complete fractures, and many can be treated by closed manipulation and an above-elbow cast. Cast treatment is generally continued for 3–5 weeks depending on the age of the child. At that stage healing is sufficiently advanced

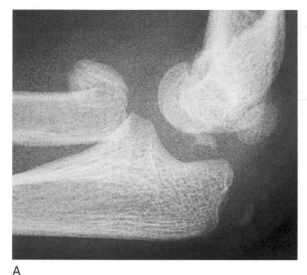

A

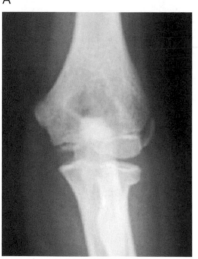

B

FIGURE 13.8 (A) Displaced radial neck fracture. (B) Satisfactory reduction after manipulation

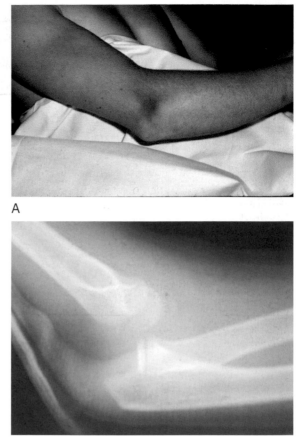

A

B

FIGURE 13.9 (A) Elbow dislocation showing visible deformity. (B) Plain radiograph showing posterior dislocation

to allow cast removal and mobilization. Complications are uncommon, but malunion occasionally occurs. Rotational malunion is poorly tolerated in the forearm particularly and results in loss of forearm rotation. To avoid this complication children should be reviewed and radiographs taken 1 and 2 weeks following reduction. Open reduction and fixation with flexible nails or plates is indicated if a satisfactory alignment cannot be achieved or if the child is approaching skeletal maturity.

Forearm fractures in adults are more often a consequence of high-energy trauma. Compartment syndrome is a well recognized complication. Most mid-shaft forearm fractures are completely displaced and are not readily amenable to non-operative treatment. Internal fixation with plates is the treatment of choice (Fig. 13.12). Failure to achieve anatomical reduction is associated with loss of the range of pronation and supination. Non-union and infection can complicate surgical treatment, but rates are usually less than 5%. Cross-union between the forearm bones after fracture complicates 2% of injuries and is more common in proximal third fractures, particularly in patients who have delayed fixation, head injury or those who develop infection.

Isolated ulnar shaft fractures are often the result of an assault when the victim sustains a blow on the forearm. If these fractures are undisplaced non-operative treatment in a cast is an acceptable form of treatment. Radiographs are required within the first 2 weeks of treatment to ensure no

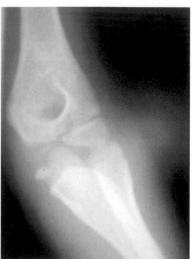

A

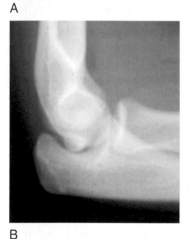

B

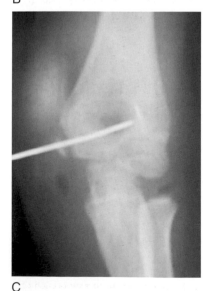

C

FIGURE 13.10   (A) Anteroposterior and (B) lateral view of elbow after reduction of dislocation showing medial epicondyle in joint, and (C) position after fixation of medial epicondyle

displacement occurs. Displaced ulnar fractures are best treated by internal fixation as this allows early mobilization.

Two patterns of forearm fracture dislocation occur and are eponymously known as the Monteggia fracture dislocation and the Galeazzi fracture dislocation. The Monteggia is the more common pattern and is characterized by an ulnar shaft fracture and a radial head dislocation. The Galeazzi pattern is a radial shaft fracture and a dislocation of the distal radio-ulnar joint. Good-quality radiographs including elbow and wrist joints are necessary in all forearm injuries to avoid missing associated dislocations at these joints. These patterns are also seen in children (Fig. 13.13) and, although internal fixation is indicated in all forearm fracture dislocations in adults, it is possible to manage these fracture patterns in children conservatively, provided that a reduction of the radial head in the Monteggia fracture and the radio-ulnar joint in the Galeazzi fracture can be obtained and maintained. If this is not possible, surgical management is required. Closed reduction of radial head dislocations may be possible, but open reduction

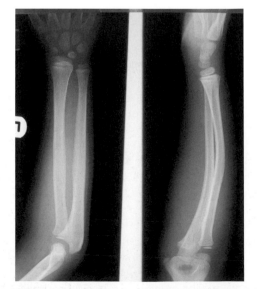

FIGURE 13.11   (Left) anteroposterior and (right) lateral radiograph of forearm in a child showing plastic deformity

and soft-tissue repair is indicated if a stable closed reduction cannot be achieved. For distal radio-ulnar dislocations additional fixation of the joint may be required. Typically the ulna has dislocated dorsally with respect to the radius. Kirschner wire fixation of the ulna to the radius should be used in patients who have an unstable joint following reduction. These wires require removal at 6 weeks to allow the patient to restore forearm rotation.

FRACTURES AT THE WRIST

Distal radial fractures are the most common fracture seen in clinical practice and are the consequence of a fall on the outstretched hand. In adults these fractures are most commonly seen in older female patients and are often associated with osteoporosis. Some eponymous terms are still in common use with these injuries. The most widely used term is Colles' fracture. This refers to an extra-articular fracture of the distal radius with dorsal angulation, displacement and shortening. The term Smith's fracture refers to an injury in a similar location but with volar displacement. Barton's fracture refers to a partial articular fracture usually associated with volar displacement.

The majority of distal radial fractures are characterized by dorsal displacement, dorsal angulation, dorsal comminution, and radial deviation of the distal fragment. These radiographic features are characterized clinically by a typical appearance of the wrist termed 'dinner-fork' deformity. Most of these fractures are isolated injuries in elderly patients, but a small percentage includes high-energy injuries in younger adults. Median nerve compression is an occasional early complication and may require urgent decompression of the nerve and reduction of the fracture.

Distal radial fractures are usually treated by closed reduction and plaster cast application for 5–6 weeks. Patients require radiography at 1 and 2 weeks following reduction to detect any loss of reduction. Approximately 30% of distal radial fractures are unstable and a satisfactory reduction cannot be maintained in a plaster cast. In patients with limited functional demands, including demented patients or high-dependency patients in institutional care, a non-anatomical reduction and malunion can be accepted. However, independent patients tolerate malunion poorly and it is often associated with wrist pain, stiffness and reduced grip strength. Operative treatment is

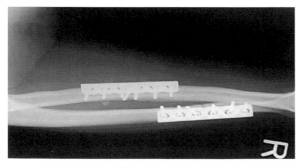

FIGURE 13.12 Post-operative view of forearm fracture in adult treated by plating

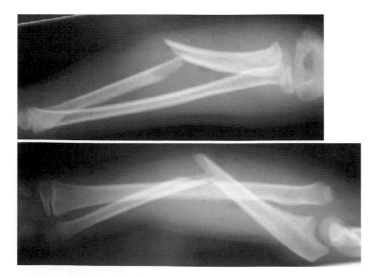

FIGURE 13.13 Monteggia fracture dislocation of forearm in a child. Note radial head dislocation. This was managed by closed reduction of the radial dislocation and application of a full arm cast

indicated in these patients when a satisfactory reduction cannot be maintained in a cast. Treatment choices include internal or external fixation or a combination of the two methods. Internal fixation using plating is mainly indicated for partial articular fractures. A small buttress plate is used. For other patterns external fixation is often employed. The most common complication of treatment is malunion. Typically this results in shortening of the radius in relation to the ulna with impingement of the ulna into the carpus, which results in limitation of wrist motion and pain. If there is significant incongruity of the distal radio-ulnar joint there is often restriction of forearm rotation. Corrective osteotomy of malunion can be carried out in fit patients.

Carpal tunnel syndrome is also a complication of distal radial fractures. It is more common in patients who heal in a significant degree of malunion. Carpal tunnel decompression is the usual treatment, but malunion may also need to be corrected.

In children the equivalent injuries are fractures through the distal metaphysis and physeal injuries, the commonest of which is the Salter–Harris II pattern. All the typical fracture patterns are seen in this region (see Chapter 12 on children's injuries). Median nerve symptoms may be seen in the bayonet fracture pattern (Fig. 13.14) where there is an overlap of the fragments.

Fractures of the carpus

Scaphoid fractures

Fractures of the scaphoid bone are the commonest carpal bone fracture and typically affect young adult males. The scaphoid bone links the proximal row with the distal row of the carpus and is vulnerable to fracture as a consequence of falls on the outstretched hand, which result in hyperextension at the carpus. Scaphoid injuries are seen in children, but the diagnosis is not always straightforward when the bone is not fully ossified. In these circumstances it is reasonable to treat the injury as a suspected fracture.

The history of a fall on the wrist is common, but very few physical signs may be present. The key clinical finding is of well localized tenderness in the anatomical snuffbox of the wrist. The fracture may be difficult to pick up on standard AP and lateral views and two additional oblique 'scaphoid views' should be obtained as a routine when fracture is suspected. Most fractures are located in the middle third (80%), but proximal pole fractures account for 15% and distal pole fractures for 5% of cases. The blood supply of the scaphoid enters distally and consequently avascular necrosis is a risk, particularly with proximal pole or displaced fractures.

Undisplaced fractures can be treated non-operatively in a cast. The usual 'scaphoid' cast is similar to that used for a distal radial fracture, but incorporates the thumb as far as the interphalangeal joint. Eight weeks of immobilization is required and some authors recommend 12 weeks. Union can be expected in 95% of undisplaced fractures.

Displaced fractures are best treated surgically. Some scaphoid fractures are associated with lunate dislocations, radial styloid fractures or other complex carpal fracture dislocation patterns. All of these should also be treated surgically. Internal fixation of the scaphoid with a small screw is the usual surgical treatment. Non-union following non-operative treatment can also be treated by internal fixation, but bone grafting is generally required.

Other carpal bones

Fractures of the other carpal bones are comparatively rare. They can usually be treated non-operatively in a cast if undisplaced. Fractures with displacement or those associated with carpal dislocations should be treated by internal fixation. Diagnosis may be difficult and computed tomography (CT) scanning is helpful in doubtful cases.

Fractures of the metacarpals and phalanges

History and clinical assessment

Fractures of the small bones of the hand are very common injuries. Many of these injuries are comparatively minor and a very satisfactory result can be expected from non-operative treatment. However, mismanagement can result in disabling deformity and stiffness. A careful history is the first step, taking note of hand dominance and occupation. The mechanism of injury may be of considerable significance, particularly with industrial injuries, where there may be crushing or penetrating trauma that will influence management decisions. Radio-

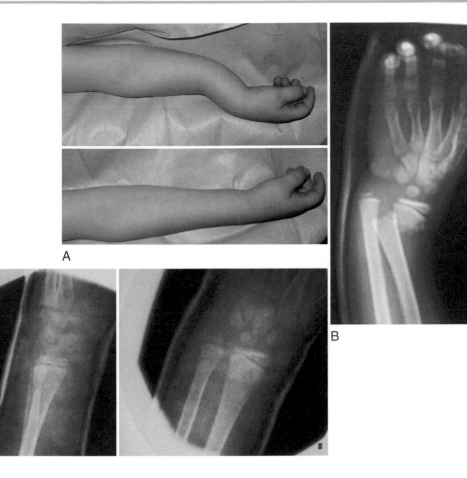

FIGURE 13.14 Completely displaced distal radial fracture in a child with (A) marked 'dinner-fork' deformity (top), and after reduction (bottom), (B) radiographs showing the fracture, and (C) anteroposterior and lateral views after closed reduction and application of a cast

graphs are not a good guide to the extent of rotational or angular deformity. In most injured hands the patient will hold the fingers in an extended position. Flexion of the fingers is necessary to judge the degree of angular and rotational deformity. In the flexed position, the middle and distal phalanges should point towards the scaphoid region of the wrist. Injuries sustained as a consequence of penetrating trauma may result in tendon or nerve injury and clinical assessment should evaluate these structures also.

Most hand fractures can be diagnosed without difficulty with radiographs. These need to include AP, oblique and true lateral views for a full assessment of the extent of injury and the need for treatment.

Management of metacarpal and phalangeal shaft fractures

Most of these fractures heal reliably and quickly and non-operative treatment in some form of splintage is the treatment of choice for the majority. The position of immobilization is important. In a position of extension the collateral ligaments of the metacarpophalangeal (MCP) joints are at their shortest length. If immobilized in this position, stiffness is the usual result, and may be very difficult to overcome. The correct position of immobilization is with the MCP joints flexed to 90° with the interphalangeal joints in full extension. In the case of the thumb, it should be immobilized in abduction and palmar opposition to minimize stiffness due to adduction contracture.

Fractures with angulation or rotation can be manipulated and reduced under anaesthesia. A splint or short cast can then be applied. Immobilization for 2–3 weeks is more than adequate for most stable metacarpal and phalangeal shaft fractures.

Unstable and intra-articular fractures

Some patterns of injury are inherently unstable and displaced intra-articular fractures, as described elsewhere, usually require surgical treatment. Angulation of more than 10° in any plane or rotational deformity causing overlapping of the fingers in flexion may require operative treatment if a stable reduction cannot be maintained by closed reduction and splintage. The exception to this rule is a fracture of the neck of the little finger metacarpal, where up to 45° of sagittal displacement can be accepted. Instability is more common with comminution or complete displacement of the fracture.

Usually Kirschner wires are used for fixation, and these are often inserted percutaneously. This has the advantage of being minimally invasive and wires may be inserted in a variety of directions and combinations. Screws and plates are available for use in small bones and are most suitable for use in intra-articular injuries. They require more invasive surgery and are technically demanding to use. Mini-external fixators are occasionally used in the hand. They are most useful in high-energy injuries with comminution and bone loss where standard methods of fixation may be technically impossible.

These principles also apply to fractures and dislocations of the hand and wrist in children. Greenstick and physeal injuries of the phalanges and metacarpals are seen in children as well as complete fractures. The same principles of management in the adults apply to children and these injuries heal rapidly. It is essential that any rotational malalignment is corrected as this does not remodel. Plates are rarely used in the child's hand as most fixations can be achieved with wires.

In the case of the thumb metacarpal a partial articular fracture at the base of the thumb metacarpal is called a Bennett's fracture and is an unstable pattern of injury. The palmar oblique ligament is attached to the small volar fragment, and the first metacarpal when detached from this

fragment is subluxed or dislocated out of the joint by the abductor pollicis longus. Reduction and Kirschner wire fixation is the most commonly used treatment.

TENDON AND NERVE INJURIES IN THE HAND

Tendon injuries

Extensor tendon injuries

These injuries may be closed or open (associated with a wound). The former can usually be treated by splinting, but open injuries require surgical exploration and repair.

A mallet finger injury is usually closed. The extensor tendon is torn from its insertion when the distal interphalangeal joint is flexed forcibly. The terminal phalanx assumes a flexed position, but can be passively extended, i.e. there is an extension lag. The injury is treated by a special splint to keep the distal interphalangeal joint extended for around 6 weeks (Fig. 13.15), and thereafter by night splinting for a further 2 weeks.

When there is a closed tear of the central slip of the extensor apparatus over the proximal interphalangeal joint, the injury may not immediately be apparent. Over the course of a few weeks the finger assumes a fixed position of flexion at the proximal interphalangeal joint and hyperextension of the distal interphalangeal joint, called a boutonnière deformity. This develops because the lateral bands in the extensor apparatus gradually slip anterior to the axis of flexion of the proximal interphalangeal joint. Suspecting the injury and keeping

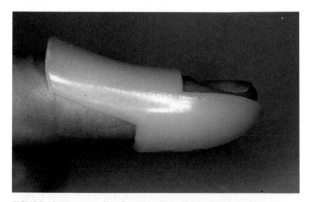

FIGURE 13.15 A mallet finger splint. The splint is held in place by wrapping tape around the part overlying the middle phalanx

the finger splinted at the proximal interphalangeal joint for 4–6 weeks can avoid this problem, which is very difficult or impossible to correct once established.

Open injuries of the extensor tendons at any level on the hand or wrist should be treated by careful suturing and post-operative splinting, followed by mobilization under the care of a physiotherapist to minimize the effect of any local adhesions.

Flexor tendon injuries

Injuries to these tendons are usually the result of cuts from knives or glass. All such injuries should be explored under general anaesthesia in an operating theatre by an experienced surgeon, as the damage may be more extensive than suspected by clinical examination. Surgical repair of flexor tendons is often followed by adhesions, especially in the region of the flexor sheath in the digit. Such adhesions limit the active movement of the digit and may result in marked impairment of hand function. They can be minimized by special techniques of suturing and post-operative mobilization.

Nerve injuries

Apart from compression neuropathies, which are discussed elsewhere, nerve damage in the hand is the result of penetrating injuries from sharp objects, and may be associated with damage to other structures, such as tendons and arteries. In the circumstances a detailed neurological examination may be impossible or misleading. It is important to suspect that there might be a nerve injury from the position of the wound, which should be explored under ideal circumstances. The ends of a completely divided nerve tend to retract. Since regeneration of a nerve relies on the ends being in contact, surgical treatment involves bringing the ends together without tension in the correct orientation. Very fine sutures that will not excite any significant tissue response are used, inserted under magnification. Any tension at the repair or reaction to foreign material will increase local fibrosis within the nerve and prevent recovery, which, even in ideal circumstances, is seldom complete.

The nerves that are commonly injured are the digital, median and ulnar nerves. Division of a digital nerve in the palm or digits causes a variable area of sensory loss distal to the injury. Division of the median nerve is commonly at the wrist, causing loss of function in most of the thenar muscles and loss of sensation in the thumb, the index, and the long and radial side of the ring finger on the palmar aspect. The ulnar nerve is also most often damaged at the wrist, causing loss of function in the hypothenar, interossei and adductor pollicis muscles, together with loss of sensation in the small finger and the ulnar half of the ring finger. It is important to realize that anatomical variations and overlap from the territories of adjacent nerves may result in some variation of these clinical signs.

LOWER LIMB INJURIES

PELVIC AND ACETABULAR FRACTURES

Pelvic fractures

Disruption of the pelvis is the result of high-energy trauma usually as a result of a motor vehicle accident. Other injuries are present in 70% of cases. Clinical assessment along Advanced Trauma Life Support (ATLS) guidelines is, therefore, required in all patients. The perineum must be carefully examined – occasionally open wounds in this region communicate with the pelvic fracture. Signs of urethral disruption (blood at the urinary meatus, perineal or scrotal haematoma and high-riding prostate on rectal examination) indicate the need for imaging of the urethra and bladder. Rectal examination is essential to detect rectal perforation, an absolute indication for faecal diversion. A neurological evaluation of the lower limbs is important, although an accurate assessment is often difficult in patients with multiple injuries.

Plain radiographs will identify most fractures. If the patient can be stabilized haemodynamically, a CT scan is the most useful additional diagnostic investigation. This allows rapid evaluation of the head, chest, abdomen and pelvis, and is the most accurate method of identifying associated injuries.

Some pelvic fractures are stable (e.g. isolated pubic ramus fractures in elderly patients). Unstable pelvic fractures are usually characterized by rotational or vertical displacement of one side of the pelvis in relation to the other side. Pelvic injuries are seen in children as a result of high-energy trauma and the same principles of management apply (Fig. 13.16).

Management

In patients who remain hypotensive despite fluid resuscitation, urgent intervention is required. External fixation is often used to reduce pelvic volume with tamponade of the expanding pelvic haematoma and provision of some bony stability. Adults treated with pelvic external fixation alone should have the frame left on for 8 weeks if possible.

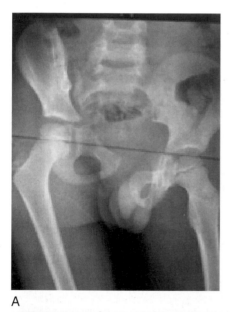

A

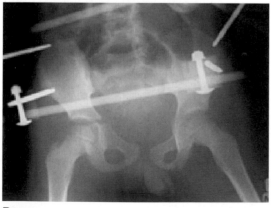

B

FIGURE 13.16 Unstable pelvic fracture in a child knocked down by a car. (A) There is disruption of the left sacro-iliac joint and symphysis, and a fracture of the inferior pubic ramus and distal displacement of the left hemipelvis. (B) The injury has been treated with an external fixator

Non-operative treatment of displaced unstable pelvic fractures has been associated with a high incidence of pelvic malunion in adults. This is associated with gait and seating problems, and disabling pelvic and lumbar back pain. The use of external fixation has been associated with a reduction in mortality and late morbidity, but it is not sufficiently rigid to maintain the reduction in more unstable patterns of injury. Internal fixation is now being used more commonly to treat these injuries.

The outcome after major pelvic disruption is often poor. This is partly due to the severity of associated injuries to other regions of the body. Mortality rates vary between 10% and 20%. Death is mainly due to uncontrollable haemorrhage or severe head injury. In general, a satisfactory anatomical result is reflected in an improved clinical outcome. Persistent pain is present in 25–35% of patients following major pelvic fracture.

Acetabular fractures

The most common accidents leading to acetabular fractures are falls from a height (40%) and motor vehicle accidents (30%). One-quarter of these patients have multiple injuries. These injuries are very unusual in children.

Since 25% of these patients have multiple injuries, a careful general assessment is required. A history of the mechanism of injury and site of pain should alert the surgeon to the diagnosis.

Bruising and abrasions on the thigh or buttock regions are common and there may be considerable degloving of skin in these areas. Leg length discrepancy due to displacement of the acetabulum is common. A shortened leg held in flexion, adduction and internal rotation suggests posterior dislocation of the hip, which is commonly associated with acetabular fractures. Weakness of dorsiflexion and numbness on the dorsum of the foot indicate sciatic nerve injury, the most common associated neurological lesion (15% of cases).

Radiology

Plain radiographs and oblique views of the acetabulum should be obtained. CT scanning with 3D reconstruction images is now very helpful for interpretation of complex fracture patterns (Fig. 13.17A). The most common pattern of injury is a posterior wall acetabular fracture with an associated posterior hip dislocation.

Management

Stable undisplaced fractures can be treated non-operatively. Patients can be mobilized partially weight-bearing on crutches progressing to full weight-bearing at 6 weeks. Serial radiographs at 1, 3 and 6 weeks should be taken to ensure healing without displacement occurs. The main indications for surgical treatment are incongruity or instability of the hip joint. Plating is the method of choice (Fig. 13.17B). Some displaced fractures can be treated non-operatively if they do not involve the major weight-bearing dome of the acetabulum.

Sciatic nerve palsy will recover completely in 50% of cases. Partial recovery occurs in 40% and no recovery in 10%. Post-operative wound infection complicates up to 5% of cases and may result in septic arthritis, which is inevitably associated with a poor outcome. Avascular necrosis is a particular risk in fractures associated with posterior dislocation, where it occurs in 20–25% of cases. Post-traumatic osteoarthritis is the major late complication and affects 20% of displaced fractures.

HIP FRACTURES

Fractures of the proximal femur involving the intertrochanteric and neck regions of the femur are very common injuries. They typically occur in elderly female patients. Most require surgical treatment.

Anatomy, classification and epidemiology

Fractures of the hip are divided into two main groups depending on their relationship to the capsule of the hip joint. Fractures of the subcapital and mid-cervical region of the femoral neck are *intracapsular* fractures (Fig. 13.18). Fractures at the base of the neck or in the trochanteric region are *extracapsular* fractures (Fig. 13.19). Intracapsular fractures may affect the blood supply of the femoral head, particularly if displaced. Complications of fracture union are common. Extracapsular fractures do not affect the blood supply of the femoral head and, since they occur in well vascularized, cancellous bone, healing complications are uncommon. Intracapsular fractures are usually described as displaced or undisplaced. Extracapsular fractures are usually considered to be stable or unstable. The main radiographic hallmark of instability is the presence of a detached lesser trochanter fracture fragment.

The demographic features of both injuries are similar – they usually occur in older female patients. The mean age is 75 years and the female:male ratio is 4:1. Dementia or some degree of cognitive impairment is common and typically

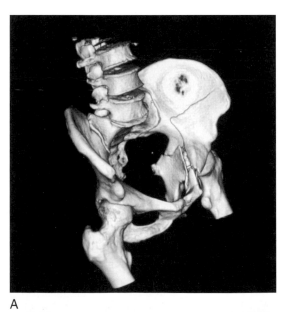

A

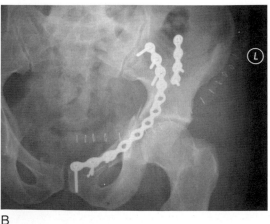

B

FIGURE 13.17 (A) 3D CT reconstruction of complex acetabular fracture of the left acetabulum; (B) position after plate fixation

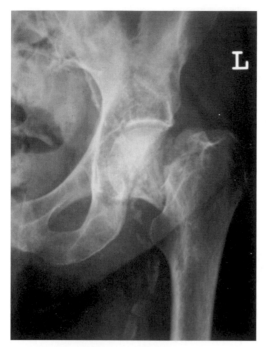

FIGURE 13.18 Displaced subcapital hip fracture. This is an *intracapsular* fracture and endangers the blood supply to the femoral head

present in 25–30% of cases. Significant medical co-morbidities are present in 70% of patients.

Femoral neck fractures in children are unusual, but carry a high risk of avascular necrosis of the femoral head even if the fracture is reduced and fixed (Fig. 13.20).

Clinical findings

There is usually a history of a fall. In displaced intracapsular or extracapsular fractures the leg is typically shortened and externally rotated. Neuro-vascular injury is very rare, but about 10% of patients will have an additional fracture, usually a proximal humeral or distal radial fracture.

Management

In the past some of these fractures were treated non-operatively in traction, but in modern ortho-paedic practice there is no role for this unless the patient is moribund on admission and not expected to survive.

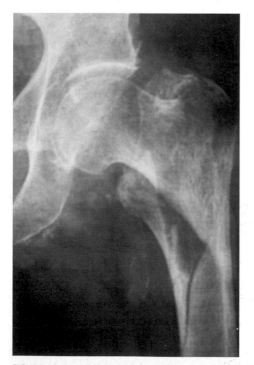

FIGURE 13.19 Displaced intertrochanteric fracture with subtrochanteric extension. This is an *extracapsular* fracture and will usually heal reliably after internal fixation

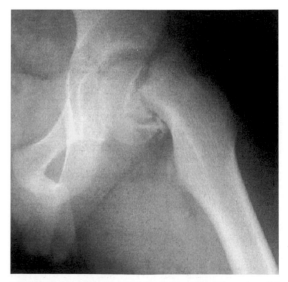

FIGURE 13.20 Salter–Harris II fracture of the femoral neck in a 10-year-old who fell from a height. An avascular necrosis of the femoral head occurred later

Intracapsular fractures

Undisplaced intracapsular fractures are generally treated by internal fixation using screws. Although they can be treated non-operatively, 15% will displace and it is safer to treat these injuries surgically. Avascular necrosis occurs in 5% of cases and conversion to arthroplasty may be required later if this is symptomatic.

Displaced intracapsular hip fractures are almost always in the subcapital region of the femoral neck. Reduction and fixation is possible, but there is a high rate of early non-union and fixation failure. Avascular necrosis affects about 15% of those that do unite. Overall, 40% of patients treated in this way will require conversion to some form of hip arthroplasty at a later stage. Most surgeons, therefore, choose to treat the majority of these patients with an arthroplasty in the first instance. Reduction and fixation should be considered in younger patients (<60 years). However, many younger patients with these injuries have risk factors that predispose to osteoporosis (alcohol abuse, steroid treatment, epilepsy treatment, renal or other metabolic bone disease). If risk factors are present then arthroplasty should be considered.

For most displaced intracapsular hip fractures, hip arthroplasty is the treatment of choice. The choices are either some form of hemi arthroplasty or a total hip arthroplasty.

Extracapsular fractures

Extracapsular hip fractures encompass fractures in the trochanteric region of the proximal femur. The clinical features are the same as for subcapital hip fractures. Characteristically, the fracture occurs in an elderly female and the leg is shortened and externally rotated at presentation.

Since the blood supply of the femoral head is not endangered, internal fixation is the treatment of choice. The most commonly used device is a sliding hip screw and plate. Alternative devices that involve intramedullary fixation are also commonly used, particularly for subtrochanteric fractures, especially if they extend a long way down the femoral shaft.

The main complications of surgery are failure of fixation (<5%), non-union (1–2%) and infection (<5%).

Outcome after hip fracture

Irrespective of the location of the hip fracture, the outcome is frequently poor. This is more a reflection of the frail medical state of these patients, rather than the nature of the surgery required. The 1-year mortality rate for all hip fractures is 30%, but in demented patients it is 50%. Rehabilitation in a non-acute institution is required in 35–40% of patients. Ultimately 70% of patients return home, but the remainder require some form of residential care.

FEMORAL SHAFT FRACTURES

Fractures of the shaft of the femur are usually the result of high-energy trauma in children and typically occur in younger male patients after motor vehicle accidents. However, an increasing number are seen in older patients after simple falls.

Clinical and radiographic assessment

The diagnosis is usually obvious with deformity and shortening of the leg. In adults approximately 10% are open injuries with a wound on the thigh communicating with the fracture (Fig. 13.21). Neurovascular injuries are uncommon, but are

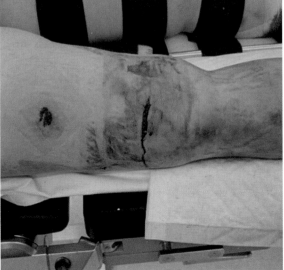

FIGURE 13.21 Compound wounds on thigh associated with high-energy femoral shaft fracture

present in 1–2% of cases. Careful assessment of distal pulses and sciatic nerve function is necessary. Compartment syndrome can occur in the thigh, but is uncommon. Many patients have additional injuries, often in the same limb. Patellar fractures, pelvic fractures and acetabular fractures with hip dislocations are the most common associated injuries. Careful assessment of the knee, hip and pelvis should be routine, and these areas all need to be included in the radiographic examination.

Treatment

Non-operative treatment was formerly common, but is rarely used now in adults. For open or closed femoral diaphyseal fractures the treatment of choice is early stabilization with an interlocking intramedullary nail (Fig. 13.22). This treatment has been associated with a very low risk of complications and high rates of union. For closed femoral shaft fractures non-union and infection rates should be no higher than 1%. The rate of malunion is also very low and is generally less than 5%. Fat embolism syndrome or acute respiratory distress syndrome (ARDS) can occur, but is more common in multiple trauma patients who have a delay to surgery. The risk is very low in patients with isolated femoral shaft fractures who are treated within 24 h of injury. Open fractures require a thorough debridement in addition to fixation.

Other surgical treatments, such as external fixation or plating, can be considered, but are used only in exceptional cases. External fixation may be useful in patients with multiple long-bone fractures and other injuries when there may not be time safely to carry out definitive internal fixation of all long-bone fractures. Plating is sometimes considered for patients with ipsilateral femoral shaft and femoral neck fractures, but has a higher rate of non-union and implant failure than intramedullary nailing.

Femoral shaft fractures in children may be managed according to the age and size of the patient. An initial assessment is required following the same guidelines for adults. If a femoral fracture is suspected it is very useful to insert a femoral nerve block, which makes further assessment more comfortable for the child who can then be placed on a Thomas splint in relative comfort. A Thomas splint may be used as definitive management for children aged between 3 and 7 years, depending on their size, family preferences and local practices. If this method is chosen, it is important that daily skin and pressure care occurs and attention is paid to maintain correct alignment of the lower limb and adequate femoral length. Shortening of about 1 cm is acceptable, as there is often an acceleration of growth of the femur after a fracture (Fig. 13.23).

Children over the age of 7 years, and younger children not suitable for traction, may have their fracture stabilized with flexible intramedullary nails. Locked intramedullary nails that cross physeal plates are not appropriate before skeletal maturity because of reports of avascular necrosis of the femoral head. Younger children may be treated in gallows traction if under 12 kg or in an immediate spica cast (Fig. 13.24). A femoral shaft fracture in a non-walking child should be considered as possible non-accidental injury and appropriate advice sought (see Chapter 12). Segmental femoral fractures, multiple injuries and a

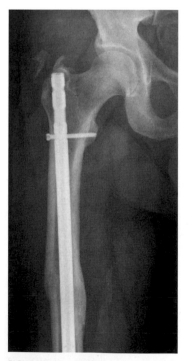

FIGURE 13.22 Healed femoral shaft fracture after fixation with intramedullary nail

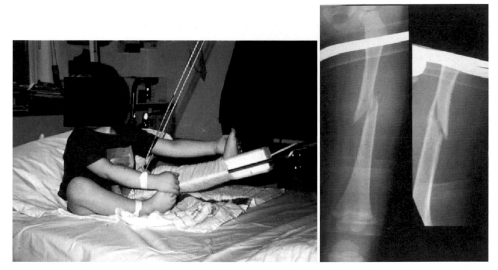

FIGURE 13.23   Management of a femoral shaft fracture on a Thomas splint in a 4-year-old

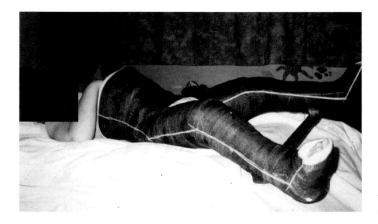

FIGURE 13.24   Bivalving of a hip spica following treatment of a fracture of the right femur in a 3-year-old

significant head injury are relative indications for fixation irrespective of the child's age. Open fractures can be managed with an external fixator. Anatomical reduction of the femur is required as the child approaches skeletal maturity. As rule of thumb, a fracture of the femur in a child will take about 1 week per year of life to heal up to the age of 5.

DISTAL FEMORAL FRACTURES

Fractures of the distal femur are less common than femoral shaft fractures and often occur in elderly female patients with osteoporosis. The diagnosis is obvious in most cases with swelling and deformity in the supracondylar region of the femur. Neurovascular injuries can occur, but are rare. A proportion of these fractures communicate with the knee joint. The diagnosis is confirmed with plain radiographs. Additional imaging is not required in most cases.

Treatment of distal femoral fractures is almost always operative unless the fracture is an undisplaced, stable injury in the distal femur with no intra-articular involvement. In distal fractures or those with intra-articular involvement, intramedullary nailing is often not technically feasible. Plating of these injuries is the treatment of choice. Fractures that are well reduced can be expected to heal in 3–6 months. Non-union complicates 5% of injuries in this area. The risk is increased in higher-energy fractures with more comminuted patterns.

In children, physeal fractures of the distal femur are not common, but an accurate reduction of types III and IV is essential to restore continuity of the joint surface and physeal plate. Growth arrest may occur (Fig. 13.25).

SOFT-TISSUE KNEE INJURIES

Sporting and occupational injuries account for the majority of soft tissue knee problems. A history of the actual event often yields information useful to make a provisional diagnosis. For patients who present with ongoing knee problems, four mechanical symptoms should be asked about: pain, locking, swelling and instability. If there has been an acute injury then the history of the actual accident, and the speed and degree of swelling are useful in making a diagnosis. If the knee became swollen immediately or within a few hours it strongly suggests the development of a haemarthrosis. The presence of an acute haemarthrosis is associated with a complete anterior cruciate ligament (ACL) tear in 70% of cases.

Swelling developing, for example, at 24 h or later, suggests a synovial effusion, which is much less specific, but it makes an acute ACL tear very unlikely. The most common soft-tissue injuries are ligament sprains or tears, meniscal tears and patellar instability.

Ligament injury

ACL and medial collateral ligament (MCL) tears are the most common knee ligament injuries and often occur in combination. Isolated MCL sprains are frequent. Posterior cruciate ligament (PCL) and lateral ligament complex injuries are rare by comparison. Collateral ligament injuries alone rarely require surgery as they heal spontaneously. They are usually treated by 6 weeks in a hinged knee brace and a programme of knee rehabilitation. Cruciate ligament injuries do not heal and are frequently associated with development of instability of the knee. ACL tears are 20 times more common than PCL tears. If symptomatic instability occurs it can be treated by ACL reconstruction using hamstring tendons or the middle third of the patellar tendon. The operation is successful in 90% of patients in restoring normal or near normal stability to the knee. The main complications are stiffness (up to 10%) and graft failure (5–10%).

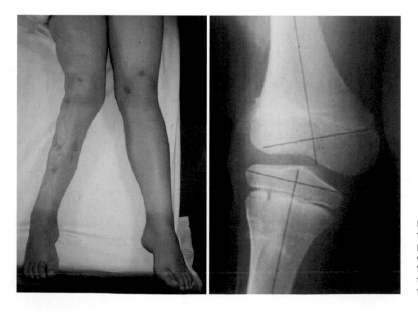

FIGURE 13.25 Post-traumatic arrest of the lateral half of the distal femoral physeal plate. The child had a severe open fracture of the left knee and a Salter–Harris IV injury of the physis. Note the valgus angulation clinically and on the X-ray due to the growth arrest

Meniscal tears

These are very common, but frequently present without a history of acute injury. Medial meniscal tears are more common than lateral meniscal tears. Degenerate flap tears involving the posterior third of the medial meniscus are more common in older patients (>35 years). They are often the result of minor twisting injuries. Bucket-handle tears of the meniscus are more common in younger patients. They are often associated with ACL tears, but the ACL tear occurs first. The instability of the knee as a consequence of the ACL tear allows the bucket-handle tear of the meniscus to occur. Diagnosis may not always be obvious on clinical examination. In doubtful cases, MRI scanning will confirm the diagnosis. The appropriate treatment is arthroscopic meniscectomy or meniscal repair. Resection of a large amount of meniscus in younger patients is associated with an increased risk of osteoarthritis. Meniscal repair is, therefore, often considered for these patients with large bucket-handle tears.

Patellar dislocation

Dislocation of the patella is most common in adolescent females, particularly if there is any generalized ligamentous laxity. Dislocation is virtually always to the lateral side. Closed reduction under sedation may be needed, but many dislocations spontaneously reduce. Initial management is conservative with a programme of knee rehabilitation. Surgical stabilization can be considered for patients with recurrent troublesome instability.

TIBIAL PLATEAU FRACTURES

Fractures of the tibial plateau are more common in older patients. Most of these injuries occur as isolated fractures and less than 2% are associated with multiple trauma. Most tibial plateau fractures involve the lateral plateau. Valgus deformity of the knee is, therefore, the most common clinical finding. In medial plateau fractures varus deformity is present. Fractures involving both the medial and the lateral plateau (bicondylar fractures) account for 10% of plateau fractures and are consequences of high-energy trauma. Extensive swelling and bruising is commonly associated with this fracture pattern. Medial tibial plateau fractures occur as a result of forced varus deformity and are associated with common peroneal nerve palsy in 10% of cases. Antero-medial plateau fractures may have disruption of the PCL and posterolateral corner ligaments. Vascular injury is not frequent, but should be considered in higher-energy patterns of injury.

Imaging

Plain radiographs are sufficient in most cases to establish the diagnosis. In cases where the extent of displacement is uncertain or in complex injury patterns then a CT scan is the most useful additional investigation.

Management

Undisplaced plateau fractures are infrequent, but if there is no articular surface displacement they can be treated non-operatively in a plaster cast or hinged knee brace, touch weight-bearing for 6 weeks. Radiographs are carried out in the first 2 weeks to ensure no displacement occurs.

Fractures with articular displacement are an indication for operative treatment in a fit patient. Internal fixation using screws or plates is the usual treatment method. External fixation can be used and may be a safer choice in patients with extensive soft-tissue injury (Fig. 13.26).

The clinical outcome is satisfactory in most patients. Wound complications affect 5% of

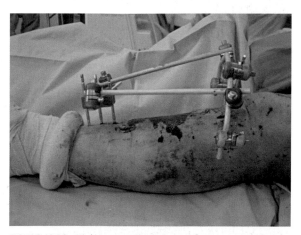

FIGURE 13.26 High-energy tibial plateau fracture treated with external fixation due to extensive soft-tissue swelling and contusions. Internal fixation with plating would be risky in this situation

patients. Deep venous thrombosis is an occasional problem also. Stiffness will occur in 5% of patients and may require a manipulation under anaesthesia to restore knee flexion after fracture union. The main long-term risk is osteoarthritis of the knee. Some degree of post-traumatic degenerative change is observed in 50–70% of patients within 10 years of injury, but total knee replacement is required in only 5% of cases.

In children fractures of the tibial spine are the commonest intra-articular fracture of the proximal tibia and correspond to a rupture of the ACL in the adult (Fig. 13.27). A fall on the flexed knee is a common mechanism of injury. The ACL stretches before the tibial spine is avulsed. The child presents with a large haemarthrosis and treatment depends on the degree of displacement as seen on the lateral X-ray of the knee. An undisplaced fracture can be managed non-operatively, but significant displacement is an indication for internal fixation of the avulsed fragment.

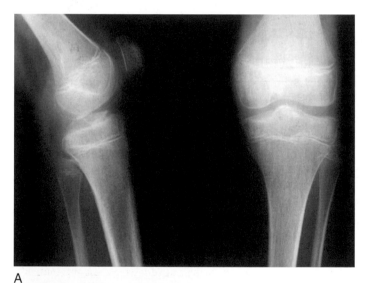

A

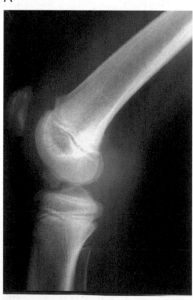

B

FIGURE 13.27 Avulsion of the tibial spine (A). This was treated conservatively. Compare the appearances in (B) where the spine is completely displaced. This was treated by reduction and fixation with a screw

TIBIAL SHAFT FRACTURES

Epidemiology

Fractures of the tibial shaft are the commonest long-bone fracture encountered in the adult. It is also the long bone most commonly complicated by open fracture. The injury occurs most frequently in young adult males, but does occur in all age groups.

Clinical and radiographic assessment

The majority of tibial shaft fractures are closed injuries that occur at the junction of the middle and distal third of the bone. Clinical diagnosis is based on the history and the clinical findings, which are usually obvious. Compartment syndrome complicates 2% of closed fractures and is present in 5–8% of open fractures. Compartment pressure monitoring facilitates earlier diagnosis. Vascular injuries are rare, but usually occur in association with open tibial fractures. They carry a very poor prognosis for limb salvage.

Management

Closed tibial shaft fractures can be treated non-operatively or operatively. Non-operative treatment was formerly the most common mode of management, but is less popular now. Patients have a closed reduction of the fracture and a long leg cast is applied. This is converted to a below-knee cast at 3–4 weeks. Casting is maintained until the fracture has united. Functional bracing is an alternative to conventional casts. Union of closed tibial shaft fractures in adults generally occurs 12–20 weeks after injury but may take longer. Malunion is a frequent complication of this method of treatment.

Plating was often used in the past, but the technique has been associated with a significant rate of soft-tissue complications, leading to deep infection and osteomyelitis. This is a difficult complication to treat in the tibia. External fixation has been used even for closed injuries but is also associated with troublesome pin-track infection and a high malunion rate.

Interlocking intramedullary nailing is now the treatment of choice for most tibial shaft fractures (Fig. 13.28), and particularly those that are consid-

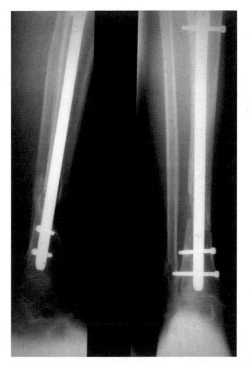

FIGURE 13.28 Tibial shaft fracture treated with interlocking intramedullary nail

ered unstable with any shortening, displacement or angulation at presentation. The nail can be inserted using minimally invasive surgery. The union rate is high and other complications are low. Non-union in closed fractures should be no higher than 2% and malunion is reported as less than 5%. Infection is a potential complication, but in closed nailing the rate is 1.5%.

Open fractures of the tibia are more of a challenge to treat. The soft-tissue injury may be severe and plastic surgery is often required to obtain reliable wound closure or coverage. Intramedullary nailing is now the most common treatment method for these injuries. Non-operative treatment in a cast is impractical in open fractures due to the complexity of the soft-tissue injury. Plating has been associated with a high rate of infection and is not recommended. External fixation is a safe method of treatment, but complicates soft-tissue management by limiting wound access.

In open fractures the wound is excised and debrided at the time of fracture stabilization. The compound wound is left open at the end of the procedure and re-inspected at 48 h to assess the need for further debridement. Wound coverage or closure (flap cover or split skin graft) should be carried out within 5–7 days of injury to minimize the risk of deep infection.

Open fractures of the tibia are characterized by more prolonged union times. These vary from 15 to 35 weeks depending on the presence and degree of bone loss. Infection after open tibial fractures is a significant risk, but with modern methods of management rates should be no higher than 10%.

In children the fracture of the tibial shaft may be associated with an intact or fractured fibula. The aim of treatment is to avoid significant shortening or angulation in the transverse and coronal planes (rotation and varus/valgus respectively). Isolated fractures of the tibial shaft usually result from rotational forces and are seen in children usually below 10 years of age (Fig. 13.29). If the fibula is intact the tibial fracture does not shorten significantly, but may angulate. Fractures of both bones may be treated in cast or, if unstable, by flexible intramedullary nailing (Fig. 13.30). As for the femur, rigid nails are not used and should not cross physeal plates. Open fractures are usually managed with an external fixator to enable access for soft-tissue coverage (Fig. 13.31). Non-union of the tibia

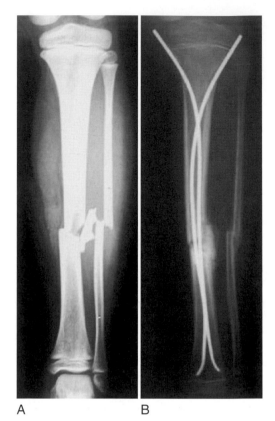

A   B

FIGURE 13.30   Unstable closed tibial fracture (A) treated by flexible intramedullary nails (B). The entry points of the nails avoid the physeal plate

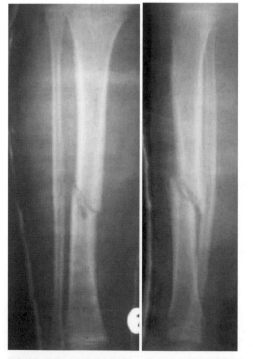

FIGURE 13.29   Isolated oblique fracture of the mid-shaft of the tibia treated in a cast

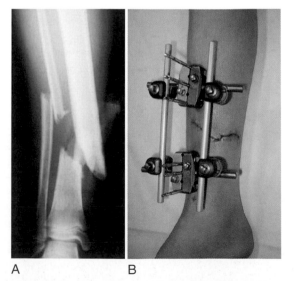

A   B

FIGURE 13.31   Open fracture of the tibia (A) treated with an external fixator (B). The skin was closed 48 h after the initial injury

is unusual in children and residual angulation may remodel if the deformity lies in the plane of motion of the adjacent joint (see Chapter 12).

DISTAL TIBIAL FRACTURES

Distal tibial fractures involving the weight-bearing surface of the distal tibia are referred to as tibial 'pilon' or 'plafond' fractures. These usually occur as a fall from a height. The talus is driven directly into the lower articular surface of the tibia causing a fracture (Fig. 13.32). The degree of articular damage and involvement of the lower third of the shaft is proportional to the energy of the injury.

Treatment of these injuries is determined by the condition of the soft tissues and the extent of comminution. Fractures with a limited number of articular fragments and a modest degree of bruising and swelling can be treated by internal fixation and plating. However, the more comminuted injuries with extensive soft-tissue involvement are often treated with limited internal fixation and external fixation, or external fixation alone. This approach reduces the risk of deep infection and wound breakdown. The long-term prognosis depends on the degree of articular comminution and the quality of articular reconstruction. Post-traumatic osteoarthritis is the most common complication and may require late ankle arthrodesis (fusion).

Distal tibial fractures in children will involve the metaphysis and physeal plate. The principles of management of these injuries are the same as at other anatomical sites.

The triplane fracture of the distal physis (Fig. 13.33) is an intra-articular fracture that occurs in early-to-mid adolescence as the distal tibial physis begins to close. It requires an accurate reduction and fixation.

ANKLE FRACTURES

Fractures of the ankle refer to injuries involving the malleolar segments of the tibia and fibula. The term

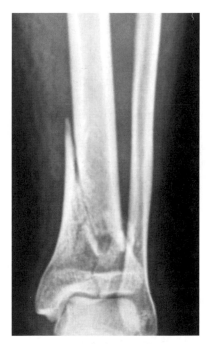

FIGURE 13.32 Pilon fracture of distal tibia caused by axial force driving talus against the articular surface of the tibia

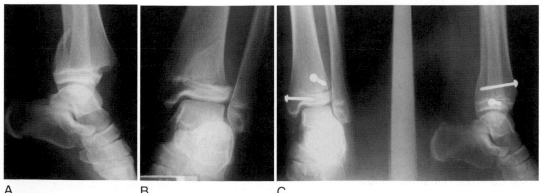

A   B   C

FIGURE 13.33 Triplane fracture of the distal tibia treated by internal fixation

excludes injuries mainly characterized by involvement of the tibial pilon or plafond already referred to above.

Epidemiology

Ankle fractures are a common injury in all adult age groups, although they exhibit a typical bimodal distribution in relation to age with a peak in young adults and a second peak in later life. Most of these injuries are sustained in low-energy accidents and most are an isolated fracture.

Clinical and radiographic assessment

Fractures of the ankle occur as a result of twisting injuries that result in rotation of the talus in the ankle mortise. As the talus rotates it abuts against the malleoli and causes a malleolar fracture or ligament disruption. In the most common pattern lateral rotation of the talus results in a lateral malleolar fracture associated with either a medial deltoid ligament disruption or a medial malleolar fracture. The instability caused results in subluxation or dislocation of the talus from the ankle.

Fractures are often described as being isolated malleolar fractures, bimalleolar (usually medial and lateral malleolar fractures) and trimalleolar fractures (medial, lateral and posterior malleolus). Clinical examination reveals tenderness with deformity and swelling.

If the ankle has been dislocated or significantly displaced it commonly results in extensive swelling, bruising and blistering of the skin. The degree of soft-tissue damage is related to the displacement, but also the duration of time before reduction is achieved. Major neurovascular disruption is rare, but local skin problems are not. They are more frequent in diabetics, patients with occlusive arterial disease and venous problems.

Plain radiographs are all that are required in the majority of cases. In the AP view the fibula is situated 30° posterior to the plane of the tibia and a clear view of the joint space is not obtained. The mortise view is a slightly oblique view obtained by internally rotating the ankle until the malleoli are in the same plane. On this view the relationship of the talus to the mortise can be easily judged.

Management

Simple ankle sprains can be treated symptomatically with strapping, elevation, ice packs and anti-inflammatory analgesia. Severe sprains can be treated for 3–4 weeks in a below-knee cast. Stable ankle fractures with an isolated lateral malleolus, but no additional disruption, can be treated in a cast for 5–6 weeks. Judgement of the stability is not completely reliable and radiographs at 1 and 2 weeks after injury in the cast are advisable to detect any loss of reduction.

Unstable fractures with displacement are best treated by internal fixation using plate-and-screw fixation of the displaced fragments. Although additional cast treatment is not mandatory, it is commonly used, particularly in older patients with osteoporotic bone or patients who are judged to be unreliable.

More severe patterns of injury occur, notably those with high fibular fractures above the level of the inferior tibio-fibular syndesmosis. These are often associated with a disruption of this joint (termed a diastasis) and a diastasis screw linking the fibula to the tibia is required as a component of the fixation. This screw is often removed 8 weeks after injury to minimize any loss of function at the inferior tibio-fibular syndesmosis.

Outcome

In stable fractures, or those that have been anatomically reduced, the functional outcome is good, and normal function can be anticipated. However, recovery is often slow with prolonged stiffness and swelling being the most common complications. Diabetic patients have a higher complication rate with infection being a particular problem. If this occurs it may be very difficult to treat and amputation is not an unusual result. Post-traumatic osteoarthritis is a well recognized problem, but fortunately is not frequent. Ankle arthritis is treated by ankle fusion if symptomatic. Ankle arthroplasty is an option, but few patients are suitable due to age, post-traumatic deformity and soft-tissue problems.

Similar injuries occur in children and the principles of anatomical reduction of fractures involving physeal plates apply as well as the need to reduce talar shift. Smooth wires may be passed across a physeal plate to stabilize a fracture. Post-traumatic ankle stiffness in children is not usually a problem.

HINDFOOT AND FOREFOOT INJURIES

Talus fractures

These are rare fractures in adults and children. They are usually a result of forced dorsiflexion of the foot with impingement of the neck of the talus on the distal tibia resulting in fracture of the talar neck. Road traffic accidents are now the most frequent cause, but falls from a height are also a well recognized cause.

Clinically, there is a lot of hindfoot and ankle swelling but no deformity unless there is considerable displacement or talar dislocation. Diagnosis is established by plain radiographs, but a CT scan may give useful additional information regarding the degree of displacement and comminution. The main risk with talar neck fractures is the potential loss of blood supply to the body of the talus. The risk of this in severely displaced fractures may be as high as 90%.

Undisplaced fractures may be treated non-operatively in a cast for 6 weeks. Displaced fractures should be treated by open reduction and fixation, as this has been associated with lower risks of avascular necrosis (AVN) than non-operative management. Patients are immobilized in a cast after surgery for 6 weeks. AVN can develop at any time within 2 years of injury and patients should be followed for this period with regular radiographs.

CALCANEUS FRACTURES

Fractures of the calcaneus typically occur as the result of a fall from a height and are common in building site workers, particularly roofers. Bilateral fractures are present in 10% of cases. Other injuries do occur and there is an association with fractures in the lumbar spine. These are unusual injuries in children. Clinical assessment reveals swollen heels, with loss of heel height, marked swelling and bruising, and skin blistering in severe cases. Diagnosis is confirmed by plain radiographs. In 75% of cases the subtalar joint is involved. CT scanning is necessary in these cases to determine the degree of joint involvement and displacement and to make a decision regarding treatment.

Extra-articular fractures can be treated non-operatively in most cases unless there is a large displaced fragment with the insertion of the Achilles tendon. Non-operative treatment entails cast immobilization for 4–6 weeks. Less severe crack fractures with no displacement can be treated partially weight-bearing without the use of a cast.

The treatment of displaced fractures remains controversial. The outcome of displaced fractures of the calcaneus with subtalar involvement has often been reported as very poor, irrespective of the mode of treatment. However, in the past two decades, modern methods of internal fixation have been associated with much better outcomes, although disappointing functional results with heel stiffness, pain and subtalar arthritis are still common. Poor prognostic features are: age over 40 years, severe comminution, smoking and diabetes. Patients who develop painful subtalar arthritis after injury are treated with subtalar arthrodesis.

MID-FOOT INJURIES

Injuries of the tarsal bones are very uncommon in adults and children. Minor undisplaced injuries can be treated non-operatively in a cast for 4 weeks. More severe injuries are usually the result of high-energy trauma, often with a crushing component (Fig. 13.34). These may be difficult to treat, but some form of internal fixation and, occasionally, external fixation may be necessary. With more extensive joint damage the outcome is poor with pain and stiffness. Late fusion may be needed.

Mid-foot dislocations through the tarso-metatarsal joint are referred to as a Lisfranc dislocation. The metatarsals typically displace laterally in relation the midfoot. This injury is best treated by internal fixation with a combination of screws and wires, which are placed across the dislocated joints after open reduction. They are removed once healing is complete. Non-operative treatment leads to poor results with valgus deformity of the forefoot and a flattened medial plantar arch.

METATARSAL AND PHALANGEAL INJURIES

The majority of these fractures occur as a result of low-energy trauma and they can usually be treated non-operatively in adults and children. For

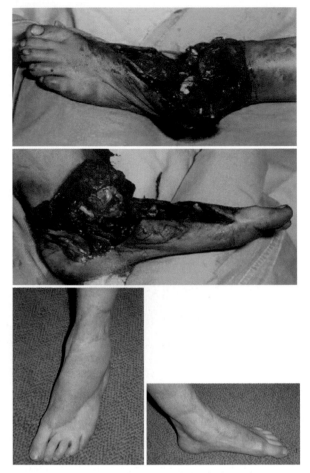

FIGURE 13.34 Severe crush injury to the right foot of an 8-year-old girl. The foot had been run over by a motor vehicle. The injuries were treated by a combination of orthopaedic and plastic surgery and the final outcome is shown above. She had no active dorsiflexion of the ankle due to the loss of all tendons over the dorsal aspect of the foot. There was normal sensation and circulation in the sole of the foot as the posterior tibial nerve and artery were intact

isolated metatarsals a padded dressing may be all that is required. Multiple injuries or those associated with a lot of pain may require a short period of cast immobilization. Most phalangeal fractures of the toes are treated with analgesia only. There

are a few exceptions that merit consideration of operative treatment.

Displaced fractures of the first metatarsal are very uncommon because the bone is very strong and only fractures as a result of significant force. Because of the importance of this bone in maintaining the medial arch and in weight-bearing in the foot, displaced fractures are best treated operatively with plating. Multiple metatarsal neck fractures are occasionally seen in high-energy injuries. They often result in plantar displacement of the metatarsal heads. Healing in this position can result in troublesome metatarsalgia later. Open reduction and wire fixation is recommended. Finally, fractures of the proximal third of the 5th metatarsal (Jones' fracture) have a propensity to non-union. They can be treated non-operatively, but careful follow-up is required to detect non-union, which may require internal fixation.

Compartment syndrome of the foot may result from a crushing injury with little bony damage, as the foot has musculo-fascial compartments. The diagnosis should be considered in any patient who has sustained a high-energy fracture or crush injury. Fasciotomy and decompression through dorsal and medial incisions is the treatment of choice to avoid an ischaemic contracture developing.

FURTHER READING

Dharmarajan TS, Banik P 2006 Hip fracture. Risk factors, preoperative assessment, and postoperative management. Postgrad Med 119(1): 31–38.

Giannoudis PV, Schneider E 2006 Principles of fixation of osteoporotic fractures. J Bone Joint Surg Br 88(10): 1272–1278.

Ivins D 2006 Acute ankle sprain: an update. Am Fam Physician 74(10): 1714–1720.

Tejwani NC, Hak DJ, Finkemeier CG, Wolinsky PR 2006 High-energy proximal tibial fractures: treatment options and decision making. Instr Course Lect 55: 367–379.

RHEUMATOLOGY

14

GENERALIZED MUSCULOSKELETAL PROBLEMS

A. K. Clarke, Julia L. Newton and Raashid Luqmani

Cases relevant to this chapter

21, 83, 85, 98, 99

●Essential facts

1. Non-specific musculoskeletal pains, especially back or neck related, are common and become more prevalent with age.

2. Pain is a neuropsychological phenomenon.

3. In most cases of chronic pain, patients need help in managing their symptoms.

4. Fibromyalgia is a pain syndrome characterized by trigger points, sleep disturbance and frequently by a precipitating painful condition.

5. Fibromyalgia is managed by improving sleep quality and teaching the patient pacing techniques, but compliance is low and the outcome remains unsatisfactory.

6. Chronic fatigue syndromes are common and disabling.

7. Pacing, psychological and physical support, provided by a dedicated multidisciplinary team, offer a significant opportunity for recovery.

8. Endocrine and rheumatic diseases are overlapping phenomena.

9. A patient may have more than one endocrine deficiency state.

10. Musculoskeletal manifestations of endocrine disease are dependent on age and underlying disease duration.

11. Recognition of an undiagnosed endocrinopathy may prevent the development of irreversible damage and significantly improve the outcome.

CHRONIC PAIN

Aches and pains are an everyday accompaniment of the human condition. Children run about and fall over. Young men play contact sports. Pregnant women get back pain. Digging the garden leads to muscular pain. Osteoarthritis affects the majority of the population. For a small minority of the population musculoskeletal symptoms are due to serious, progressive disorders, such as rheumatoid arthritis. One of the major challenges of modern medicine is that group of patients who do not have a major rheumatic disorder, but whose symptoms are in excess of what can be described as 'the aches and pains of everyday life'. It can be argued that in our modern consumerist society there is a basic intolerance of *any* symptoms. This does not explain the large number of people who regularly attend their general practitioners (GPs) and rheumatology departments complaining of disabling symptoms that interfere with work, household duties and leisure activities. At least 5 million people in Britain suffer from disabling chronic pain. It is usually precipitated by one or more episodes of acute pain that does not resolve as one would expect following the passage of time or with appropriate treatment.

In this chapter the features of the commonly seen conditions and their management are described, using an evidence-based approach. There are a number of recognized chronic pain syndromes, including:

- Fibromyalgia
- Chronic fatigue syndromes
- Complex regional pain syndrome (CRPS) (previously algodystrophy, Sudek's atrophy or sympathetic dystrophy)
- Causalgia
- Phantom limb pain
- Post-herpetic neuralgia
- Inappropriate pain (otherwise pain augmentation).

Although the physical signs may vary, the main feature is unremitting pain that interferes with normal activities. The pain is often described by the sufferer as burning or crushing. The pain may be modified by analgesics, but is rarely abolished and is often more sensitive to drugs aimed at neurogenic pain, such as carbamazepine.

Type I complex regional pain syndrome is idiopathic and was formerly known as reflex sympathetic dystrophy, Sudek's atrophy or algodystrophy. Type II complex regional pain syndrome follows a nerve injury and was formerly referred to as causalgia. CRPS type I is characterized clinically by severe prolonged pain out of proportion to any injury, allodynia (pain on light touch to the skin), cold, clammy skin and loss of function (Fig. 14.1). Typically the skin is red and has a shiny appearance, with hypersensitivity. The exact cause of the condition is unknown. A variety of physiological abnormalities have been described including autonomic dysfunction, microcirculation abnormalities and muscle mitochondrial changes, among others. Radiographs will often show osteoporosis, which is frequently patchy. Bone scanning shows increased turnover. Inflammatory markers are not normally raised.

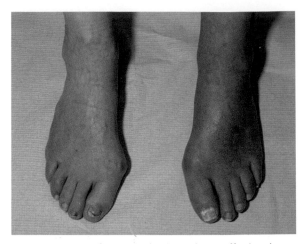

FIGURE 14.1 Complex regional pain syndrome affecting the lower limb. Note the dusky discoloration

Causalgia (CRPS type II) is very similar to CRPS type I in the intensity of the pain, but usually without the obvious physical signs. Most cases of CRPS are treated by intensive physiotherapy and usually resolve slowly over a period of months.

A common management problem is actually abolishing the pain. Many patients spend considerable time and energy looking for a cure, which is not attainable. For many, the best approach is to assist the patient to adapt and cope with the pain, using cognitive behavioural therapy.

IMPORTANCE OF A POSITIVE DIAGNOSIS

Many diseases present with aches and pains, general malaise and fatigue. Common ones include hypothyroidism, malignant disease and connective tissue disorders, such as systemic lupus erthythematosus (SLE). It is essential when confronted by a patient with such symptoms to take a full history, paying particular attention to such factors as weight loss, change in bowel habit and the red flags associated with serious back pain (see Chapter 22).

A careful clinical examination will ensure that inflammatory arthritis and hypothyroidism *are* excluded and the typical signs of fibromyalgia, for instance, are present. Appropriate investigations may be necessary. It is particularly important that in suspected inappropriate pain and chronic fatigue syndromes a full medical screening is undertaken.

FIBROMYALGIA

Fibromyalgia is a relatively new condition. Although rheumatism, fibrositis and lumbago are terms of some antiquity, fibromyalgia only became a recognized rheumatological diagnosis in the early 1980s. It is important to emphasize that fibromyalgia is *not* a disease. It can be precipitated by any condition that causes sleep disturbance and can be induced by deliberate sleep deprivation. The diagnosis depends upon the presence of three criteria: 1) a precipitating cause; 2) sleep disturbance and 3) trigger points.

Typically, the patient reports that they wake in the very early hours of the morning. This means they miss out on the critical phase of sleep – that part which includes rapid eye movement (REM) sleep and Delta wave sleep. The trigger points occur at very specific places. For research purposes the definition of fibromyalgia requires that there should be 11 out of the 15 recognized points to be tender and that all four quadrants of the body be involved. What is more there should not be tenderness in other parts of the body. Other features may include blushing and brisk tendon reflexes. Typically fibromyalgic patients report that on some days they feel good and full of energy, while on others they are very achy and feel exhausted. The obvious response to this is to cram as much into the good days as possible. Inevitably the patient suffers extreme symptoms for the next 2 or 3 days.

Management includes improvement in the sleep pattern, attention to the underlying precipitating cause and pacing. Typically, the sleep is improved by the use of small doses of a tricyclic antidepressant. The most popular is amitriptyline. Usually it is started in very low dose, 10 mg, given 2–3 h prior to retiring for the night. The dose is then slowly increased (i.e. every 7–10 days) by 10 mg until a dose is found that produces a good, refreshing, sleep pattern, without hangover. In the absence of clinical depression it is rare to have to go above 30 or 40 mg daily. Hangover is signifi-cantly reduced by giving the drug well before going to bed.

Once a good sleep pattern starts to emerge the underlying cause can be addressed. *In many cases the cause will have resolved spontaneously,* especially if it is a simple mechanical spinal problem. However, if the condition is complex, such as rheumatoid arthritis, then this needs to be brought under control.

Pacing is the key to a successful outcome. Because of the typical peaks and troughs of the condition it is important that on the good days only normal activities are pursued, i.e. the amount that the individual can cope with on a bad day. This allows for a steady improvement in the physical capacity.

Caught early and treated vigorously, fibromyalgia is a treatable condition, with a good prognosis. If left, then the likelihood of improvement reduces, especially if the patient holds specific beliefs about the origins of the symptoms, based on the probability of serious organic disease. This form of illness behaviour is a poor prognostic factor.

CHRONIC FATIGUE SYNDROMES

There are few conditions that carry more emotional baggage than chronic fatigue syndrome (CFS). For a number of years there has been almost open warfare between sufferers and the medical profession. Many doctors dismissed the diagnosis (especially when described as myalgic encephalomyelitis [ME]). Doctors often felt that the condition was a form of neurosis, with no physical basis. Sufferers refused to believe that there were any psychological factors influencing their condition. Many maintained that there was a specific pathological entity due to a disturbance of the immune system, despite the lack of any good evidence for such a process. Although this is still a controversial area, a truce has been declared because of the emergence of considerable common ground. Firstly, it is recognized that we are looking at a group of disorders rather than a single entity. There are likely to be several of causes of CFS. No-one doubts the existence of CFS as a complication of certain well defined viral illnesses, such as influenza or glandular fever. Similarly, severe, longstanding fibromyalgia frequently develops into CFS. Other precipitants do appear to include surgical operations and debilitation associated with severe medical illnesses. Some cases appear to arise spontaneously. The condition is much commoner in women and there is a significant subgroup of adolescents.

Fatigue is the primary symptom. This is not just tiredness, nor the type of almost pleasant fatigue felt after heavy physical activity, but an overwhelming sensation that makes the sufferer feel physically ill. It is not relieved by sleep and, indeed, many patients complain that even when they do sleep properly (sleep is often disturbed, with early morning waking) it is not refreshing. Other symptoms include arthralgia and myalgia (which is why many patients are referred for rheumatological opinions), low-grade fever, irritable bowel syndrome, visual disturbance, and poor concentration and memory. There are usually good days and bad days and, as with fibromyalgia, there is a very strong temptation to overdo things on the good days. There are no specific clinical signs.

Wherever possible a positive diagnosis of CFS should be made, rather than seeing it as a diagnosis of exclusion. Other causes of fatigue, such as hypothyroidism and severe anaemia, do need to be considered in the differential diagnosis, but it is unusual for a good history and examination not to spot these types of problems and simple screening tests, such as thyroid function and a full blood count, should be undertaken. Once a positive diagnosis is made, the temptation to 'do just one more round of investigations' should be resisted.

Treatment consists of reassurance that the diagnosis has been positively made, that the condition is treatable and that a programme is available. That programme should include carefully paced activity, help with sleep disturbance and cognitive behavioural therapy. There are a number of support organizations in the UK and elsewhere, and, recently, an initiative by the Department of Health has seen a network of cooperative centres for the management of CFS come into being.

RHEUMATIC MANIFESTATIONS OF METABOLIC AND ENDOCRINE DISEASES

Many endocrine disorders have musculoskeletal manifestations. A rheumatological complaint may, therefore, be indicative of an undiagnosed endocri-

nopathy. An endocrine history will uncover common symptoms that suggest an endocrine cause (Box 14.1). Because endocrine and rheumatic diseases often coexist, it is important to ask about endocrine symptoms in a patient with an established rheumatological diagnosis.

In this section the common rheumatic manifestations of metabolic and endocrine disease will be discussed (Table 14.1). The more common diseases are concentrated upon, but some rarer disorders have been included if musculoskeletal symptoms are particularly prominent.

Diabetes mellitus

Both type 1 and 2 diabetes mellitus (DM) are associated with rheumatological complaints (Table

---

Box 14.1
Endocrine history questions

- Weight change
- Hair loss/dryness
- Infertility
- Reduced libido
- Mood changes
- Fatigue
- Heat/cold intolerance
- Constipation/diarrhoea
- Family history
- History of other endocrine problems

Table 14.1 Endocrine and metabolic diseases with musculoskeletal manifestations

Endocrine disorders	Metabolic disorders
Diabetes mellitus	Hyperlipidaemia
Hyperthyroidism	Renal failure
Hypothyroidism	Ochronosis
Hyperparathyroidism	Haemochromatosis
Acromegaly	Lysosomal storage disorders
	Glycogen storage metabolic myopathies

Table 14.2 Musculoskeletal manifestations of diabetes mellitus

Specific to diabetes mellitus	Increased prevalence in diabetes mellitus	Possible association with diabetes mellitus
Limited joint mobility	Dupuytren's contracture	Osteoarthritis
Diabetic amyotrophy	Palmar flexor tenosynovitis	
Diabetic muscle infarction	Carpal tunnel syndrome	
	Adhesive capsulitis	
	DISH*	
	Scleroedema	
	Neuropathic arthropathy	
	Bone and joint infection	

*Diffuse idiopathic skeletal hyperostosis.

14.2). These disorders are either unique to diabetic patients or are known to occur in the general population, but have an increased incidence in patients with DM. Musculoskeletal problems in DM are becoming increasingly common due to the increased life expectancy of diabetic patients. The pathophysiology of these disorders in DM is poorly understood.

The presence of one musculoskeletal problem in DM increases the likelihood of developing other musculoskeletal complications; there is an increased incidence of adhesive capsulitis (AC), Dupuytren's contracture (DC) and limited joint mobility (LJM) occurring together than would be expected. Treatment may include corticosteroid injection, which in DM should be used with caution as hyperglycaemia may follow.

Limited joint mobility (aka diabetic cheiroarthropathy, diabetic hand syndrome)

This condition produces a generalized non-painful stiffness and puffiness of the hands with flexion contractures of all the fingers so that the patient is unable to place the palmar surfaces of the hands and fingers flatly together ('prayer sign'). It begins with the little finger and progresses laterally. Some 8–50% of patients with DM develop limited joint mobility (LJM); it occurs in both types 1 and 2 DM. On biopsy there is a loss of elastic fibres in the skin. There is an association between the presence of LJM and microvascular and macrovascular compli-

cations in DM. There is no effective therapy, but good diabetic control and exercises concentrating on finger extension may help to prevent further deterioration of the condition.

Dupuytren's contracture

Dupuytren's contracture (DC) is due to thickening and tethering of the palmar fascia resulting in digital contracture (see p. 283). This condition occurs more commonly in diabetic patients, but is also common in the general population; it affects 5–13% of the general population and 12–63% of diabetic patients. It initially affects the ring and little fingers in the general population, but the ring and middle fingers in diabetics. Sixty-five per cent are bilateral and men are affected more than women overall, but there is an equal sex incidence when present in association with DM. It is usually less progressive in the diabetic population and there is less need for surgery. Although often idiopathic, there are other known associations in addition to diabetes (Table 14.3).

Treatment includes occupational therapy, physiotherapy, steroid injections and surgical fasciectomy, but the latter is the only treatment supported by evidence.

Palmar flexor tenosynovitis

This common condition is due to fibrous proliferation of the tendon sheath preventing the normal smooth movement of the tendon. There is often an

Table 14.3 Associations of Dupuytren's contracture

Association	Frequency
Familial	27–68%
Diabetes	20–63%
Prior hand trauma	13%
Alcohol	10%
Epilepsy	2%
Smoking	unknown
Manual labour	unknown
Ischaemic heart disease	unknown
HIV infection	unknown

associated 'trigger finger'. It affects less than 1% of the general population compared to 11% of diabetic patients. The underlying reason for this increased prevalence is not known. Treatment includes good glycaemic control, hand exercises, local corticosteroid injections and surgery if these conservative measures fail.

Adhesive capsulitis

This normally common condition (see p. 282) has a significantly increased prevalence in the diabetic population of 11–30%. It is characterized by progressive painful restriction of glenohumeral movement. The pathology involves inflammation and then fibrosis resulting in adherence of the joint capsule to the humeral head. There are three stages to adhesive capsulitis; painful, adhesive and resolution. The process takes up to 2 years. Although physiotherapy, non-steroidal anti-inflammatory drugs (NSAIDs) and local corticosteroid injections may help with pain and range of motion to a degree, no treatment appears to shorten the cycle. In diabetics adhesive capsulitis tends to occur at a younger age and is often less painful, but the cycle to resolution often takes longer.

Osteopenia

Osteopenia and osteoporosis occur in type 1 DM. The longer standing the DM, the greater the bone loss and increased fracture risk. Insulin and insulin-like growth factor 1 (IGF-1) have anabolic effects, including the promotion of osteoblastic activity. The lack of these proteins in type 1 DM, but the excess presence in type 2 DM, helps to explain the normal bone density of type 2 diabetic patients. Type 2 DM is also associated with obesity, which again is associated with a lower incidence of osteopenia/osteoporosis. Despite the reassuring nature of DEXA results in type 2 DM, some studies do still suggest an increase in fracture risk. The exact mechanisms of these findings are not known.

Carpal tunnel syndrome

This is a common entrapment neuropathy affecting the median nerve as it passes through the carpal tunnel at the wrist under the transverse carpal ligament (see p. 285). Some 11–16% of patients with DM develop carpal tunnel syndrome (CTS). Typically, the patient develops pain and paraesthesia in the median nerve distribution: the palmar and dorsal aspects of the thumb, index and middle fingers and the radial half of the ring finger. The exact distribution may vary from person to person and the pain may radiate to the forearm. The pain and paraesthesia is typically worse at night. Weakness may develop affecting the muscles supplied by the median nerve: the thenar eminence of the thumb. The ideal muscles to test are abductor pollicis brevis and opponens pollicis. There may be muscle atrophy of the thenar eminence. Tinel's test, tapping over the median nerve at the wrist, and Phalen's test, prolonged palmar flexion of the wrist for 60 s, may reproduce the symptoms. Diagnosis is based on history and examination and electrophysiology studies. Treatment includes splinting, corticosteroid injection and surgical release but, where it is a secondary phenomenon, treatment of the underlying disorder is most important. Some 5–8% of patients with CTS have diabetes, highlighting the importance of a high index of suspicion at the patient's first presentation.

Diffuse idiopathic skeletal hyperostosis (aka Forestier's disease)

Diffuse idiopathic skeletal hyperostosis (DISH) is a condition where calcification of the anterior longitudinal ligament of the spine occurs with hetero topic ossification of joint capsules, tendon entheses and ligaments (Fig. 14.2). It is often asymptomatic or may present with spinal pain and stiffness. In the normal population DISH is a disease of the elderly and has a prevalence of 2–13%. In diabetics it typically occurs at a younger average age and the prevalence is increased to 13–49%. It is more common in type 2 DM. It is hypothesized that the increase in IGF-1 in type 2 DM promotes osteoblast proliferation and ossification.

Diabetic amyotrophy

Diabetic amyotrophy is characterized by painful severe muscle wasting and weakness, typically affecting the proximal lower limbs. It is a subset of diabetic neuropathy and reflexes are absent. It usually affects older men with type 2 DM. The aetiology is unknown and, although there is usually spontaneous improvement, this is often incomplete.

Scleroedema

This is a rare condition that has an association with DM, usually longstanding type 1 disease, but it does occur with type 2 DM. Other associations include blood dyscrasias and post-infection. It is of unknown cause and characterized by non-pitting induration of the skin. In diabetic patients it classically affects the upper back and tends to spare the extremities, but it may contribute to the development of limited joint mobility. Generally, it is a benign self-limiting skin disease. On histological examination there is excess mucopolysaccharide deposition in the dermis and it is clearly distinguishable from scleroderma. There is no proven effective treatment.

Neuropathic arthropathy (aka Charcot's joint)

This is a destructive arthropathy that affects the tarsal and metatarsal joints in the foot. The exact mechanism of neuropathic arthropathy is not fully understood. There is increased osteoclastogenesis and osteopenia, and hypervascularity of bone in these patients. The bone is weakened and susceptible to fracture and collapse. The universal presence of a sensory neuropathy combined with arterial disease, trauma and infection is thought to predispose to the characteristic painless chronic deformity of a 'Charcot's joint'. The affected limb may become swollen, warm and red, often without a history of trauma. There may be associated skin ulceration and infection, sometimes requiring amputation. The main differential diagnoses are shown in Box 14.2.

Good diabetic control and foot care are of prime importance in all diabetic patients and prevention is the main aim of management. Instability or deformity may limit the use of standard footwear. The foot should be kept plantigrade with orthoses to maintain a normal gait pattern. Early diagnosis of neuropathic arthropathy will help to prevent further deterioration. Bisphosphonates have been used to halt the aggressive osteoclast activity. In advanced cases surgery may be required.

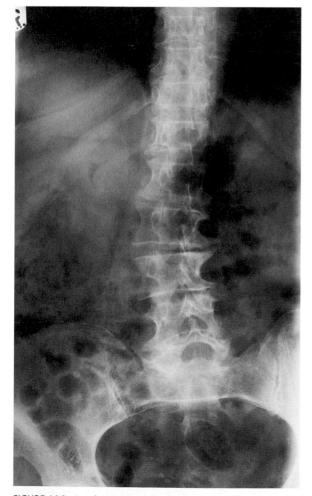

FIGURE 14.2 Lumbar spine radiograph showing flowing osteophytes in a patient with diffuse idiopathic skeletal hyperostosis

Box 14.2
Differential diagnosis of neuropathic osteoarthropathy

- Osteomyelitis
- Erosive inflammatory arthritis
- Osteoarthritis
- Tumour

Table 14.4 Musculoskeletal manifestations in thyroid disease

Arthralgia	hypo- and hyper-
Myalgia	hypo- and hyper-
Raised creatine kinase	hypo-
Proximal painless myopathy	hypo- and hyper-
Carpal tunnel syndrome	hypo-
Chondrocalcinosis	hypo-
Osteoporosis	hyper-
Increased fracture risk	hypo- and hyper-
Osteonecrosis	hypo- and hyper-
Thyroid acropachy	hyper- (specifically Grave's disease)

Bone and joint infection

The prevalence of both septic arthritis and osteomyelitis is increased in DM. There is an increased incidence of soft-tissue infection and ulceration, particularly in association with neuropathic arthropathy. This provides a route from which bone and joint infection could develop by direct invasion from an overlying soft-tissue infection or haematogenous spread to a distant joint.

Investigation of a suspected septic arthritis must include synovial fluid aspiration. Magnetic resonance imaging (MRI) is very useful in differentiating neuropathic arthropathy from osteomyelitis in the diabetic foot, but bone biopsy may be required. Treatment is with appropriate antibiotics and washout of the affected septic joint. For more details on bone and joint infection see p. 88.

Diabetic muscle infarction

This is a rare phenomenon and usually occurs in the thigh. Diagnosis is by MRI and biopsy demonstrates muscle necrosis and an associated microvasculopathy.

Osteoarthritis

There is an increased rate of osteoarthritis (OA) in diabetic patients, but this is not well characterized and may be due to the increased level of obesity rather than the diabetes. For more details on OA see Chapter 15.

Thyroid disease

Both hypo- and hyperthyroidism have rheumatological associations (Table 14.4).

Congenital absence of thyroid hormone occurs as an autosomal recessive trait in 1 in 4000 births. The phenotypic picture includes growth retardation, delayed dental development and delayed skeletal maturation. A well described skeletal abnormality is deformity of the 12th thoracic and the 1st lumbar vertebrae, known as a gibbus deformity. In developed countries this condition is routinely tested for at birth, but in cases of delayed epiphyseal closure or growth retardation, thyroid function tests should be carried out. Acquired hypothyroidism, most commonly due to the autoimmune condition Hashimoto's thyroiditis, is most prevalent in middle-aged women and is often subclinical.

The effects on the musculoskeletal system in hyperthyroidism may be due to excess thyroid hormone, either from primary hyperthyroidism or from excess replacement therapy.

Osteoporosis

The highly organized process of bone remodelling is explained in Chapter 2. Thyroid hormone is known to be a stimulator of bone remodelling and increased bone turnover. Excess thyroid hormone causes a decrease in cancellous bone. There is a direct relationship between the length of the excess thyroid hormone production and the severity of the osteoporosis.

Thyroid acropachy

Thyroid acropachy is a rare condition characterized by the development of painless soft-tissue swelling of the fingers and toes in association with clubbing and periostitis. This condition is unique to longstanding Grave's disease; an autoimmune condition characterized by the presence of thyroid autoantibodies.

Effects of treating thyroid disease on the musculoskeletal problems

With treatment of the underlying thyroid disease, the arthralgia, muscle disorders and CTS resolve. Thyroid acropachy is due to the circulating antibodies and is, therefore, unresponsive. Osteoporosis and osteonecrosis are not reversible with treatment of the underlying thyroid disorder.

Hyperparathyroidism

Primary hyperparathyroidism is due to an excess production of parathyroid hormone (PTH) by the parathyroid glands. Secondary hyperparathyroidism occurs when there has been prolonged stimulation of the parathyroid glands due to a low serum calcium. Secondary hyperparathyroidism is most commonly seen in renal failure and in malabsorption syndromes. The main consequences of hyperparathyroidism are hypercalcaemia and osteopenia/osteoporosis. Primary hyperparathyroidism is the commonest cause of hypercalcaemia and 80–90% of cases are due to an adenoma. Rheumatic manifestations of hyperparathyroidism are shown in Box 14.3.

Classic parathyroid bone disease occurs in both primary and secondary subtypes and is called oste-

---

> ## Box 14.3
> ### Rheumatoid manifestations of hyperparathyroidism
>
> - Bone pain
> - Arthralgia
> - Osteopenia/osteoporosis
> - Insufficiency fractures
> - Calcium pyrophosphate deposition disease/chondrocalcinosis
> - Metastatic calcification
> - Renal failure
> - Proximal myopathy with normal creatine kinase
> - Osteitis fibrosa cystica

---

itis fibrosa cystica (OFC). OFC is characterized by osteopenia, subperiosteal bone resorption and cyst formation, and the commonest areas to be involved are the distal phalanges, the distal clavicle and the skull. A cyst-like area with associated swelling is known as a Brown tumour. Due to early diagnosis, OFC is now a rare phenomenon.

An elevated or inappropriately normal PTH level in the presence of raised serum calcium confirms hyperparathyroidism. This is in contrast to the hypercalcaemia of malignancy, the second commonest cause of a raised calcium, where the PTH will be suppressed. Phosphate levels will be in the low normal or low range and bone alkaline phosphatase will be raised.

Hyperadrenocortisolism

This can either be congenital, acquired or iatrogenic from corticosteroid treatment. Before epiphyseal closure, hypercortisolism leads to growth retardation and a reduction in peak bone mass. The clinical picture in adults is called Cushing's syndrome (CS). The most important musculoskeletal manifestation in CS is bone loss and increased fracture risk. Myopathy with a normal creatine kinase is common in CS and may be severe. With treatment, the majority of the musculoskeletal manifestations are reversible. The bone mass may take up to 10 years to recover, during which fracture risk remains increased, and recovery may be incomplete.

Acromegaly

The clinical syndrome associated with acromegaly is due to an excess of growth hormone (GH). This is usually secondary to a pituitary tumour. GH, via stimulation of insulin-like growth factor 1 (IGF-1), stimulates protein synthesis and, therefore, growth of all tissues producing characteristic changes in the bone and soft tissue of the musculoskeletal system. The overall impact on bone depends upon what other hormone deficiencies may be present. The musculoskeletal manifestations of acromegaly are shown in Box 14.4.

The arthritis in acromegaly is a biphasic process. Initially, there is joint pain in association with ligament laxity and cartilage overgrowth. This produces widened joint spaces on X-ray. The second stage is the development of premature and severe

> **Box 14.4**
> **Musculoskeletal manifestations of acromegaly**
>
> - Enlargement of the hands and feet
> - Arthralgia
> - Ligament laxity
> - Cartilage overgrowth
> - Osteoarthritis
> - Myalgia
> - Carpal tunnel syndrome
> - Chondrocalcinosis
> - Diffuse idiopathic skeletal hyperostosis
> - Spinal cord compression, nerve root compression and cauda equina syndrome
> - Kyphosis
> - Proximal myopathy with normal creatine kinase

> **Box 14.5**
> **Main musculoskeletal features of alkaptonuria**
>
> - Connective tissue pigmentation, 'ochre' in colour, visible in the sclera and pinna
> - Degenerative arthritis of spine and large joints
> - Acute inflammatory exacerbations of arthritis
> - Dense calcification of intervertebral discs

OA. Early OA in acromegaly gives the unusual pathognomonic X-ray appearance of osteophytes and a widened joint space compared to the narrow joint space usually associated with OA. Advanced acromegalic arthropathy is typical of advanced OA, but the distribution is unusual with frequent involvement of the non-weight-bearing joints. The most commonly affected joint is the hip.

An increased bone mineral density is recognized in acromegaly. Osteoporosis and insufficiency fractures also occur at an increased rate, but the osteoporosis occurs late in the disease and is secondary to hypogonadism, which is caused by the pituitary tumour.

Alkaptonuria (aka ochronosis)

Alkaptonuria is a rare autosomal recessive disease affecting 1 in 200 000 of the population and causing a deficiency of homogentisic acid oxidase. The disease manifests itself in the second and third decades. A classic sign is the oxidation of urine to a dark colour on standing. The main musculoskeletal features of alkaptonuria are shown in Box 14.5.

The main differential diagnoses are OA, ankylosing spondylitis (AS) and calcium pyrophosphate dihydrate (CPPD) deposition disease, which may co-exist. The lack of osteophytes and small-joint involvement in combination with major involvement of the non-weight-bearing joints helps to differentiate ochronotic arthropathy from OA. The absence of the classical syndesmophytes and sacroiliitis of AS helps to differentiate ochronotic arthropathy from AS. There is no specific treatment for the arthritis.

Osteoarticular disorders of renal origin

Patients with renal failure and on long-term dialysis are surviving for longer and musculoskeletal conditions (Table 14.5) are an important cause of morbidity and reduced quality of life.

β2-Microglobin amyloidosis

This is a consequence of chronic renal failure, not just long-term haemo- or peritoneal dialysis. β2-microglobulin amyloid is deposited in and around joints and tendons causing a spectrum of problems.

Diagnosis is by history and examination in combination with typical radiological findings and the classic Congo red staining of amyloid tissue on biopsy. A non-invasive test using ^{123}I-labelled serum amyloid P component (^{123}I-SAP) demonstrates increased radio-tracer uptake in the presence of amyloid deposition.

Treatment is mainly symptomatic. Successful renal transplantation can lead to an improvement in symptoms and a degree of regression of amyloid deposits. There is return with graft failure and recommencement of dialysis.

Table 14.5 Musculoskeletal manifestations in renal failure

Manifestation	Description
β2-microglobulin amyloidosis	Carpal tunnel syndrome (CTS), adhesive capsulitis (AC), symmetrical erosive arthropathy of small and large joints, erosive spondyloarthropathy often with cervical spine involvement, flexion contractures, bone cysts, pathological fractures within amyloid deposits in bone
Crystal arthropathies	Calcium phosphate, calcium pyrophosphate dihydrate (pseudogout), calcium oxalate, monosodium urate (gout)
Bone and joint infection	Septic arthritis, osteomyelitis, discitis
Erosive arthropathy	A painless erosive arthritis in dialysis patients without amyloidosis. A separate entity to osteoarthritis and rheumatoid arthritis
Carpal tunnel syndrome	37% of renal failure patients with CTS do not have amyloidosis. The underlying cause for the increased incidence is not known
Osteonecrosis	A small increase in osteonecrosis in patients on dialysis. A large increase after transplantation due to the high-dose corticosteroids
Secondary hyperparathyroidism	See hyperparathyroidism section

Crystal arthropathies

A variety of crystal deposition may occur in renal disease. The commonest crystal is calcium phosphate and, as well as producing an acute arthritis, periarticular deposition is frequent and usually asymptomatic. CPPD deposition disease is only slightly higher in patients with renal failure than in the general population. The X-ray appearance of chondrocalcinosis in renal failure may be produced by both CPPD and calcium oxalate deposition. Gout is common in patients with renal failure, but this risk returns to normal once dialysis is commenced.

Bone and joint infections

Renal failure, dialysis and immunosuppressive treatment for transplants all increase the risk of infection. The presence of pre-existing joint disease further increases the risk; patients with amyloid arthropathy are particularly susceptible. Septic arthritis is more often polyarticular in DM.

Primary hyperlipidaemia

The primary hyperlipidaemias are a common collection of disorders affecting 1 in 500 people. Musculoskeletal problems, although benign, are often the initial or an early complaint of familial hypercholesterolaemia. Early diagnosis has obvious cardiovascular benefits for the future.

The main musculoskeletal problem is tendon xanthomas typically of the Achilles tendon. In homozygotes these appear in childhood and in heterozygotes in early adulthood. An oligoarthritis and a non-deforming polyarthritis, often flitting in nature, may also occur.

Treatment is symptomatic; NSAIDs as required, but the use of these should be the minimum dose for the shortest duration to control the symptoms. This is to minimize the potential increase in a population that already has a significant risk of cardiovascular events. Rarely, excision is necessary. Aggressive treatment with lipid-lowering drugs can lead to regression in xanthoma size.

Lysosomal storage disorders

The lysosomal storage disorders include the glyco-sphingolipidoses and the mucopolysaccharidoses. The commonest type within each of the two groups is Gaucher's disease and Hurler's syndrome respectively (Table 14.6). These are a rare collection of genetic disorders, but have been included because the musculoskeletal manifestations are important causes of extraneurological morbidity. These disorders have a combined prevalence of 8–14 per 100 000 live births.

Table 14.6 Musculoskeletal manifestations of the common lysosomal storage disorders

Disorder	Enzyme deficiency	Manifestation
Gaucher's disease	β-glucosidase	Osteopenia, increased fracture risk, focal lytic/sclerotic lesions, osteonecrosis
Hurler's syndrome	α-L-iduronidase	Short stature, dyostosis multiplex*, craniofacial abnormalities, entrapment neuropathies, spondylolisthesis, degenerative arthritis

*Encompasses the radiological findings of large skull, hypoplastic vertebrae, gibbus deformity of the vertebrae, paddle-shaped ribs

Table 14.7 Glycogen storage disease types with prominent muscle symptoms

Glycogen storage disease type	Name	Enzyme deficiency	Manifestation
II (adult-onset subset)	Pompe disease (acid maltase deficiency)	α-1,4-glucosidase	Proximal myopathy and respiratory muscle weakness
V	McArdle disease	Myophosphorylase	Muscle fatigue, muscle cramp, weakness and rhabdomyolysis
VII	Tauri disease	Phosphofructokinase	

Recent developments in enzyme replacement therapy have altered the course of the diseases and the musculoskeletal complications.

Glycogen storage disease

These are a rare collection of genetic diseases, glycogen storage disease (GSD) I to VII with an overall incidence of 1 in 25 000 live births. Although the involvement of muscle is present in all types, the clinical picture is often dominated by other features including liver failure and severe hypoglycaemia. The only types likely to present to a rheumatologist are patients with GSD II (adult-onset subset), V and VII (Table 14.7). In these types the involvement of skeletal muscle dominates the clinical picture.

Haemochromatosis

Haemochromatosis is an autosomal recessive disease with an approximate incidence of 1 in 300.

Pathogenesis

There is increased iron absorption leading to iron deposition in the tissues and viscera. Chronic iron overload leads to tissue damage and subsequent fibrosis.

Clinical features

It has an equal sex incidence with onset in middle age in men, but is delayed to post-menopausal age in women. The symptoms and signs of the organ systems involved are listed in Box 14.6. The arthropathy is one of the commonest manifestations of haemochromatosis and is present in 40–60% of patients. It typically involves the metacarpophalangeal (MCP) joints of the index and middle fingers. Some 15–30% of patients suffer acute inflammatory episodes of arthritis secondary to CPPD deposition usually affecting the wrist and knees. The associated chondrocalcinosis can also be seen in the intevertebral discs and the symphysis pubis. One of the common mutations to cause haemochromatosis is also associated with porphyria cutanea tarda.

Investigations

Abnormal liver function tests (LFTs) support the diagnosis, which is confirmed by demonstrating iron overload with a high serum ferritin. Liver biopsy also demonstrates excess iron in the parenchymal cells. Plain X-ray demonstrates typical

> **Box 14.6**
> **Clinical manifestations of haemochromatosis**
>
> - Porphyria cutanea tarda
> - Skin pigmentation
> - Chronic arthropathy
> - Chondrocalcinosis
> - Cardiomyopathy
> - Hepatic cirrhosis
> - Hepatocellular carcinoma
> - Diabetes
> - Hypogonadism

changes of OA with joint space narrowing, osteophytes and sclerosis.

Differential diagnosis

Secondary iron overload from repeated transfusions, for example for thalassaemia. Alcoholic liver disease can cause abnormal liver function tests (LFTs) and a raised ferritin.

Treatment

Excess iron is removed by regular venesection. Menstrual blood loss is the reason presentation is delayed in women. Iron chelating agents may be used. The arthropathy does not respond to venesection and is managed symptomatically with analgesia and NSAIDs. The latter should be used with caution in liver disease. Diagnostic awareness of the arthropathy associated with haemochromatosis may allow early diagnosis and instigation of effective treatment in the pre-cirrhotic stage, which then has a good prognosis. Once cirrhosis has developed there is a 200-fold increased risk of hepatocellular carcinoma.

FURTHER READING

Ardic F, Soyupek F, Kahraman Y, Yorgancioglu R 2003 The musculoskeletal complications seen in type II diabetics: predominance of hand involvement. Clin Rheumatol 22: 229–233.

Birklein F 2005 Complex regional pain syndrome. J Neurol 252: 131–138.

Carnevale V, Romagnoli E, D'Erasmo E 2004 Skeletal involvement in patients with diabetes mellitus. Diabetes Metab Res Rev 20: 196–204.

Guzman J, Esmail R, Karjalalainen K et al 2001 Multidisciplinary rehabilitation for chronic low back pain: systematic review. BMJ 322: 1511–1516.

Jacobs-Kosmin D, DeHoratius RJ 2005 Musculoskeletal manifestations of endocrine disorders. Curr Opin Rheumatol 17: 64–69.

Kay J, Bardin T 2000 Osteoarticular disorders of renal origin: disease-related and iatrogenic Baillieres Clin Rheumatol 14(2): 285–305.

Lemstra M, Olszynski WP 2005 The effectiveness of multidisciplinary rehabilitation in the treatment of fibromyalgia: a randomized controlled trial. Clin J Pain 21: 166–174.

Mannerkorpi K 2005 Exercise in fibromyalgia. Curr Opin Rheumatol 17: 190–194.

Ong BN, Evans D, Bartlam A 2005 A patient's journey with myalgic encephalomyelitis. BMJ 330: 648–650.

Roberts CGP, Ladenson PW 2004 Skeletal involvement in patients with diabetes mellitus. Lancet 363: 793–803.

Sandstrom MJ, Keefe FJ 1998 Self-management of fibromyalgia: the role of formal coping skills training and physical exercise training programs. Arthritis Care Res 11: 432–447.

15

OSTEOARTHRITIS AND CRYSTAL ARTHROPATHIES

George Nuki

Cases relevant to this chapter

68, 70–72, 76, 86, 92, 98

● Essential facts

1. Osteoarthritis (OA) is the clinical and pathological outcome of a range of factors that lead to pain, disability and structural failure in synovial joints.

2. By the age of 65, 80% of people have radiographic evidence of OA affecting the spine, hips, knees, hands and feet, but only one in four are symptomatic.

3. There is only a weak relationship between symptoms and radiographic evidence of structural changes of OA.

4. Structural failure of articular cartilage, bone and periarticular tissues results from abnormal mechanical stresses in normal joints or normal forces in abnormal joints.

5. OA is a dynamic process of remodelling and proliferation of new bone, cartilage and connective tissues, as well as focal degeneration of articular cartilage.

6. Insidious pain occurs as a result of increased pressure or microfractures in the subchondral bone, low-grade synovitis, inflammatory effusions, capsular distension, enthesitis or muscle spasm, and nocturnal aching may be associated with hyperaemia in the subchondral bone.

7. Consider a predisposing underlying condition in patients with OA before the age of 40 or if OA develops in unusual sites.

8. Focal joint space narrowing and the presence of osteophytes are the main radiographic features of OA.

9. Medical treatment of OA is to relieve symptoms, maintain and improve joint function, and minimize disability and handicap; optimal management requires a combination of non-pharmacological and pharmacological modalities.

10. Surgical management of OA is indicated where medical therapy has failed; joint replacement is effective and cost-effective irrespective of age.

11. Calcium pyrophosphate dihydrate crystals are deposited at entheses, in hyaline cartilage and fibrocartilage, and are associated with chondrocalcinosis and degenerative changes; shedding of crystals into joints can provoke acute synovitis (pseudogout) or chronic pyrophosphate arthropathy.

12. Calcific periarthritis is due to periarticular deposition of hydroxyapatite.

13. Acute gout usually presents as monoarthritis in a distal joint of the foot or hand.

14. Recurrent attacks of gout cause progressive cartilage and bone erosion, deposition of palpable masses of urate crystals ('tophi'), and an asymmetrical erosive inflammatory polyarthritis.

15. Allopurinol is the drug of choice for the long-term management of recurrent acute attacks, or chronic gout.

Table 15.1 Subsets of osteoarthritis

Primary (idiopathic)	Secondary
Localized • Hands and feet • Knee • Hip • Spine	Post-traumatic Congenital/developmental Localized • Hip disease, e.g. Perthes' • Mechanical and local factors, e.g. obesity, hypermobility, varus–valgus
Other Generalized (three or more joints)	Generalized • Bone dysplasia • Metabolic Calcium deposition disease • Calcium pyrophosphate deposition disease • Hydroxyapatite arthropathy • Destructive arthropathies Other bone and joint disorders • Avascular necrosis • Rheumatoid arthritis • Paget's disease Miscellaneous other diseases • Endocrine, e.g. acromegaly, neuropathic

192

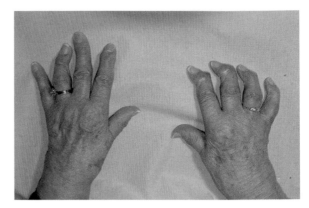

FIGURE 15.1   Hand osteoarthritis

OSTEOARTHRITIS

Osteoarthritis (OA), also sometimes called osteoarthrosis or degenerative joint disease, is not a single disease, but rather the clinical and pathological outcome of a range of disorders and conditions that lead to pain, disability and structural failure in synovial joints. OA is conventionally classified as being *primary* (idiopathic) or *secondary,* when it follows some clearly defined predisposing disorder or disease (Table 15.1), but it is becoming increasingly apparent that the development of all types of OA is associated with multiple aetiological factors.

EPIDEMIOLOGY

OA is the commonest type of arthritis. Radiographic and autopsy surveys show a steady age-related increase in prevalence from the age of 30. By the age of 65, 80% of people have some radiographic evidence of OA, although only one in four is symptomatic. The joints most frequently affected are the spine, hips, knees and some of the small joints of the hands and feet (Fig. 15.1). Community-based studies in the UK have shown that 10% of the population over the age of 55 have troublesome knee pain and, of those, 25% are severely disabled. OA is the leading cause of physical disability in people over the age of 65. The prevalence of both radiographically defined OA, and of OA-related disability, is greater in women than in men. Although disability associated with OA also increases steadily with age, the majority of people with OA-related disability in the community are between the ages of 55 and 75.

Risk factors for OA include constitutional factors such as age, gender, the shape and alignment of joints, obesity and some genetic determinants, but there are also important environmental triggers, such as previous injury or the repetitive trauma associated with certain recreational activities, such as weightlifting or long-distance running, and with some occupations, such as mining and farming. Mechanical factors play a role in the pathogenesis of all types of primary, as well as secondary, OA. Joint failure occurs when mechanical stresses overwhelm the capacity of articular tissues to resist and repair the damage. Structural failure of the *articular* cartilage, bone and periarticular tissues can result from abnormal mechanical stresses damaging previously normal tissues, or from the failure of pathologically impaired joint tissues in response to physiologically normal mechanical forces (Fig. 15.2). Obesity, joint malalignment, occupational trauma and muscle weakness are all important, potentially modifiable, biomechanical risk factors, which determine the site and severity of the disease. *Race and ethnicity*

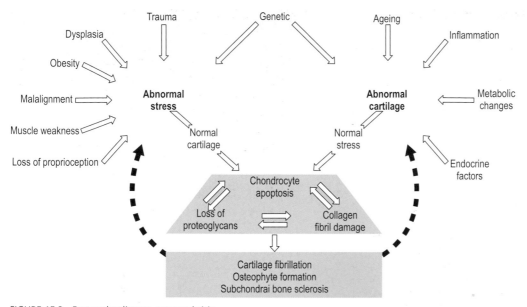

FIGURE 15.2   Factors leading to osteoarthritis

have some influence on the probability of developing OA at different sites. While OA of the knee is prevalent in all ethnic groups (particularly frequent in black women), hip, hand and generalized OA are seen predominantly in Caucasians. *Genetic factors* are known to be important determinants. Twin studies suggest hereditability of up to 65% in primary OA of the hand and knee, but the susceptibility genes themselves still remain largely undefined.

Progress has been made in identifying mutations in collagen genes that are associated with different types of bone and cartilage dysplasia where OA is part of a more complex phenotype, but none of these single gene mutations in genes that code for structural matrix proteins appears to be important in determining susceptibility to the common types of OA. Recently, however, there has been some progress in identifying polymorphisms in genes that code for signalling proteins involved in the development and maintenance of articular cartilage, which do appear to be associated with susceptibility to hip OA in certain ethnic groups (see Chapter 3).

PATHOLOGY AND PATHOGENESIS

OA involves all tissues of the joint (subchondral bone, ligaments, capsule and synovial membrane) as well as the articular cartilage, but inflammatory changes in the synovium are usually minor and secondary. To a variable extent OA is always a dynamic process characterized by remodelling of the anatomy of the joint and *proliferation* of new bone, cartilage and connective tissues in the form of *osteophytes*, as well as by focal *degeneration* of articular cartilage. While in many cases these processes reach a state of non-progressive equilibrium, in others there is symptomatic failure of the joint characterized by progressive degeneration of the articular cartilage with fibrillation, fissuring, ulceration and, eventually, full-thickness, focal loss of the cartilage at sites of joint loading. In addition, with wear, there is compaction and sclerosis ('eburnation') of the adjacent subchondral bone and the formation of bone cysts (Fig. 15.3). The biomechanical properties of the cortical and subchondral bone play an important role in protecting articular cartilage following impact loading. It is suggested that the pathogenesis of OA in some cases may be initiated by an increase in the density and stiffness of the subchondral bone following the healing of microfractures caused by unprotected impulsive loading of joints. The consequent loss of bone viscoelasticity results in steep stiffness gradients in the bone. This in turn results in stretching and fibrillation of the overlying articular cartilage, as well as focal osteonecrosis and the formation of bone cysts. In support of this hypothesis patients with hip and knee OA have higher than normal bone mass and there is evidence that focal increases in subchondral bone density can precede and predict future cartilage loss in patients with OA of the knee. The sequence of pathological and biochemical changes in the articular cartilage in OA follows a characteristic pattern (Table 15.2), whether primary or secondary to changes in the subchondral bone. Early increases in matrix hydration and articular cartilage thickness follow disruption of the collagen fibre network, loss of tensile strength in the superficial zone of the articular car-

tilage and swelling of the negatively charged, high-molecular-weight proteoglycan, aggrecan. Initially, chondrocyte activation and proliferation of clusters of chondrocytes are associated with an *anabolic* response with increased synthesis and turnover of matrix collagens and proteoglycans, but in the later stages of OA, *catabolism* of cartilage matrix proteins outstrips the capacity for cartilage repair. Anabolic mediators include growth factors, such as the insulin-like growth factor (IGF-1), fibroblast growth factor (FGF) and transforming growth factor β (TGFβ), and the bone morphogenetic proteins (BMPs): the anti-inflammatory cytokine interleukin-4 and proteinase inhibitors, such as tissue inhibitors of metalloproteinases (TIMPs) and plasminogen activator inhibitor (PAI). Catabolic mediators include nitric oxide, prostaglandins and the pro-inflammatory cytokines interleukin-1 (IL-1β), tumour necrosis factor (TNFα), IL-6 and IL-17; as well as metalloproteinases (MMPs 1,8,13) and aggrecanases (ADAM-TS 4, 5).

CLINICAL FEATURES

Pain is the presenting symptom in the majority of patients. Usually insidious in onset and intermittent at first, the pain is typically aching in character. Initially, it is provoked by weight-bearing or movement of the joint, and relieved by rest, but as the disease progresses the pain may be more prolonged and experienced at rest, and may become

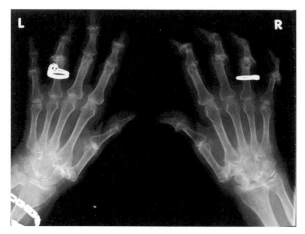

FIGURE 15.3 Radiographic appearances of osteoarthritis, showing loss of joint space and sclerosis in both hands especially at the first carpometacarpal joint

Table 15.2 Structural, cellular and biochemical changes in articular cartilage in osteoarthritis

Structural change	Cellular change	Biochemical change
Early changes		
↑ Cartilage thickness	Collagen fibre network disrupted, leading to: ↓ Collagen fibrillogenesis ↑ Chondrocyte activation ↑ Chondrocyte proliferation	↑ PG synthesis and content ↑ Chondroitin sulphate ↓ Keratan sulphate ↑ Water content ↑ Cartilage oligomeric protein ↓ Aggrecan size ↑ Collagen synthesis Chondroitin sulphate neoepitopes re-expressed
Later changes		
↓ Cartilage thickness Fibrillation	Chondrocyte apoptosis	↓ PG synthesis and content ↓ Aggrecan ↓ Chondroitin sulphate ↓ Collagen synthesis

severe enough to wake the patient at night. Prolonged early morning stiffness is not a feature as it is in rheumatoid arthritis and other predominantly inflammatory joint diseases, but a few minutes of early morning stiffness and transient stiffness (gelling) after rest are common. Pain in OA can emanate from all the tissues of the joint, except the articular cartilage, which is aneural. Pain may result from increased pressure or microfractures in the subchondral bone, from low-grade synovitis, inflammatory effusions, capsular distension, enthesitis or muscle spasm, and nocturnal aching may be associated with hyperaemia in the subchondral bone. Associated anxiety and depression are not uncommon, and these can amplify pain and disability. There is only a weak relationship between symptoms and radiographic evidence of structural changes of OA at all joint sites, although the correlation between pain and structural changes is somewhat stronger in the weight-bearing joints (hip>knee) than in the small joints of the hands. Functional impairment as a result of restriction of movement can be the presenting complaint in patients with OA of the hands, hip or knee, even in the absence of pain. Physical signs associated with osteoarthritis include: restriction of movement of joints as a result of capsular fibrosis or blocking by osteophytes, palpable bony swelling, periarticular or joint-line tenderness, deformities with or without joint instability, muscle weakness and wasting in addition to occasional joint effusions, and palpable or even audible joint crepitus.

COMMON CLINICAL PRESENTATIONS

The salient features of the common types of hip, knee, hand and nodal generalized OA are summarized in Table 15.3.

Hip OA commonly affects the superior pole of the joint. Typically, patients present with pain in the groin on exercise, but referred pain in the buttock, anterior thigh, the knee and even the lower leg are not uncommon. With increasing severity it radiates down to the knee, is constant on exercise, and begins to cause stiffness and inability to reach down to tie shoe-laces. Pain begins to disturb sleep. Enjoyment of active hobbies is curtailed and eventually life becomes a misery. The natural history often ends in bony ankylosis in flexion.

Characteristically, examination reveals an antalgic gait with painful restriction of internal rotation

Table 15.3 Common clinical types/patterns of osteoarthritis

Knee osteoarthritis	Hip osteoarthritis	Hand osteoarthritis
Patello-femoral and medial joint compartments	Supero-lateral or central (medial or polar)	Distal interphalangeal and proximal interphalangeal joints, carpometacarpal (CMC) joints of the thumbs
Knee pain Pain on walking ↑uneven ground ↑stairs Antalgic gait Difficulty rising from chairs	Groin pain → thigh/medial side of the knee → buttock Antalgic gait Difficulty with socks and toenails	Pain/swelling/stiffness + Restricted movements Symptoms often settle Hand function preserved Frequent family history
Bilateral>unilateral	Unilateral>bilateral	Usually bilateral
Women>men	Women>men	Women≫men Perimenopausal onset
Varus>valgus or Fixed flexion deformities Joint-line tenderness Joint-line bony swelling Crepitus Quads muscle wasting	Pain/restricted movements: internal rotation (early), external rotation/abduction (later) Fixed flexion/ext. rotation Limb shortening Quads/gluteal muscle weakness and/or wasting	Heberden's nodes ± Bouchard's nodes Subluxation 1st CMC Squaring of hand Associated with OA in other joints (especially knees and medial OA of the hips)

with the hip in flexion. Medial pole OA is less common. It occurs more frequently in women, is more frequently bilateral and less frequently progresses. In patients with nodal generalized OA, the pattern of hip involvement is usually also medial or concentric. Bony destruction of the acetabulum or femoral head may lead to a 'bobbing' short-leg gait. A Trendelenburg gait is rare, but a coxalgic (Duchenne) gait is more common due to a desire to off-load the hip abductor muscles and hence reduce the joint reaction force, which is often three times body weight in single-leg stance. There is little to see apart from thigh wasting and, perhaps, fixed flexion. Tenderness is rare. Range of movement reveals a global deficit and fixed flexion, reduced adduction and internal rotation are often seen. Rotation is often the most 'irritable' of the movements.

Anteroposterior radiographs of the hip and pelvis should be carefully inspected to detect cardinal features of osteoarthritis. Destructive arthropathy and avascular necrosis may be associated with non-steroidal anti-inflammatory drug (NSAID) therapy.

Knee OA commonly affects the medial and patello-femoral compartments of the joint, but may affect any of the three compartments. The medial compartment in most frequently affected, and leads to a varus deformity. Forces that occur on weight-bearing will pass medial to the knee and this increases point-loading in the medial compartment. Typically, patients present with anterior or medial knee pain aggravated by walking on uneven ground and by ascending or descending stairs. On examination they frequently have a characteristic antalgic gait and bilateral, symmetrical varus deformities. In some patients knee OA is associated with nodal generalized OA. Unilateral knee OA, especially in men, may be a consequence of a previous injury, meniscus tear or complete meniscal resection.

Nodal osteoarthritis is a clinically distinct form of primary generalized OA, with a strong genetic component. It is much more frequent in women than in men and characteristically affects the interphalangeal (IP) joints of the fingers (DIPs>PIPs) and the carpometacarpal joints of the thumbs. The onset, which is sometimes subacute with considerable pain, swelling and local inflammation, is often in the perimenopausal period, and may be triggered by oestrogen withdrawal and other endocrine changes at this time. Although multiple joints in both hands are frequently affected, the onset is typically episodic and additive in pattern, with each joint going through a sequence of changes over a number of months. Pain, soft-tissue swelling and tenderness are followed by the gradual development of hard, bony swellings on either side of the extensor tendons on the dorsal aspect of the fingers in relationship to the IP joints. Heberden's nodes at the DIPs are more frequent than Bouchard nodes at the PIPs. After the inflammation has settled patients are left with relatively pain-free, knobbly fingers. Although the lesions can be associated with considerable deformity and subluxation, serious disability is unusual. In nodal generalized OA osteophyte formation and subluxation of the 1st carpometacarpal joints results in characteristic 'squaring' of the hands, and the knees and other joints may be also affected. Rarely, in cases with a more acute onset ('hot Heberden's nodes'), the initial soft-tissue inflammation is associated with the development of cysts containing hyaluronate. *Erosive OA* is the name sometimes given to describe a rarer variant of nodal osteoarthritis, which is characterized by similar episodic symptoms and signs of local inflammation followed by the development of more destructive subchondral erosions associated with florid proliferation of bone, instability and subluxation in the proximal and distal interphalangeal joints.

ATYPICAL AND 'SECONDARY' OSTEOARTHRITIS

The possibility of some defined predisposing underlying condition (see Table 15.1) needs to be considered, particularly in patients who develop typical symptoms and signs of OA before the age of 40, in those that develop OA in joints that are usually not affected, and in those with certain characteristic patterns of joint involvement. A history of major preceding trauma, such as a fracture that resulted in articular cartilage damage or subsequent malalignment, is often found to be the cause of monoarticular OA developing at an early age or in a joint, such as the ankle, that is seldom otherwise affected. Nearly 50% of patients have knee OA 21 years after open meniscectomy and the average time to develop hip OA following a fracture dislocation is 7 years. Early-onset OA with prominent involvement of the 2nd and 3rd metacarpophalangeal joints is very characteristic in patients with haemochromatosis and may be an early clinical clue that leads to establishment of the diagnosis. Although deposition of calcium pyrophosphate dihydrate (CPPD) and basic calcium phosphate (BCP or apatite) crystals is common in articular cartilage in OA, the possibility of familial CPPD disease should always be considered in patients presenting with premature knee OA. This is especially important when the knee OA is accompanied by frequent inflammatory episodes or prominent hypertrophic radiographic features and in patients presenting with OA in relatively atypical joints, such as the shoulder, elbow or radiocarpal joints in the wrists.

INVESTIGATIONS

Plain radiographs are widely used to assess the severity of the structural changes in patients with OA. Because radiographic evidence of OA is so frequent in asymptomatic middle-aged and elderly persons, radiographs are much less useful in the differential diagnosis of arthritis in patients presenting with articular symptoms. Focal, rather than uniform, joint space narrowing and the presence of osteophytes are the main radiographic features, with subchondral bone sclerosis and cysts in more advanced cases. Ossified synovial loose bodies and chondrocalcinosis can also sometimes be detected on plain radiographs. In order to assess the extent to which joint space narrowing reflects loss of articular cartilage in the tibiofemoral joints, standing radiographs are required.

Magnetic resonance imaging (MRI) is being developed for the earlier and more quantitative detection of articular cartilage changes, including changes in hydration and proteoglycan composition, but has yet to be refined and validated sufficiently to make it useful in clinical practice. This is also true of isotope scans with ^{99}Tc-labelled bisphosphonate, which in research studies have been proved to show increased uptake of isotope in OA joints that subsequently go on to develop progressive structural changes. MRI is, however, useful for detecting intra-articular soft-tissue lesions, such as meniscus tears, and for the diagnosis of osteonecrosis. Bone scintigraphy is indicated for the detection of osteonecrosis, stress fractures and bone metastases.

Blood tests are not helpful in the diagnosis or management of OA and are largely used to exclude other diseases associated with systemic inflammation or metabolic abnormalities. For example, measurements of serum calcium and alkaline phosphatase are critical for the diagnosis of primary hyperparathyroidism and hypophosphatasia; measurement of serum ferritin is required for the diagnosis of haemochromatosis; and detection of homogentisic acid in the urine will confirm a diagnosis of ochronosis.

Although cartilage degradation products, such as hyaluronan, keratan sulphate and cartilage oligomeric protein, and cartilage synthesis markers, such as Type II collagen c-propeptide, have been shown to be increased in the plasma, synovial fluid or urine of patients with OA, there are currently no biochemical or molecular markers that have clinical utility for diagnosis, monitoring the progress of structural changes or assessing the prognosis of OA in clinical practice.

Synovial fluid analysis in OA is really only indicated to exclude bacterial joint infection. The fluid is usually clear and viscous with a low cell count. Detection of crystals by polarizing light microscopy is not helpful in distinguishing OA from primary crystal deposition disorders, as crystals of CPPD and BCP are each detected in up to half of all effusions from patients with knee OA.

MANAGEMENT

Treatment is predominantly directed at relieving symptoms, maintaining and improving joint function, and minimizing disability and handicap. Optimal management of patients with all types of OA requires a combination of non-pharmacological and pharmacological modalities.

Non-pharmacological modalities of therapy

- All patients should be provided with access to information and education about the objectives of treatment and the importance of changes in life-style, exercise, weight reduction, and in other measures to unload the damaged joint. The initial focus should be on self-help and patient-driven treatments, rather than on passive therapies delivered by health professionals.
- All patients with lower limb OA should be given advice about appropriate footwear with

thick, soft soles. Laterally wedged insoles can give symptomatic relief to some patients with medial tibio-femoral compartment knee OA.

- Patients with symptomatic OA of the hip or knee can benefit from referral to a physiotherapist for: a) assessment and instruction in appropriate exercises to reduce pain and improve functional capacity, and b) assessment and provision and instruction in the use of a stick or walker in appropriate circumstances.
- Patients with hip and knee OA should be encouraged to undertake and continue with regular aerobic, muscle-strengthening and range-of-movement exercises. Pool exercises can be effective in patients with symptomatic hip OA associated with muscle spasm.
- Patellar taping can provide short-term symptom relief in some patients with patello-femoral OA.
- A knee brace can reduce pain, improve stability and reduce the risk of falls in patients with knee OA associated with mild/moderate varus or vagus instability.
- Heat packs, ice packs, acupuncture and transcutaneous electrical nerve stimulation have all been shown to be effective modalities for helping with short-term pain control in some patients with knee OA in controlled trials.

Pharmacological modalities of therapy

- Paracetamol (up to 4 g daily) should be the analgesic of first choice for patients with symptomatic OA.
- In patients who do not respond adequately to a trial of paracetamol, the choice of alternative or additional analgesics needs to take into account both the relative efficacy and safety of the drug or drug combination being considered as well as concomitant medication and co-morbidities.
- In some patients who do not respond adequately to paracetamol, NSAIDs at the lowest effective doses can be added or substituted, but long-term use of NSAIDs should be avoided if possible. In patients with increased gastrointestinal risk, a COX2 selective agent or a non-selective NSAID with

co-prescription of a proton pump inhibitor or misoprostol for gastroprotection can be considered.

- All NSAIDs (including COX2 selective agents) should be used with caution in patients with cardiovascular risk factors.
- Topical NSAIDs or topical capsaicin can be effective as adjuncts or alternatives to oral analgesics in some patients with symptomatic knee OA.
- Intra-articular injections with corticosteroids can be considered in patients with moderate-to-severe pain who are not responding adequately to oral analgesic/anti-inflammatory agents and in patients with symptomatic knee OA with effusions or other physical signs of local inflammation.
- Intra-articular injections of hyaluronate can be helpful in some patients with knee OA who are unresponsive to, or intolerant of, repeated injections of intra-articular corticosteroids.
- Treatment with glucosamine and/or chondroitin sulfate may provide symptomatic benefit in patients with knee OA. If no response is apparent within 6 months, treatment should be discontinued. The evidence that these agents may also have structure-modifying effects in slowing the progression of articular cartilage loss remains inconclusive.
- The use of opioids and narcotic analgesics can be considered in exceptional circumstances for the treatment of severe, refractory pain where other pharmacological agents have been ineffective or are contra-indicated. Non-pharmacological therapies should be continued in such patients and surgical treatments should be considered.

Surgery

Patients with hip or knee OA, who are not obtaining adequate pain relief and functional improvement from a combination of non-pharmacological and pharmacological treatment, should be considered for joint replacement surgery. Replacement arthroplasties are effective and cost-effective interventions for patients with significant symptoms and/or functional limitations associated with a reduced health-related quality of life, despite conservative therapy, irrespective of age. Patients unfit for general anaesthesia can sometimes be considered for surgery using a regional anaesthesia, but active sepsis, leg ulcers and significant peripheral vascular disease are important contra-indications.

By far the commonest surgical procedure for hip OA is total hip replacement (arthroplasty). Over 50 000 are performed annually in the UK. Patient-derived outcome measures for locomotor disease (for example the Short Form (SF) 12 questionnaire) reveal that the quality of life improves dramatically after a successful total hip arthroplasty. The first durable hip replacement, the Charnley low-friction arthroplasty, was developed by Sir John Charnley in the early 1960s and some of his patients still have their implants to this day. His solution to the difficult problem of developing a durable surface with little wear-debris and a low coefficient of friction was to articulate a metal ball within a polyethylene (plastic) socket. Most hip replacements in the UK are cemented into the bone (Fig. 15.4), although uncemented components, which rely on a strong bond between elastic bone and a tightly fitting metal surface, are frequently used in Europe and the USA. In recent years younger patients have been deemed suitable for metal-on-metal hip replacements, which simply resurface the joint (Fig. 15.5).

For a new type of hip replacement to be introduced in the UK it has to be shown to have a 3-year survival rate of 97%. This is the minimum achieved by current generations of hip replacements. The elderly have the best chance of their hip replacement outliving them. Younger patients will have a high chance of revision surgery at some time in the future as the bearing surface wears down or the implant's fixation to bone loosens. Overall, about one-quarter of hip replacement surgery is for revision of an implant.

Counselling a patient about a hip replacement before surgery is essential. OA of the hip can be distressing and disabling, but is not directly life-threatening. On the other hand, surgery can be fatal. The usual indication is for failure of non-surgical management of hip arthritis. About 90% of patients achieve a pain-free hip once recovery from the operation is complete. Overall, the risks of surgery are: death 1%, infection 1–2%, dislocation 1–2% and loosening 1% per annum to 10 years. Individual surgeon, implant and patient factors will greatly modify these broad figures.

Infection after joint arthroplasty is a major concern and is often impossible to eradicate. It is possible that almost every joint is colonized by bacteria at the time of implantation, but frank infection occurs only on the rare occasions when the balance of host response to pathogen virulence favours infection. Hospital-acquired infections, such as MRSA (methicillin-resistant *Staphylococcus aureus*) and VRE (vancomycin-resistant enterococcus), have well known tenacity. Almost equally

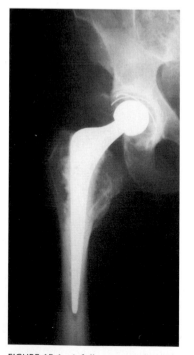

FIGURE 15.4   A fully cemented metal-on-polyethylene total hip replacement

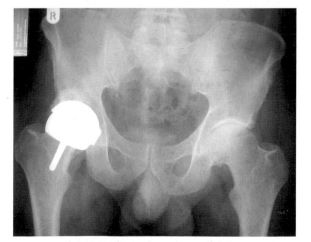

FIGURE 15.5   A resurfacing metal-on-metal total hip replacement

difficult to treat is the skin-borne *Staphylococcus epidermidis*, which now contributes to more than half of infected arthroplasties. Early infections (within 2 weeks) can often be treated with joint debridement. Later infections cause loosening of the implant or cement interface with bone, and these need to be revised. This may be done in one stage (less morbidity, lower infection eradication rate), in two stages separated by 6 weeks or by implant removal, known as a 'Girdlestone' excision arthroplasty (greater morbidity, higher infection eradication rate).

In young and physically active patients with significant symptoms from unicompartmental knee OA, high tibial osteotomy may offer an alternative intervention that can delay the need for joint replacement for about 10 years. Osteotomy and joint-preserving surgical procedures should be considered in young adults with symptomatic hip or knee OA, especially when there is dysplasia or varus/valgus deformity. Total joint replacement, however, results in pain relief and improved function within 4 months of surgery, but the range of movement may not be improved. Over 90% of these prostheses will survive for 15 years. Infection is difficult to eradicate in total joint arthroplasty and very occasionally transfemoral amputation is undertaken for intractable infection. The risk–benefit analysis is otherwise very similar to that for total hip arthroplasty. Lateral compartment OA occurs less commonly. Reasons should be sought, which include a congenitally hypoplastic lateral femoral condyle, inflammatory arthritis and an arthritic hip causing an adducted thigh. Where hip and knee arthritis occur together, the hip is usually replaced first. Early patello-femoral arthritis can respond well to physiotherapy. In patients with unicompartmental disease, unicompartmental knee replacement is effective, although a total knee replacement may prove more durable. In patients with OA of the knee, joint fusion can be considered as a salvage procedure when joint replacement has failed.

NATURAL HISTORY AND PROGNOSIS

Progression and prognosis in patients with OA is to some extent joint specific, with subsets of patients with knee, hip and hand OA that progress at different rates. Structural changes in knee OA

usually evolve slowly over a number of years with some patients remaining stable for years at a time. Clinical and radiographic deterioration does, however, occur in one- to two-thirds of patients followed up for 15 years despite frequent early improvement in pain and mobility.

Knee pain and radiographic evidence of OA in the contralateral knee are both predictors of disease progression. One-half to two-thirds of patients with hip OA also progress over 10 years, but patients with medial or concentric pattern OA hip, which is sometimes associated with nodal generalized OA, generally have a better prognosis. Rapid progression of hip disease was formerly thought to be associated with osteonecrosis and consumption of NSAIDs ('analgesic hip'), but other groups of patients who have not taken analgesics have been found to have an identical clinical course and pathology. Fifty per cent of patients with hand OA and DIP joint involvement also show evidence of radiographic progression over 10 years, despite early improvement in symptoms. Progression of structural deterioration is generally slower in the PIP joints and the CMC joint of the thumb. The presence of nodal OA has been found to be associated with a sixfold increase in the risk of progression of knee OA and it also increases the likelihood of developing OA following meniscectomy considerably. Other risk factors associated with *progression* of knee OA include obesity, low bone density, chondrocalcinosis, knee effusions and low intakes of vitamins C and D, as well as mechanical determinants, such as injury, joint instability and varus–valgus malalignment.

CRYSTAL ARTHRITIS AND DEPOSITION-ASSOCIATED DISEASE

A variety of crystals can be associated with acute and chronic arthritis, bursitis, tendonitis, periarthritis and deposition in connective tissues (Table 15.4).

CRYSTAL FORMATION AND PATHOGENESIS (Fig. 15.6)

Crystals form in tissues when the concentration of their chemical constituents exceeds their solubility

Table 15.4 Common associations with crystal deposition

Crystal	Association
Calcium pyrophosphate dihydrate (CPPD)	Acute pseudogout Sub-acute/chronic arthritis Chondrocalcinosis
Basic calcium phosphates	Calcific periarthritis/tendonitis Sub-acute/chronic arthritis Calcinosis
Calcium oxalate	Acute arthritis in renal dialysis patients
Monosodium urate monohydrate (MSU)	Acute gouty arthritis Sub-acute/ chronic arthritis Tophi Renal calculous disease

Less common associations include acute arthritis/renal calculi with xanthine crystals in patients with xanthinuria and cholesterol crystals in patients with rheumatoid arthritis and chronic joint effusions.

threshold, but many tissues sustain supersaturated levels of relevant solutes for long periods without crystallization because of the presence of inhibitory proteins and ions. Crystal formation is also favoured by falls in local temperature, pH and by the presence of crystal *nucleators.* Microcrystals usually stimulate inflammation only after being shed into synovial joints or bursae following loosening in the adjacent connective tissue matrix. This can follow trauma, complex changes in the matrix during intercurrent illness or surgery, or, in the case of gout, after partial dissolution following the initiation of uric acid-lowering drug therapy. The microcrystals have a highly negatively charged, reactive surface that can be directly membranolytic, as well as having the capacity to activate leucocytes and bind numerous serum and cell membrane proteins. Although crystal-induced inflammation is largely a neutrophil-dependent process, driven by the capacity of protein-coated crystals to activate and recruit leucocytes, there is evidence to suggest that the initial interaction may be with resident macrophages through Toll-like receptors. Subsequent activation of

201

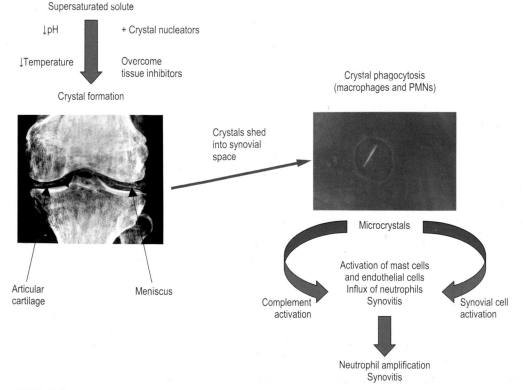

FIGURE 15.6 Mechanisms involved in crystal formation and crystal-induced inflammation

complement and vascular endothelial cells leads to vasodilatation, increased blood flow and ingress of polymorphonuclear leucocytes with release of cascades of inflammatory mediators. These include the pro-inflammatory cytokines IL-1, IL-6 and TNFα, prostaglandins, neutrophil chemotactic chemokines, such as IL-8, in addition to kinins and calgranulins that act as amplification factors.

CALCIUM PYROPHOSPHATE DIHYDRATE CRYSTAL DEPOSITION

Calcium pyrophosphate dihydrate (CPPD) crystals are deposited at entheses as well as in hyaline and, particularly, in fibrocartilage, where they are associated with chondrocalcinosis and degenerative changes. Shedding of crystals into the joint can provoke an attack of acute synovitis (pseudogout) and also a more chronic pyrophosphate arthropathy.

Epidemiology

Autopsy and radiographic surveys indicate that chondrocalcinosis is a common age-related phenomenon. The menisci and articular cartilage of the knees are most frequently affected, but radiographic chondrocalcinosis can also be seen in the triangular cartilage of the wrists, the intervertebral discs, the symphysis pubis and the labrum of the acetabulum of the hip, and occasionally at other sites The prevalence of radiographic chondrocalcinosis in the knees increases from less than 5% in people under the age of 70 to nearly 30% in those over the age of 85. Although the presence of chondrocalcinosis is usually unassociated with symptoms of joint disease, the age-adjusted prevalence of OA of the knee is modestly increased (women>men). Pyrophosphate arthropathy is two to three times more common in women than in men and usually presents in patients over the age of 70.

Causes and associations

While chondrocalcinosis and pseudogout are most frequently sporadic and idiopathic, crystal formation can follow the changes in matrix proteins and proteoglycans that occur with ageing and OA. Chondrocalcinosis, pseudogout and many cases of chronic pyrophosphate arthropathy can, however, be secondary to a range of inherited or acquired disorders associated with changes in pyrophosphate metabolism (Table 15.5). Overproduction of

Table 15.5 Causes of calcium pyrophosphate dihydrate crystal deposition, and associated disorders

	Association/metabolic cause
Sporadic	Ageing changes in matrix. ↑ Extracellular PPi due to *ANKH* mutations in some cases
Osteoarthritis	Changes in cartilage matrix
Metabolic diseases Haemochromatosis	Crystal nucleation and ↓ ALP and PPi degradation by iron
Wilson's disease	Crystal nucleation and ↓ ALP and PPi degradation by copper
Hypophosphatasia	↓PPi degradation due to absence of ALP
Hypomagnesaemia	Chronic diarrhoea, dietary deficiency, Bartter's disease, Gitelman's syndrome→ ↓Mg, co-factor for crystal solubility
Primary hyperparathyroidism	↑ Adenylate cyclase and PPi production
Gout	Crystal nucleation/co-precipitation by urate crystals
Familial disease	CCAL 1 (chondrocalcinosis 1) is associated with mutations in chromosome 8q CCAL 2 (chondrocalcinosis 2) is associated with mutations in the *ANKH* gene on chromosome 5p Spondyloepiphyseal dysplasia and CPPDD are associated with *COL2a* mutations

ALP, alkaline phosphatase; PPi, pyrophosphate; OA, osteoarthritis; CPPDD, calcium pyrophosphate dihydrate deposition disease.

inorganic pyrophosphate (PPi), the anionic component of crystals of CPPD, by hypertrophic chondrocytes, is a feature of some of these disorders. Extracellular PPi is generated by the ectoenzyme nucleoside triphosphate pyrophosphohydrolase (NTPPH) and the transmembrane pyrophosphate transporter ANKH. Mutations of the *ANKH* gene, which result in increases in extracellular PPi, have been found to be associated with some sporadic cases of pyrophosphate arthropathy, as well as with families with CPPD deposition. Paradoxically, PPi is also a potent inhibitor of crystallization of basic calcium phosphates (BCP), so that increased levels of PPi found in patients with hypophosphatasia lead to both CPPD deposition in the form of chondrocalcinosis and defective mineralization of bone with the BCP crystal hydroxyapatitite. Conversely, polymorphisms of NTPPH, which lead to markedly reduced extracellular PPi, have been associated with severe BCP crystal arthropathy.

Clinical presentation

CPPD is most frequently brought to clinical attention by the incidental finding of chondrocalcinosis on skeletal radiographs (Fig. 15.7).

Pseudogout is a common cause of acute inflammatory monoarthritis in the elderly. The knee is the site of more than half of all attacks, the duration of which can vary from a few days to 4 weeks. As its name implies, pseudogout can resemble acute gout with severe joint pain, swelling, tenderness and effusion associated with erythema of the overlying skin and systemic symptoms, so it is always important to consider the possibility of joint sepsis in the differential diagnosis. Subacute or 'petite' attacks are not uncommon and there is sometimes polyarticular clustering of acute episodes. Pseudogout occurs more frequently in men than in women.

Chronic pyrophosphate arthropathy is more common than pseudogout and occurs more frequently in elderly women. Symptoms and signs vary according to the intensity of the associated inflammation. A few patients have a persistent subacute inflammatory oligoarthritis lasting for months, that can be mistaken for rheumatoid arthritis, while more than half of all those affected have a much more indolent arthritis resembling osteoarthritis, punctuated in some cases by superimposed acute or subacute attacks. The knees are most frequently

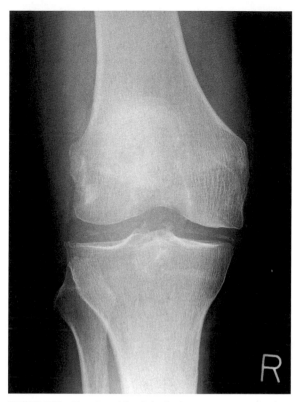

FIGURE 15.7 Chondrocalcinosis in the knee

affected, but chronic pyrophosphate arthritis may also involve the wrists, shoulders, elbows and metacarpophalangeal (MCP) joints in the hands, as well as the hips and the mid-tarsal joints in the feet. An arthritis resembling OA in the 2nd and 3rd MCP joints commencing before the age of 50 should alert one to the possibility of a haemochromatotic arthropathy associated with CPPD. In a minority of patients severe destructive changes associated with CPPD and subluxation of a knee or shoulder may resemble a neuropathic arthropathy (Charcot joint), without any associated neurological deficit.

Investigations

Examination of synovial fluid by compensated, polarizing light microscopy allows CPPD crystals to be detected and distinguished from crystals of monosodium urate monohydrate (Fig. 15.8). Gram stain and culture are required to exclude bacterial infection. Radiographs may show evidence of chondrocalcinosis in fibrocartilage or hyaline articular cartilage (see Fig. 15.7), but absence of visible

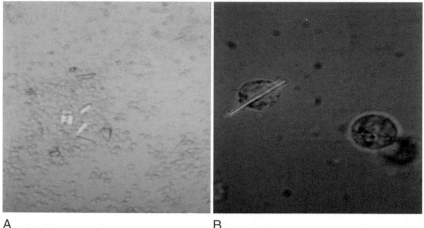

A   B

FIGURE 15.8 Compensated polarized light microscopy of synovial fluid. (A) Positively birefringent crystals of calcium pyrophosphate dihydrate (CPPD) from patient with pseudogout. (B) Negatively birefringent crystal of monosodium urate monohydrate from a patient with gout

chondrocalcinosis does not rule out the possibility of pseudogout or pyrophosphate arthritis.

Treatment

Joint aspiration and intra-articular injection of corticosteroids are the most effective means of treating an acute or sub-acute attack of pseudogout. NSAIDs and colchicine are less effective than they are in the treatment of classical gout, and great care must be taken when using them in elderly people.

BASIC CALCIUM PHOSPHATE (BCP) CRYSTAL DEPOSITION

Regulated deposition of the BCP crystal hydroxyapatite (HA) is essential for the formation of bones and teeth. However, pathological deposition of BCP crystals of hydroxyapatite, octacalcium phosphate, tricalcium phosphate and magnesium whitlockite in musculoskeletal tissues is associated with calcific periarthritis, the very destructive Milwaukee shoulder syndrome and many cases of OA. They are also responsible for *metastatic* calcification in a number of metabolic disorders and for ectopic, *dystrophic* calcification in a number of connective tissue diseases and in many situations where there has been damage to the connective tissue matrix (Table 15.6).

Calcific periarthritis results from periarticular inflammation in association with deposition of HA microcrystals. Acute episodes are characterized by local pain, heat, swelling and tenderness, sometimes accompanied by reddening of the overlying skin, and by systemic features of inflammation, such as fever and a raised C-reactive protein (CRP) and erythrocyte sedimentation rate (ESR). The shoulder region (supraspinatus tendon) is most frequently affected in middle-aged men or women, but monoarticular and polyarticular attacks can also occur in the region of the hip, knee, ankle, elbow or wrist. Attacks can be spontaneous or can follow trauma. Rarely, calcific periarthritis is familial, or secondary to metabolic disorders, such as chronic renal failure or hyperparathyroidism. In most cases, however, there is no serum biochemical abnormality. Radiographs show evidence of tendon-associated calcinosis, which sometimes disappears spontaneously following an acute attack. Aspiration of the subacromial bursa may reveal cloudy white fluid containing masses of HA crystal aggregates that stain for calcium with Alizarin red. Definitive crystal identification involves X-ray diffraction, infrared spectroscopy or electron microscopy, but is not required in clinical practice.

Acute attacks usually respond to symptomatic treatment with analgesics or NSAIDs. Aspiration and/or corticosteroid injection are seldom necessary and surgical excision is only very rarely required if massive deposits are the cause of painful impingement.

Table 15.6 Disorders associated with basic calcium phosphate crystal deposition

Musculoskeletal syndromes	Metabolic disorders with metastatic calcification	Ectopic dystrophic calcification
Calcific periarthritis	Vitamin D intoxication	Dermatomyositis and polymyositis
Milwaukee shoulder syndrome	Chronic renal dialysis	Systemic sclerosis and CREST syndrome
Ossification of posterior longitudinal ligament (OPLL)	Hyperparathyroidism	Prolapsed intervertebral discs
Osteoarthritis	Pseudohyperparathyroidism	Hip arthroplasties
		Myositis ossificans
		Paraplegia
		Atherosclerotic plaques
		Damaged heart valves
		Scarring of lungs, lymph nodes and adrenals
		Tumoral calcinosis

Supraspinatus tendon deposits of HA, unassociated with symptoms, can be seen in shoulder radiographs in 3–4% of the population.

Apatite-associated destructive arthropathy (cuff tear arthropathy; 'Milwaukee' shoulder/knee syndrome) is a relatively uncommon but distinctive type of destructive arthritis seen in the elderly. Women are affected more frequently than men. The shoulders and knees are the main joints involved, but the wrists, hips and mid-tarsal joints are occasionally affected. Sudden onset of pain and swelling in a shoulder associated with the presence of a large cool effusion and the rapid development of joint subluxation and destruction are characteristic. Ultrasound or radiographs show evidence of rotator cuff defects with upward migration and destruction of the humeral head, with relatively little osteophyte formation or bone remodelling. Some, but not all, cases are associated with calcific periarthritis, but synovial fluid analysis reveals large volumes of a relatively non-inflammatory fluid with numerous crystals of HA and CPPD, as well as elevated levels of metalloproteinase activity.

Treatment is with analgesics, NSAIDs and supportive physiotherapy as well as with joint aspiration and injection of intra-articular corticosteroids. Occasionally, surgical intervention with a shoulder spacer or replacement arthroplasty is required.

GOUT

Gout results from tissue deposition of microcrystals of monosodium urate monohydrate (MSUM) from hyperuricaemic body fluids. Clinical manifestations include acute arthritis, bursitis, tenosynovitis and cellulitis, tophaceous deposits, chronic arthritis, renal disease and urolithiasis.

Prolonged hyperuricaemia is necessary but not sufficient for the development of gout. Hyperuricaemia is usually defined as a serum uric acid (SUA) greater than two standard deviations above the population mean (>0.42 mmol/l in men and >0.36 mmol/l in women), although the theoretical solubility threshold for MSUM in tissue fluids is approximately 0.4 mmol/l in both sexes. Gout and hyperuricaemia can be *primary* or *secondary* to drugs or disorders that interfere with uric acid excretion or augment the production of uric acid (Table 15.7).

The epidemiology of gout and that of hyperuricaemia are closely related. SUA concentrations are distributed in the community as a continuous variable. Levels are influenced by age, sex, body bulk, ethnicity and genetic constitution as well as by dietary intake of purines and alcohol. SUA levels are higher in men than in women, rising after puberty in males and only after the menopause in

Table 15.7 Some factors contributing to the development of hyperuricaemia and gout

Primary	Secondary
Diminished renal excretion of uric acid	
Isolated renal tubular defect in fractional clearance of uric acid (most patients)	Renal insufficiency
Familial juvenile hyperuricaemic nephropathy	Hypertension
	Drug administration: • Any diuretic (but particularly thiazides) • Low-dose salicylates • Ciclosporin • Pyrazinamide
	Lactic acidosis: • Alcohol • Fasting or vomiting • Severe exercise
	Volume depletion
	Lead toxicity
	Glucose-6-phosphatase deficiency
Increased production of urate	
Increased purine synthesis *de novo*: • Idiopathic • Hypoxanthine–guanine phosphoribosyl transferase deficiency • Phosphoribosyl pyrophosphate synthetase superactivity	Increased turnover of purine nucleotides: • Myeloproliferative disorders, e.g. polycythaemia rubra vera, chronic granulocytic leukaemia • Lymphoproliferative disorders, e.g. chronic lymphocytic leukaemia • Severe exfoliative psoriasis
	Accelerated catabolism of purine nucleotides: • Cytotoxic drug therapy ('tumour lysis syndrome') • Alcohol ingestion • Fructose ingestion/intolerance • Glucose-6-phosphatase deficiency (GSD type I) • Myogenic (GSD types III, V and VII)

females. The overall incidence of gout is about 1.4 per 1000 per year and the overall prevalence in general practice is about 1%. Asymptomatic hyperuricaemia is 10 times more common. *Primary* gout occurs predominantly in men and gouty arthritis is exceptionally rare in women before the menopause. Gout in older women is usually *secondary* and often associated with renal insufficiency, hypertension and/or diuretic drug therapy. *Primary* gout is the most common cause of inflammatory arthritis in men over the age of 40 years. It is age related,

with a peak onset in men between 40 and 50 years of age. The incidence and prevalence of gout increase with the level of the SUA. The risk of developing gout in men rises from 0.5% per annum when the SUA is 0.42 mmol/l to 5.5% per annum in those with SUA of 0.54 mmol/l. Recent evidence suggests that the incidence and prevalence of gout and hyperuricaemia are increasing as the age structure of the population changes and also probably as a consequence of rising levels of SUA associated with obesity and affluent life-styles. Seventy-five per cent of patients with gout have features of the metabolic syndrome (central obesity, hypertension, hyperglycaemia, hypertriglyceridaemia and low levels of high-density lipoprotein (HDL)) and recent epidemiological studies have confirmed that alcohol consumption (especially beer) and diets high in red meat and shellfish are risk factors for the development of gout, while diets rich in dairy products, which are uricosuric, are protective.

Aetiology

Purine nucleotide synthesis and degradation are regulated by a balanced interaction of biochemical pathways (Fig. 15.9). Uric acid is the end product of

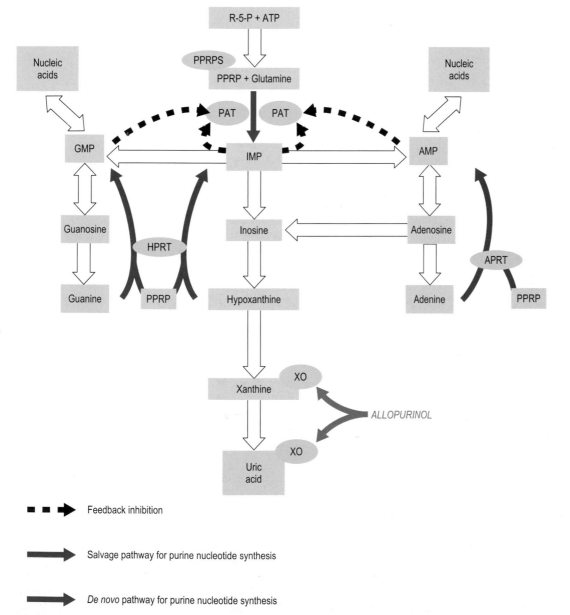

FIGURE 15.9 Pathways of purine synthesis and degradation. AMP, adenosine monophosphate; APRT, adenine phosphoribosyl transferase; GMP, guanosine monophosphate; HPRT, hypoxanthine–guanine phosphoribosyl transferase; IMP, inosine monophosphate; PAT, phosphoribosyl pyrophosphate amidotransferase; PPRP, phosphoribosyl pyrophosphate; PPRPS, phosphoribosyl pyrophosphate synthetase; R-5-P, ribose-5-phosphate; ATP, adenosine triphosphate; XO, xanthine oxidase

purine metabolism in humans, who lack the enzyme uricase that degrades uric acid to allantoin in most mammals. The miscible pool of uric acid in normal individuals is about 1200 mg. More than half of this is derived from endogenously synthesized purine nucleotides and the rest from ingested dietary purines. Sixty per cent of the uric acid pool is replenished daily from the catabolism of purine nucleotides and bases. Two-thirds of the uric acid formed each day is excreted by the kidney and one-third is eliminated via the gastrointestinal tract (Fig. 15.10). Renal clearance of uric acid follows three main processes: filtration at the glomerulus; proximal tubular reabsorption facilitated by the membrane urate transport protein URAT 1; and active tubular secretion in various parts of the renal tubule mediated by the organic anion transporter OAT, the sodium-dependent phosphate co-transporter NPT 1 and the urate-channelling protein UAT.

Genetic and environmental factors lead to gout and hyperuricaemia by increasing the production of uric acid and/or reducing its excretion (see Table 15.7). In about 90% of patients with *primary* gout hyperuricaemia is associated with a genetically determined renal tubular defect in which the capacity to increase uric acid excretion in response to a purine load is impaired. A similar, but more profound, defect in fractional clearance of uric acid occurs in Maoris and Polynesians, and in a rare form of familial juvenile hyperuricaemic nephropathy associated with mutations in uromodulin (the Tamm–Horsfall urinary protein). In 10% of patients with gout there is increased production of uric acid, usually as a result of increased turnover of cellular nucleoproteins. In less than 1% of mutations in the purine salvage enzyme hypoxanthine–guanine phosphoribosyl transferase (HPRT), the *de novo* purine pathway enzyme phosphoribosyl pyrophosphate synthetase (PPRPS) or the glycogenolytic enzyme glucose-6-phosphatase (G-6-P) leads to accelerated *de novo* purine nucleotide synthesis and overproduction of uric acid (see Fig. 15.9 & Table 15.7).

Clinical features

Acute gout most frequently presents as an acute monoarthritis in one of the distal joints of the foot or hand. The metatarsal joint of the great toe is the first joint affected in more than 50% of patients ('podagra') (Fig. 15.11), but attacks may also occur in the ankle, subtalar or mid tarsal joints, the knee, wrist, elbow or small joints of the hands. The hips, shoulders and joints of the axial skeleton are not affected. The onset may be insidious, but more typically is explosively sudden, frequently waking the patient from sleep. The affected joint becomes hot, red, swollen and extremely tender to any touch. Very acute attacks may be accompanied by

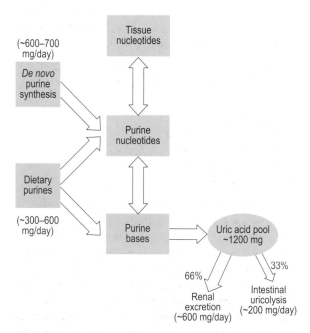

FIGURE 15.10 The uric acid pool. Origin and fate of uric acid in normal humans

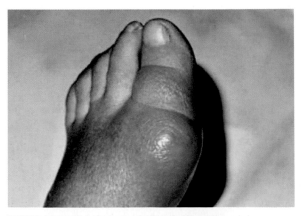

FIGURE 15.11 Acute gouty arthritis ('podagra')

Box 15.1
Events responsible for provoking attacks of acute gout

- Alcohol
- Dietary excess
- Drugs:
  - diuretics (especially thiazides)
  - initiation of uric acid-lowering drug therapy with allopurinol or uricosurics
  - cytotoxics
- Fasting or severe dieting
- Surgery
- Systemic illness
- Trauma
- Unusual physical exercise

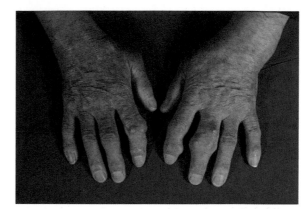

FIGURE 15.12   Chronic tophaceous gout

fever and systemic symptoms of inflammation, and are sometimes preceded by prodromal symptoms of anorexia, nausea or change in mood. Untreated first attacks will typically resolve spontaneously and completely in 1–2 weeks, sometimes with pruritus and desquamation of the overlying skin. Some patients suffer a single attack or experience another only after many years, but most patients will have a second attack within 12–18 months. If left untreated patients tend to suffer recurrent acute or sub-acute attacks with increasing frequency. These may be more prolonged with progressive shortening of the symptom-free 'intercritical' period between attacks. In such individuals, polyarticular acute gouty arthritis, bursitis and cellulitis are not uncommon and can lead to diagnostic confusion. Acute attacks of gout may be precipitated by a number of factors (Box 15.1).

Chronic tophaceous gout

First attacks of gouty arthritis are seldom associated with residual deformity or disability, but recurrent attacks are followed by progressive cartilage and bone erosion, deposition of palpable masses of urate crystals ('tophi') and an asymmetrical inflammatory polyarthritis in the feet, hands or wrists, with secondary OA and disability associated with deformities and restriction of joint movements (Fig. 15.12). Tophi develop in the helix of the ear as well as in bursae, tendon sheaths and periarticular tissues. The severity of the joint damage and the speed with which tophi develop are related to the level of the SUA. While tophi are usually observed only after about 10 years of recurrent gout in untreated, or inadequately treated, patients, they can develop much more rapidly in the hands or feet in patients with *secondary* gout, such as transplant patients receiving ciclosporin or post-menopausal women with heart failure and renal insufficiency receiving diuretic drugs.

A history of renal colic associated with uric acid calculi is found in about 10% of patients with gout attending hospital clinics in the UK. Uric acid urolithiasis is also associated with:

- Hot climates, dehydration and low urine flow
- Low urine pH (e.g. chronic diarrhoeal diseases or ileostomy)
- Hyperuricosuria
- Purine overproduction
- High intake of dietary purines
- Treatment with uricosuric drugs
- Defects in tubular resorption of uric acid.

Chronic renal disease can complicate chronic tophaceous gout, as a result of MSUM crystal deposition in the renal medulla variably combined with the effects of renal tubular obstruction with crystals of uric acid, hypertension, glomerulosclerosis and secondary pyelonephritis in patients with gout and prolonged, uncontrolled hyperuricaemia. In treated patients minimal renal insufficiency is largely age related, and proteinuria is mild and non-progressive.

Acute crystal nephropathy can result from sudden obstruction of the collecting ducts and ureters with uric acid crystals following treatment of leukaemia or lymphoma with cytotoxic drugs ('tumour lysis syndrome'). The problem can usually be avoided by prophylaxis with allopurinol, high fluid intake and urine alkalinization before chemotherapy, but care needs to be undertaken to discontinue alkalinization of the urine in hyperphosphataemic patients to avoid precipitation of calcium phosphate crystals in the renal tubules.

Investigations

Certain diagnosis requires the identification of MSUM crystals from tophi, synovial or bursal fluid by compensated, polarizing light microscopy (see Fig. 15.8). Synovial fluid from patients with acute gouty arthritis is frequently turbid with a high polymorphonuclear leucocyte count, and Gram stain and culture are required to exclude bacterial infection. Blood tests usually show evidence of a systemic inflammatory response with a raised CRP and ESR, and sometimes a moderate neutrophil leucocytosis and reactive thrombocytosis. The SUA should be measured, but has very limited diagnostic value as asymptomatic hyperuricaemia is very common and the SUA is raised at the time of an acute attack of gout in only about 60% of patients.

Radiographs are seldom helpful at the time of the first attack, but can be used to assess joint damage in patients who have had recurrent episodes. Patients with chronic tophaceous gout may have periarticular soft-tissue swelling flecked with calcification on plain radiographs as well as characteristic 'punched out' erosions with sclerotic margins, overhanging edges and relatively little periarticular osteoporosis (Fig. 15.13), but in many cases the radiographic appearances are similar to those in patients with other types of inflammatory joint disease and osteoarthritis.

All patients with gout should have measurements of blood pressure and renal function, and be further assessed for cardiovascular risk, with screening tests for diabetes mellitus, hyperlipidaemia and the metabolic syndrome.

When a diagnosis of gout has been established, possible causes of primary and secondary hyperuricaemia should be considered (see Table 15.7).

If there is reason to suspect overproduction, rather than underexcretion, of uric acid, this can be established, in the absence of renal impairment, by finding a 24-h urine uric acid excretion of >1 g (6 mmol) while on a low purine diet. The possibility of specific enzyme defects associated with an increase in *de novo* purine synthesis should be suspected:

- in the absence of disorders associated with increased turnover or breakdown of purine nucleotides
- if gout develops before the age of 20 years
- when there is a family history of gout commencing at an early age
- when uric acid lithiasis is the presenting feature in a young person.

Treatment

Patient education and understanding the rationale for therapy are vital for the successful management of gout.

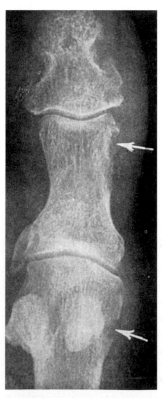

FIGURE 15.13 Chronic tophaceous gout. Radiograph showing characteristic punched-out erosions with overhanging margins

Acute gout

Rest and prompt treatment with full doses of a rapidly acting oral NSAID, such as naproxen or indometacin, are the treatment of choice for acute attacks, provided that there are no contra-indications. NSAIDs should be avoided in patients with heart failure, renal insufficiency or a recent history of gastrointestinal ulcer, bleed or perforation, and they should be used with great circumspection in frail, elderly patients with multiple pathology and in patients with cardiovascular disease. In patients with increased risk of development of peptic ulcers, bleeds or perforation, the use of a NSAID with co-prescription of a gastroprotective agent, or the use of a highly selective COX2 inhibitor, such as etoricoxib 120 mg od, can be considered for treating acute gout. However, selective COX2 inhibitors should not be used in patients with established ischaemic heart disease, cerebrovascular disease or peripheral vascular disease.

Colchicine, which inhibits neutrophil phagocytosis, can be used as an effective alternative to NSAIDs for the treatment of acute gout. Despite being slower to act, it is best given in a relatively low oral dose (e.g. 0.5 mg 8-hourly), as it has a low therapeutic index, and nausea, diarrhoea or abdominal cramps commonly supervene before resolution of the acute arthritis. Intravenous colchicine has been associated with a number of sudden deaths and should not be used.

If oral therapy is precluded, a parenteral NSAID or NSAID suppository can be used if NSAIDs are not otherwise contra-indicated. Alternatively, joint aspiration, intra-articular injection of a corticosteroid or a short course of systemic corticosteroids can be safe and effective.

Treatment with uric acid-lowering drugs should not be started until the acute attack has completely settled, because they can prolong the acute attack or trigger further episodes. Treatment with very low doses of aspirin for cardiovascular prophylaxis should be continued, and has very little effect on SUA levels, but patients should be advised to avoid aspirin and salicylate-containing medicines for analgesia as these can interfere with uric acid excretion and precipitate an attack of gout.

Recurrent, intercritical and chronic gout

Treatment is aimed at reducing the SUA level to 0.30–0.36 mmol/l (i.e. well below the solubility threshold of urate) in order to prevent crystal formation and optimize dissolution of existing MSUM crystals in tissues. Initially, attention should be given to the avoidance of modifiable risk factors and to life-style modifications when these are appropriate, e.g.:

- Avoid or discontinue diuretic drugs when these are not absolutely required for the control of cardiac failure
- Gradual weight loss in obese patients
- Restriction of alcohol (especially beer) consumption
- Avoid high intake of foods with high purine content (especially shellfish, red meat and offal).

Prolonged administration of uric acid-lowering drugs should be started in the following circumstances:

- The patient has suffered recurrent acute attacks
- There is evidence of tophi or chronic gouty arthritis
- There is associated renal disease or urate lithiasis
- The SUA is very elevated (>0.54 mmol/l)
- The patient needs to continue to take diuretic drugs
- Normal levels of SUA cannot be achieved by risk factor/life-style modification.

Allopurinol is the drug of choice for the long-term management of gout because of its efficacy, safety and convenience. It lowers the SUA by inhibiting the enzyme xanthine oxidase that converts the purine bases xanthine and hypoxanthine to uric acid (see Fig. 15.9). Renal function should be checked before commencing therapy. In patients with normal renal function, oral treatment should be commenced at 100 mg daily with a NSAID, or colchicine 0.5 mg 12-hourly to prevent 'breakthrough' attacks of acute gout that otherwise often follow the commencement of treatment with uric acid-lowering drugs. The SUA should be measured monthly and the dose of allopurinol increased by 100-mg increments to a maximum of 900 mg/day to optimize the reduction of SUA. If renal function is impaired, lower doses of allopurinol should be used (creatinine clearance

60 ml/min – 200 mg daily; creatinine clearance 20 ml/min – 100 mg/day). Side effects of allopurinol include mild rashes in about 2% of patients and much rarer, severe and even life-threatening hypersensitivity reactions, as well as potentially dangerous drug interactions with oral anticoagulants and azathioprine. Allopurinol desensitization can be undertaken in patients who have developed mild hypersensitivity rashes, but should not be attempted in those who have suffered more severe reactions, epidermal necrolysis or drug-induced vasculitis. The allopurinol metabolite oxypurinol can be tried carefully as an alternative.

Another approach to treating transplant recipients and those with severe tophaceous gout who are unable to tolerate allopurinol has been the use of a recombinant uricase (rasburicase) as a uricolytic agent. This agent, and a purified non-recombinant uricase (uricozyme), can also be used for the prevention and treatment of acute uric acid nephropathy following chemotherapy for malignant disease.

More frequently, the uricosuric drug sulfinpyrazone (100 mg 8-hourly with colchicine 0.5 mg 12-hourly po) is used as an alternative to allopurinol to lower the SUA in patients with *primary* gout if renal function is normal. It is, however, contraindicated in patients with impairment of renal function, in whom it is ineffective, and in patients with urate urolithiasis or overproduction of uric acid associated with heavy uricosuria.

Gout is frequently associated with hypertension and hyperlipidaemia, which require treatment to reduce cardiovascular risk. Losartan, an angiotensin-1 receptor antagonist, which is effective in hypertension, and the hypolipidaemic agent fenofibrate, both have uricosuric properties. Although they are not recommended as substitutes for allopurinol or standard uricosuric drugs for lowering the SUA, they can be considered as an option for the treatment of hypertension or hyperlipidaemia in patients with gout.

Asymptomatic hyperuricaemia

Most people with asymptomatic hyperuricaemia never develop gout and, in those that do, renal complications rarely precede the first attack of gouty arthritis. Consequently, it is unnecessary to treat the majority of people with asymptomatic hyperuricaemia before they have experienced a first attack of gout. Uric acid-lowering treatment should, however, be considered from the outset in young people with persistently very high SUA levels (>0.6 mmol/l), especially when there is a strong family history of gout, renal disease or urolithiasis; or in persons known to have inborn errors of purine metabolism associated with increases in *de novo* purine synthesis, as renal damage may precede joint pathology in these patients.

Aside from gout there is compelling epidemiological evidence to suggest that hyperuricaemia is associated with a poor outcome in patients with hypertension, heart failure, cerebrovascular disease and glomerulonephritis. However, evidence that hyperuricaemia is the cause, rather than the consequence, of the underlying pathology is inconclusive, as is evidence to suggest that raised levels of SUA may be an independent risk factor for ischaemic heart disease. Although there is insufficient evidence at the present time to suggest that treatment of asymptomatic hyperuricaemia would reduce cardiovascular risk, the finding of persistent hyperuricaemia should not be ignored. Rather it should stimulate a search for secondary causes of hyperuricaemia (see Table 15.7), careful examination and investigation of the patient for features of the metabolic syndrome, and a detailed assessment for other, established, cardiovascular risk factors.

FURTHER READING

Abramson SB, Attur M, Yazici Y 2006 Prospects for disease modification in osteoarthritis. Nat Clin Pract Rheumatol 2: 304–312.

Hawker GA 2006 Who, when, and why total joint replacement surgery? The patient's perspective. Curr Opin Rheumatol 18: 526–530.

Jordan KM, Cameron JS, Snaith M et al 2007 British Society for Rheumatology and British Health Professionals in Rheumatology guideline for the management of gout. Rheumatology (Oxford) 46: 1372–1374.

Pandit H, Aslam N, Pirpiris M et al 2006 Total knee arthroplasty: the future. J Surg Orthop Adv 15: 79–85.

Rosenthal AK 2006 Calcium crystal deposition and osteoarthritis. Rheum Dis Clin North Am 32: 401–412, vii.

Teng GG, Nair R, Saag KG 2006 Pathophysiology, clinical presentation and treatment of gout. Drugs 66: 1547–1563.

Zhang W, Moskowitz RW, Nuki G et al 2007 OARSI recommendations for the management of hip and knee osteoarthritis, part I: critical appraisal of existing treatment guidelines and systematic review of current research evidence. Osteoarthritis Cartilage 15: 981–1000.

INFLAMMATORY ARTHRITIS

Hill Gaston and Mark Lillicrap

Cases relevant to this chapter

16, 21, 68, 70–72, 75, 77–82, 85, 86, 100

●Essential facts

1. Rheumatoid arthritis (RA) is a common destructive inflammatory polyarthritis affecting 1% of the population.

2. Patients with persistent early morning stiffness with pain or swelling in at least three joint areas should be investigated for an inflammatory arthropathy.

3. In all cases of RA, disease-modifying anti-rheumatic therapy should be started as soon as possible.

4. Multidisciplinary management of RA helps patients to maintain long-term function.

5. Surgery may be required in RA to improve function and to relieve pain.

6. A diagnosis of ankylosing spondylitis is often delayed by 8–10 years, because back pain is very common.

7. Reactive arthritis is a form of spondyloarthritis triggered by infections of the gastrointestinal or genitourinary tract.

8. Post-infectious arthritis (distinct from reactive arthritis) is associated with viral or bacterial infections.

9. In many patients with inflammatory arthritis, pregnancy exerts an immunosuppressive effect, with the exception of systemic lupus erythematosus (SLE), which typically flares during pregnancy.

RHEUMATOID ARTHRITIS

DEFINITION

Rheumatoid arthritis (RA) is a common systemic inflammatory disease affecting approximately 1% of the population, characterized by a destructive inflammatory polyarthritis. The arthritis has a predisposition for the hands and feet, particularly proximal interphalangeal (IP) joints, metacarpophalangeal (MCP) joints and wrists, but can affect any synovial joint. Although synovitis is the characteristic feature, RA is a multi-system disease potentially involving the lungs, heart, eyes, vascular tree, haematopoietic system and the nervous system. Eighty per cent of adults affected by RA will have a positive rheumatoid factor (RF) (IgG or IgM autoantibodies recognizing IgG) at some point during the disease, although up to 60% of patients may be RF negative at presentation and up to 10% of the normal population have RF, usually at low titre (see Chapter 4). Classification criteria for RA were defined by the American College of Rheumatology in 1987 (Box 16.1). RA is defined as the presence of four or more of the seven criteria. RA as defined by this classification is probably a

> **Box 16.1**
> **1987 American College of Rheumatology criteria for classification of rheumatoid arthritis**
>
> - Early morning stiffness
> - Arthritis affecting three or more joint areas
> - Hand joint arthritis
> - Symmetrical arthritis
> - Rheumatoid nodules
> - Rheumatoid factor
> - Bone erosions.
>
> The presence of at least four of the above criteria is required to classify a patient as having rheumatoid arthritis.

heterogeneous syndrome rather than a single disorder and the variability of the disease – pattern of presentation, prognosis, response to treatment and extra-articular manifestations – reflects this. Whether some of the more recently described autoantibodies, such as those to citrullinated peptides, will define more homogeneous patient groups remains to be seen.

AETIOLOGY AND PATHOGENESIS

The cause of RA is unknown. Genes play a part: individuals with certain HLA types are at increased risk and having an identical twin with the disease markedly increases risk (discussed in detail in Chapter 3). Several alleles of the HLA-DRB1 gene (e.g. HLA-DRB1*0401 and 0404) have been shown to be associated with disease in different populations; these alleles share a common amino acid sequence (residues 70–74, the 'shared epitope'), although how this is involved in disease aetiology remains an active research question. However, carrying an HLA genotype associated with RA or having an identical twin affected does not inevitably mean that disease will develop. Thus, environmental factors, as yet undefined, must also be important. Perhaps the most likely hypothesis, given the association with HLA-DR alleles, is that an aberrant T-lymphocyte response to an environmental antigen results in an autoimmune inflammatory response focused on the synovium.

However, as yet, no such antigens have been identified, and the T-lymphocyte model remains a hypothesis. Furthermore, the presence of RF and other autoantibodies, such as those directed against citrullinated peptides, in the majority of patients suggests significant B-lymphocyte involvement in disease pathogenesis. Autoreactive T cells may drive autoantibody production.

Whatever triggers the initial immune activation there is clear evidence of an active downstream immune response in patients with RA. It is this chronic inflammatory response, within the synovium, that accounts for the musculoskeletal clinical features. It also causes the destructive changes in the cartilage and bone that are characteristic of the disease. Treatment with disease-modifying agents aims to control this process. In the majority of patients with RA, the inflammation is associated with a pro-inflammatory cytokine milieu in the synovium dominated by tumour necrosis factor (TNFα), which is produced by macrophage-like synoviocytes. This production may be driven by either autoreactive T cells or immune complexes containing RF and other autoantibodies. One of the most dramatic recent developments in RA has been the use of anti-TNFα therapies; these show marked efficacy, not only in reducing symptoms, but also in slowing disease progression.

CLINICAL FEATURES

History

The characteristic feature of any inflammatory arthritis is early morning stiffness present for at least 30 min, and usually for several hours on waking. It is often better in the afternoon, but recurs with immobility and towards the evening (diurnal variation). Any patient who spontaneously offers a history of early morning stiffness needs thorough investigation to exclude an inflammatory arthropathy. The stiffness is characteristically accompanied by pain and swelling, most commonly of the wrists and the small joints of the hands and feet, in a symmetrical distribution in the initial stages. However, the arthritis can affect any synovial joint and, although patients frequently present with hand symptoms, presentation with other joints does not exclude the diagnosis. Symptoms may be acute or insidious in onset. A useful indicator that symptoms reflect an underlying inflammatory arthritis is their responsiveness to non-steroidal anti-inflammatory drugs (NSAIDs). This should be explored in the history, but note that over-the-counter doses of ibuprofen are not anti-inflammatory. RA causes significant functional limitation and it is important to enquire about impairment of activities of daily living (ADLs) and occupational issues in all patients. Extra-articular manifestations can occur early and a thorough review of all systems is required.

Examination

If allowed appropriate opportunity, the patient will usually give the clinician enough information to make the diagnosis from the history. Examination then allows the clinician to confirm the diagnosis. The GALS screen (see Chapter 1, p. 5) is a validated screening examination of the musculoskeletal system and identifies involved joints that can then be assessed further with appropriate regional examination routines. The characteristic features in a patient presenting with RA are swelling, warmth and joint-line tenderness of affected joints. Erythema is unusual. The pattern of joint involvement (Fig. 16.1) most frequently includes the wrists (carpi and distal radioulnar joints), the proximal IP joints (particularly index and middle fingers) and the MCP joints (again index and middle fingers). In the hands the distal IP joints are generally spared. The feet should be examined because early foot involvement is associated with a worse prognosis and would indicate a need for more aggressive

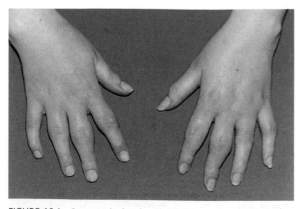

FIGURE 16.1 Symmetrical polyarthritis in a patient with rheumatoid arthritis. The wrists, metacarpophalangeal and proximal interphalangeal joints are symmetrically involved

early treatment. MCP and metatarsophalangeal (MTP) squeeze tests, in which the heads of the metacarpals and metatarsals are squeezed gently by the examiner between thumb and middle finger (until the fingernail just blanches), are sensitive indicators of underlying synovitis. The 'textbook' changes of RA, such as boutonnière and swan-neck deformities, ulnar deviation of the metacarpals, and radial deviation of the wrist, are seen late and will not be present in early disease.

A systemic examination looking for rheumatoid nodules (characteristically seen on the elbows) and other extra-articular features should be undertaken. RF-seropositive patients and those who are also homozygous for the HLA-DR shared epitope are at increased risk of extra-articular manifestations of the disease; these are also generally associated with a poorer prognosis and an increased mortality. These are discussed in Chapter 18 on systemic complications of rheumatic diseases.

EARLY RHEUMATOID ARTHRITIS

One of the problems with the American College of Rheumatology criteria (Box 16.1) is that symptoms need to be present for at least 6 weeks for a diagnosis to be made. The difficulty is that the differential diagnosis of an arthritis that lasts less than 6 weeks is very broad, including a large number of self-limiting conditions (e.g. post-viral arthritis), many of which would fulfil the classification criteria transiently. Indeed, it is not until symptoms have been present for 12 weeks that the clinician can be confident of the diagnosis. However, there is increasing evidence that treatment needs to be given early to prevent joint damage from occurring. It is, therefore, not appropriate to wait for patients to fulfil classification criteria before initiating therapy. One of the challenges is to try to identify which of the patients with a short duration of symptoms will go on to develop chronic disease. At presentation a good proportion of patients who go on to develop chronic RA will have normal radiographs and a negative rheumatoid factor. Some patients may not have an elevated C-reactive protein (CRP) or erythrocyte sedimentation rate (ESR). A fast-track referral is recommended for patients with possible inflammatory arthritis to allow early specialist involvement. Unfortunately, due to limited resources, this is not always achieved. The pattern of disease, involvement of the feet, a rising CRP, and a positive rheumatoid factor (or antibodies to citrullinated peptides) have all been shown to have predictive value in determining prognosis. There is also evidence that the presence of the shared epitope (especially homozygosity) predicts the development of more severe disease (see Chapter 3). Currently, these are research findings and routine investigation does not include HLA typing.

TESTS

Although the diagnosis of RA can be made largely through appropriate history and examination, investigations are frequently confirmatory and contribute to subsequent management decisions. Blood tests should include a full blood count, renal and hepatic biochemistry, inflammatory markers (ESR and CRP), RF and anti-nuclear antibodies (ANAs). There is increasing use of anti-CCP antibody testing, and this may ultimately prove to be more effective than RF testing. A full blood count may show a normochromic, normocytic anaemia and, less frequently, an elevated platelet count, in keeping with a systemic inflammatory response. Hepatic biochemistry can show a depressed albumin and an elevated alkaline phosphatase, again due to the systemic inflammatory response. RF, as mentioned above, is not diagnostic of RA, being found in otherwise healthy individuals and may be negative in RA (particularly in early disease). However, a positive RF correlates with more severe disease and is seen much more frequently in those patients with extra-articular manifestations. Inflammatory arthritis is a feature of systemic lupus erythematosus (SLE) and, although the pattern of joint involvement is different, ANAs should be checked. If the ANA test is positive there is some evidence that sulfasalazine is a less effective treatment. In early disease a viral arthritis screen should also be undertaken, particularly looking for evidence of recent exposure to parvovirus B19, which can cause a transient symmetrical polyarticular synovitis clinically indistinguishable from RA.

Imaging studies should include hand and foot radiographs, looking for periarticular osteopenia or erosions (Fig. 16.2), and a chest X-ray – paraneoplastic arthritis can be similar to RA, sarcoidosis can cause an inflammatory arthritis, particularly of the ankles, and latent tuberculosis (TB) or undiag-

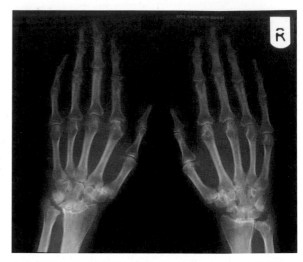

FIGURE 16.2 Radiographs of hands to show erosive arthritis affecting metacarpophalangeal joints and wrists

nosed interstitial lung disease are relative contraindications to certain treatments. Current research is exploring the role of ultrasound and MRI in early inflammatory arthritis to predict progression to chronic disease but, like shared epitope testing, these are currently research investigations.

TREATMENT

Once a diagnosis has been confirmed, treatment should be initiated. It is clear that both erosive damage and functional impairment occur early and can be controlled more effectively by initiating disease-modifying anti-rheumatic drug (DMARD) therapy early in the disease. This emphasizes the need for a fast-track referral system for patients with possible RA.

Non-steroidal anti-inflammatory drugs

NSAID responsiveness is frequently seen in RA, but this is only symptomatic therapy. Monotherapy with NSAIDs has no impact on progression of rheumatoid damage. Therefore, even if symptoms are controllable with NSAIDs, additional therapy with DMARDs is still required. There is no difference in efficacy with COX2-specific therapies, although the side-effect profile with regard to the gastrointestinal tract is preferable. Given the requirements for long-term therapy at high doses, COX2-specific treatments may be preferable, but only in those without cardiovascular risk factors.

Corticosteroids

Corticosteroids can, like NSAIDs, significantly improve inflammatory symptoms. Pulses of intramuscular steroids can be helpful in controlling symptoms, but have not been shown to modify disease progression. By contrast, and unlike NSAIDs, low-dose prednisolone (7.5 mg per day) has been reported to reduce both the rate of progression of erosive disease and the chances of developing erosive damage in the early years of the disease. Prednisolone is, therefore, both symptom relieving and disease modifying. However, although no significant adverse events were seen in the cohort on treatment, osteoporotic prophylaxis is required, and some clinicians have understandable reservations about the risks of long-term steroid use. The duration of steroid treatment required and whether the benefits are lost on stopping remain unknown.

For actively inflamed joints, intra-articular injection of long-acting corticosteroids (e.g. methylprednisolone) can be very useful in producing powerful local anti-inflammatory effects whilst decreasing the less desirable systemic effects of steroids. This is a helpful option whilst awaiting the action of disease-modifying drugs.

Disease-modifying anti-rheumatic drugs

DMARD therapy should be initiated promptly. Weekly methotrexate (up to 25 mg/week) is a common first-line treatment, although daily sulfasalazine (up to 3 g/day) is another option. Both of these treatments are known to be efficacious, although the evidence base for methotrexate is stronger and longitudinal studies show it is better tolerated. Folic acid (5 mg weekly) has been shown to reduce the side effects of methotrexate (mouth ulcers, gastrointestinal upset and possibly hepatic and haematological disturbance). The authors' practice is to prescribe *M*ethotrexate on a *M*onday and *F*olic acid on a *F*riday to aid compliance.

Other DMARDs include leflunomide, hydroxychloroquine, intramuscular gold, ciclosporin and azathioprine. All of these DMARDs take between 6 and 12 weeks to take effect, and all patients need to be educated about both the need to take medication regularly and the risks associated with them (see Chapter 5). With the exception of hydroxy-chloroquine, all these treatments require regular blood test monitoring and, if possible, all should be avoided in pregnancy. There is increasing evidence that combination therapy with DMARDs is efficacious. Regimens usually include methotrexate as standard, and have used a variety of different additional DMARDs. Whether these should be used in a step-up fashion (rapidly adding treatments to get control) or a step-down fashion (start with all drugs and gradually reduce/remove once control is achieved) remains an area of active research. Although the pharmacology of the DMARDs is understood, exactly why they are efficacious in RA is not entirely clear. They probably have an effect at a number of levels of the inflammatory cascade.

Biologic therapy

Patients who fail to respond to the conventional DMARDs are being managed with biologic therapies. TNFα had been shown to be a critically important cytokine in RA pathogenesis, and was thus an attractive target for anti-cytokine therapy. Three anti-TNFα therapies – infliximab, adalimumab (chimeric antibodies targeting TNFα) and etanercept (recombinant-soluble TNF receptor) – are currently licensed and all have shown efficacy in randomized controlled trials. They reduce signs and symptoms of disease, preserve function, reduce radiological progression, and improve patients' quality of life. The major risk of anti-TNFα treatments seems to be reactivation of latent infection, particularly tuberculosis, since TNFα is an important cytokine in maintenance of the granulomata, which confine mycobacteria. Pre-treatment screening and vigilance during treatment is, therefore, critical. Treatment with anti-TNFα is not curative and the drugs must be administered indefinitely, although the possibility that their use in very early disease might result in long periods of remission is under investigation. Other biologic treatments include rituximab, a B cell-depleting antibody and cytotoxic T-lymphocyte antigen-4-immunoglobulin, which reduces stimulation of T cells and may affect antigen presenting cells. These agents are now licensed for use and the new challenge will be deciding when and how to use these newer and, inevitably, costly treatments most appropriately.

Further discussion on the medical management of RA can be found in Chapter 5.

Non-pharmacological therapy

Treatment of RA is not solely pharmacological; patient education, physiotherapy and occupational therapy are also core aspects of management. All patients should have access to therapy services at an early stage and throughout their disease; multi-disciplinary management improves the chances of patients maintaining long-term function. Surgery may also be required for both functional and pain-relieving purposes.

Chapter 6 provides more detailed information on the non-pharmacological management of RA and Chapter 7 on surgical management.

PROGNOSIS

Although current treatments have undoubtedly improved the control of RA symptoms and reduced the rate of progression of erosive damage, the disease is still associated with significant mor-bidity (with decreased quality of life scores on validated instruments) and a significant risk of unemployment and disability. Standardized employment ratios are reduced to about 0.8 (1.0 for general population) for patients with RA even with current treatments. RA is also associated with a significant mortality. Standardized mortality rates for patients with RA are increased to approximately 1.5. Part of this increased mortality is attributable to an increased risk of cardiovascular disease. The cardiovascular risk is independent of conventional risk factors, such as smoking and cholesterol, sug-gesting that RA is itself a risk factor. The standard-ized mortality rates are greatest in those patients with increased disease activity at baseline and in those with extra-articular disease. Further studies will address whether current treatment of RA mod-ifies the mortality rates.

SPONDYLOARTHRITIS

The spondyloarthritides have a prevalence slightly lower than that of RA. Spondyloarthritis can be sub-divided into five conditions (Box 16.2).

ANKYLOSING SPONDYLITIS

Definition

Ankylosing spondylitis (AS), whose prevalence is between 0.5% and 1%, is the principal inflamma-tory disease of the axial skeleton.

> **Box 16.2**
> **Diseases classified as forms of spondyloarthritis**
>
> - Ankylosing spondylitis
> - Psoriatic arthritis
> - Reactive arthritis
> - Arthritis associated with Crohn's disease or ulcerative colitis
> - Undifferentiated spondyloarthritis: arthritis that fulfils criteria for spondyloarthritis, but does not fall into any of the other four categories

Aetiology/pathogenesis

This remains unknown; the association with HLA-B27 is striking as >90% of patients are positive. Although discovered more than 30 years ago, the explanation for the association remains elusive. The initial assumption was that B27 must act by performing its usual physiological role of present-ing antigenic peptides to CD8+ T lymphocytes. However, arthritogenic peptides, from infectious agents or autoantigens, have not been defined. More recent theories have implicated unusual fea-tures of HLA-B27, such as expression of the B27 heavy chain on the cell surface without its usual partner, β2-microglobulin, or as heavy chain homodimers (which consist of two identical copies of the heavy chain).

Clinical features

History

The typical presentation is one of insidious low back pain in a male in their twenties; a family history is often reported. There are associated inflammatory features, particularly early morning stiffness and stiffness after immobility. Symptoms improve during the day and with exercise, unlike mechanical back pain. Sacroiliac joint involvement produces buttock pain, and alternating buttock pain with walking is well recognized. As the disease progresses, symptoms from involvement of cervical and thoracic spine may become more prominent. Peripheral joints, particularly the hips and shoulders, are frequently involved. Enthesitis (inflammation at points of insertion of ligaments

220

and tendons) is characteristic of spondyloarthritis and occurs as heel, plantar and chest pain.

Extra-articular features may give rise to symptoms; iritis is common (25–40%) and may predate spinal symptoms, and HLA-B27 incidence is increased even in patients with acute anterior uveitis and no joint symptoms. The eye is red and painful. The patient has photophobia and requires prompt examination by an ophthalmologist. Local steroid drops are usually adequate to treat the condition, but inflammation of the iris can result in its adhesion to the cornea or lens ('synechiae') leading later to glaucoma and cataract. Less common extra-articular features include aortic incompetence and cardiac conduction abnormalities, apical lung fibrosis and cauda equina syndrome.

Examination

The range of movement in the lumbar spine is measured, looking for restriction in all planes. Schober's test is a useful (see Chapter 1) and reproducible measure of lumbar flexion, and can aid assessment of disease progression as well as diagnosis. Cervical spine movement should also be assessed and the distance between the occiput or tragus and a wall, when the patient stands as close as possible to a wall. Normally the occiput will readily touch the wall whilst the tragus–wall distance varies from individual to individual. The measurement is useful for assessing an increasing kyphosis. Chest expansion is measured to assess involvement of the thoracic spine and costovertebral joints (<2.5 cm is abnormal). Sacroiliac joint tenderness is assessed by stressing the joint, e.g. by compression of the pelvis or forcibly flexing the hip towards the contralateral iliac crest. These tests have relatively low sensitivity and specificity for sacroiliitis. Extra-articular features should be sought.

Tests

Diagnosis is too often delayed by 8–10 years, mainly because of the high prevalence of back pain in the community, and is often missed in women who have milder disease. The delay is potentially serious since patients may have an irreversible loss of spinal mobility by the time the diagnosis is made.

Few tests are helpful; ESR and CRP are not always elevated, and radiographs will be normal in early disease. HLA-B27 status is not helpful diagnostically – it is present in 8% of the population, many of whom will have back pain and, therefore, the B27 status is potentially misleading. However, if the patient is B27 *negative* the risk of AS is considerably less, and this may be helpful. Isotope scintigraphy may show increased uptake in the sacroiliac (SI) joints before changes become apparent on X-rays, and CT shows erosive changes better than plain films. MRI with gadolinium enhancement is the most sensitive technique to detect SI joint and lumbar spine inflammation (Figs 16.3 & 16.4).

Treatment

Regular exercises are important for maintaining range of movement and all patients require instruction by physiotherapists. Patients should have regular follow-up to document any loss of movement and to provide incentives to continue daily exercise, which improves long-term outcome. Most patients require high doses of the more powerful NSAIDs; some patients will only respond to phenylbutazone, an NSAID not otherwise used due to its unacceptable toxicity in some patients. Etoricoxib seems to be the most effective of the

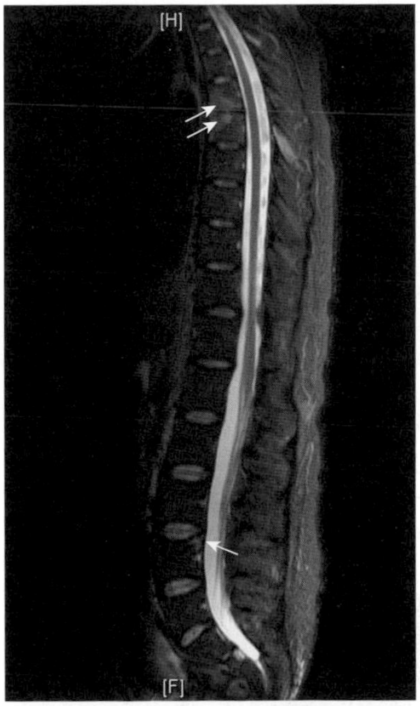

FIGURE 16.3 MRI appearances of spine in ankylosing spondylitis to show Romanus lesions – these 'shiny corners' indicate localized bone oedema at the site of the entheses

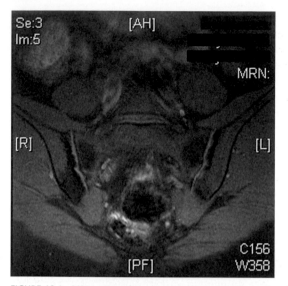

FIGURE 16.4   MRI scan to show bone oedema in the sacral and iliac bones in a patient with active ankylosing spondylitis

COX2-selective NSAIDs. Sulfasalazine is some-times useful for the peripheral arthritis associated with AS, but it has no effect on spinal disease. Anti-TNFα therapies have proven remarkably effective in controlling fatigue and malaise along with joint symptoms, and have transformed some patients' lives. Whether treatment with anti-TNFα therapy can be continued for many decades must remain questionable. Other agents that have shown some efficacy include intravenous bisphosphonates.

Prognosis

AS appears to be most active for the first decade of the disease and low-grade activity is thought to persist for many decades. The chronic changes of patients with AS involve reduced standardized employment rates (0.9) and reduced quality-of-life scores compared to the general population. Poor prognostic factors for AS include early hip involve-ment, persistent elevation of the ESR, hyper-gammaglobulinaemia and early limitation of spinal movements. Like those with RA and psoriatic arthritis, patients with AS have an increased cardio-vascular mortality and morbidity, and an increased standardized mortality rate of approximately 1.5. This is not entirely attributable to orthodox cardio-vascular risk factors.

PSORIATIC ARTHRITIS

DEFINITION

Psoriasis (PsA) is a common condition affecting 1–3% of the population, so that many people with psoriasis also suffer various rheumatic disorders. However, the incidence of inflammatory arthritis is significantly higher in patients with psoriasis than in non-psoriatic control populations. More recent investigations show consistent differences in syno-vial histology between PsA and RA, with more prominent angiogenesis, a less expanded lining area and increased neutrophilia in PsA. Likewise, even in patients with symmetrical polyarthro-pathy, rheumatoid factor is not present at high titres and antibodies to citrullinated peptides (more specific for RA) are generally absent in PsA.

AETIOLOGY/PATHOGENESIS

The pathogenesis of PsA is unknown. One hypoth-esis is that it represents an intra-articular 'Koebner' phenomenon, i.e. the equivalent of the lesions that develop in skin at sites of trauma. Joints commonly undergo trauma and could be susceptible. Psoriasis also affects the normal relationship with skin bac-teria and abnormal responses to bacterial antigens may play a role in PsA, as in other forms of spon-dyloarthritis. Genes in the HLA region have been associated with disease – alleles of HLA-C and MICA.

CLINICAL FEATURES

Several features are particularly characteristic of PsA (Box 16.3).

Classifications of different forms of PsA have been attempted, but patients commonly have dif-ferent combinations of features, e.g. distal IP involvement (Fig. 16.5), sacroiliitis and oligoarthri-tis, and these may evolve from oligoarthritis to polyarthritis, for example. Some patients have arthritis that is clinically indistinguishable from RA, but, as noted above, it is usually RF seronega-tive and in most cases should be considered a sepa-rate disorder. Spinal involvement may be identical to AS.

The skin lesions of psoriasis are often obvious, but may be mild and very limited, and possibly not known to the patient – check scalp, umbilicus and natal cleft. Nail changes are common, including dystrophy, pitting, ridging and onycholysis; nail changes may be the only evidence of psoriasis. In some patients arthritis precedes the development of skin disease ('psoriatic arthritis sine psoriasis'), but the diagnosis is then based on features that are typical of spondyloarthritis (e.g. dactylitis and enthesopathy) and/or a strong family history of psoriasis. In children, joint disease often precedes skin disease and a family history of psoriasis is included as a minor criterion for diagnosis.

TESTS

Apart from an acute-phase response and the absence of rheumatoid factor or other autoantibodies, there is little help from the laboratory. HLA-B27 is present in 50% of those with spinal involvement. Synovial biopsies are not generally useful in an individual case, even though statistically significant differences can be found in features such as vascularity when groups of RA and PsA synovial biopsies are compared. In later stages, radiographs may show the characteristic osteolysis involving the digits, leading to a characteristic 'pencil-in-cup' appearance. Signs of enthesopathy, such as plantar spurs, may be present, together with sacroiliitis, which may be asymmetrical.

TREATMENT

The treatment follows the same guidelines as those for RA, or for AS if spondylitis is the dominant feature. Leflunomide is often the DMARD of choice, but methotrexate will also help the skin disease; conversely hydroxychloroquine is generally avoided because of exacerbations in skin disease. The evidence base for DMARDs in PsA is much less extensive; anti-TNFα therapies have been impressive in improving both skin and joint disease.

PROGNOSIS

Like RA, PsA patients show reduced quality of life scores and reduced standardized employment rates

> **Box 16.3**
> **Clinical features of psoriatic arthritis**
>
> - Dactylitis
> - Oligoarthritis, particularly in weight-bearing joints
> - Distal interphalangeal joint involvement, usually in association with psoriatic nail disease
> - Sacroiliitis
> - Osteolysis, leading to 'telescoping' of digits following the loss of bone from phalanges

223

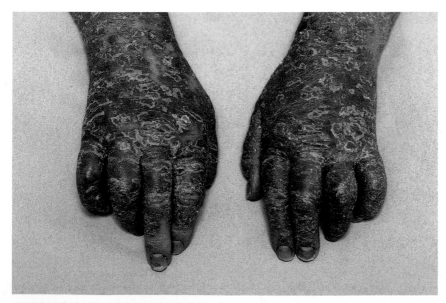

FIGURE 16.5   Distal and proximal interphalangeal joint inflammation in a patient with psoriatic arthritis

(0.9 for psoriatic arthritis compared to 0.8 for RA). Although not studied as extensively as in RA, the limited available data suggest a similar increase in the standardized mortality rate for PsA patients at 1.6. Like RA patients, the main contributor to mortality is cardiovascular disease and, again, severe disease at presentation is a major risk factor along with the presence of erosive disease.

REACTIVE ARTHRITIS

DEFINITION

Reactive arthritis is a form of spondyloarthritis that is usually triggered by specific infections of the gastrointestinal or genitourinary tract. The incidence is ~40–50 per million for reactive arthritis triggered by either enteric infection or by *Chlamydia*. Although it is a form of post-infectious arthritis, it is useful to distinguish reactive arthritis from diseases such as post-viral arthritis and post-streptococcal arthritis (see below), since they have different clinical features and are not part of the spondyloarthritis group.

AETIOLOGY AND PATHOGENESIS

The disease is caused by specific bacteria in a susceptible host. The principal organisms involved are *Salmonella* spp., *Campylobacter jejuni* and *C. coli, Yersinia enterocolitica* and *Y. pseudotuberculosis, Shigella* spp. and *Chlamydia trachomatis.* Other organisms, such as *Clostridium difficile* and *Chlamydia pneumoniae*, are sometimes implicated. Only a few per cent of those infected develop arthritis and the proportion varies. It is higher in HLA-B27+ subjects, but B27 also predisposes to more severe and long-lasting arthritis.

The aetiology is not fully understood; organisms cannot be cultured from affected joints, but their antigens and, particularly in the case of *C. trachomatis,* the organism itself reaches the synovium, but is in a non-dividing state. Vigorous immune responses to the infection are detectable in the joint. It has been suggested that autoimmune responses develop in chronic disease ('molecular mimicry' – an immune response to the bacterium cross-reacting with something in the joint), but this is unproven.

CLINICAL FEATURES

The arthritis is acute and is usually oligoarticular, with a predilection for weight-bearing joints. Inflammatory backache and/or sacroiliac joint tenderness are seen. Fever and malaise are common. Joints are usually obviously swollen and hot so that septic arthritis and crystal arthritis become the principal differential diagnoses. Diagnosis relies heavily on a history of previous infection. Note that symptoms from reactive arthritis-inducing enteric infection can be surprisingly mild, particularly in *Yersinia* infection. Likewise *Chlamydia* infection is commonly asymptomatic, so that a history of a new sexual partner should be sought. In addition extra-articular features may be very helpful in reaching a diagnosis (Table 16.1).

TESTS

ESR and CRP are elevated, often grossly, and there may be neutrophilia. Autoantibodies are not present. Synovial fluid contains numerous white cells, but is sterile. Other tests can identify the preceding infection responsible for triggering reactive arthritis: stool and urethral culture and PCR/LCR tests for *Chlamydia* in urine are required. *Shigella* should be sought, particularly in those who acquired enteritis abroad. IgM antibodies or a rising titre of IgG and IgA antibodies for enteric pathogens such as *Yersinia* and *Campylobacter* are useful. Radiographs are not helpful in acute diagnosis. Typing for HLA-B27 may be useful in estimating prognosis.

Table 16.1 Extra-articular features of reactive arthritis

Site	Manifestation
Skin	Keratoderma blennorrhagica (a psoriatic rash) on the soles Circinate balanitis on the prepuce
Mucous membranes	Painless palatal ulcers
Eyes	Conjunctivitis, often transitory, or rarely uveitis
Entheses	Check the plantar fascia and Achilles tendon insertion for pain

TREATMENT

Full-dose NSAIDs and additional analgesics are required acutely. Affected joints should be aspirated to exclude other diagnoses; when infection is excluded, intra-articular steroids should be given and repeated as needed. Disease-modifying drugs are not usually required, but when disease persists sulfasalazine or methotrexate is a reasonable choice, although there are no controlled trial data. Long-term antibiotics have been used assuming that the arthritis is maintained by persistent infection, but controlled trials have not supported their use. Patients with *Chlamydia* infection require adequate conventional treatment.

The prognosis is generally favourable; many patients have mild arthritis, inflammatory back pain or enthesopathy, which does not come to medical attention. Those seen in hospital still have an 80% chance of being symptom-free with no residual joint damage at 1 year and a further 10% resolve in the next year. However, 10%, mainly those who are HLA-B27 positive, have a persistent oligoarthritis or evolve into AS or undifferentiated spondyloarthritis.

ARTHRITIS ASSOCIATED WITH INFLAMMATORY BOWEL DISEASE

DEFINITION

Many patients with inflammatory bowel disease (IBD) also have an inflammatory arthritis, usually with features that are associated with other forms of spondyloarthritis. Approximately 10% have peripheral arthritis, and a further 5% AS-like disease.

AETIOLOGY/PATHOGENESIS

This is unknown, but may be similar to reactive arthritis with gut flora playing the role attributed to the specific pathogens in reactive arthritis. Spondylitis and IBD seem closely linked: a proportion of AS patients have asymptomatic IBD, whilst B27-transgenic rats, which develop AS-like disease, display a Crohn's-like bowel disease at an even higher frequency than spondylitis.

CLINICAL FEATURES

The peripheral arthritis has been subdivided into types I and II. Type I is oligoarticular, asymmetrical, and associated with active bowel disease. This is conceptually similar to reactive arthritis triggered by enteric infection. Type II arthritis is symmetrical and polyarticular (more than five joints), and is not related to the activity of the bowel disease. There are distinct differences in the frequencies of HLA antigens in these two forms, which support the clinical distinction. Enthesopathy is common in both subtypes. Extra-articular features include iritis and skin lesions, such as erythema nodosum and pyoderma gangrenosum.

TESTS

The presence of IBD in a patient with spondyloarthritis is confirmed by radiological and endoscopic examination; technetium scans and indium-labelled leucocyte scans are also sometimes useful to demonstrate occult IBD. Biopsies distinguish between ulcerative colitis and Crohn's disease.

TREATMENT

Treatment is broadly similar to that for other forms of spondyloarthritis, except that sulfasalazine is the DMARD of first choice because of its additional effect on IBD. Note that drugs that do not have a sulphonamide component are effective against IBD, but not against arthritis, so patients receiving these agents for IBD may need to switch to sulfasalazine. NSAIDs can exacerbate IBD, so the treatment requirements of the arthritis and IBD may conflict. Methotrexate can exacerbate IBD, though in many patients it is an effective treatment for both conditions. Lastly, anti-TNFα drugs are useful for the arthritis and for Crohn's disease, but ineffective in ulcerative colitis. Patients with ulcerative colitis who require total colectomy will have improvement in type I peripheral arthritis, but this may flare if they develop 'pouchitis' – inflammation in the ileal reservoir that is usually fashioned after colectomy.

POST-INFECTIOUS ARTHRITIS

DEFINITION

The principal post-infectious arthritides (distinct from reactive arthritis) are associated with viral or bacterial infections. These arthritides are not associated with the other features common to spondyloarthritis (enthesitis, sacroiliitis, etc.), or with HLA-B27.

Viral infections

Arthritis commonly follows parvovirus or rubella infection in adults, but can occur after many viral infections including HIV, EBV and CMV. Some countries have endemic arthritis-inducing α-viruses, e.g. Ross River virus in Australia, and O'nyong-nyong and Chikungunya virus in East Africa. In these cases the virus can be detected in affected joints.

Bacterial infections

Diseases in which the organism can be detected in the joint include Lyme disease and Whipple's disease, but, as in reactive arthritis, the joints do not appear conventionally septic. This is either because the number of organisms present is very small, as in Lyme disease, or the bacterium cannot be cultured, e.g. *Tropheryma whippelii*, which causes Whipple's disease.

Infections by *Streptococcus* and *Neisseria* (gonococcus and meningococcus) are triggers of inflammatory arthritis, but the features of spondyloarthritis including its extra-articular manifestations are absent. Both organisms can also cause septic arthritis as well as post-infectious arthritis. In Western countries rheumatic fever is very rare, but should still be considered in patients with arthritis and a streptococcal infection. Cardiac involvement or erythema chronicum migrans should be looked for, but a 'pure' post-streptococcal arthritis is a much commoner sequel to infection, especially in adults.

CLINICAL FEATURES

History

It is useful to enquire about: recent throat infections; new sexual partners; fever; lymphadeno-
pathy or weight loss; travel to areas where Lyme disease or viral arthritides are endemic; and contact with small children and, if so, whether there has been a recent outbreak of 'slapped cheek' disease in their school, indicating parvovirus exposure.

Examination

In addition to the arthritis, there may be features associated with the primary infection. Rashes may be evident particularly in gonococcal disease where small pustules on peripheries are characteristic but easily missed. The rash of Lyme disease is not usually present by the time arthritis begins.

TESTS

Streptococcus and *Neisseria* can be cultured from appropriate sites, and IgM antibodies for viral infections should be sought. Note that the majority of adults will have IgG antibodies to parvovirus, rubella, EBV and CMV, so only IgM antibodies are helpful. The anti-streptococcal antibodies (anti-streptolysin O and anti-DNase), which may persist for long periods, should be measured, as well as antibodies to *Borrelia,* which causes Lyme disease. Currently, Whipple's disease is best diagnosed by using the polymerase chain reaction for the uncultivable *T. whippelii* on intestinal biopsies or synovial fluid or tissue.

TREATMENT

Treatment is directed at the underlying infection and in most cases the arthritis requires only symptomatic measures, since it will be self-limiting once the infection has been treated. An exception is post-streptococcal arthritis, which may pursue a chronic course, and a proportion of Lyme disease patients also have arthropathy that is resistant to antibiotics.

PREGNANCY AND THE RHEUMATIC DISEASES

Approximately 50% of all pregnant women experience back pain during pregnancy. Significant back pain occurs in about 25%, and severe disability in about 8% of patients. After pregnancy, problems are serious in about 7%. Connective tissue diseases frequently affect women during childbearing years. Fertility may be reduced in some cases, but for the majority of patients monitoring and treatment in pregnancy is complicated and best managed by close collaboration between gynaecologists, rheumatologists and paediatricians.

INFLUENCE OF PREGNANCY ON AUTOIMMUNE DISEASES

In many patients with inflammatory arthritis pregnancy exerts an immunosuppressive effect and patients may go into remission. Typically, this is short lived, and flares occur in the post-partum period. SLE and antiphospholipid antibody syndrome may develop during pregnancy and should be considered in the differential diagnosis for any pregnant woman with a new onset of arthritis. Maternal flares may occur in one-third of patients, especially in the second trimester and post partum. The risk is highest for women with active lupus at the time of conception and those who have antiphospholipid antibody and hypertension. By contrast, if SLE is in remission at conception, the risk of flare is <15%.

Fetal cells can persist in the circulation of women who have been pregnant (microchimaerism); there have been suggestions that this could be a possible cause of autoimmune disorders in women.

EFFECTS ON THE FETUS

Fetal loss is a recognized risk in SLE and antiphospholipid antibody syndrome. Untreated primiparas who have SLE or SLE-like disease and antiphospholipid antibody have an approximately 30% probability of losing a pregnancy, often in the second trimester. Mothers who have circulating anti-Ro and anti-La antibodies may be completely asymptomatic, but there is a 1% risk of fetal heart block, as these antibodies are able to cross the placenta and bind to fetal heart tissue. Antiphospholipid antibody syndrome is a major cause of fetal loss, pre-eclampsia and premature birth.

DRUGS IN PREGNANCY

NSAIDs are not teratogenic, but if given in late pregnancy can induce renal and cardiac side effects in the fetus. NSAIDs should, therefore, be stopped by gestational week 32. Corticosteroids are frequently necessary to control rheumatic disease flares and for prevention of serious organ manifestations. However, due to an increased risk of cleft palate, high doses (1–2 mg/kg) should be avoided in the first trimester. Among disease-modifying drugs, sulfasalazine, azathioprine and antimalarials have the safest record. Ciclosporin can be given throughout pregnancy if necessary. Insufficient data exist for treatment of pregnant patients with TNF inhibitors. There are reports of infliximab being used as a treatment for infertility and some women having children whilst continuing to receive anti-TNF treatment to control their arthritis. The severity of the disease under treatment determines whether continuation of one of these drugs is justified. Prophylactic withdrawal of drugs before pregnancy is mandatory for leflunomide and the cytotoxic agents, methotrexate and cyclophosphamide. It is essential to ensure effective contraception during treatment and to discontinue drugs before conception is planned. There may be fertility problems for patients who have received significant accumulated doses of cyclophosphamide. Most drugs are secreted into milk and, therefore, any treatment offered to a mother post partum can carry risks to the child and may influence the decision on breast- or bottle-feeding. Ideally, mothers should be encouraged to breast-feed, but if they are suffering a flare of disease it would be better to stop breast-feeding so that they can receive appropriate therapy without potential harm to the child.

FURTHER READING

American College of Rheumatology Subcommittee on Rheumatoid Arthritis Guidelines 2002 Guidelines for the management of rheumatoid arthritis: 2002 Update. Arthritis Rheum 46(2): 328–346.

Braun J, Brandt J, Listing J et al 2002 Treatment of active ankylosing spondylitis with infliximab: a randomised controlled multicentre trial. Lancet 359: 1187–1193.

Gaston JSH, Lillicrap MS 2003 Arthritis associated with enteric infection. Best Pract Rheumatol 17: 219–239.

Orchard TR, Thiyagaraja S, Welsh KI et al 2000 Clinical phenotype is related to HLA genotype in the peripheral arthropathies of inflammatory bowel disease. Gastroenterology 118: 274–278.

WEBSITE

Arthritis Research Campaign. Rheumatoid Arthritis – An Information Booklet. Online. Available: *http://www.arc.org.uk/arthinfo/ patpubs/6033/6033.asp*

228

SYSTEMIC DISEASES

17

Ian N. Bruce, Nick Wilkinson, Julia L. Newton and Raashid Luqmani

Cases relevant to this chapter

84, 85, 87–90, 93, 94, 99

●Essential facts

1. Systemic lupus erythematosus (SLE) is mediated by immune complex deposition or the effects of pathological antibodies.

2. The symptoms and signs of SLE are diverse; non-specific constitutional upset characterized by malaise, low-grade fever, fatigue and unexplained weight loss is common.

3. The long-term survival for patients with SLE has improved from a 5-year mortality of 50% in the 1950s to <15% mortality currently after 10 years.

4. The antiphospholipid syndrome is characterized by recurrent thrombosis (arterial or venous) and/or pregnancy morbidity, and persistently elevated levels of antibodies to phospholipid-related proteins.

5. Proximal muscle weakness is the typical presenting feature of myositis.

6. There is a risk of malignancy in patients with dermatomyositis, particularly in the 2–3 years before and after the diagnosis of myositis is made.

7. Pulmonary hypertension is a complication of limited cutaneous scleroderma affecting 5–35% of patients.

8. Interstitial lung disease occurs in most patients with scleroderma, but progression to severe disease occurs in less than 20%.

9. Vasculitis is inflammation of blood vessels with occlusion leading to tissue damage, usually of unknown aetiology, with an incidence of >100 per million per year.

10. Untreated multi-system vasculitis is fatal without cytotoxic drugs and delay in diagnosis significantly affects morbidity and mortality.

11. Anti-neutrophil cytoplasm antibody testing is helpful in supporting a diagnosis in patients who have suggestive clinical and/or pathological features of vasculitis.

12. Clinical distinction between active vasculitis and infection may be difficult and requires careful multi-specialty management (if in doubt treat for infection first).

SYSTEMIC LUPUS ERYTHEMATOSUS

The connective tissue diseases represent a family of conditions that can be broadly defined as: multi-system inflammatory diseases of autoimmune origin associated with the anti-nuclear antibody (ANA) family of autoantibodies. There are a number of conditions that fall within this family and connective tissue diseases often show elements of overlap and similarity. These conditions have certain underlying pathological features that they

Table 17.1 Relative occurrence of specific pathological features that underlie the connective tissue diseases

Pathology	SLE	DM/PM	Sjögren's syndrome	Scleroderma	APS
Inflammation	+++	+++	++	+/–	–
Fibrosis	+	++	++	+++	–
Vasospasm	++	+	+	+++	–
Thrombosis	++	+/–	+/–	+	+++

These pathological features explain many of the clinical features of these conditions.
APS, antiphospholipid syndrome; DM/PM, dermatomyositis/polymyositis; SLE, systemic lupus erythematosus.

share, but that occur relatively more frequently in some of the subgroups compared to others (Table 17.1). The four key pathological processes that underlie the connective tissue diseases are inflammation, fibrosis or scarring, vasospasm and vascular thrombosis. The primary clinical features and many of the complications associated with these conditions can be deduced from these underlying pathological processes. Certain clinical/pathological features of these diseases are also more frequent with particular autoantibody subtypes. The presence of particular autoantibody subtypes may alert the clinician to investigate a particular organ or system for clinical features of relevance (Fig. 17.1).

SLE is the 'model' connective tissue disorder. It presents as a multi-system inflammatory disease with a wide range of clinical manifestations. Most of the clinical manifestations can be explained on the basis of excess production of pathogenic autoantibodies. These autoantibodies either cause tissue injury directly or mediate the production of immune complexes that deposit in target organs to provoke tissue inflammation. However SLE is associated with the production of a range of other autoantibodies whose significance is unclear.

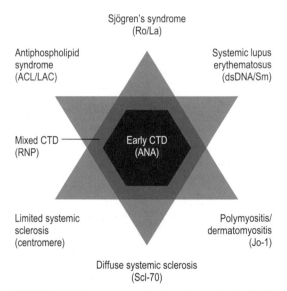

FIGURE 17.1   The spectrum of anti-nuclear antibody (ANA)-associated connective tissue diseases (CTD) showing the association of disease classification and autoantibody subtypes. The overlapping spectrum of connective tissue disease and associated antibodies in serum are shown in parentheses. ACL, anti-cardiolipin antibody; LAC, lupus anticoagulant; RNP, anti-ribonucleoprotein antibody; dsDNA, double-stranded DNA antibody; Ro/La, anti-Ro/La antibodies; Scl-70, anti-Scl-70 antibody; Jo-1, anti-Jo-1 antibody; Sm, anti-Sm antibody. (Adapted from Ahmad Y, Bruce IN 2000 Connective tissue disease and the role of the general practitioner. In Practice Series, arc Publications)

EPIDEMIOLOGY

SLE, while uncommon, is not a rare condition. In UK studies the prevalence is approximately 1 in 4000 individuals but there is a marked female preponderance with a female:male ratio of 9–13:1, meaning that SLE affects approximately 1 in 2000 females in the UK. There are also differences in prevalence according to ethnic background.

Compared to white Caucasians, the prevalence is approximately two to three times higher in Asians from the Indian subcontinent and five to 10 times higher in Africans and Afro-Caribbeans. SLE can present at any age from childhood through to elderly. The peak age at onset is in the late third, early fourth decade of life, with a second peak in the sixth decade.

AETIOLOGY

The cause of lupus remains unclear, but there is a strong genetic predisposition with first-degree family members being 50 times more likely to develop the disease than the background population. Additional factors known to cause or influence the development of lupus include UV light exposure, female sex hormones and certain drugs, e.g. chlorpromazine, hydralazine and isoniazid. It is known that anti-DNA antibodies are directly toxic to the kidney, but it is not certain what role, if any, is played by the numerous other autoantibodies produced in SLE.

CLINICAL FEATURES

The symptoms and signs of SLE are diverse, but as indicated in Table 17.1 inflammation is the predominant pathology associated with many of the key clinical features. Non-specific constitutional upset characterized by malaise, low-grade fever, fatigue and unexplained weight loss are common in SLE. More specific inflammatory features include a malar or 'butterfly' rash, which is often light sensitive, and other cutaneous lesions including alopecia, mucosal ulceration and digital vascular changes such as nail-edge infarcts and splinter haemorrhages. Arthritis (small joint symmetrical polyarthritis) is also a common presenting feature. The arthritis is non-erosive, but in some cases ligamentous laxity can result in deformities similar to those seen in rheumatoid arthritis (RA) (Jaccoud's arthropathy; Fig. 17.2). In contrast to RA, however, these deformities are reducible. Importantly, SLE is also associated with inflammation in other organ systems, including serositis, nephritis and involvement of the central nervous system. Renal disease is often asymptomatic and can affect up to 25% of patients, although a higher occurrence is noted in Afro-Caribbean, Chinese and Indo-Asian patients. Careful clinical assessment and regular urine examination is, therefore, necessary to alert the clinician to this possibility. A wide range of neuropsychiatric presentations have been described. Currently, the classification of SLE is based on a combination of clinical and laboratory investigations and patients should have four of 11 criteria to confirm the classification of SLE (Box 17.1).

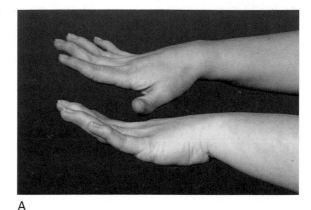

A

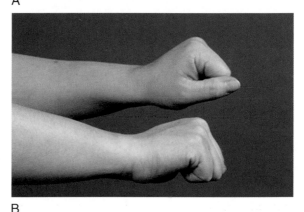

B

FIGURE 17.2 Jaccoud's arthropathy in a patient with systemic lupus erythematosus. There are swan neck deformities on several digits (A). These are, however, fully reducible and the patient is still able to make a complete fist (B). This deformity is a result of ligamentous laxity rather that joint subluxation

Thrombosis represents an important cause of clinical manifestations in lupus. The propensity to thrombosis is related to the presence of antiphospholipid antibodies, which reflect a pro-coagulant state. In addition, blood vessel inflammation can impair the normal anticoagulant properties of the blood vessel lining. As a result, patients with SLE are at increased risk of venous thromboembolism, arterial thrombosis and adverse pregnancy outcomes (see antiphospholipid syndrome).

Up to 50% of patients with SLE also describe Raynaud's phenomenon, although this is usually less severe and less likely to cause digital ulceration compared to patients with scleroderma. Typical skin changes include scarring or fibrosis and a subgroup of patients with SLE present with discoid lupus lesions (Fig. 17.3), which are often discrete lesions, associated with scaling, hypo- or

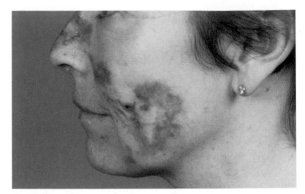

A

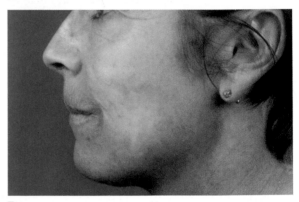

B

FIGURE 17.3   (A) Actively inflamed discoid lupus eruption on the light-exposed skin of the cheek and bridge of nose. (B) Even after successful treatment there is still residual atrophy and depigmentation of the affected area

hyper-pigmentation and loss of associated skin appendages. If discoid lesions occur on the scalp this results in scarring alopecia.

OTHER COMPLICATIONS

Infection is a common complication in patients with SLE. Active disease is associated with complement consumption, relative hyposplenism, neutropenia and lymphopenia. In addition to low absolute counts, leucocyte function is also impaired. In addition, drugs such as corticosteroids and immunosuppressive agents increase the propensity to infection. It is also not unusual for infection to co-exist with a flare-up of the underlying inflammatory disease and, therefore, sepsis needs to be carefully considered in most clinical settings. It is also increasingly recognized that SLE is associated with an accelerated onset of atherosclerosis. The early development of atherosclerosis coupled with the increased thrombotic risk seen in SLE means that atherosclerosis should be considered in the differential diagnosis of relevant presentations, e.g. acute chest pain, acute focal neurological event.

LABORATORY ABNORMALITIES

Simple investigations can be extremely informative in SLE patients. Anaemia may be present due to chronic disease, but haemolytic anaemia (positive Coombs' test) may also occur. Leucopenia, in particular lymphopenia, is characteristic and thrombocytopenia can occur either as a chronic, stable, low platelet count or as an acute profound thrombocytopenia, which is associated with bruising and bleeding complications. Urine abnormalities may be detected on dipstick (haematuria, pyuria and proteinuria). Any such abnormality requires further investigation to exclude infection and significant renal involvement. Patients can have significant glomerulonephritis requiring immunosuppressive therapy even when the serum creatinine is within normal limits and, therefore, persistent microscopic haematuria/proteinuria usually requires a renal biopsy to determine further management. Serologically, patients with active lupus often have reduced C3 or C4 complement concentrations due to immune complex-driven consumption. Hypocomplementaemia may also be due to an underlying hereditary complement deficiency, which itself is a risk factor for developing SLE. ANA testing is positive in >90% of SLE patients; however, the titre does not reflect underlying disease activity. In contrast, antibodies to double-stranded DNA (dsDNA) are highly specific for SLE, although they may be positive in only 60% of all cases. In some patients, the titres of dsDNA antibodies do reflect underlying disease activity and in such cases rising titre may portend a future flare of clinical disease.

CLINICAL COURSE AND PROGNOSIS

SLE classically runs a relapsing and remitting course. With treatment, initial clinical manifestations are often suppressed; however, as treatment is tapered a further flare can occur. Certain triggers for flares can sometimes be recognized, such as psychosocial stress, intercurrent infection, UV light exposure or exposure to exogenous oestrogens. While a clinical flare-up is often associated with recurrence of the previous clinical features, it is not unusual for new clinical features to develop or for a flare-up to be characterized by an entirely new organ/system involvement. Obviously, as the disease and its treatment can cause chronic morbidity, additional complications can also mimic a flare of the disease. For example, a patient with SLE presenting with acute chest pain may have an inflammatory serositis such as pericarditis. However, acute chest pain may also be caused by a pulmonary embolus, acute myocardial infarction or bacterial pneumonia, all of which are more common in SLE patients.

The long-term survival for patients with SLE has improved considerably over the past 50 years. In the 1950s the 5-year mortality was 50%. Currently the 10-year survival is greater than 85% in most series. There is increased mortality in patients of Afro-Caribbean or African-American background. Mortality is also higher in patients who have renal or pulmonary involvement as well as patients with thrombocytopenia.

MANAGEMENT OF SYSTEMIC LUPUS ERYTHEMATOSUS

In the management of patients with SLE the aim is to make a clear diagnosis and to determine the extent of involvement. It is also important to determine if specific clinical features can be attributed to inflammation, thrombosis or other disease mechanisms, as well as to exclude specific complications such as infection. For mild non-life-threatening disease, topical therapies, NSAIDs and general life-style advice, such as avoidance of sun exposure, may be sufficient. For mild-to-moderate disease antimalarial drugs (hydroxychloroquine or chloroquine phosphate), methotrexate, leflunomide, azathioprine and/or low-dose corticosteroids are frequently used. In patients with significant organ involvement, e.g. proliferative glomerulonephritis, severe neuropsychiatric involvement or uncontrolled generalized disease, immunosuppressive drugs, such as cyclophosphamide or mycophenolate mofetil, are indicated. Because of the risks of long-term toxicity from cyclophosphamide, most patients are switched to maintenance azathioprine or mycophenolate following successful initial disease control. More recently, novel therapies, such as anti-CD20 monoclonal antibodies, have shown promise in refractory disease. In addition to these therapies, other specific agents to control symptoms and/or to prevent complications are commonly required (Table 17.2). These therapies include anticonvulsants, anticoagulants, antihypertensives, lipid-lowering drugs and bone protective agents.

234

Table 17.2 Examples of drugs commonly used in the management of patients with systemic lupus erythematosus, including the indication and disease process being treated

Indication	Pathological process	Drug class	Examples
Disease process	Inflammation	Antimalarials	Hydroxychloroquine Chloroquine Mepacrine
		Steroids	Prednisolone Deflazacort
		Immunosuppressants	Azathioprine Methotrexate Cyclophosphamide
	Raynaud's phenomenon	Vasodilators	Nifedipine Amlodipine Prostacyclin
	Clotting risk	Anti-platelet drugs	Aspirin Clopidogrel
		Anticoagulants	Warfarin Heparin
Associated symptoms	Depression	Antidepressants	Fluoxetine Paroxetine Amitriptyline
	Seizures/epilepsy	Anticonvulsants	Sodium valproate Phenytoin Carbamazepine
	Peptic ulceration	Ulcer healing drugs	Ranitidine Lansoprazole Omeprazole
Prevention of late complications	Osteoporosis	Bone protective agents	Calcium Vitamin D Risedronate Alendronate Calcitriol
	Hypercholesterolaemia	Lipid-lowering drugs	Simvastatin Pravastatin Fenofibrate
	Hypertension	Antihypertensives	Bendroflumethazide Captopril Losartan Amlodipine

ANTIPHOSPHOLIPID SYNDROME

BACKGROUND

The antiphospholipid syndrome (APS) is defined as a clinical syndrome characterized by a tendency to recurrent thrombosis (arterial or venous) and/or pregnancy morbidity associated with persistently elevated levels of antibodies to phospholipid-related proteins.

Antiphospholipid antibodies have been formally studied and delineated as recently as the early 1980s. However, an associated test for the lupus anticoagulant (LAC) was described in the early 1950s. This functional test is an in vitro assay in which a phospholipid-dependent coagulation test is prolonged (e.g. activated partial thromboplastin time, Russell's viper venom test, etc.). This prolongation cannot be corrected by the addition of normal plasma (which excludes a clotting factor deficiency). In contrast, however, adding phospholipid in excess to the mixture will normalize the test. While the in vitro phenomenon is that of prolongation of a clotting time, the lupus anticoagulant test actually reflects a prothrombotic tendency. It is also increasingly recognized that, while it was first described in the context of SLE, the lupus anticoagulant can also be observed in patients who do not have SLE.

CLINICAL FEATURES (Table 17.3)

Vascular thrombosis

Thrombosis associated with antiphospholipid syndrome can occur in any part of the circulation. The most important thrombotic complications include deep vein thrombosis and pulmonary embolism as well as stroke (Fig. 17.4), myocardial infarction and retinal artery occlusion. Untreated, there is a high risk of recurrent thrombotic events and, indeed, a careful clinical history may reveal previous unexplained thrombotic episodes in the distant past. APS patients can experience thrombosis on the venous and arterial side of the circulation, although

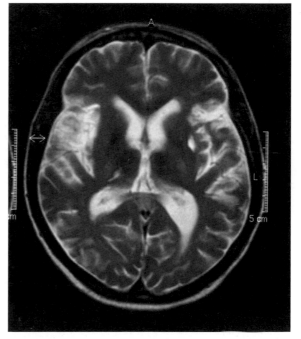

FIGURE 17.4 Magnetic resonance image of the brain in a patient with systemic lupus erythematosus and secondary antiphospholipid syndrome. The scan demonstrates significant cerebral atrophy as well as several areas of infarction from previous thrombotic episodes (strokes)

Table 17.3 Summary of the Sapporo criteria for the diagnosis of antiphospholipid syndrome

Clinical criteria	Laboratory criteria*
Vascular thrombosis – objectively confirmed, single or recurrent episode(s) Arterial thrombosis OR Venous thrombosis	Anticardiolipin antibodies IgG or IgM
Pregnancy morbidity (any of): • Three or more unexplained spontaneous abortions before 10 weeks' gestation • One or more unexplained death of a fetus after 10 weeks' gestation • One or more premature delivery due to pre-eclampsia/eclampsia before 34 weeks' gestation	Lupus anticoagulant

*Needs to be positive on two occasions at least 6 weeks apart.
Antiphospholipid syndrome (APS) when one clinical AND one laboratory criteria are fulfilled.

it is more common for recurrent thrombosis to occur on the same side of the circulation as the previous thrombosis.

Pregnancy morbidity

APS often presents initially as a poor obstetric history. This can be either as unexplained spontaneous abortions before the 10th week of gestation or one or more unexplained deaths of a morphologically normal fetus after the 10th week of gestation. Other pregnancy morbidity, e.g. severe pre-eclampsia or severe placental insufficiency resulting in premature birth before 34 weeks' gestation, can also be part of this syndrome. The mechanism of pregnancy morbidity is believed to be thrombosis of the placental circulation resulting in failure of the placenta to develop adequately. In some cases frank placental infarction is seen.

Other clinical features

Approximately one-third of patients with APS have thrombocytopenia, which is usually a chronic stable thrombocytopenia ($50-150\times10^9$/l). In addition, about 15% also have a Coombs-positive haemolytic anaemia. Cutaneous features associated with APS include livedo reticularis (Fig. 17.5), superficial thrombophlebitis and chronic leg ulcers. On careful screening, patients with APS frequently have thickening of cardiac valves and 20–30% may have clinical evidence of mitral valve prolapse. In the central nervous system, clinical syndromes, such as transverse myelitis, chorea and migraines,

have also been noted. It is, however, unclear whether these are primarily thrombotic in nature or whether they represent a separate pathogenic mechanism. Occasionally patients can present with thrombosis in multiple vascular beds. This 'catastrophic' antiphospholipid syndrome is difficult to recognize clinically and is associated with a high mortality rate.

CLASSIFICATION

The initial descriptions of APS occurred in the context of SLE. APS may also be a complicating feature of other autoimmune diseases, e.g. rheumatoid arthritis, Sjögren's syndrome, etc. In this context the term secondary APS is usually employed. It is becoming increasingly recognized, however, that the majority of patients with APS do not have any other systemic autoimmune condition, and these are described as primary APS.

MANAGEMENT

APS is only one cause of recurrent thrombosis or miscarriages. Careful evaluation should, therefore, be undertaken to identify other causes of thrombosis, e.g. Factor V Leiden, protein C and protein S deficiencies. Similarly, for recurrent miscarriage other causes, e.g. hormonal, anatomical and chromosomal causes, should be actively excluded. APS will constitute anything from 5% to 30% of such cases.

Positive antiphospholipid antibodies without clinical thrombosis or pregnancy loss

There is no clear consensus as to how this group of patients should be managed. There is no high-quality clinical trial evidence on which to base any recommendations, but it is recognized that these patients are at increased risk of future thrombosis and many authorities would recommend low-dose aspirin as well as general advice on stopping smoking, avoiding oestrogen-containing contraceptives, and maintaining good control of cholesterol and blood pressure. Low-molecular-weight heparin is sometimes offered for patients undergoing surgery, long-haul flights (>4 h duration) and in patients who have a plaster cast applied.

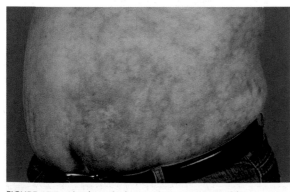

FIGURE 17.5 Livedo reticularis rash in a patient with antiphospholipid syndrome. The rash has a bluish purple reticular pattern, which does not improve in a warm environment

Recurrent pregnancy loss

In women who have had previous pregnancy morbidity associated with APS, randomized trials demonstrate that the optimum therapy is low-dose aspirin combined with low-molecular-weight heparin. This regimen can increase the live birth rate from <30% to approximately 80%. In view of the fact that the mother will also be at increased risk of venous thrombosis for up to 6 weeks postpartum, this treatment regimen may be continued until this point. It should, however, be noted that in women who have had a previous vascular thrombosis and who are already taking warfarin outside of pregnancy special planning for pregnancy is required. Since warfarin is teratogenic, this will need to be stopped prior to 6 weeks' gestation and the mother transferred to a full therapeutic treatment regimen of heparin until after delivery.

Management of thrombotic complications

Patients with APL who experience a thrombotic event have a significant risk of recurrent thrombosis if left untreated. As a result, for the majority of patients life-long anticoagulation is recommended with warfarin. The target international normalized ratio (prothrombin ratio) (INR) is usually kept at 2.0–3.0, although in cases where further events occur a higher-intensity anticoagulation (INR > 3.0) may be indicated. In patients who are fully anticoagulated there is little evidence that the addition of aspirin confers any further risk reduction. It is also useful to give general advice about maintaining good cardiovascular health. The use of oestrogen-containing contraceptives and hormone replacement therapies is contraindicated in these patients.

ADULT MUSCLE DISORDERS

Idiopathic inflammatory muscle disease comprises a group of conditions that are characterized by inflammation of striated muscle. These myositis syndromes fall within the family of connective tissue diseases and they can occur on their own or overlap with other connective tissue diseases, as outlined previously. Myositis is a rare condition with an annual incidence of approximately five to seven new cases per million. The aetiology remains unknown.

CLASSIFICATION AND DIAGNOSTIC CRITERIA

The commonly described subtypes are outlined in Table 17.4. In addition, there are classic criteria for the diagnosis of the two most frequently described syndromes, polymyositis and dermatomyositis (Table 17.5). The commonest presenting feature

Table 17.4 Classification of common inflammatory myositis syndromes

Adult-onset syndromes	Childhood-onset syndromes
Polymyositis	Childhood-onset myositis
Dermatomyositis	
Malignancy-associated myositis*	
Myositis overlapping with other connective tissue disease	
Inclusion body myositis	

*Malignancy more frequently associated with dermatomyositis.

Table 17.5 Summary of Bohan and Peter criteria for the diagnosis of polymyositis and dermatomyositis

Criteria
Symmetrical proximal muscle weakness
Biopsy evidence of myositis
Electromyographic changes consistent with myositis
Raised muscle enzymes on serum testing
Typical rash of dermatomyositis

Diagnosis
Polymyositis (definite/probable): at least three of the first four criteria present
Dermatomyositis (definite/probable): typical rash PLUS at least two of the first four criteria

is with proximal muscle weakness, which usually evolves over a 3–6-month period, but can be more insidious, or in some cases an acute presentation can be observed. In a small proportion of patients, the presenting feature is with the classic rash. The usual muscle groups involved include the proximal musculature of the upper and lower limbs, which will cause difficulty in functions requiring limb strength. Simple tasks, such as arising from a low chair, stepping into trousers as well as brushing hair, etc., can become difficult. Patients sometimes walk with a 'waddling' gait. Other striated muscle is also involved and weakness of the neck flexors, as well as abdominal muscle weakness, can be observed causing difficulties getting out of bed, etc. Since the upper oesophagus has significant amounts of striated muscle, dysphagia can occur. The myocardium may also be involved and involvement of the respiratory muscles can cause exertional dyspnoea.

Cutaneous involvement in dermatomyositis

The classic rash involves linear scaling papules on the dorsum of the hand (Gottron's papules), as well as a purple erythematous rash around the eyelid (heliotrope rash; Fig. 17.6). Patients with myositis may also experience photosensitivity with associated facial erythema and erythema of the 'V' of the neck. Nailfold capillaries can be extremely abnormal with giant capillary loops and a 'ragged nailfold' appearance.

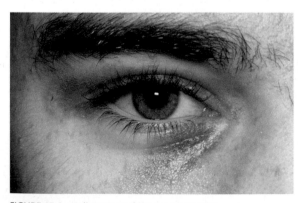

FIGURE 17.6 Heliotrope rash in a patient with dermatomyositis showing the typical erythematous periorbital rash. The name is derived from the heliotrope flower, which is a purple colour

Other clinical features

Patients with myositis may also have a polyarthritis. In addition to involvement of the respiratory muscles, the lung parenchyma can be involved with a diffuse interstitial pneumonitis that can also result in dyspnoea. This is particularly common in patients with antibodies Jo-1.

CHRONIC COMPLICATIONS

The initial clinical features of myositis in the muscles, skin and lungs reflect an underlying inflammatory disorder. Secondary fibrosis/scarring can also occur. In the lungs this can result in pulmonary fibrosis, and in the muscle this can result in long-term weakness and the failure to restore muscle strength to the pre-morbid levels. Scarring and fibrosis within muscle is particularly disabling in childhood-onset dermatomyositis where areas of muscle damage can be complicated by soft tissue calcinosis and the failure of the muscle to grow adequately, resulting in flexion contractures.

MYOSITIS AND THE ASSOCIATION WITH MALIGNANCY

Patients with myositis, especially patients with dermatomyositis, have been found to have an increased risk of developing an underlying malignancy. This increased risk of malignancy persists throughout the patient's lifetime, but the risk is particularly high in the 2–3 years before and after the diagnosis of myositis is made. The common sites of malignancy include the gastrointestinal tract, lungs, ovaries and the lymphatic system. As a general rule, the malignancies associated tend to be those of relevance to the age, gender and ethnicity of the patient. Vigilance is, therefore, required throughout the follow-up period for patients with dermatomyositis in particular, and initial screening for such cancers should be included in the management plan.

INVESTIGATIONS

Routine laboratory tests often reveal a low-grade anaemia of chronic disease associated with an elevated erythrocyte sedimentation rate (ESR). Biochemical tests show elevated creatine phosphokinase (CK) in the majority of patients, and in patients with extreme elevations in CK, myoglobulinuria may occur that can lead to renal impairment. An electromyograph is a sensitive test for myositis. At the point of needle insertion spontaneous fibrillation can be observed, as can polyphasic potentials on muscle contraction. A muscle biopsy can provide important information by confirming the presence of an inflammatory cell infiltrate. The inflammatory pattern in polymyositis tends to be scattered throughout the muscle tissue. By contrast, dermatomyositis is frequently characterized by perivascular infiltration. The muscle biopsy is useful to exclude other non-inflammatory muscle diseases and to identify patients with inclusion body myositis, which is less responsive to conventional therapy. In addition to these investigations, magnetic resonance imaging (MRI) is increasingly being employed as a sensitive test to pick up muscle inflammation. It can be a useful modality to decide on which muscle groups to biopsy.

MANAGEMENT

High-dose corticosteroids remain the mainstay of treatment in inflammatory myositis. Corticosteroids (1–2 mg/kg per day) can be used for the initial few weeks until significant clinical improvement occurs and the CK has fallen to within the normal range. There is evidence that intravenous immunoglobulin may be effective.

Other immunosuppressive agents, such as azathioprine, methotrexate and cyclophosphamide, have also been used. Such agents can be used for their 'steroid-sparing' properties. This can be particularly useful in patients who require moderate to high doses of steroids to control their disease adequately. These agents are indicated in patients who have an associated interstitial pneumonitis (note: methotrexate would be relatively contraindicated for such patients). In the medium term, management of these patients is often complicated by the development of steroid myopathy. This can be difficult to distinguish from the primary disease. In most cases, however, steroid myopathy will be associated with a normal CK concentration and the EMG may be useful to distinguish ongoing chronic inflammation from simple mild myopathic changes. In some cases, however, a repeat muscle biopsy may be indicated to distinguish a flare from steroid myopathy.

In addition to medical management it is important to encourage patients to rehabilitate their muscles after an episode of myositis towards their premorbid levels. In addition, one should have a low threshold for re-evaluating the patient to rule out an underlying malignancy, should the clinical circumstances suggest this.

RAYNAUD'S PHENOMENON AND SCLERODERMA

Raynaud's phenomenon is a condition resulting from vasospasm, characterized by intermittent colour changes of pallor, cyanosis and subsequent hyperaemia in response to cold and/or emotional stress. Although most typically noted in the fingers, the circulation of the toes, ears, nose and tongue may be affected. Raynaud's phenomenon is more common in women than men, with prevalence estimates ranging from 4% to 30%. Geographic variations in the prevalence relate to differences in climate. Raynaud's phenomenon may be a primary or a secondary process. In the primary form, attacks affect all digits in a symmetrical fashion, but do not result in tissue necrosis, ulceration or gangrene; no cause of Raynaud's can be detected, ANAs are not present, the nailfold capillaries look normal and the ESR is not raised. In the secondary form of the disease, symptoms commence at an older age (usually over 30 years), giving rise to painful and asymmetrical episodes, sometimes causing ischaemic skin lesions and typically associated with positive autoautoantibodies and capillaroscopic abnormalities, often with clinical features suggestive of connective tissue diseases, especially systemic sclerosis.

Raynaud's is distinct from acrocyanosis, where there is continuous cyanosis of the hands or feet aggravated by cold temperature. Patients should be advised to stop smoking and to avoid medication that can induce vasospasm, such as β-blockers. Patients should avoid sudden changes in temperature where practical. This may mean wearing warm clothing, and gloves and socks, even in moderate weather. Medication used for Raynaud's includes calcium-channel blockers (such as nifedipine up to 80 mg daily). Alternatively, a sympatholytic agent (prazosin), an angiotensin II receptor type I antagonist (losartan) or a selective sertonin-reuptake inhibitor (fluoxetine) may be useful.

Systemic sclerosis, or scleroderma, is a systemic autoimmune disease that is mediated by vascular damage and fibrosis within the skin and visceral organs. The term scleroderma includes localized skin fibrosis (previously termed morphoea) and generalized forms with inflammatory, vascular and fibrotic pathology. The two main forms are limited cutaneous scleroderma and diffuse cutaneous scleroderma. Localized skin fibrosis may appear as an area of increased or reduced pigmentation, typically with some erythema and skin thickening. Over time, the central area of skin may become pale, whilst the edge of the lesion, representing the active area of fibrosis, may spread further. Patches of scleroderma can occur at any site, typically on the trunk and limbs. In childhood forms, the patches may be linear and can have a significant effect on growth of the affected area, leading to hematrophy. Treatment is largely supportive.

Limited cutaneous scleroderma is typically associated with anti-centromere antibodies. It is defined by the extent of skin involvement (peripheral skin involvement distal to the elbows). There is a tendency to develop Calcinosis, oEsophageal dysmotility, Sclerodactyly and Telangiectasia in many patients, leading to the previous description of CREST syndrome. Diffuse cutaneous scleroderma involves more widespread skin changes proximal to the elbows, and may, in advanced cases, cover almost the whole body surface. There is an association with the presence of anti-Scl-70 antibodies.

Although scleroderma has a significant mortality, there have been major improvements in the management of renal and pulmonary disease. With longer survival, we are increasingly aware of the effects of progressive fibrosis in many organs, such as the gastrointestinal tract, resulting in problems such as acid reflux, malabsorption and faecal incontinence. Angiotensin-converting enzyme inhibitors for scleroderma renal crisis, proton pump inhibitors for reflux oesophagitis and advanced therapies for severe pulmonary arterial hypertension are now established. Better understanding of the underlying mechanisms means that, in future, cytokine-directed treatments may modify the course of the disease. At present, however, systemic sclerosis remains one of the least treatable of the autoimmune rheumatic diseases.

Pulmonary hypertension is a recognized complication of limited cutaneous scleroderma in 5–35% of patients. It may respond to vasodilatation using high doses of calcium channel antagonists, continuous intravenous prostacyclin or endothelin-1 antagonists. In severe cases, lung transplantation should be considered. Interstitial lung disease occurs in most patients with diffuse cutaneous scleroderma, but progression to severe restrictive lung disease occurs in less than 20%, many of whom will die. The histological changes are of non-specific interstitial pneumonia. The most effective initial treatment is with cyclophosphamide and low-dose corticosteroid therapy, but progression to lung fibrosis may be resistant to therapy.

SJÖGREN'S SYNDROME

Dry eyes and mouth are the main features of Sjögren's syndrome, which may occur as a primary disease, typically in association with autoantibodies (anti-Ro or anti-SSA, and anti-La or anti-SSB). The exocrine glands are affected in a destructive, fibrosing process leading to failure of gland function. The pathological findings are of focal lymphocytic infiltration in the exocrine glands. Skin lesions may occur in up to 10% of patients, typically a cutaneous vasculitis, but patients may also develop photosensitive rashes identical to those seen in SLE, suggesting a common pathogenesis, but creating diagnostic confusion in some cases. Bronchial and bronchiolar dysfunction is the main lung manifestation rather than interstitial lung disease (more commonly seen in SLE and RA). Up to 13% of patients suffer from Raynaud's phenomenon. Both tubular interstitial nephritis and glomerulonephritis have been described. Neurological involvement is usually characterized by peripheral sensory neuropathy (not responsive to immunosuppression), and in some cases sensorineural hearing loss. Autonomic neuropathy is reported in patients with long-standing disease, but is rarely symptomatic. Sub-clinical myositis may occur in over 25% of patients, with histological abnormalities similar to those seen in inflammatory myositis. Around 20% of patients have anaemia, cytopenias and a raised ESR, along with hypergammaglobulinaemia. The feared risk of transformation to lymphoma is lower than previously thought. Recent studies suggest that the incidence is less than 10%. Overall, Sjögren's is a slowly progressive condition with a much better prognosis than most inflammatory rheumatic diseases. Therapy is usually directed to supporting the failing exocrine glands (artificial tears and saliva) or stimulating residual gland function via muscarinic receptors (for example with pilocarpine or cevimeline). For those patients with extraglandular disease, which is mainly mediated by cryoglobulinaemia, immunosuppression with steroids and cytotoxic agents may be necessary. Female patients with anti-Ro and/or anti-La antibodies who are of child-bearing years may need counselling with regard to the possible risks of congenital heart block.

SYSTEMIC VASCULITIS

Vasculitis means inflammation of blood vessel walls with narrowing and occlusion leading to tissue or organ damage. Primary vasculitis is diagnosed if there is no underlying connective tissue disease; if vasculitis occurs in a patient with RA or SLE, for example, it is regarded as secondary. Vasculitis may be important in atherosclerosis where inflammation is responsible for plaque rupture and vessel occlusion. There are more than 100 new cases of primary vasculitis per million per year. Many patients have skin vasculitis only. The more serious forms of vasculitis, such as Wegener's granulomatosis and microscopic polyangiitis, are less common; between 2.4 and 9.7 cases per million per year with a prevalence of between 30 and 53 per million per year.

AETIOLOGY

Most forms of vasculitis have no known cause. Table 17.6 summarizes factors known to cause vasculitis or associated with it. Infection can trigger episodes of disease (e.g. nasal carriage of *Staphylococcus aureus* increases risk of relapses of Wegener's granulomatosis). There is a seasonal variation in Wegener's granulomatosis (more cases are seen during spring and winter compared to autumn or summer). Hepatitis B is a cause of polyarteritis nodosa (PAN), but as a result of better public health and an immunization campaign the incidence of hepatitis B-related diseases is falling. Identifying a cause is a very important basis for treatment, and most patients with hepatitis B-related PAN can be cured by eradication of the virus. Unfortunately, it is more difficult to eradicate hepatitis C, a known cause of mixed essential cryoglobulinaemia. Other environmental factors that have been implicated are silica exposure, possibly by acting as a stimulant or adjuvant. Living in a farming or rural community has been linked to increasing risk of developing Churg–Strauss syndrome.

Genetic factors are important and may increase the risk or severity of disease. $\alpha1$-Anti-trypsin deficiency increases the risk of developing Wegener's granulomatosis. $\alpha1$-Anti-trypsin is the natural factor to neutralize proteinase-3, a toxic neutrophil enzyme that digests bacteria. One form

Table 17.6 Factors that have been associated with the development or severity of vasculitis

Factor	Association	Effect
Hepatitis B virus	Definite	Some cases of polyarteritis nodosa
Hepatitis C virus	Definite	Most (>90%) patients with mixed essential cryoglobulinaemia
HIV virus	Definite	Undifferentiated vasculitis
Anti-thyroid drugs	Definite	Reversible forms of vasculitis similar to microscopic polyangiitis and Wegener's granulomatosis
Streptococcus pneumonia	Definite	Rheumatic fever and bacterial endocarditis
$\alpha1$-Anti-trypsin deficiency	Probable	Increases the risk and severity of Wegener's granulomatosis
Silica exposure	Possible	Increases risk of small vessel vasculitis
Farming and exposure to farm animals	Possible	Increases risk of Churg–Strauss syndrome

of anti-neutrophil cytoplasm antibody (ANCA), often found in patients with Wegener's granulomatosis, is directed against proteinase-3 (see later).

PATHOLOGY

Some patients have intense inflammatory infiltration around blood vessels, invading through the vessel wall, causing necrosis of surrounding tissue. In other cases there is a granulomatous infiltrate, sometimes with giant cells (as seen in temporal arteritis or occasionally in Wegener's granulomatosis). Figure 17.7 shows a section from a temporal artery biopsy in a patient with temporal arteritis. In the kidney, pathological abnormalities are similar in different forms of vasculitis, suggesting that the kidney has a limited response to poor blood flow through its capillaries and venules. The typical renal lesion of a small-vessel vasculitis is focal segmental necrotizing glomerulonephritis (focal because it affects only a few glomeruli and not all of them, segmental because it may only affect a part of the glomerulus, and necrotizing implying tissue destruction). This may occur in Wegener's granulomatosis, microscopic polyangiitis, Churg–Strauss syndrome or other conditions such as SLE or bacterial endocarditis. The result is that you need to interpret the pathological findings together with the clinical and serological abnormalities.

CLASSIFYING DIFFERENT TYPES OF VASCULITIS

A precise diagnosis of vasculitis has implications for treatment and outcome. Patients with leucocytoclastic skin vasculitis often require no treatment apart from supportive management, and the outcome is very good. By contrast, patients with microscopic polyangiitis may present with lung haemorrhage and glomerulonephritis; they need aggressive chemotherapy and the outcome may be poor despite best management (mortality of up to 20–40% despite treatment). The pathology findings in vasculitis can be helpful, but because of greater awareness of vasculitis, patients increasingly present with less severe abnormalities. Patients should be investigated and treated at an early stage rather than to let the condition develop into a full-blown form, by which time organ failure may have occurred. The pathological findings may be shared by different types of vasculitis. For example, granulomatous inflammation may be seen in patients with Wegener's granulomatosis as well as patients with Churg–Strauss syndrome.

Classification of systemic vasculitis is based on the size of the smallest vessel to be affected by the vasculitic process. The distinction is between large-vessel disease, where large vessels alone are affected; medium-vessel disease, where medium-sized vessels such as small arterials are predominantly affected, although in some circumstances

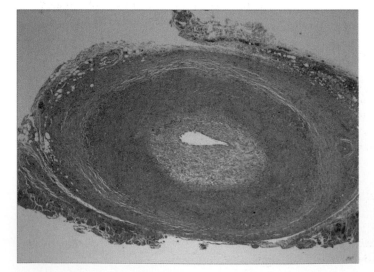

FIGURE 17.7 A low-power view of a temporal artery biopsy. The lumen is oedematous resulting in stenosis of the lumen. The internal elastic lamina has been destroyed by a cellular infiltrate, which extends through the media

242

larger vessels may also be affected; and small-vessel vasculitis, where capillaries can be involved, although, confusingly, these patients can also have medium- and large-vessel disease. However arbitrary this system might seem, it is probably the most useful guide to therapy because often the smaller sized vessel involved determines which organs can be affected and, therefore, which treatment you will wish to give to patients. Table 17.7 summarizes the different forms of vasculitis according to vessel size.

Anti-neutrophil cytoplasm antibody (ANCA) defines a subgroup of patients with small-vessel vasculitis who have a predilection for renal disease (typically Wegener's granulomatosis and microscopic polyangiitis) and who require similar treatment.

AN APPROACH TO DIAGNOSIS

Making a diagnosis of vasculitis requires a thorough history and physical examination because many abnormalities are apparent from this simple basic clinical evaluation. Patients with multisystem disease should be assessed for the possible diagnosis of vasculitis. There are very few conditions that cause such widespread organ involvement. In fact, the more organ systems involved, the narrower the differential diagnosis becomes. Vasculitis may be secondary to an underlying connective tissue disease. Infection and drugs can cause vasculitis; you need to take a full history and examination. Rarely, malignancy may cause vasculitis, but usually the primary tumour is obvious. The clinical presentation of some primary forms of vasculitis can overlap with each other.

In a patient with multi-organ disease, we need to look for raised inflammatory markers, abnormal serological tests such as ANCA, and try to confirm the diagnosis with a biopsy from an affected organ, or by imaging the vessels to show the abnormalities (usually smooth tapered narrowing or aneurysms, or both). However, investigating patients at an early stage of their disease may produce inconclusive results.

EVALUATION OF PATIENTS WITH AN ESTABLISHED DIAGNOSIS

A comprehensive assessment of patients with systemic vasculitis is essential as a basis for deciding appropriate therapy. Initial evaluation should include assessment of both active vasculitis and the presence of pre-existing damage, which may have occurred following episodes of previous vasculitis or even as a result of treatment of previous vasculitis. It is important to make this distinction, because treatment needs to be appropriate to the needs of the individual patient. For example, if the patient has established renal failure from previous episodes of disease activity, then it is unlikely to respond to aggressive immunosuppression, whereas if renal failure has developed more rapidly and there are signs of active nephritis then there is every reason to act quickly and offer immunosuppressive treatment. A full history should be taken and peripheral vasculature examined. Typically such patients would have full examination of the upper airways; the eyes; skin; nail beds; chest and cardiovascular, abdominal, neurological and locomotor systems. Blood pressure must be measured in every patient and urine should be routinely tested for the presence of blood and protein. Weight is very useful as a baseline.

The initial blood test should measure renal function and liver function, haematology, acute-phase reactants and autoantibody screen. Viral studies may be relevant, especially for hepatitis B and C, and occasionally for HIV. Diagnostic imaging may be necessary or further assessment of organ function, such as lung function testing, may be helpful. In most instances, however, a chest X-ray is a useful part of the initial diagnostic workup (Fig. 17.8) mainly to exclude other pathologies, such as neoplastic disease or infection. Remember to consider previous episodes of treated or untreated tuberculosis (TB), which may have an important bearing on further management (if the patient actually has TB as a cause of their vasculitis, then you would want to treat the TB; if patients have active vasculitis and the presence of partially treated or previously untreated TB, you may need to consider anti-TB prophylaxis). Clinical evaluation of patients' progress remains the cornerstone of management and cannot be superseded by any routine blood monitoring. The same checklist of symptoms and signs of active vasculitis serves a useful role in monitoring patient disease state. It is also useful to document disease damage more formally and systems are available to record this. A useful checklist is shown in Table 17.8.

Table 17.7 Primary vasculitides

Disease	Epidemiology	Symptoms, signs and investigations	Treatment and outcome
Giant cell arteritis or temporal arteritis (large-vessel vasculitis)	Elderly. Annual UK incidence 13 per million or 42 per million over 60	Headaches, scalp tenderness, visual disturbance, jaw claudication often with polymyalgia High erythrocyte sedimentation rate (ESR), granulomatous inflammation on temporal artery biopsy	Corticosteroids. Relapse rates vary (30–80%). Steroid taper over 1 to 4 years Methotrexate may be useful additional therapy
Takayasu's arteritis (large-vessel vasculitis)	Females under 50 especially in Eastern countries. UK incidence 0.1 per million/year	Chronic ischaemia, new loss of pulses, bruits, systemic upset. Angiography – vessel narrowing or post-stenotic dilatation. MRA – wall oedema, carotid Doppler flow	Corticosteroids 5–10-year survival 80–90%, but 47% have permanent disability
Polyarteritis nodosa (medium-vessel vasculitis)	Adults. UK incidence 0–4.6 per million/year	Multi-system organ involvement No glomerulonephritis Hepatitis B virus positive in some cases. Biopsy of affected area or angiography, especially mesenteric, can show aneurysms or vessel narrowing	Corticosteroids plus antiviral agents (for hepatitis B +ve disease) or cyclophosphamide (for hepatitis B -ve disease) Mortality 23% (non-HBV PAN), 33% (HBV PAN); relapse 8% HBV PAN, 20% non-HBV PAN
Kawasaki disease (mucocutaneous lymph node syndrome) (medium-vessel vasculitis)	Endemic and epidemic forms with seasonal variation. UK incidence 34 million/year in children under 5 years vs 900 million/year in Japan	Fever, mucocutaneous inflammation; cervical lymphadenopathy; polymorphous exanthema Desquamation of skin 10 days after onset. Coronary arteries often involved Diagnosis on clinical findings plus coronary artery dilatation on echocardiography	High-dose aspirin and intravenous gammaglobulin decreases incidence of coronary artery aneurysms Coronary artery lesions occur in 15–25% of untreated patients, but less than 10% of those given IVIG
Wegener's granulomatosis (small-vessel vasculitis)	Adults mainly, can occur in children. Annual incidence in UK 8.5 per million	Upper and lower airways, often with renal involvement Granulomatous inflammation in airways, focal segmental necrotizing glomerulonephritis in the kidney, C-ANCA positive in most cases against PR3	Localized upper airway disease cotrimoxazole plus or minus prednisolone or methotrexate with prednisolone Mupirocin useful for eradicating nasal *Staphylococcus* Systemic disease requires prednisolone and cyclophosphamide and plasma exchange for rapid progressive renal impairment

Table 17.7 Continued

Disease	Epidemiology	Symptoms, signs and investigations	Treatment and outcome
Churg–Strauss syndrome (small-vessel vasculitis)	Adults mainly, although can occur in children. Annual UK incidence 2.4 per million	Respiratory tract features dominant – asthma, allergic rhinitis, pulmonary infiltrates Multiple drug allergies, mononeuritis multiplex; cardiac involvement is serious Eosinophilia; may be ANCA positive, usually P-ANCA (myeloperoxidase)	Corticosteroids; cyclophosphamide for serious disease (especially cardiac or renal involvement) Mortality low, but relapse rate and morbidity high
Microscopic polyangiitis (small-vessel vasculitis)	Adults mainly, but can occur in children. Annual UK incidence 2.4 per million	Haematuria, pulmonary haemorrhage, systemic upset with multi-system involvement Renal biopsy shows FSNGN P-ANCA usually positive (myeloperoxidase)	Corticosteroids and cyclophosphamide; plasmapheresis for renal failure Mortality 10–40%; relapse 20%
Henoch–Schönlein purpura (small-vessel vasculitis)	Predominantly in children but adults may be affected (they have worse prognosis). Annual UK incidence 1.2 per million in adults	Purpuric rash, flitting arthritis, abdominal pain, rectal bleeding, haematuria Skin biopsy or gastrointestinal tract biopsy may show IgA-dominant immune deposits, especially on basement membrane	Self-limiting in childhood, but if renal involvement present carries adverse prognosis Adults – more indolent course Steroids may be used for arthralgia and rash
Leucocytoclastic vasculitis (small-vessel vasculitis)	Adults and children	Skin involvement only with purpura or occasional ulcers or bullae	Symptomatic treatment with antihistamines; colchicine, steroids for resistant cases
Essential mixed cryoglobulinaemia (small-vessel vasculitis)	Adults mainly but can occur in children. Annual UK incidence 1.2 per million	Purpura, arthralgia, urticaria, ulcers and renal involvement Type II cryoglobulinaemia, strong association with hepatitis C virus	Antiviral therapy and steroids and plasmapheresis
Uncertain or unclassified	Annual UK incidence 4.8 per million	As above	May be any of the above

SEROLOGICAL MARKERS OF DISEASE ACTIVITY

Basic biochemical and haematological parameters and measurements of acute-phase response help to differentiate active disease from irreversible

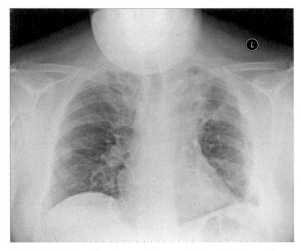

FIGURE 17.8   Lung involvement in a patient with Wegener's granulomatosis. There is an extensive shadowing from granulomatous infiltration into the lungs

damage. The ANCA test has improved our awareness of vasculitis by identifying patients who appear to have a vasculitis, but it is not a useful screening tool on its own. It must be used with clinical judgement in patients in whom there is a suspicion of vasculitis.

DIFFERENTIATING VASCULITIS FROM INFECTION

There is a close relationship between infection and vasculitis. Some infectious diseases cause certain types of vasculitis, for example hepatitis B and hepatitis C. *Staphylococcus aureus* can exacerbate episodes of Wegener's granulomatosis, but has not been shown to cause the disease. In patients who have an established diagnosis of vasculitis who become ill, it is important to differentiate the deterioration caused by intercurrent infection from that caused by vasculitis. This can be difficult because the clinical presentation may be exactly the same and it is very important to suspect infection, especially as most patients are on immunosuppressive drugs, which may mask obvious features of sepsis.

Table 17.8 Symptoms, signs and investigations that may occur in the context of active systemic vasculitis

Symptom	Sign/investigation
Systemic	Malaise, myalgia, arthralgia/arthritis, headache, fever and weight loss
Cutaneous	Infarct, purpura, ulcer, gangrene and other skin vasculitis
Mucous membranes/eyes	Oral ulcers, genital ulcers, proptosis, conjunctivitis, episcleritis, scleritis, visual disturbances with visual loss, uveitis, retinal exudates and retinal haemorrhages
Ear, nose and throat	Nasal obstruction, bloody nasal discharge, crusting, sinus involvement, new deafness, hoarseness/stridor, subglottic stenosis and adnexal inflammation
Respiratory	Persistent cough, dyspnoea, wheeze, haemoptysis, pulmonary haemorrhage, nodules, cavities, infiltrate, pleurisy, pleural effusion and respiratory failure
Cardiovascular	Bruits, new loss of pulses with or without threatened loss of limbs, aortic incompetence, pericardial pain/rub, ischaemic cardiac pain and congestive cardiac failure
Gastrointestinal	Severe abdominal pain, bloody diarrhoea, intestinal perforation/infarct and acute pancreatitis
Renal	Hypertension (diastolic >95 mmHg), proteinuria >0.2 g/24 h, haematuria >10 red cells per high power field, renal impairment/failure, rise in creatinine >30% or fall in creatinine clearance >25%
Neurological	Organic confusion/dementia, seizures (not hypertensive), stroke, cord lesion, sensory peripheral neuropathy, cranial nerve palsy, motor mononeuritis multiplex

In many cases it is necessary to start empirical antibiotic therapy at the same time as, or just prior to, introducing more immunosuppression, in case the problem is infection plus active vasculitis.

MANAGEMENT

Although there are different forms of vasculitis, there is a lot of overlap in organ involvement, and it is the organ involvement that primarily dictates the type of treatment that is most appropriate. For example, patients with ANCA-associated vasculitis involving the kidney will be given the same treatment whether the diagnosis happens to be Wegener's granulomatosis, Churg–Strauss syndrome or microscopic polyangiitis. We have summarized the drug treatments according to disease severity in Table 17.9.

The management of systemic vasculitis is very complex and we would strongly advise the involvement of physicians with experience in these diseases. Careful attention to important details, such

Table 17.9 Summary of therapies for systemic vasculitis

Therapy	Specific drugs	Disease
Mild	None or colchicine or dapsone	Cutaneous leucocytoclastic vasculitis and some cases of Henoch–Schönlein purpura
Moderate	Prednisolone/prednisone	Giant cell arteritis, Takayasu's arteritis, resistant or severe cutaneous vasculitis
	Co-trimoxazole (trimethoprim–sulfamethoxazole)	Non-renal Wegener's granulomatosis
	Methotrexate + steroids	Non-renal Wegener's granulomatosis, resistant giant cell arteritis and resistant Takayasu's arteritis
	Azathioprine + steroids	Remission maintenance in microscopic polyangiitis, Wegener's granulomatosis, polyarteritis nodosa, Churg–Strauss syndrome, resistant giant cell arteritis and resistant Takayasu's arteritis
	Ciclosporin A + steroids Ciclosporin A or azathioprine or α-interferon ± steroids	Resistant giant cell arteritis Behçet's syndrome
Standard	Cyclophosphamide and steroids	Microscopic polyangiitis, Wegener's granulomatosis, polyarteritis nodosa (hepatis B negative), necrotizing vasculitis, Churg–Strauss syndrome with internal organ involvement (not just asthma)
Severe	Plasmapheresis + cyclophosphamide + steroids	Microscopic polyangiitis, Wegener's granulomatosis, polyarteritis nodosa, Churg–Strauss syndrome with life-threatening or severe organ involvement
Specific	Intravenous gamma-globulin and aspirin	Kawasaki disease
	Antiviral drugs/plasmapheresis	Hepatitis B-related PAN, cryoglobulinaemic vasculitis related to hepatitis C
Experimental	Mycophenolate mofetil and steroids	ANCA-associated systemic vasculitis
	Leflunomide with steroids Infliximab Deoxyspergualin Rituximab (anti-CD20) Immune ablation with autologous bone marrow transplantation	Wegener's granulomatosis Wegener's granulomatosis Wegener's granulomatosis Wegener's granulomatosis Severe Wegener's granulomatosis

as pre-treatment blood counts, renal function, and regular checks on haematology and biochemistry, can prevent inappropriate use of immunosuppression and limit toxicity from drug treatment. Supportive treatments alongside the standard immunosuppression outlined in the tables helps to prevent side effects from the primary immunosuppressive therapy. Damage as a result of systemic vasculitis may need separate management, such as the management of hypertension from renal involvement or the use of bone protection for osteoporosis and fracture.

A rational basis for managing systemic vasculitis depends heavily on appropriate diagnosis, accurate staging and assessment of disease activity prior to initiating treatment. In some patients specific therapy is available, but for the majority non-specific interference with the immune system is the most appropriate treatment. Small-vessel vasculitis with multi-system involvement requires intense immunosuppression with cyclophosphamide and steroid, regardless of diagnosis. By contrast, larger-vessel vasculitis usually responds to steroids alone and many types of cutaneous vasculitis need no treatment at all. Improvements in treatment will only come through better understanding of the underlying mechanisms of systemic vasculitis.

Drug toxicity remains a significant issue, as does the problem of relapsing disease, and this has been the basis for developing new strategies that are both more effective and less toxic for patients with systemic vasculitis. We hope that new agents will be introduced within the next decade.

SARCOIDOSIS

Sarcoidosis is a chronic inflammatory multi-system disease of unknown aetiology. It affects both sexes, all ages, all races and all geographical locations. The prevalence is 10–40/100 000. It is characterized by the presence of non-caseating granulomas.

CLINICAL FEATURES
(see Table 17.10)

Sarcoidosis may be completely asymptomatic or constitutional symptoms of fever, weight loss and fatigue may be prominent. Pulmonary manifestations are the most common feature, but musculo-

Table 17.10 Clinical features of sarcoidosis

Organ	Frequency	Manifestation
Respiratory	90%	Hilar lymphadenopthy, pulmonary infiltrates and cor pulmonale
Bone and joints	13–38%	Arthralgia, acute arthritis, chronic arthritis, enthesitis, dactylitis, cystic bone lesions and periosteal reaction
Skin	30%	Erythema nodosum, hyperpigmented papules and lupus pernio
Eyes	20%	Uveitis, conjunctival granulomas and interstitial keratitis
Muscle	5–15%	Myopathy and, rarely, a raised creatine kinase
Neurological	5–10%	Headaches, cranial neuropathies, meningeal disease, mass, hypothalamic dysfunction, seizures and papilloedema
Salivary glands	3–9%	Sicca symptoms and parotid swelling
Liver	8%	Hepatomegaly
Spleen	6%	Splenomegaly
Kidney	5–10%	Nephrocalcinosis, hypertension, proteinuria, haematuria, renal failure
Cardiac	Reported	Conduction defects, arrhythmia, sudden death, cardiomyopathy and pericardial effusion
Vascular	Reported	Large- and medium-vessel vasculitis

skeletal symptoms are prominent and varied, and can mimic many other rheumatological conditions. The onset is either acute or subacute and then follows either a self-limiting or chronic recurring course.

The acute arthritis typically affects the ankle joints; this is a combination of an arthritis, tenosynovitis and soft-tissue oedema. This is usually non-erosive and self-limiting. The triad of arthritis, erythema nodosum (EN) and hilar lymphadenopathy is called Löfgren syndrome. The chronic arthritis is much less common and usually polyarticular. Bone involvement occurs in long-standing disease and is often asymptomatic.

DIFFERENTIAL DIAGNOSIS

The differential diagnosis is wide and specific to the presentation. The most important differential for the bilateral hilar lymphadenopthy (with and without EN) is tuberculosis.

PATHOGENESIS

The pathogenesis of sarcoidosis is due to stimulation of the host immune response to an unknown foreign antigen. There is evidence of community, seasonal and geographical clustering.

INVESTIGATION

The typical pathological finding is of non-caseating epithelioid and giant cell granulomas are demonstrated, combined with a compatible clinical and radiographic picture. Angiotensin converting enzyme (ACE) is produced by the epithelioid cells in granulomas. The serum ACE may be raised, but the sensitivity and specificity of this test is only 47–55% and 77% respectively. Hypercalcaemia occurs in 5–7%, but is usually transient. The sarcoid macrophage is able to synthesize 1,25-dihydroxyvitamin D and parathyroid hormone-related protein.

TREATMENT

The drugs used in the treatment of sarcoidosis are shown in Table 17.11. Mild disease requires no treatment or symptomatic treatment only.

The most important aspect of treatment is the early recognition of features compatible with sarcoidosis for an early diagnosis and instigation of appropriate treatment.

Table 17.11 Drugs used for sarcoidosis treatment

Drug	Indication
Non-steroidal anti-inflammatory drugs (NSAIDs), simple analgesics	Symptom control
Systemic corticosteroids	Parenchymal lung involvement, arthritis unresponsive to NSAIDs
Topical corticosteroids	Eye disease
Hydroxychloroquine	Cutaneous disease
Methotrexate and azathioprine	Steroid-sparing agents for more severe disease
Ciclosporin and cyclophosphamide	Refractory neurosarcoidosis
Anti-tumour necrosis factor	Severe refractory disease (case reports only)

RHEUMATIC FEVER

Rheumatic fever (RF) is a clinical syndrome in which inflammation of the skin, joints, heart and brain is attributed to cross-reaction with certain strains of group A streptococci. Today RF remains a leading cause of acquired heart disease in children and young adults in many parts of the world and, although uncommon in industrialized countries, there is evidence of a resurgence of RF activity, possibly due to changes in community strains of streptococci.

Diagnosis of RF is based upon Jones' criteria (Table 17.12), a list of clinical manifestations compiled to avoid inaccurate diagnosis and now used to avoid morbidity from unnecessary antibiotic use and unwarranted anxiety. The probability of acute RF is high when there are *either* two major manifestations *or* one major and two minor manifestations *plus* laboratory evidence of antecedent group A streptococcal infection *sine qua non*. Suspicion arises at the presentation of an acutely inflamed joint, typically a flitting polyarthritis, or the presence of a new mitral or aortic regurgitant murmur at times of fever or sore throat. Other major criteria occur far less frequently; patients with Sydenham's chorea have involuntary, spasmodic, purposeless movements, are emotionally labile and have

Table 17.12 Diagnosis of rheumatic fever using Jones' criteria

Requires laboratory evidence of group A streptococcal infection plus either two major manifestations or one major and two minor manifestations from:

Major manifestations	Minor manifestations	Evidence of antecedent streptococcal infection
Carditis	Arthralgia	Positive throat culture
Polyarthritis	Fever	Positive rapid streptococcal antigen test
Chorea		Raised or rising ASOT ± antiDNAse B
Erythema marginatum	Raised acute-phase reactants (erythrocyte sedimentation rate, C-reactive protein)	
Subcutaneous nodules	Prolonged PR interval	

changes in personality; erythema marginatum occurs typically on the trunk and has a pink serpigenous border, with central clearing, that changes shape before the observer's eyes; easily overlooked subcutaneous nodules are small, painless and localized over bony prominences (such as the spine) and in tendon sheaths. Evidence of streptococcal infection includes cultured growth from throat swabs, high antistreptolysin O titres (ASOT) (>800 Todd units), or raised anti-DNAse B titre in the presence of moderately raised ASOT. Patients with a high suspicion of RF should have a cardiological assessment including echocardiography.

Management of RF involves treatment of the acute inflammatory episode with NSAIDs (aspirin or ibuprofen) and antibiotics (penicillin), avoidance of recurrent episodes of RF with prophylactic antibiotics, and cardiac follow-up and intervention as required. The duration of prophylactic antibiotics is debated, but as a guide intramuscular benzathine penicillin (1.2 million units every 3 or 4 weeks) or oral penicillin (250–500 mg twice daily) may be given until the end of full-time education or 5 years after the last acute attack. If carditis occurs it is often mild and resolves spontaneously in about 80% of patients. If there is valvular involvement prophylactic antibiotics are required at times of dental and surgical intervention to avoid bacterial endocarditis. The need for valve replacement is based upon the severity of cardiac failure.

FURTHER READING

Anderson R, Malmvall BE, Bengtsson B-A 1986 Long-term corticosteroid treatment in giant cell arteritis. Acta Med Scand 220: 465–469.

Denton CP, Black CM 2004 Scleroderma: clinical and pathological advances. Best Pract Res Clin Rheumatol 18: 271–290.

Dhillon R, Newton L, Rudd PT et al 1993 Management of Kawasaki disease in the British Isles. Arch Dis Child 69: 631–638.

Gayraud M, Guillevin L, le Toumelin P et al 2001 Long-term follow up of polyarteritis nodosa, microscopic polyangiitis, and Churg-Strauss syndrome: analysis of four prospective trials including 278 patients. Arthritis Rheum 44: 666–675.

Gonzalez-Gay MA, Garcia-Porrua C 1999 Systemic vasculitis in adults in Northwestern Spain, 1988–1997: clinical and epidemiologic aspects. Medicine 78: 292–308.

Jennette JC, Falk RJ, Andrassy K et al 1994 Nomenclature of systemic vasculitides: proposal of an international consensus conference. Arthritis Rheum 37: 187–192.

Ramos-Casals M, Tzioufas AG, Font J 2005 Primary Sjögren's syndrome: new clinical and therapeutic concepts. Ann Rheum Dis 64: 347–354.

Van der Woude FJ, Rasmussen N, Lobatto S et al 1985 Autoantibodies against neutrophils and monocytes: tool for diagnosis and marker of disease activity in Wegener's granulomatosis. Lancet 1: 425–429.

SYSTEMIC COMPLICATIONS OF RHEUMATIC DISEASES AND RARE ARTHROPATHIES

Raashid Luqmani and Nick Wilkinson

Cases relevant to this chapter

78, 89–91, 94, 100

●Essential facts

1. Many inflammatory rheumatic diseases are associated with systemic features, including weight loss, malaise, weakness and fever.

2. Long-standing rheumatoid arthritis (RA) predisposes to sensory peripheral neuropathy.

3. Lung alveolitis and fibrosis are common long-term complication of RA, systemic lupus erythematosus (SLE) and diffuse cutaneous scleroderma.

4. Cardiovascular morbidity and mortality are increased in all inflammatory rheumatic diseases, especially SLE.

5. Gastrointestinal complications of non-steroidal anti-inflammatory drugs are common and may cause anaemia.

6. Anaemia due to active inflammatory disease will not respond to oral iron.

7. The risk of developing malignancy, especially non-Hodgkin's lymphoma, is five times higher in patients with inflammatory rheumatic disease, compared to healthy individuals.

8. Patients with ankylosing spondylitis should be advised of the 20% risk of acute anterior uveitis.

9. Joint infection is more likely in patients with inflammatory joint disease than in patients with previously normal joints.

10. Kawasaki disease should be considered in children with a high spiking pyrexial illness (39–40°C) with negative blood cultures and no response to antibiotics.

11. SLE occurs in childhood in 20% of patients with similar clinical features and management to adults.

The inflammatory arthritides, the connective tissue diseases, and their treatment may have significant effects outside the bones and joints. Table 18.1 gives some examples and outlines the systems that might be affected. Some of this information is expanded on in other chapters of the book. This chapter provides a brief overview of problems to consider in everyday practice.

SYSTEMIC FEATURES

Many inflammatory rheumatic diseases are associated with significant systemic features, which may be responsible for weight loss, malaise, weakness and fever. This makes the differential diagnosis wider, with concerns over whether or not patients have malignancy, infection or drug toxicity.

Table 18.1 Summary of systemic complications of rheumatic diseases and their management

System	Problems	Examples
Systemic	Weight loss, fever, malaise	Many inflammatory diseases
Cutaneous	Drug reactions; rashes; vasculitis; Raynaud's; skin fibrosis	Most drugs; RA, SLE, psoriatic arthritis; scleroderma, connective tissue disease, vasculitis
Neurological	Peripheral sensory and motor neuropathies; mononeuritis multiplex; compression of nerves or spinal cord; cerebral infarction; cranial nerve palsies	RA, SLE and connective tissue diseases; vasculitis
Pulmonary	Pulmonary fibrosis/alveolitis; pleurisy and pleural effusions; pulmonary infiltrates/bleeding; nodules; bronchial ulceration; bronchial dryness	RA, SLE, connective tissue diseases, vasculitis
Cardiovascular	Increased atherosclerosis leading to premature coronary artery disease and cerebrovascular disease; vascular inflammation of all sizes of blood vessel; valvular heart disease; thrombotic events in arteries or veins	SLE and RA, vasculitis. Effect of non-steroidal anti-inflammatory agents; antiphospholipid antibody syndrome
Gastrointestinal	Peptic ulcer disease; liver fibrosis; liver function abnormalities; overlap between inflammatory bowel disease and arthritis	NSAID use; methotrexate and sulfasalazine; Crohn's disease-related arthritis
Genitourinary problems	Renal impairment; nephritis; renal tract infections; dyspareunia; infertility; pregnancy loss	Vasculitis, SLE and other connective tissue diseases; drug effects; antiphospholipid antibody syndrome
Eyes/mucous membranes	Oral/genital ulcers, dryness of mouth and eyes; uveitis; cataracts	Behçet's syndrome; SLE, RA, Sjögren's and other connective tissue diseases; ankylosing spondylitis, juvenile arthritis; steroids
Haematological	Anaemia of chronic disease or gastrointestinal blood loss; neutropenia; thrombocytopenia; splenomegaly	RA, SLE and connective tissue diseases; NSAID effects
Lymphoma risk/ cancer risk	Increased risk of lymphoma; connective tissue diseases presenting with tumours; risk of immunosuppressive agents	RA, SLE and all connective tissue diseases; all immunosuppressive agents
Infection	Joint infections usually derived from bacteraemia, local spread form osteomyelitis or direct trauma to the joint. Usually affects single joint. Patients with rheumatoid arthritis are more likely to suffer infections, especially if treated with immunosuppressive agents	Patients with pre-existing inflammatory joint disease are at highest risk
Amyloid	Chronic inflammation leading to deposition of inert protein which interferes with affected organ function	Long-standing uncontrolled inflammation in juvenile arthritis, rheumatoid arthritis and spondyloarthritis

NEUROLOGICAL PROBLEMS

Long-standing rheumatoid arthritis (RA) predisposes to sensory peripheral neuropathy (glove and stocking distribution). Chronic peripheral nerve injury may occur from synovitis in the wrist compressing the median nerve resulting in carpal tunnel syndrome. Acute cord compression is a feature of long-standing RA with instability of the cervical spine, due to erosive disease of the odontoid peg, ischaemic pressure from pannus and compounded by instability of the atlantoaxial articulation. Mononeuritis multiplex results from rheumatoid vasculitis causing nerve injury. The brain may be at risk in systemic lupus erythematosus (SLE) as a result of ischaemia through vasculitis, clotting of vessels by anti-cardiolipin antibody syndrome, or the vasculopathy of SLE. Mechanical problems in the spine may lead to nerve or cord compression depending on the level of injury and its severity. Careful evaluation of the nervous system is important in any patient with back pain, especially if they have a history of pain or numbness in a peripheral limb.

PULMONARY PROBLEMS

Lung alveolitis and fibrosis are common long-term complications of RA, SLE and scleroderma (especially diffuse cutaneous scleroderma). The pleural sac may be inflamed as part of a generalized polyserositis. In SLE and the vasculitides this is often acute with painful pleuritic pain, but in RA it is often more insidious leading to quite large pleural effusions and, eventually, to breathlessness on exertion. Rheumatoid lung nodules may be seen as isolated peripheral shadows on a chest radiograph raising suspicion of tumour; they may even liquefy in the centre giving rise to a fluid level and concern about possible abscess; occasionally lung nodules occur prior to the onset of joint symptoms causing considerable diagnostic confusion. Patients with systemic vasculitis affecting small vessels may develop alveolar inflammation and haemorrhage, typically in microscopic polyangiitis and Goodpasture's syndrome. Haemorrhage may also occur in Wegener's granulomatosis and Churg–Strauss syndrome; however, diffuse infiltrates and/or nodules are more common; bronchial and tracheal ulceration and inflammation leading to stenosis are characteristic findings in Wegener's granulomatosis. Patients with Sjögren's syndrome can develop dryness in the trachea and bronchi, leading to cough, and predisposing to chest infections through impaired clearance of secretions.

CARDIOVASCULAR PROBLEMS

Cardiovascular risk of hypertension and cardiac failure on drug therapy, especially non-steroidal anti-inflammatory drugs (NSAIDs), is well recognized and has led to a re-evaluation of the role of NSAIDs in the long-term management of rheumatic diseases. Cardiovascular morbidity and mortality in all rheumatic diseases, especially SLE, is mediated via accelerated atherosclerosis. Atherosclerosis itself is recognized as an inflammatory condition. The risk of myocardial infarction in some patients with RA is higher than for patients with type 2 diabetes.

GASTROINTESTINAL PROBLEMS

Gastrointestinal complications of NSAIDs and other drugs used to manage RA are common. Peptic ulcer, bleeding and perforation are highest in elderly patients or those also receiving steroid therapy, and NSAIDs should be avoided or used with caution in this group. Liver function abnormalities are common in patients treated with methotrexate, leflunomide and sulfasalazine. Liver fibrosis is much less common. Small bowel inflammation may be caused by NSAIDs leading to abdominal pain, anaemia with an iron-deficient blood picture and normal upper gastrointestinal endoscopy. Small bowel examination of these patients may reveal ulcers or scarred areas with membrane formation (NSAID enteropathy).

GENITOURINARY PROBLEMS

Urinary tract infections are common in female patients with rheumatic diseases, especially if they are on immunosuppressive drugs. Dyspareunia due to dryness of the vagina is relatively common in patients with Sjögren's syndrome, but patients may not raise the issue through embarrassment, or thinking that it is not connected to their rheumatic disease. It can be managed with simple lubricant creams. Small-vessel systemic vasculitides and SLE can involve the glomeruli, leading to kidney inflammation and loss of function. All such patients should have their blood pressure checked, urine tested for blood and protein, and renal function assessed regularly. Unexplained haematuria should be thoroughly investigated in patients who have been treated with cyclophosphamide to look for evidence of urothelial cancer.

HAEMATOLOGICAL PROBLEMS

A low haemoglobin is often secondary to either bleeding due to NSAID therapy, or active inflammatory disease (in which case it will not respond to oral iron). Haemolysis may occur in connective tissue diseases especially SLE. SLE may induce neutropenia or thrombocytopenia. In some cases, resistant to systemic immunosuppression, spleno-megaly is justified, but patients will need pneu-moccocal vaccine prior to splenectomy followed by lifelong penicillin V. Thrombocytopenia typi-cally occurs in primary antiphospholipid antibody syndrome. A small number of patients with RA develop splenomegaly, thrombocytopenia and neutropenia (Felty's sydrome).

LYMPHOMA RISK/ CANCER RISK

All patients with inflammatory rheumatic disease are at a five times higher risk of developing a malig-nancy, especially non-Hodgkin's lymphoma, com-pared to controls. If patients are treated with immunosuppressive drugs, such as azathioprine, the risk may double (i.e. to 10 times normal). More potent immunosuppressive agents such as cyclo-phosphamide increase the risk of other tumours, especially bladder cancer, because one of the main metabolites of cyclophosphamide, acrolein, is excreted via the kidneys.

EYES/MUCOUS MEMBRANES

Oral and genital ulceration occurs as a result of disease, such as SLE or Behçet's syndrome. Oral ulcers may also be caused by drug therapy such as methotrexate. Dry eyes and mouth are common in primary and secondary Sjögren's syndrome. Patients with ankylosing spondylitis should be advised of the 20% risk of acute anterior uveitis; patients with juvenile idiopathic arthritis (JIA) (especially anti-nuclear antibody (ANA)-positive oligoarthritis) should be screened for chronic uveitis. Long-term steroid use predisposes to cata-ract formation.

INFECTION RISK

Joint infection is more likely in patients with inflammatory joint disease than in patients with previously normal joints; it is important to con-sider the possibility of infection in patients with RA presenting with a flare of arthritis affecting a single joint. Immunosuppressive drugs used for treating rheumatic diseases carry a significant risk of infection, especially the more potent agents. Use of specific cytokine inhibitors, such as anti-TNF, is a particular concern, and has been associated with an increased incidence of tuberculosis (TB) in pre-disposed individuals.

AMYLOID RISK

Systemic amyloidosis is characterized by produc-tion and deposition of inert insoluble protein in vessels and organs eventually leading to failure. Primary (AL) amyloid (usually due to multiple myeloma, rarely congenital amyloidosis) is caused by excessive deposition of immunoglobulin light chains and is a form of monoclonal gammopathy. Secondary (AA) amyloid is produced from inflam-matory (such as serum amyloid A protein) and non-inflammatory proteins, hormones or apolipo-proteins (with genetic predisposition in Alzheim-er's disease). AA amyloid previously accounted for organ failure and death in cases of JIA and RA. Better management of arthritis has resulted in sub-stantial improvement in overall survival, including a significant fall in the number of cases of amyloid. The most common cause (in 64%) of amyloid in Turkey is familial Mediterranean fever (FMF); 16% is due to infectious diseases, such as TB and other chronic lung infections such as bronchiectasis, RA accounts for 4% of cases and spondylarthropathy is the cause in 3%. Most patients present with peripheral oedema and proteinuria. Enlargement of the liver or spleen may be present in 11–17%. In 38% of cases there is progression to end-stage renal disease.

RARE ARTHROPATHIES

Adult Still's disease is a rare inflammatory disorder resulting in typical features of fever, arthralgia, rash and leucocytosis. Other clinical manifesta-tions include sore throat, lymphadenopathy and/or splenomegaly, liver dysfunction. Patients do not have rheumatoid factor or ANA, and systemic markers of inflammation are elevated and ferritin levels are characteristically very high. Treatment is usually with steroids for systemic manifesta-tions, and methotrexate or anti-TNF therapy for arthritis.

SYSTEMIC INFLAMMATORY CONDITIONS IN CHILDHOOD

Although individually many of the multi-system inflammatory diseases are rare in childhood, each with an incidence of 0.1–1 in 10 000, collectively they form a significant proportion of the paediatric rheumatology workload. This is attributable to complex presentation and, at times, a relentless progression requiring constant screening of renal, pulmonary, cardiovascular and cerebral function, along with complications from long-term therapy. Furthermore, since presentation may mimic other childhood diseases, both common, such as infectious diseases, and sinister, such as leukaemia and lymphoma, general physicians are frequently involved in the diagnostic challenge.

For ease of consideration, these diseases have been classified by a characteristic feature of pyrexia or rash. Overlap between these diseases is common, to such an extent that the diagnostic label may change with time as the true nature of the disease becomes apparent. As a result, it is essential for regular monitoring of symptoms, signs and laboratory screening tests to challenge early diagnoses and re-evaluate therapy. To avoid repetition this section focuses on paediatric aspects of inflammatory disease and where relevant the reader is referred to other sections for a more general account of the disease.

PYREXIAL PRESENTATION

Differentiating this group of non-infectious inflammatory diseases, identified in Table 18.2, from self-limiting paediatric infectious disease relies upon suspicion, and a detailed history and examination to identify characteristic features and symptom complexes.

Kawasaki disease should be considered early in a high spiking pyrexial illness (39–40°C) with negative blood cultures and unresponsive to antibiotics. This is because timely treatment with intravenous immunoglobulins and aspirin will avert life-threatening coronary aneurysms. The diagnosis is made when there are four of five diagnostic criteria in addition to 5 days of fever: i) conjunctivitis and ii) oral mucosal changes each occur in 90% of cases, iii) rash in 80%, and iv) lymphadenopathy and v) palmar erythema occur in 70%. In an infant, the criteria may be incomplete, but inconsolable irritability in the absence of meningitis should raise suspicion.

Other important diagnoses to consider are leukaemia, lymphoma and neuroblastoma, which may present with fever and constitutional disturbance. A blood count and film discussed with the haematologist may help in the diagnosis of leukaemia, the commonest childhood malignancy to result in musculoskeletal pain and arthritis, but a bone marrow aspirate is definitive.

In systemic-onset juvenile idiopathic arthritis (JIA) there is a quotidian fever, which spikes to >39°C once or twice a day and always returns to normal. It may be accompanied by a salmon-pink or urticarial rash and may precede the polyarthropathy by months. A rare and life-threatening association with systemic-onset JIA, SLE, and disorders of infectious and neoplastic origin is macrophage activation syndrome, characterized by abnormalities of liver function, a rapid fall in erythrocyte sedimentation rate (ESR) and bleeding diathesis. Periodic fever syndromes and vasculitic syndromes may also present with fever, rash and arthritis. They are often distinguished by the key features and investigations identified in Table 18.2, although many such diagnoses remain undifferentiated. Of the microbiological investigations the throat swab is important in determining the presence of streptococcus.

The periodic fever syndromes are rare, but important, systemic conditions that cause intermittent episodes of systemic inflammation, with organ involvement, especially in the abdomen, joints and skin. They occur predominantly in children and young adults. They are inherited disorders of the immune system, due to defects in the genes that control cytokine function. FMF is the most common variant; others in this group include hypergammaglobulinaemia D and periodic fever syndrome (HIDS), TNF receptor-associated periodic syndrome (TRAPS), Muckle–Wells syndrome, familial cold urticaria (FCU), familial cold autoinflammatory syndrome (FCAS) and chronic infantile neurological cutaneous and articular syndrome (CINCA).

SKIN PRESENTATION

Diagnoses typically associated with a characteristic rash (Table 18.3), such as Henoch–Schönlein purpura, SLE and juvenile dermatomyositis (JDM), also present with constitutional symptoms of sustained fever, fatigue, anorexia and weight loss.

Table 18.2 Pyrexial presentation of multi-system inflammatory disease in childhood

Diagnosis	Characteristic features	Investigation
Kawasaki disease	High spiking fever (39–40°C) >5 days 4 of 5 criteria (*see text*) (± irritability in infant) Coronary artery aneurysms if untreated	Suspicion Platelets, ECHO
Systemic-onset juvenile idiopathic arthritis (SoJIA)	Quotidian fever and evanescent rash may precede polyarthritis by months (*see text and Chapter 28*). Serositis, hepatosplenomegaly, lymphadenopathy	Platelets, ECHO
Neoplasia (leukaemia, lymphoma, neuroblastoma)	Always consider if multi-system disease of indeterminate cause, and if normal/low platelets	Blood film; bone marrow aspirate; abdominal USS/CT
Reactive illnesses • Arthritis & eye disease • Rheumatic fever • Lyme disease	 Preceding enteric infection Jones' criteria (*see Chapter 16*) Rash & arthritis following a tick bite (*Chapter 16*)	Stool culture Throat swab, ASOT Anti-DNAse b Borrelia

Other vasculitides
• Polyarteritis nodosa
• Wegener's granulomatosis
• Microscopic polyangiitis
• Churg–Strauss syndrome
• Takayasu's arteritis
• Behçet's disease
	See text in Chapter 17
	} Fever, weight loss, fatigue,
	} *plus one of:*
	  – skin lesions
	  – focal neurological deficit
	  – myositis & arthritis
	  – nephritis/hypertension
		Renal angiography
		MRI/MRA
		Tissue biopsy
		ANCA

Periodic fever syndromes • Familial Mediterranean fever • Hyper-IgD syndrome • TRAPS • Muckle–Wells syndrome • PFAPA	*60% of periodic fevers are unclassifiable* 1–3 d fever, peritoneal/pleuropericardial pain, arthritis 3–7 d fever, erythema, aggressive arthritis >7 d fever and ocular signs Prolonged fever, urticaria and deafness **P**eriodic **F**ever, **A**phthous ulcer, **P**haryngitis, **A**denitis	 Genetic analysis IgD; *MVK* analysis TNFα receptor study Hearing test
Macrophage activation syndrome (*haemophagocytic lymphohistiocytosis*)	Life-threatening complication of systemic onset JIA, SLE, virus. Persistent fever, lymphadenopathy, hepatic failure and purpura; with sudden fall in ESR & platelet count and marked rise in LFTs and ferritin	Bone marrow aspiration

The onset of SLE occurs in childhood in 20% of patients and in the young has similar clinical features and management to those in adults (see Chapter 17). A malar rash is also seen in JDM, but the violaceous heliotrope of the upper eyelid, Gottron's papules and periungual erythema are classical. MRI of the thigh is used to confirm the inflammatory myopathy. A recurrent polycyclic course is observed in 60% of patients with JDM and may involve the joints, gastrointestinal tract, lungs and central nervous system. Treatment includes steroids and methotrexate, but in severe cases cyclophosphamide is used.

The rash of juvenile sarcoid, distinct from sarcoid in adolescents and adults, is described as 'sago', and localized scleroderma, more common in children than adults, is typically of a linear rather than morphoea form of distribution. Sarcoid and scleroderma may respond to steroids and methotrexate.

Of the two inflammatory illnesses peculiar to the first few months of life, inflammation in CINCA (see Table 18.3) is progressive whereas in neonatal lupus, attributable to transplacental passage of maternal autoantibodies, is transient. However, the heart block from neonatal lupus can be permanent.

Table 18.3 Skin presentation of multi-system inflammatory disease in childhood

Diagnosis	Characteristic features	Investigation
Henoch–Schönlein purpura	Palpable purpura of classic distribution (*see Chapter 17*). Possible intussuseption, arthralgia, nephritis	Urinalysis; blood pressure
Post-streptococcal vasculitis (*cutaneous polyarteritis*)	Palpable purpura with palmar involvement; may be associated with arthritis and transient neuropathy	Throat swab, ASOT Anti-DNAse b
Systemic lupus erythematosus	(*see Chapter 17*) Rash in 75% of patients; malar rash in 50% of patients Lupus nephritis and CNS disorder determine outcome	ANA, dsDNA, complement, ESR, lymphocyte count, urinary protein
Juvenile dermatomyositis	Violaceous heliotrope on upper eyelids, Gottron's papules, periungual erythema and proximal inflammatory myopathy. Also synovitis; GI ulceration; pulmonary fibrosis; CNS disease (rare)	MRI/USS of thigh Muscle enzymes (Endoscopy, CT chest)
Juvenile sarcoid	'Sago' rash, boggy arthritis, eye disease	Biopsy
Scleroderma	Linear waxy thickened skin resulting in limb deformity Also morphoea; systemic sclerosis very rare	Thermography Capillaroscopy
Mixed connective tissue disease	Raynaud's and arthropathy	Anti-RNP
Neonatal lupus erythematosus	Inflammation of skin, liver and haematological complications. Heart block permanent	ECG, ECHO
CINCA (chronic infantile neurological, cutaneous and articular syndrome)	Onset in infancy of triad of rash, symmetrical arthropathy & chronic meningitis	MRI, lumbar puncture

257

FURTHER READING

Grateau G 2003 Musculoskeletal disorders in secondary amyloidosis and hereditary fevers. Best Pract Res Clin Rheumatol 17: 929–944.

Grateau G 2004 Clinical and genetic aspects of the hereditary periodic fever syndromes. Rheumatology 43: 410–415.

Tuglular S, Yalcinkaya F, Paydas S et al 2002 A retrospective analysis for aetiology and clinical findings of 287 secondary amyloidosis cases in Turkey. Nephrol Dial Transplant 17: 2003–2005.

19

BONE DISORDERS

Julia L. Newton and Raashid Luqmani

Cases relevant to this chapter

37, 41, 45, 51, 53, 63, 64, 73, 82, 92, 95, 98

● Essential facts

1. Osteoporosis is the most common bone disorder.

2. It is important to look for underlying causes of osteoporosis.

3. The aim of treatment of osteoporosis is to prevent fragility fractures.

4. Bisphosphonates with calcium and vitamin D supplementation are first-line treatment of osteoporosis.

5. Osteomalacia is under-diagnosed in the UK.

6. The commonest cause of osteomalacia is vitamin D deficiency.

7. Paget's disease is due to overactivity of the osteoclast; it is often asymptomatic.

8. Osteonecrosis causes morbidity in young active people; the signs and symptoms are non-specific and often mild.

9. Causes of osteonecrosis include increased intraosseous pressure, fat emboli, external compression of blood supply, direct osteocyte death, mechanical stress and increased thrombotic tendency.

10. Magnetic resonance imaging is the most sensitive investigation for early osteonecrosis.

11. Early diagnosis of osteonecrosis significantly improves outcome.

OSTEOPOROSIS

Osteoporosis is the most common bone disorder and the pathophysiology is discussed in detail in Chapter 2. It is a significant cause of morbidity, increased disability and mortality, and imposes a major economic burden on the NHS. There is a 10–20% increase in mortality in the 12 months following a hip fracture. Osteoporosis is defined as a condition of skeletal fragility characterized by reduced bone mass and microarchitectural deterioration predisposing a person to an increased risk of fracture. It is due to one, or a combination, of three mechanisms: a failure to reach peak bone mass, an increase in bone resorption and a reduction in bone formation. It is more common in women and in the Caucasian population. Post-menopausal bone loss is the most significant cause of osteoporosis (Box 19.1).

CLINICAL FEATURES

Osteoporosis is asymptomatic. Fragility fractures are the main consequence of osteoporosis, resulting in the need for medical attention, either as pain or loss of height with development of a thoracic kyphosis (Fig. 19.1). If the osteoporosis is secondary to another disorder, for example, Cushing's syndrome, features of the underlying disease may be the initial presenting complaint. The bones most

Box 19.1
Causes of osteoporosis

- Post-menopausal oestrogen deficiency
- Amenorrhoea – eating disorder, exercise induced
- Hyperparathyroidism
- Malabsorption, e.g. coeliac disease
- Osteomalacia
- Hyperthyroidism
- Cushing's disease
- Hypopituitarism, hypogonadism
- Multiple myeloma

Box 19.2
Risk factors for the development of osteoporosis

- Previous fracture
- Family history
- Excess alcohol
- Smoking
- Corticosteroid treatment
- Amenorrhoea for 6 months (excluding pregnancy)
- Late menarche
- Early menopause including surgical menopause
- Low body weight
- Immobility/physical inactivity
- Drugs – heparin, phenytoin
- Inflammatory arthritis – rheumatoid arthritis, ankylosing spondylitis
- Gastrectomy

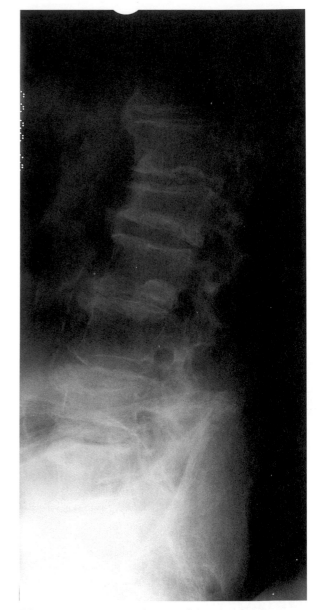

FIGURE 19.1   Osteoporotic fracture of the spine showing vertebral collapse

frequently affected by a fragility fracture are the hip, vertebra and wrist. The risk is directly related to age and due to a combination of age-related bone loss and increased rate of falls (Box 19.2).

AETIOLOGY

As described in Chapter 2, bone remodelling is a dynamic process, and the resorption and laying down of new bone are tightly coupled processes. In osteoporosis there is an imbalance of osteoclast and osteoblast activity. There may also be an increase in the initiation of new bone remodelling cycles (activation frequency). The resorption phase is faster than the formation phase, which can further contribute to osteoporosis when the activation frequency is high. Genetic factors contribute strongly to peak bone mass and to the rate of bone loss after peak mass has been achieved. Oestrogen (OE) has a central role in both men and women,

Table 19.1 Underlying mechanisms of osteoporosis

Disease	Mechanism
Post-menopausal osteoporosis	Increased rate of remodelling, uncoupling of bone formation and resorption, increased osteocyte apoptosis, low OE increases T-cell production of IL-1 and TNFα (both are osteoclastogenic), low OE reduces osteoprotegerin (a regulator of bone turnover)
Hyperparathyroidism	Increased bone turnover
Hyperthyroidism	Increased bone turnover
Cushing's disease	Uncoupling of bone resorption and formation
Corticosteroid treatment	Uncoupling of bone resorption and formation; increased osteocyte apoptosis, renal calcium loss and secondary hyperparathyroidism
Vitamin D deficiency	Secondary hyperparathyroidism
Calcium deficiency	Secondary hyperparathyroidism

Box 19.3
Investigations for osteoporosis

- Thyroid function tests
- Bone turnover markers
- Bone profile (calcium, phosphate, alkaline phosphatase, parathyroid hormone)
- Vitamin D
- Multiple myeloma screen (erythrocyte sedimentation rate, serum immunoglobulins and protein electrophoresis, urinary Bence Jones protein)
- Consider cortisol, testosterone, oestradiol

Table 19.2 Bone turnover markers

Resorption	Serum C- and N-telopeptides of type 1 collagen crosslinks (urine)
Formation	Bone-specific alkaline phosphatase, osteocalcin, C- and N-terminal propeptides of type 1 collagen

but men do not have the same dramatic changes in sex hormone levels during middle age as women do (Table 19.1).

DIAGNOSIS

Bone mineral density (BMD) is measured using dual-energy X-ray absorptiometry (DEXA) scanning. A T score of less than −2.5 indicates osteoporosis and a T score of between −1.0 and −2.5 indicates osteopenia.

INVESTIGATIONS

Box 19.3 outlines the investigations for osteoporosis.

Bone turnover markers

Bone turnover marker levels (Table 19.2) are affected by a number of factors:

- Significant inter- and intra-individual variation
- Turnover parallels growth velocity
- Circadian rhythm
- Seasonal variation (follows vitamin D levels through seasons)
- Medication (bisphosphonates, corticosteroids)
- The presence of other disease, overt or subclinical, that affects bone turnover (Paget's disease, thyroid disease, hyperparathyroidism, osteomalacia)
- Renal failure causes a false increase in bone turnover markers.

TREATMENT

The aim of treatment is to reduce the incidence of fragility fractures. Life-style modification measures should be discussed with all patients, including improving calcium intake (equivalent of 1 pint of milk a day or 1200–1500 mg/day), supplemental vitamin D (800 iu/day), weight-bearing exercise, smoking cessation and reduction of alcohol consumption if excessive. Exercise promotes increased bone density, but also helps in fall prevention. Hip protectors have been advocated, but compliance is poor. Current drug options below (Table 19.3) reduce fracture risk by up to 50%, but patients can, therefore, still fracture despite appropriate treatment.

Monitoring treatment includes the use of bone turnover markers to assess if remodelling rates have been significantly supressed by anti-resorptive medication.

OSTEOMALACIA

Osteomalacia and rickets are due to vitamin D deficiency, which causes an accumulation of osteoid and poor mineralization of bone. The clinical picture is called rickets or osteomalacia, depending upon whether it is before or after cessation of growth respectively.

VITAMIN D METABOLISM

Vitamin D is a pro-hormone formed by the action of ultraviolet radiation on its precursor (7-dehydrocholesterol) in the skin. It undergoes two hydroxylation steps to become an active hormone. The first, the 25-hydroxyaltion step to become 25-hydroxycholecalciferol, occurs in the liver, and the second, in which the 25-hydroxycholecalciferol is converted to 1,25-dihydroxycholecalciferol (calcitriol), takes place in the kidney.

CLINICAL FEATURES

In rickets, the areas of bone most severely affected are the metaphyses of long bones leading to a characteristic clinical and radiological picture (Box 19.4).

The signs and symptoms of osteomalacia are often vague and the diagnosis may be missed unless specifically considered (Fig. 19.2). These clinical features and the typical radiological findings are listed in Table 19.4. There is a considerable differential diagnosis for osteomalacia (Box 19.5).

Box 19.4
Clinical features of rickets

- Craniotabes of the skull
- Enlarged epiphyses of wrists
- 'Rickety rosary' of osteochondral junctions
- Harrison's sulcus in the rib cage
- Bow, knock knee or windswept leg deformities
- Floppy baby
- Dental abnormalities
- Delayed growth

Table 19.3 Drugs for osteoporosis, with mechanism of action and side effects

Drug	Mechanism of action	Side effects
Calcium and vitamin D	Reduces hyperparathyroidism of increasing age	Hypercalcaemia
Bisphosphonates	Inhibition of osteoclast activity, increased osteoclast programmed cell death, slowing of the remodelling cycle allowing full mineralization of new bone to occur	Oesophagitis
PTH (teriparatide) – synthetic N-terminal portion of PTH	Large increase in bone formation (anabolic) and a modest increase in resorption, increased periosteal apposition (deposition of bone on the surface to increase strength)	Hypercalcaemia, nausea, leg cramps
Strontium ranelate	Mechanism is not fully understood. Has anti-resorptive and anabolic effects	Headache, nausea, deep vein thrombosis (DVT)
HRT (hormone replacement therapy)	Reduces bone resorption by blocking cytokine signalling to the osteoclast	Risk of breast cancer, DVT, increased cardiovascular risk
SERMs (selective (o)estrogen receptor modulators)	Reduces bone resorption	Increased DVT risk and hot flushes (no increase in breast cancer risk)
Biologic therapies	e.g. antibody to RANKL	Experimental at present

INVESTIGATIONS

The typical biochemical findings for osteomalacia and other disorders of bone are shown for comparison in Table 19.5. As well as a bone profile (calcium, phosphate, parathyroid hormone, alkaline phosphatase), urea and electrolytes and serum ferritin will identify any evidence of renal failure or malabsorption as an underlying cause for osteomalacia.

AETIOLOGY

Osteomalacia is usually caused by vitamin D deficiency, but there are other rarer causes to consider (Table 19.6). The main cause of hypovitaminosis D is a lack of sun exposure; the two largest at-risk groups are women and children screened from the

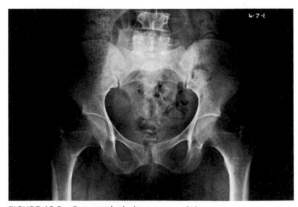

FIGURE 19.2   Osteomalacia in a young Asian woman complaining of pain in the hips – note the Looser zone in the right femoral neck

Table 19.4 Features of osteomalacia

Symptoms	Bone pain, proximal myopathy with normal creatine kinase, pain from a pathological fracture, polyarthralgia
Signs	Bone tenderness, waddling gait, proximal weakness, tetany (hypocalcaemia)
Radiology	Looser's zone (cortical fractures on the compression side of the bone), pathological fractures, demineralization, features of hyperparathyroidism – chondrocalcinosis, subperiosteal erosions
Biochemistry	Calcium – normal or low; phosphate – normal or low; bone-specific alkaline phosphatase – normal or increased; 25-hydroxyvitamin D – low; 1,25-hydroxyvitamin D – normal or low; PTH – high
Histology	Excessive osteoid and reduced mineralization. Caution as similar picture in disorders with increased bone turnover (hyperparathyroidism, Paget's disease, hyperthyroidism)

Box 19.5
Differential diagnosis of osteomalacia

- Osteoporosis
- Fibromyalgia
- Polymyalgia rheumatica
- Polymyositis
- Rheumatoid arthritis
- Multiple myeloma
- Metastatic bone disease

Table 19.5 Typical biochemical findings in common bone diseases

	Ca^{2+}	PO_4	ALP	PTH	U & Es	25-(OH) Vit D	1,25-$(OH)_2$ Vit D
Osteomalacia	ln/↓	ln/↓	↑	↑	n	↓	ln/↓
Osteoporosis	n	n	n	n	n	n	n
Primary hyperparathyroidism	↑	ln/↓	↑/hn	↑	n/↑	n	n
Renal osteodystrophy	ln/↓	↑/hn	↑	↑	↑	ln/↓	ln/↓
Paget's disease	n*	n	↑	n	n	n	n

n=normal, ln=low normal, hn=high normal, ALP=alkaline phosphatase, U & Es=urea and electrolytes, PTH=parathyroid hormone, 25-(OH) Vit D=25-hydroxyvitamin D, 1,25-$(OH)_2$ Vit D=1,25-hydroxyvitamin D.
*High if immobility or secondary osteosarcoma.

Table 19.6 Causes of vitamin D deficiency

Hypovitaminosis D	Lack of sun exposure, poor dietary intake
Malabsorption	Coeliac disease, gastrectomy, pancreatic insufficiency
Renal disease	Hypophosphataemic renal disease (hereditary and acquired forms), Fanconi syndromes (hereditary and acquired forms), distal renal tubular acidosis, renal osteodystrophy
Others	Anticonvulsants – phenytoin, carbamazepine (catabolize vitamin D to inactive metabolites), aluminium, heavy metal poisoning, bisphosphonates

Table 19.7 Clinical features of Paget's Disease

Common	Rare
Bone pain	Osteosarcoma
Deafness	Vascular steal phenomenon
Pathological fractures	High-output cardiac failure
Bone deformity	
Headache	
Nerve root compression	

sun by clothing for religious reasons and the elderly in institutions.

Renal osteodystrophy encompasses the spectrum of bone disease in association with chronic renal failure. The main components are hyperparathyroidism and osteomalacia.

MANAGEMENT

Management consists of education to prevent osteomalacia, particularly in at-risk populations, e.g. the elderly, and replacement therapy. Vitamin D is abundant in oily fish and supplemented in certain cereals. Fifteen minutes of sunshine to the face and hands/forearms three times a week between April and September is sufficient sun exposure. Darker skin requires longer sun exposure to generate the same amount of vitamin D. Protocols for vitamin D replacement depend upon the severity of the deficiency and the compliance of the patient. Mild deficiency can be replaced with 800 iu orally a day; more severe deficiency should be treated with high-dose bolus therapy and then 800 iu daily maintenance. Rarely, parenteral vitamin D is given. Calcium supplementation of 1500 mg a day should routinely be given.

PAGET'S DISEASE

Paget's disease of bone (PD) is the second most common bone disorder after osteoporosis affecting 5.4% of the population over 55 years of age in the UK. The prevalence is highly variable between races and countries. The highest rate is in the UK and it is rare in Japan, China, India and Scandinavia. The normal, highly regulated process of bone remodelling is disturbed. There is excessive bone resorption and, due to the tightly coupled nature of osteoclast and osteoblast activity, this is followed by the rapid laying down of disorganized, weak, abnormal bone. For a review of the normal bone remodelling cycle read Chapter 2.

CLINICAL FEATURES

The frequency of PD increases with age. It is rare at less than 50 years and affects both sexes with a slight predominance in men. It is often asymptomatic and discovered incidentally from a raised alkaline phosphatase (ALP) in the blood or an X-ray performed for an unrelated reason. Only 10–30% of people with PD are symptomatic and the commonest presentation is pain (Table 19.7). Osteosarcoma is a frequently quoted complication of PD, but it is becoming rarer and occurs in less than 1% of patients. PD has a predilection for certain bones, but may affect anywhere in the skeleton (Box 19.6).

Seventeen per cent of patients have a single site of PD. Once diagnosed it is rare for new sites to develop during a patient's lifetime. The lesions are highly localized and progress slowly, but relentlessly, once present.

AETIOLOGY

The aetiology is incompletely understood. There is a genetic and an environmental component to the disease. Current hypotheses are based around an environmental insult in a genetically predisposed

> ### Box 19.6
> **Most frequently affected bones in Paget's disease (descending order of frequency)**
>
> - Pelvis
> - Lumbar spine
> - Femur
> - Thoracic spine
> - Sacrum
> - Skull
> - Tibia
> - Humerus

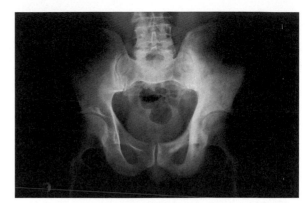

FIGURE 19.3   Paget's disease of the hemipelvis

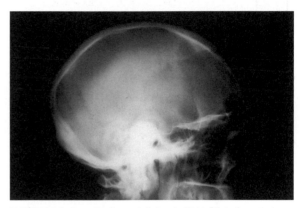

FIGURE 19.4   Paget's disease of the skull showing the phenomenon of osteoporosis circumscripta

individual. The primary abnormality lies within the osteoclast. Osteoclasts in PD are increased in number and size and multinucleated. Osteoclast precursors are also abnormal and are hypersensitive to factors that stimulate their differentiation into mature osteoclasts, including RANKL and $1,25\text{-}(OH)_2D_3$. Osteoblasts are normal, but have increased activity due to increased stimulation from factors released by the osteoclasts. The initial lesion is, therefore, osteolytic followed by the rapid laying down of weak disorganized bone.

INVESTIGATIONS

A raised bone-specific ALP, a marker of bone formation, is often the first clue. Other markers of bone turnover are increased including osteocalcin (formation) and N-telopeptide of type 1 collagen in the urine (resorption). Calcium is usually normal unless there has been a recent fracture or prolonged immobility. An X-ray will show the typical appearances of thickened, coarse cortical bone (Fig. 19.3) and in some cases, during phases of highly increased osteoclast activity, the appearance of localized osteoporosis, called osteoporosis circumscripta (Fig. 19.4).

TREATMENT

Who and when to treat is the main question. Pain is the most common reason for treating. Other reasons for medical treatment include sequelae of the disease: fractures and nerve root compression from the expanded bone. Prior to surgery, treatment may be indicated because pagetic bone is more vascular and consequently bleeds more.

Bisphosphonates inhibit osteoclast activity and promote osteoclast apoptosis and are the mainstay of treatment. Before bisphosphonates were available salmon calcitonin, another inhibitor of osteoclasts, was used, but patients rapidly developed antibodies.

OSTEONECROSIS (AKA AVASCULAR NECROSIS, ASEPTIC NECROSIS, BONE INFARCTION OR OSTEOCHONDRITIS DISSECANS)

Osteonecrosis (ON) is the final common pathway of a number of conditions that result in bone death. The pathophysiology of ON is discussed in Chapter 2.

AETIOLOGY

The aetiology is multifactorial, but the final stage of ON is bone death due to a compromised blood supply. Trauma and sickle cell disease are the two most common causes of ON worldwide. There are many identified risk factors and associated conditions (Table 19.8) for atraumatic ON, but there is still a significant number of idiopathic cases. Many of the idiopathic cases occur in children, adolescents and young adults. Two of these conditions, osteochondritis dissecans and Perthes' disease, are specifically discussed.

CLINICAL PRESENTATION

Many of the patients affected by ON are young and active with a predeliction for certain bones (Box 19.7). Pain is usually the presenting complaint and may be accompanied by a limited range of movement. Up to one-third of patients are asymptomatic. There is a high incidence of bilateral

Table 19.8 Risk factors for ON and conditions associated with ON

Risk factor/associated condition	Mechanism*
Trauma	Interruption to blood supply
Corticosteroid treatment, Cushing's disease	Increased intraosseous pressure, fat emboli, inhibition of angiogenesis, increased osteoporosis and microfracture, direct osteocyte death; the cumulative dose of corticosteroids is more predictive of increased risk than the daily dose
Haemoglobinopathies – sickle cell disease, thalassaemia	Sludging of abnormal red blood cells, marrow hyperplasia and increased intraosseous pressure
Hyperlipidaemia	Increased intraosseous pressure, fat emboli, intravascular coagulation
Alcohol	Fatty liver and fat emboli, direct osteocyte death, secondary Cushing's syndrome
Autoimmune conditions – SLE, APLS	Increased thrombotic tendency
Inherited clotting cascade abnormalities – factor V Leiden, protein C and S deficiency	Increased thrombotic tendency
Marrow infiltration	Increased intraosseous pressure, increased thrombotic tendency
Infection ± disseminated intravascular coagulation	Increased thrombotic tendency
Malignancy	Corticosteroid treatment, marrow infiltration, increased thrombotic tendency
Polycythaemia rubra vera	Sluggish blood flow, increased thrombotic tendency
Hyperbaric exposure (Caisson's disease)	Intramedullary nitrogen bubbles
Pregnancy	Impaired venous drainage by gravid uterus, mechanical stress from increased weight, increased endogenous steroids
Haemophilia	External arterial compression from recurrent haemarthroses
Gaucher's disease	Sludging of abnormal red blood cells, fat emboli, increased intraosseous pressure
Radiation therapy	Dose-dependent osteocyte death, aetiology unclear
HIV infection	Unknown
Bisphosphonates	Unknown aetiology, affects the jaw

*These are proposed mechanisms, not all are proven.

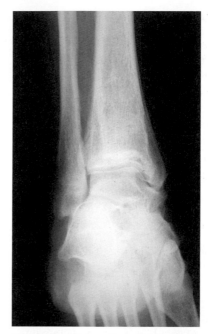

FIGURE 19.5 Plain radiograph of osteonecrosis showing an unusual osteonecrosis of the distal tibial shaft of a 41-year-old woman with an inflammatory arthritis for 2 years. Changes include subchondral sclerosis in the distal tibia at the ankle joint. Some periosteal reaction is noted along the distal aspect of the tibia. There is some narrowing of the joint space medially with sclerosis

involvement in atraumatic cases involving the femoral head, femoral condyles and humeral head. Premature degenerative disease is a common consequence of ON and a major cause of disability.

METHODS OF DIAGNOSIS

Magnetic resonance imaging (MRI) is the most sensitive method and may detect pathology before collapse is seen radiographically (Figs 19.5 & 19.6). Once osteonecrosis is well established, every imaging method, such as standard plain film, CT and isotope bone scan, will reveal it. Table 19.9 lists the various methods of imaging and their characteristic findings in osteonecrosis.

MANAGEMENT

Treatment may include avoidance of weight-bearing, analgesia and surgery, such as bone decompression and joint replacement.

OSTEOCHONDRITIS DISSECANS

This condition usually affects children and adolescents and is discussed in Chapter 26.

PERTHES' DISEASE

This condition usually affects children and adolescents and is discussed in Chapter 26.

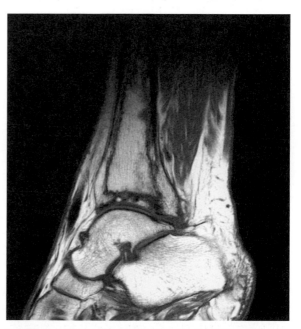

FIGURE 19.6 The corresponding MRI scan showing an extensive bone infarct within the distal tibia. There is some linear high signal within the longitudinal axis of the Achilles tendon. This may represent an area of longitudinal tearing

Table 19.9 Methods of imaging patients with suspected osteonecrosis

Imaging method	Time of diagnosis	Findings	Characteristics
MRI	Days to weeks	Decreased signal in a segmental pattern	Excellent sensitivity Good specificity
Isotope bone scan	Weeks	Early decreased uptake, late increased uptake	Good sensitivity Poor specificity
Plain X-ray	Weeks to months	Radiolucency, osteonecrosis, microfractures, subchondral collapse	Poor sensitivity Good specificity
CT	Months	Reactive sclerosis, subchondral collapse	Poor sensitivity Good specificity

Management

Prevention by the recognition and management of treatable disorders like hyperlipidaemia and alcoholism is crucial. Early diagnosis and intervention improves outcome so a high index of suspicion is important. ON is an irreversible process. Management includes conservative treatment to reduce the use of the affected joint and simple analgesics. Surgery is often required and the commonest procedures are core decompression and joint replacement. Prognosis is dependent upon the location and stage of the disease. There is the potential for biologic therapies in the future.

FURTHER READING

Assouline-Dayan Y, Chang C, Greenspan A et al 2002 Pathogenesis and natural history of osteonecrosis. Semin Arth Rheum 32(2): 94–124.
Pavelka K 2000 Osteonecrosis. Baillieres Clin Rheumatol 14(2): 399–414.

ORTHOPAEDICS

269

TUMOURS OF THE MUSCULOSKELETAL SYSTEM AND PATHOLOGICAL FRACTURES

20

Daniel Porter

Cases relevant to this chapter

1, 24, 25, 30, 73, 85, 92, 94, 95, 98, 99

●Essential facts

1. Tumours can be neoplastic (benign or malignant), inflammatory (infection, inflammatory nodules) or miscellaneous (e.g. ganglion, bursa).

2. Benign tumours of bone are slow growing and have a well defined margin.

3. Osteosarcoma particularly affects adolescent boys, especially in the metaphyses of long bones.

5. Chondrosarcoma commonly affects adults and most arise '*de novo*', but in 10% of cases there is a pre-existing enchondroma or osteochondroma.

6. A soft-tissue lump is likely to be sarcoma if it is painful, growing rapidly, larger than 5 cm in size and deep to deep fascia.

7. Metastatic bone tumours occur at any age, but are the most frequent cause of a painful lytic bony lesion in the elderly.

8. In patients with rheumatoid arthritis or gout, nodules commonly occur as part of the disease.

9. Pathological fractures occur after minimal force; they include osteoporotic fractures in the elderly, osteogenesis imperfecta in the young, fractures through infected or dead bone, and fractures through neoplastic bony lesions.

10. The matrix of a benign cystic lesion is purely lytic, and the margins well defined; malignant lesions and rapidly growing benign lesions have infiltrative edges.

11. Avoid fixation of a pathological fracture prior to obtaining a definitive diagnosis.

12. Most malignant pathological fractures will not heal; therefore, the implant should be 'load-bearing' rather than 'load-sharing'.

TUMOURS

The word *tumour* comes from the Greek word for 'swelling'. Swellings of the musculoskeletal system can be classified as neoplastic (benign), neoplastic (malignant), inflammatory or miscellaneous. In general, the lay-person's term for neoplasm is tumour. A neoplasm is an abnormal growth of cells over which control of growth has been lost. Removal of the stimulus that caused it does not stop it growing, and the tissue is clonal (has arisen from a clone – an almost identical mother cell).

NEOPLASTIC (BENIGN)

Benign neoplasms do not metastasize to other tissues beyond the local tumour. Sometimes the tumour may become malignant, but only if the classification of the tumour changes (for example, an enchondroma to a chondrosarcoma). A soft-tissue swelling that is pain-free, static or slowly growing, superficial and less than 5 cm in size has only a tiny chance of being malignant.

Important benign neoplasms of soft tissue are listed in Table 20.1; they are far more common than malignant ones.

Benign tumours of bone usually grow slowly and, therefore, tend to have a well defined margin. The bone has chance to react and often does so by expansion with cortical changes. Treatment is frequently a biopsy-cum-curettage to remove the majority of macroscopic tumour without causing morbidity. In most benign bone tumours this allows bone healing to eradicate remaining microscopic tumour. Important examples of benign bone neoplasms are listed in Table 20.2.

NEOPLASTIC (MALIGNANT)

Malignant neoplasms can metastasize to distant organs. They have invasive qualities both locally and distantly. It is this feature that makes the tumour so difficult to treat and may lead to the patient's death. Malignant tumours of the musculoskeletal system can be divided into tumours of bone or soft tissue. Primary bone tumours are usually sarcomas. Sarcomas have cells of origin that reflect the range of mesodermal tissue from which they arise (soft tissue – liposarcoma, fibrosarcoma, rhabdomyosarcoma, leiomyosarcoma, angiosarcoma, haemangiosarcoma, synovial sarcoma, malignant peripheral nerve sheath tumour; bony – osteosarcoma, chondrosarcoma, Ewing's sarcoma). Most soft-tissue sarcomas behave in a similar way independent of subtype.

Most soft-tissue sarcomas are graded according to their mitotic rate. Low-grade sarcomas have a slow growth rate and low metastatic potential. All cancers have the potential to spread locally, to regional lymph nodes and distantly. Sarcomas rarely spread to lymph nodes, so the main distant site for metastasis is the lung. This is most frequent in high-grade sarcomas.

Table 20.1 Benign neoplasms of soft tissue

Tumour	Features
Lipoma	Very common. MRI feaures usually typical fat but may be difficult to discriminate atypical lipoma from liposarcoma
Aggressive fibromatosis (desmoid tumour)	Locally difficult to resect completely. Resolution over many years. Radiotherapy, tamoxifen, vitamin C may help
Myxoma	Difficult to resect locally and may recur after many years. Occasionally de-differentiates to myxoid sarcoma
Leiomyoma	In retroperitoneum and gastrointestinal tract may have malignant potential
Haemangioma	May be congenital or acquired. Large ones in children may require multidisciplinary approach because of skin involvement
Schwannoma	Usually benign on a major nerve. Can be 'shelled' away from the nerve without damage
Neurofibroma	Integral within the nerve and cannot easily be 'shelled' away from it
Synovial chondromatosis	Forms in large joints and is difficult to eradicate. May de-differentiate to chondrosarcoma
Giant cell tumour of tendon sheath	Forms on tendons and easily 'shells' away from them

Table 20.2 Benign neoplasms of bone

Tumour	Radiographic features	Clinical features/treatment
Simple (unicameral) bone cyst	Large expanded well demarcated lytic metaphyseal lesion	Children. Heals spontaneously after fracture or may require bone graft
Aneurysmal bone cyst	Large lytic metaphyseal lesion	Blood-filled spaces. Curettage necessary
Giant cell tumour of bone	Metaphyseal to articular surface. Aggressive appearance	Solid tumour with soft-tissue involvement. Bony destruction results in extended joint replacement surgery
Eosinophilic granuloma (Langerhans' cell disease)	May have aggressive appearance	Part of a systemic disorder. Check anterior pituitary function
Osteoid osteoma	Cortical lesion. Central nidus with lytic ring and surrounding sclerosis	Children and young adults. Osteoid-producing tumour. Painful. May be curetted or ablated using heat under CT control
Osteoblastoma	Large lytic metaphyseal lesion	An osteoid osteoma over 2 cm in size
Chondroblastoma	Epiphyseal	Curettage and bone grafting
Fibrous cortical defect	Bubbly, lytic within cortex. Little change with time	Curettage if large and painful

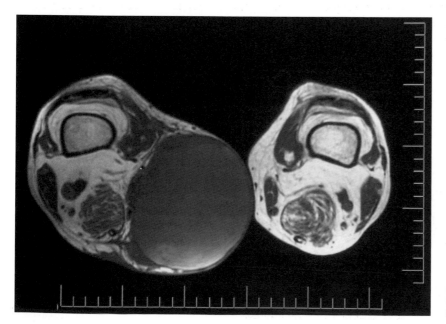

FIGURE 20.1 Magnetic resonance imaging of a large soft-tissue sarcoma in the lower thigh

A patient who presents with a soft-tissue lump has a high (>90%) risk of this being a sarcoma if it is: a) painful, b) growing rapidly, c) larger than 5 cm in size and d) deep to deep fascia. Figure 20.1 shows an MRI of a large soft-tissue sarcoma demonstrating most of these features. An X-ray may provide evidence of calcification (calcified haematoma, possibly synovial sarcoma). MRI scan defines solid from cystic and identifies a solid focus for biopsy, which should only be undertaken by the surgical team that will undertake the definitive surgery, or a competent radiologist. Nowadays these multidisciplinary teams exist in teaching hospitals accredited as national centres for sarcoma care. The histopathologist should identify the lesion through haematoxylin and eosin staining and immunohistochemistry to subtype the biopsy specimen. Cytogenetics may be useful. It should be remembered that the biopsy may not be representative of the entire specimen. Following a diagnosis of sarcoma, further 'staging' investigations would include blood tests (full blood count, clinical chemistry, clotting screen, erythrocyte sedimentation rate (ESR), C-reactive protein (CRP)) and a CT scan of chest to identify any lung metastases.

Adult soft-tissue sarcomas are relatively insensitive to radio- and chemotherapy. The mainstay of local control is, therefore, surgical resection. If possible this should be limb salvage surgery to preserve function. Invasion of important neurovascular structures may mean amputation is the only potentially curative option. Ultimately the decision on definitive treatment should be taken by a multidisciplinary team.

There is a role for radiotherapy in high-grade tumours with close surgical margins, as this reduces the risk of local recurrence. The value of chemotherapy is still under debate. Survival is dependent on grade, size, depth and initial success of treatment.

Bone sarcomas can be classified into three main types:

1. Osteosarcoma

   This is the most common of the bony sarcomas and is an osteoid-producing malignant tumour; 90% are high grade. It affects adolescents mainly and males are more commonly affected than females. It can also affect children and has a later peak in old age where it may occur in Paget's disease and after radiation for other cancers. Common sites are the long-bone metaphyses (distal femur>proximal tibia>proximal humerus>proximal femur>distal tibia). X-rays usually show a mixed sclerotic/lytic lesion that has indistinct margins (Fig. 20.2). At the margins of periosteal elevation a little triangle of new bone is evident (Codman's triangle). Radiating calcification may be seen in the sub-periosteal tumour expansion (sun-ray spiculation). Further investigations include all staging undertaken for soft-tissue sarcomas, but, in

addition, bone scintigraphy can identify osteosarcoma that may have developed in other bones. Since the 1980s survival has improved markedly to about 60% at 5 years, which is almost entirely due to chemotherapy. Local control, however, is still best gained by surgery, although the tumour is often downsized and made more amenable to resection by pre-operative (neo-adjuvant) chemotherapy. Factors determining extent of surgery are similar to those in soft-tissue sarcomas. Limb salvage surgery in children who have remaining skeletal growth will require skeletal support, which grows over time. If possible, the growth plates should be preserved, but often this is impossible. Alternatively a 'growing' metal endoprosthesis could be implanted. In adults the choice lies between a biological or a non-biological solution. The former involves allograft or autograft (e.g. a vascularized fibular graft) to create new bone within the defect. The latter utilizes an endoprosthetic implant to replace the excised tumour. The services of a plastic surgeon are often required to gain skin cover after resection and implantation or when the tumour involves skin.

2. Ewing's sarcoma

   The second most common primary malignant bone tumour again mainly affects children. Soft-tissue Ewing's sarcoma may also occur occasionally. It is always high grade and is thought to originate from neuro-ectodermal cell types. It affects diaphyses most frequently. The clinical picture is of systemic upset (weight and appetite loss, low-grade pyrexia, elevated ESR, a warm erythematous swelling). The differential diagnosis both clinically and radiographically lies between infection and eosinophilic granuloma (Langerhans' cell histiocytosis). 'Staging' investigations are as for osteosarcoma. Treatment has again been revolutionized by neo-adjuvant chemotherapy, after which either radiotherapy or surgery is required to treat residual tumour at the local disease site. Five-year survival is about 50%.

3. Chondrosarcoma

   This most commonly affects adults beyond their 5th decade and usually arises 'de novo'. Ten per cent arise from a pre-existing chondroid lesion (enchondroma or

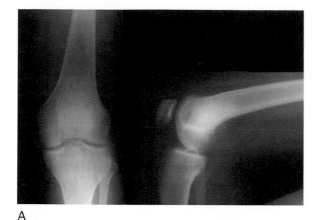

A

B

RIGHT KNEE

C

FIGURE 20.2 (A) Presenting anteroposterior and lateral X-rays of an osteosarcoma of the distal femur. Note the cortical destruction. (B) Axial MRI scan demonstrates soft-tissue extension posteriorly. (C) X-ray of the endoprosthesis, which is really an extended knee replacement

osteochondroma). Chondrosarcomas can be low, medium or high grade, and the metastatic risk is proportionate to their grade. Radiographs usually reveal calcification within the lesion. These tumours are very insensitive to adjuvant treatment, and surgical resection is the only potential for cure. Five-year survival is as high as 90% for low-grade, but only 60% for high-grade chondrosarcoma.

4. Other malignant tumours

a) Adamantinoma

This is a rare low-grade malignant tumour, which affects long-bone diaphyses in children and young adults. Treatment involves bony excision and metal or biological replacement. Metastatic rate is about 10%.

b) Multiple myeloma

This is really a haematological malignancy that may arise within the bone marrow (Fig. 20.3). The megakaryocyte undergoes malignant transformation to produce a clone of immunoglobulin. X-rays or bone scintigraphy often shows lesions throughout the skeleton or in a single site (plasmacytoma). Blood tests should include plasma electrophoresis (to seek a malignant immunoglobulin band) and Bence Jones proteins (immunoglobulins) sought on urine microscopy. Treatment is skeletal support for the bony skeleton and chemotherapy for widespread disease. Survival may be as high as 70% at 5 years, but diminishes rapidly at 10 years.

FAMILIAL NEOPLASTIC TRAITS AND MUSCULOSKELETAL NEOPLASIA

Familial traits linked to musculoskeletal neoplasia are listed in Table 20.3, together with important features. All traits are autosomal dominant. Malignancy tends to arise one or two decades earlier than in the same disease in the general population (sporadic disease).

SECONDARY TUMOURS OF BONE

Although these can occur at any age, they are the most frequent cause of a painful lytic bony lesion in the elderly. Radiographs of malignancy in bone usually reveal a lesion that is destroying the mineral content of bone without the bone having the chance to react to the tumour. Soft-tissue involvement may be inferred from surrounding soft-tissue shadows. Bone scintigraphy may demonstrate several bony lesions, suggesting widespread metastases. A solitary metastasis should be biopsied to ensure it does not represent a primary bone tumour – treatment of this would be very different.

The source of the metastasis should be sought. A clinical history of weight loss, bowel or chest symptoms is important, as is a previous history of cancer treatment. A careful examination of chest, abdomen, pelvis, breast, thyroid and prostate are recommended together with blood tests (P-SA, plasma electrophoresis together with routine blood screen as for primary tumours, as above). A chest X-ray, CT scan of chest, abdomen and pelvis should be considered for cryptic tumours and sometimes biopsy may be the only way to identify the origin of the tumour. Treatment should be determined in

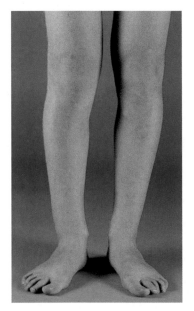

FIGURE 20.3 Hereditary multiple exostoses. Note the hard bony swellings evident over the long-bone metaphyses

Table 20.3 Familial traits linked to musculoskeletal neoplasia

Trait	Genetic mutation	Neoplasms	Comments
Li–Fraumeni syndrome	*P53* (17p)	All sarcomas	Also breast, adrenocortical, leukaemia and brain
Familial retinoblastoma	*Rb* (8p)	Osteosarcoma most common second tumour	Model from which Knudson's '2-hit' hypothesis drawn
Hereditary multiple exostosis (Fig. 20.3)	*EXT1* (8q) *EXT2* (11p)	Osteochondroma Chondrosarcoma	Lifetime risk only 1–5%
Ollier's disease (multiple enchondromatosis)	Not inherited	Enchondroma Chondrosarcoma	Risk up to 50%. Also haemangiosarcomas and granulosa cell tumours in Maffucci's syndrome
Neurofibromatosis 1 (Von Recklinghausen syndrome)	*NF1* (17q)	Malignant peripheral nerve sheath tumour, schwannoma, neurofibroma	Axillary freckles, iris Leisch nodules, spinal dural ectasia, pseudarthrosis of tibia
Gardner's syndrome	*APC* (5q)	Aggressive fibromatosis (desmoid tumour) Mandibular osteoma	Associated familial polyposis

Table 20.4 Malignances that metastasize to bone

Cancer	Features
Small round cell tumours of childhood (neuroblastoma, nephroblastoma, rhabdomyosarcoma, leukaemia)	Paediatric oncology overview for entry into clinical trial for treatment
Lung	Median survival no more than 1–2 years
Breast	Some lesions are sclerotic. Median survival up to 5 years
Prostate	90% of lesions are sclerotic. Endocrine treatment important in prolonged survival
Thyroid	Treatment with ^{131}I important for prolonged survival
Renal	A solitary metastasis can occur decades after the primary tumour. Its excision can be curative. Therefore consider treatment as if a primary bone malignancy
Lymphoma	Treatment with chemotherapy can cure
Leukaemia	An occasional cause of unexplained 'bone pain' in children

conjunction with an oncologist who has an interest in the tumour type. Principles are described later in this chapter. The British Orthopaedic Association together with the British Association of Surgical Oncology has produced guidelines on treatment.

The important malignancies that metastasize to bone are listed in Table 20.4.

INFLAMMATORY NODULES

Swelling is one of the quartet of inflammatory features. Soft-tissue inflammatory nodules are those formed as a consequence of an inflammatory process. These include rheumatoid nodules on the extensor surface of the joints, especially elbows and knees. Gout produces deposits of calcium urate crystals in tissues adjacent to superficial small joints. Small foreign bodies can stimulate intense inflammatory reaction, especially blackthorn (biological) and fibreglass (chemical). Soft-tissue infections form as a consequence of cellulitis or from a penetrating wound, which may have been unnoticed or long forgotten. Characteristic clinical signs of abscess formation should be present unless the patient is immunosuppressed. Tuberculous abscesses of the spine produce a typical deformity and discharge only rarely. Bony infections may mimic some bone tumours, such as Ewing's sarcoma and eosinophilic granuloma. Sometimes only biopsy can discriminate tumour from infection.

MISCELLANEOUS NODULES

Fibromatosis nodules form in Dupuytren's disease within the palmar and sometimes the plantar aponeurosis. Tendon xanthomata form in lipid storage disorders. Bruises within bone may sometimes liquefy rather than resolve. Alternatively they may ossify and produce myositis ossificans. Sometimes this process is congenital and causes deformity and ankylosis of joints (myositis ossificans progressiva). Old tendon avulsions can cause muscle lumps (biceps, rectus femoris) that worry patients, as may partial rupture of the Achilles tendon. Inguinal or femoral herniae will appear in the groin as a mass. Bursae may enlarge (olecranon, infra and pre-patellar, psoas). Ganglions may be small or large (Fig. 20.4) and are found typically around the wrist, feet and knee (semimembranosus, Baker's or popliteal cyst, meniscal cyst).

PATHOLOGICAL FRACTURES

A pathological fracture is one that requires minimal force to sustain. It, therefore, encompasses common fractures due to osteoporosis in the elderly, osteogenesis imperfecta in the young, fractures through infected or dead bone, and fractures through neoplastic bony lesions. It is these latter that will be discussed in this chapter.

The clue to a pathological fracture is in the history and in the radiograph. The history is

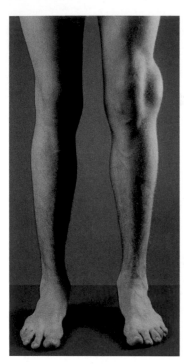

FIGURE 20.4   A large benign cyst adjacent to the knee joint

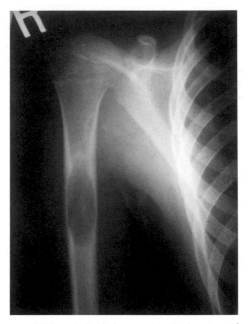

FIGURE 20.5   A simple bone cyst in the humerus of a child. Pathological fracture is likely

frequently one of minimal trauma. This sometimes leads to unjustified allegations of non-accidental injury. A past medical history of adenocarcinoma may lead to the suspicion of bony metastases. Frequently several days of pain at the site precede the fracture.

The radiographs will show a lesion at the point of fracture, which may be subtle to appreciate, especially if there are no previous images of the area before the fracture occurred. Key features to describe are matrix and margins. The matrix of a benign cystic lesion is purely lytic, and the margins well defined. By contrast, malignant lesions and rapidly growing benign lesions have infiltrative edges. A slowly growing lesion will allow the bone to respond to the tumour by expansion of its diameter in children. If rapidly growing it will not have time to react and a 'punched-out' appearance may be evident.

A key management principle in pathological fracture is to avoid fixation of the fracture prior to obtaining a definitive diagnosis. This can sometimes be assumed in a child with obvious radiographic features of a benign simple bone cyst (see below) or in an older adult with previous

history of adenocarcinoma together with bone scintigraphic evidence of multiple lesions. Otherwise it is safest to undertake a biopsy first and, whilst waiting for the result, the patient should be kept comfortable in a cast or in traction. Injudicious early fixation may disseminate malignant cells and, if the lesion proves to be a primary malignant bone tumour, then this may lead to amputation rather than limb salvage surgery. Fractures through primary malignant bone tumours (and isolated renal cell metastases) should be staged and treated in the same way as if not fractured.

In a child a lytic lesion of bone is most commonly a benign neoplasm. Most frequently this will represent a large simple bone cyst (Fig. 20.5). Characteristic childhood diagnoses associated with pathological fractures are listed in Table 20.5. In adults, increasing age makes the likelihood of metastatic bone disease more likely.

Choice of management should be centred on providing a stable fixation that will outlive the patient. It can be assumed that most pathological fractures will not heal. The implant should, therefore, be 'load-bearing' rather than 'load-sharing'. Hence intramedullary nails are preferred to plates and screws. Joint arthroplasty can be used close to major joints. Most modern implants are designed to

Table 20.5 Childhood diagnoses and the associated pathological fractures

Neoplasm	Type	Characteristics
Simple (unicameral) bone cyst	Benign	Common. Long-bone metaphyses
Aneurysmal bone cyst		Rare. Often long-bone metaphyses
Eosinophilic granuloma		Rare. May mimic Ewing's sarcoma or infection
Osteoblastoma		Rare. May be in difficult site
Enchondroma		Common in digits
Osteosarcoma	Malignant	Long-bone metaphyses. Pathological fracture alone may not impose much worse prognosis
Ewing's sarcoma		May mimic infection
Bony metastasis		Source may be leukaemia, lymphoma, neuroblastoma, Wilms' tumour

Table 20.6 Adult diagnoses and the associated pathological fractures

Neoplasm	Type	Characteristics
Giant cell tumour	Benign	Common. Often locally aggressive
Aneurysmal bone cyst		Rare. Often long-bone metaphyses
Eosinophilic granuloma		Rare. May mimic Ewing's sarcoma or infection
Enchondroma		Common in digits
Osteosarcoma	Malignant	Long-bone metaphyses. Pathological fracture alone may not impose much worse prognosis
Chondrosarcoma		Frequently in pelvis, proximal humerus or femur
Radiation-induced sarcoma		In radiation field after previous cancer treatment
Bony metastasis		Most common in elderly

weight-bear repetitively for a year or two prior to undergoing fatigue failure. This is beyond the median life expectancy of many patients with pathological fractures through bony metastases. Bone acrylic cement augmentation of the lesion after curetting the metastasis allows additional stability after fixation. Some metastatic tumours can be treated with hormonal or endocrine therapy (prostate with anti-androgens, breast with anti-oestrogens, thyroid with ^{131}I, renal carcinoma with immunotherapy). This may allow the fracture to heal rapidly and allow occasional longer-term survival. Characteristic adult diagnoses associated with pathological fractures are listed in Table 20.6.

FURTHER READING

Mannan K, Briggs TW 2005 Soft tissue tumours of the extremities. Br Med J 331: 590.

Myhre-Jensen O 1981 A consecutive 7-year series of 1331 benign soft tissue tumours. Clinicopathologic data. Comparison with sarcomas. Acta Orthop Scand 52: 287–293.

Weber KL 2005 What's new in musculoskeletal oncology. J Bone Joint Surg Am 87: 1400–1410.

UPPER LIMB

21

Geoff Hooper and Daniel Porter

Cases relevant to this chapter

14, 19–22, 96, 97, 100

SHOULDER

The function of the shoulder and elbow joints is to position the hand in space. Their dysfunction can be overcome by accommodation in the young, but this is more difficult in the elderly with degenerative disease.

OSTEOARTHRITIS

Primary shoulder osteoarthritis (OA) is much less common than that of the major joints of the lower limb. It results in a global reduction in range of movement of the glenohumeral joint, but most particularly external rotation. Secondary OA may follow a major tear of the rotator cuff tendon (see below). Radiographs confirm loss of joint space and osteosclerosis. Rheumatoid arthritis (RA) frequently affects the shoulder joint and causes destruction of humeral head, glenoid and rotator cuff. In the presence of reasonable bone stock and an intact cuff, a total shoulder replacement can be performed. Where the glenoid cavity or rotator cuff is deficient, however, it may be best simply to undertake a hemiarthroplasty in which the humeral head alone is replaced. This acts as a 'spacer' and abolishes pain, although movement is very restricted.

The sterno-clavicular joints can become arthritic. This may be difficult to discriminate from a medial end of clavicle swelling, which is usually due to an osteitis and is rarely neoplastic. Sternoclavicular arthropathy is most commonly part of an inflammatory process. A steroid injection may help in speeding resolution. At the other end the acromioclavicular joint may be arthritic. Steroid injection in rarely long lasting and surgical treatment is excision of the distal 1 cm of clavicle.

BICEPS TENDON RUPTURE

The biceps tendon has a long-head origin from the superior margin of the glenoid and its insertion is the bicipital eminence of the radius. Both tendons can be avulsed, resulting in a 'Popeye' bunching-up appearance to the biceps belly when contracted. It is only possible to repair the long head when the injury is very acute. Repair of the insertion is achieved by drilling a new insertion into the radius.

IMPINGEMENT SYNDROME AND ROTATOR CUFF DISEASE

Movement of the shoulder in rotation and initiation of abduction is produced by action of the rotator cuff – a conjoined tendon that is also a roof to the glenohumeral joint capsule described in Chapter 1. When the shoulder abducts the tendon has to contract underneath the acromion. This may result in impingement between the acromion and the cuff where it inserts into the greater tuberosity. Usually the subacromial bursa will act as a buffer to prevent a frictional reaction, but in middle age there is a tendency for inflammation to occur within the bursa after shoulder exercise. If only the bursa and cuff are inflamed, this is known as (subacromial) impingement syndrome. It is painful to elevate and abduct the arm though an arc of movement of about 45–120° (Fig. 21.1). There may be only slight tenderness just lateral to the acromion, but special tests for impingement are usually positive (Jobe's test puts the greater tuberosity under the acromion in shoulder abduction and internal rotation; forced abduction against resistance provokes pain). Resolution may be expected, but can be speeded by steroid injection into the subacromial bursa. Plain radiographs may reveal acute calcification (calcific tendonitis) within the supraspinatus tendon; if acute, chalky material may be aspirated providing instant relief. Where plain radiographs show osteophytic 'beaking' of

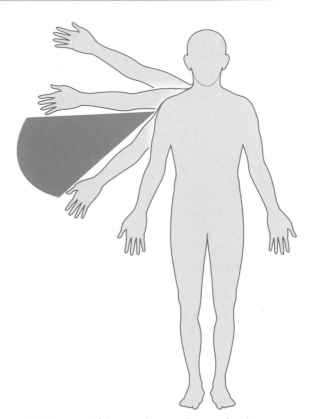

FIGURE 21.1 Painful arc syndrome – diagram showing range of painful movement between 45° and 120° of abduction. The scapula is stabilized by the examiner's hand and the patient asked to abduct the arm. The examiner observes the presence or absence of discomfort as the arm abducts

the lateral edge of the acromion or a reduced distance between the humerus and the acromion then steroid injection may help but will not provide a cure. Arthroscopic subacromial decompression of the bony spur and debridement of inflammatory soft tissue may give relief. A tear of the rotator cuff may be partial or complete. A tear of any size may inhibit abduction through pain, so a diagnostic local anaesthetic injection into the subacromial bursa, followed by assessment of active movement, may be diagnostic of the extent of a tear. Ultrasound or MRI can define its extent further. A small tear can be managed as impingement syndrome. A medium-sized tear can be repaired by open or arthroscopic means. A chronic massive tear in the elderly is rarely repairable; over time it will result in abnormal forces applied across the glenohumeral joint and secondary osteoarthritis (cuff arthropathy) will result.

FROZEN SHOULDER

Frozen shoulder (adhesive capsulitis) is seen in middle age and in the elderly. There is capsular fibrosis that results in three overlapping clinical phases: initially, the shoulder is painful and increasingly stiff; secondly it is stiff but less painful; and thirdly, the stiffness resolves. Even so a proportion of patients will have residual stiffness beyond this. Each phase lasts 6–12 months. Diagnosis is made on clinical grounds with global loss of movement (especially external rotation) without significant radiographic abnormality. It is important to reassure the patient that the condition is eventually self-limiting, but that physiotherapy is important to aid retention of movement. Arthroscopic capsular fluid distension may break down adhesions and result in a shorter clinical course.

MONONEURITIS

A mononeuritis is usually viral in origin and most frequently affects the long thoracic nerve. This causes winging of the scapula. The patient is disturbed by this new finding and cannot identify a reason. In the absence of any other positive clinical finding it is important to reassure that there will be a resolution over 6–24 months. Nerve root irritation from cervical spondylosis may cause pain referred to its dermatomal distribution. Over the shoulder this will be the C4 and C5 nerve roots. Subphrenic abscess and gall-bladder pain can also be referred to the tip of the shoulder.

ELBOW
OSTEOARTHRITIS

Secondary OA of the elbow is much more common than primary. Trauma, synovial proliferative disorders (chondromatosis, pigmented villonodular synovitis), haemoglobinopathies and RA are recognized insults. Stiffness of the elbow and reduced forearm rotation through an arthritic proximal radio-ulnar joint are usually less troublesome than pain. Arc of flexion after a total elbow replacement is rarely greater than 30°–120° and is undertaken for intractable pain. Excision of the radial head in RA can also be helpful.

EPICONDYLITIS

Tennis elbow (lateral epicondylitis) is an inflammatory process at the forearm extensor origin on the humeral lateral supracondylar ridge. The diagnosis is made by a suitable history of overuse (e.g. in tennis) of the extensor muscles of the forearm. The common extensor origin is tender and forced extension of the wrist and digits against resistance increases the discomfort. This is usually self-limiting and a period of rest and, perhaps, anti-inflammatory medication is all that is required to allow the symptoms to settle. Occasionally, the condition becomes chronic. Ultrasound treatment, steroid injection and common extensor surgical release have been tried, but recent evidence suggests that a steroid injection may impair full recovery. A similar condition affects the common flexor origin on the medial supracondylar ridge (golfer's elbow) at the common flexor origin.

NERVE ENTRAPMENT

All three major nerves can be the subject of entrapment around the elbow. Symptoms are of pain, sensory disturbance and motor dysfunction in the distribution of that nerve. Confirmation can be gained by nerve conduction studies. The ulnar nerve is most vulnerable within the ulnar groove of the ulna. It can be affected by traction produced by valgus deformities of the elbow (after elbow fractures and RA), or by direct injury. The ulnar nerve passes under myotendinous bands both above and below the elbow. Treatment is either freeing the ulnar nerve within its groove (neurolysis) or transposition of the nerve anteriorly. The median nerve dives deep to the pronator teres muscle of the forearm. Splinting may be helpful, although decompressive surgery may be necessary. The motor branch of the radial nerve (posterior interosseous branch) is prominent as it winds around the radial neck to enter the posterior forearm compartment between the two heads of supinator muscle. Here it is prone to traumatic or surgical injury. Exploratory and decompressive surgery is reserved for those in whom no recovery is seen for several months after the insult. The terminal sensory branches of the radial nerve may be compressed due to direct pressure over the nerves at the wrist, by a tight metal watchstrap or sometimes handcuffs. The resultant numbness over the dorsoradial aspect of the hand usually improves spontaneously, but slowly.

HAND PROBLEMS
DUPUYTREN'S DISEASE

This condition is characterized by thickening and shortening of the longitudinal fibres of the palmar and digital fascia. As the fascia shortens it may draw the fingers down toward the palm. The cause is unknown, but in many cases there is a strong family history. It is a very common condition in peoples of Northern European origin, but rare in most other racial groups. It is more common in men. Patients will often falsely attribute it to manual work. The presentation is very variable, from small nodules in the palm of the hand that do not progress, to a relentless and deforming condition involving several digits. Treatment is necessary if the function of the hand is affected. Surgical treatment is the only method that is effective in straightening the digits. Simple division of the cords of abnormal tissue (fasciotomy) or their excision (limited fasciectomy) is employed. It is important to realize that surgery does not 'cure' Dupuytren's disease, as the tendency to form the abnormal tissue is built into the patient. Recurrence or extension of the disease is usual and can be dealt with by a radical excision of the recurrent tissue and overlying skin, with replacement by a full-thickness skin graft (dermofasciectomy).

TRIGGER FINGER

In this condition a digit sticks in the fully flexed position and must be straightened with the other hand, often with a painful snap (Fig. 21.2). It is due to lack of free running of the flexor tendon through the tunnel at the base of the digit. It is more common in diabetics and in RA. It is treated by injecting the tendon sheath with a small volume of steroid and local anaesthetic or by surgical release of the tunnel if this is not effective.

DE QUERVAIN'S DISEASE

This condition is the result of myxoid degeneration of the wall of the tunnel in the extensor retinaculum containing the tendons of extensor pollicis brevis and abductor pollicis longus, causing it to become grossly thickened. The condition occurs most frequently in women around the menopause and less frequently in the post-partum period. Pain is felt on the radial border of the wrist especially when moving the thumb. Finkelstein's test is a provocation test inducing pain by deviating the hand into ulnar deviation with the thumb held across the palm. The condition is treated by a steroid and local anaesthetic injection around the tendons at the tunnel, or by surgical release of the tunnel.

OSTEOARTHRITIS

The most common sites for OA in the hand are the trapezio-metacarpal (first carpometacarpal) joint of the thumb ray (Fig. 21.3) and the distal interphalangeal joints. Older women are most affected. OA of the distal interphalangeal joints is seldom disabling, but bony prominences around the joints (Heberden's nodes) may be unsightly. Trapezio-metacarpal OA often causes pain when gripping or twisting, for example when opening jars. The discomfort tends to settle with time and in most cases simple analgesia is all that is required. If disabling discomfort persists, surgical treatment may be required. Removal of the trapezium relieves pain, but resultant weakness of grip may be troublesome.

RHEUMATOID ARTHRITIS

The hand is commonly involved. Examination for the integrity of individual hand tendons is

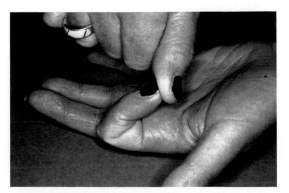

FIGURE 21.2 Unlocking a trigger finger

shown in Figure 21.4. Inflammatory synovitis causes stretching of the capsules of the small joints and damage to tendons, producing characteristic problems, such as ulnar deviation of the fingers, thumb deformities and tendon ruptures. These problems can be prevented if the disease process can be controlled by medication; otherwise complex surgical reconstruction will be necessary.

CARPAL TUNNEL SYNDROME

This extremely common condition occurs most often in middle-aged women, but it can also be a problem during pregnancy. Increased pressure on the median nerve beneath the flexor retinaculum causes characteristic symptoms of tingling, pain and numbness in the hand, usually much more troublesome at night. Typically the patient is woken at night and relieves the symptoms by some manoeuvre, such as shaking the hand, holding it dependent or running cold water over it. Nerve conduction studies show slowing of conduction in the nerve at the wrist. In milder cases symptoms may be controlled by splinting the wrist at night or an injection of steroid and local anaesthetic into the tunnel. Surgical release of the carpal tunnel provides good relief of nocturnal symptoms in most cases.

FURTHER READING

Douglas G, Nicol F, Robertson C (eds) 2005 Macleod's clinical examination, 11th edn. Churchill Livingstone, Edinburgh

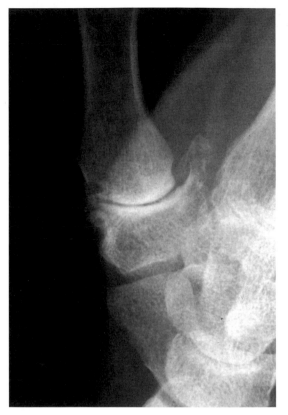

FIGURE 21.3　Osteoarthritis of the trapezio-metacarpal joint

A
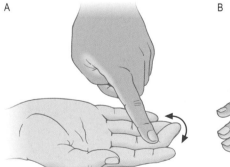

B
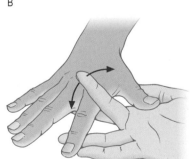

FIGURE 21.4　Testing flexor digitorum profundus (A) and superficialis (B). (From Douglas et al 2005)

CERVICAL AND LUMBAR SPINE

22

R. W. Marshall

Cases relevant to this chapter

17, 18, 24, 28–31, 33, 34, 50, 74, 78

●Essential facts

1. Degenerative conditions of the spine occur in lordotic areas; the thoracic spine is a rare source of back pain.

2. Intervertebral disc degeneration is normal over the age of 40 years; radiographic abnormalities of disc space narrowing and bone spurs around the discs and facet joints have little clinical relevance.

3. Cervical spondylosis most commonly affects C5/6, resulting in numbness in the index finger and thumb, weakness of the biceps muscle and a reduced biceps reflex.

4. Cervical cord compression can present in young to middle-aged patients due to disc herniation, but it is more likely to occur in older patients due to bone thickening around degenerate joint margins.

5. Atlanto-axial involvement occurs in 50% of patients with rheumatoid arthritis (RA) who have neck problems, but all levels can be affected, from occiput to cervicothoracic junction.

6. 'Whiplash' injuries are caused by rear-end collision in motor vehicles; the occupants have a hyperextension injury of the neck.

7. Mechanical pain or 'simple back pain' occurs in 80% of the population; 80% will resolve spontaneously within 6 weeks and in 80% no clear cause can be identified.

8. Radiological investigation of back pain is most helpful in the over 50s (looking for metastases), in the under 20s (looking for adolescent disc herniation, spondylolysis or benign tumour) or if inflammatory spinal disease is suspected.

9. Features of abnormal illness behaviour in patients with back pain include: apparent limitation of straight leg raising but no problem sitting upright with extended legs, superficial tenderness to palpation, non-dermatomal numbness, low back pain with skull pressure, back pain on simulated rotation of the spine and inappropriate verbalization during examination.

10. The following are 'red flag' features of back pain: violent trauma; constant, progressive non-mechanical pain; thoracic pain; presentation under 20 or over 55 years; previous history of carcinoma; use of systemic steroids; drug abuse or HIV; systemically unwell; weight loss; lumbar stiffness; widespread neurological signs and structural deformity.

11. Ninety per cent of disc herniations resolve spontaneously by dehydration and resorption of herniated material; the diagnosis is clinically obvious and there is no benefit in rushing to special investigations.

12. In patients with spinal stenosis, because the thick joints lie posterior to the spinal nerves, the sciatica is worse with standing and walking (lumbar extension), but relieved by sitting (lumbar flexion).

SPINAL ANATOMY

The spine consists of seven cervical, 12 thoracic and five lumbar vertebrae, plus the sacrum and coccyx. Since adopting the upright posture, the human spine has acquired secondary lordotic curves in the cervical and lumbar regions either side of the primary thoracic kyphosis. The degenerative conditions of the spine tend to occur in these lordotic areas and the thoracic spine is rarely the source of back pain. At each level of the spine there is a motion segment, comprising two adjacent vertebrae, the intervertebral disc, a pair of zygoapophyseal synovial joints (facet joints) and the supporting ligament complexes. The spinal cord occupies the adult spinal canal down as far as the L1–2 level and below this the lumbar and sacral nerves form the cauda equina (horse's tail), which floats in the cerebrospinal fluid occupying the lower end of the theca (meningeal sac).

DEGENERATIVE CONDITIONS OF THE CERVICAL SPINE

Cervical pathology is largely due to degenerative disease. Intervertebral disc degeneration is the norm over the age of 40 years and radiographic evidence of disc space narrowing and bone spurs

around the margins of the discs and facet joints has little clinical relevance. The presence of disc herniations or osteophytes on the uncovertebral joints can cause nerve root pain, which usually manifests as pain down an arm (brachialgia) with altered sensation in the corresponding dermatome and weakness in the corresponding myotome. The commonest level affected is C5/6 and this affects the 6th cervical nerve (C6) so there is numbness in the dermatome affecting the index finger and thumb, weakness of the biceps muscle and a reduced biceps reflex. The C6/7 level is the second commonest and presents with 7th cervical nerve compression symptoms and signs (Fig. 22.1). Pain is reproduced by lateral rotation to the symptomatic side (Spurling's sign) or with axial compression produced by pressure on the patient's head.

Most cervical nerve compression symptoms improve with time, but there is a place for physiotherapy, non-steroidal anti-inflammatory drugs (NSAIDs) and epidural steroid injections. The best investigation is a magnetic resonance scan (Fig. 22.2). Because pathology is common, even in subjects who have no symptoms, the scan findings must be carefully correlated with the clinical findings. In cases where the symptoms fail to improve with time and conservative treatment, a cervical discectomy can be performed. This procedure is carried out through an anterior approach, which

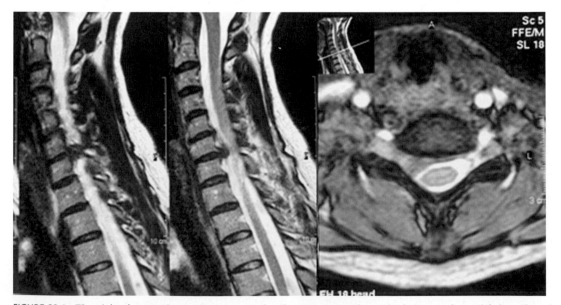

FIGURE 22.1   T2-weighted magnetic resonance images showing two consecutive sagittal views and an axial view. There is a herniated disc at C6/7 occluding the exit foramen for the right 7th cervical nerve

288

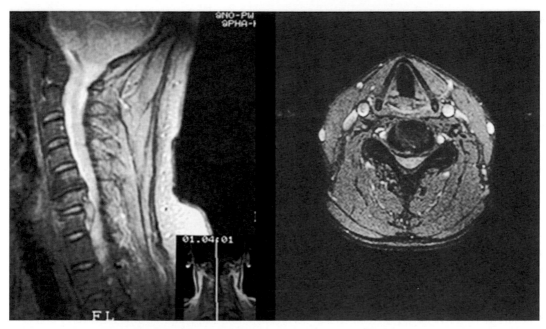

FIGURE 22.2   Magnetic resonance imaging of T2 sagittal and axial views through cervical stenotic segment showing a disc and osteophyte complex causing flattening and compression of the spinal cord

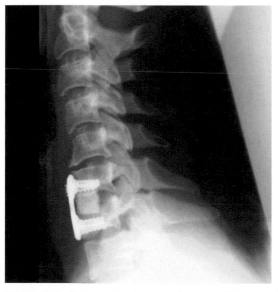

FIGURE 22.3   Post-operative lateral radiograph of the cervical spine after anterior discectomy and spinal fusion using a ceramic block as a bone substitute and a cervical plate and screws to secure the 'graft' and immobilize the C6/7 level

gives excellent access to the intervertebral disc. The disc is excised completely and, after decompression of the affected nerve, the level is usually fused using a bone graft from the iliac crest or a bone substitute, such as tricalcium phosphate (Fig. 22.3). The procedure is usually straightforward and

excellent results can be achieved. There is a risk of damage to the recurrent laryngeal nerve, which can induce hoarseness. The airway needs careful observation afterwards and a drain is used to reduce the risk of haematoma formation.

CERVICAL MYELOPATHY

Cervical cord compression can present in young to middle-aged patients due to disc herniation, but it is much more likely to occur in older patients due to bone thickening around degenerate joint margins. The stenosis develops insidiously without any pain. Unfortunately, its silent, gradual onset is often responsible for the patients presenting very late. They may have upper motor neurone weakness of all four limbs. The hands become clumsy, especially for fine tasks, such as button fastening and writing. Rapid fist clenching is impaired ('dysdiadochokinesia' or clumsiness in performing alternating rapid hand movements). Hofmann's sign may be present – thumb flexion in response to flicking the middle finger distal interphalangeal joint into extension. Lower limb involvement results in spasticity and an ataxic, scissoring gait. Sensation is impaired, reflexes are brisk, plantar reflexes are extensor and there may be clonus of ankles and knees (rhythmical contraction of muscle in response to a suddenly applied and sustained stretch stimulus). Magnetic resonance scanning confirms the presence of cord compromise due to canal narrowing. Surgical decompression is indicated to prevent the loss of hand and lower limb function. Operations for single- or double-level stenosis are usually carried out anteriorly, but multi-level stenosis may be better treated by a posterior approach involving removal of the laminae. The Japanese are genetically prone to develop ossification of the posterior longitudinal ligament (OPPL), so stenosis is common in Japan and their surgeons have led the way in devising new techniques, such as laminoplasty and skip laminectomy, to allow decompression with minimal compromise of spinal stability.

RHEUMATOID ARTHRITIS OF THE CERVICAL SPINE

Cervical rheumatoid disease (RA) occurs in patients with severe peripheral joint involvement. Proliferation of synovial pannus causes erosion and destruction of the small joints in the cervical spine. In 50% of cases with rheumatoid disease of the neck, the atlanto-axial articulation is involved, but the disease can affect all levels from occiput to cervico-thoracic junction. Pannus around the odontoid peg damages the transverse ligament and creates atlanto-axial instability. The patient may be aware of mechanical clunking in movements involving flexion and extension of the neck and may become reliant upon a collar or in the worst cases hold their own head to limit the unpleasant movements that are accompanied by pain and sometimes by electric shock sensations up into the head and down the back ('Lhermitte's phenomenon', which is not pathognomonic of spinal cord compression and can also occur in demyelinating disorders, such as multiple sclerosis). However, in others, the neck instability and spinal cord damage may be silent and impaired limb function may be erroneously attributed to the peripheral joint disease until the spinal cord damage is irreversible.

Cord dysfunction develops and manifests as impairment of hand function and heavy legs. If unchecked the patient becomes wheel-chair bound and the condition may even cause sudden death (see Chapter 1). Plain radiographs look unremarkable, but flexion/extension views (Fig. 22.4) unmask the instability and show excessive movement of the atlas on the axis (>3 mm). The condition is treated by posterior fusion of C1/2 with bone grafting and internal fixation using wires, screws or a combination of these methods.

Much less commonly there is occipito-cervical joint involvement with 'cranial settling', a condition where the skull base descends onto the

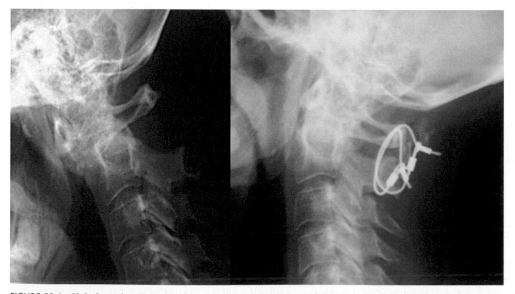

FIGURE 22.4 Plain lateral radiographs of a rheumatoid cervical spine showing atlanto-axial instability before and after reduction, posterior cable wiring and bone grafting

> **Box 22.1**
> **Ranawat grading of cervical myelopathy**
>
> - Grade I – normal neurology
> - Grade II – paraesthesiae and brisk reflexes
> - Grade IIIa – myelopathy, ambulatory
> - Grade IIIb – quadriparesis, bed and chair-bound

cervical spine and the odontoid peg penetrates through the foramen magnum causing pressure on the medulla oblongata. This condition presents with brainstem dysfunction, including dysarthria, dysphagia and diplopia due to cranial nerve disturbance. It is potentially fatal and requires occipito-cervical fusion employing metal plates and screws from the skull extending the full length of the cervical spine. Sometimes the odontoid peg and pannus have to be removed before the posterior stabilization can be performed safely and this is done through a trans-oral approach to C1 and C2.

The Ranawat grading of myelopathy is the most commonly used method of assessing the severity of cervical spine involvement and the outcome after treatment (Box 22.1). Operative treatment does not reverse the neurological effects fully, but it is often possible to produce improvement by one Ranawat grade. Whilst myelopathy is the most compelling reason to operate on the cervical spine, cases without neurological compromise may require operative treatment for painful instability.

The subaxial parts of the cervical spine are frequently involved and rheumatoid erosion of these joints gives rise to neck pain, cervical nerve root compression syndromes, subluxation of the joints causing a 'staircase' appearance due to a number of levels with spondylolisthesis, and spontaneous ankylosis with ensuing neck stiffness. A rigid collar may be enough to control these symptoms and operative treatment can usually be avoided between C3 and T1.

'WHIPLASH' INJURIES

These injuries have a few common characteristics: they are caused by rear-end collision in motor vehicles, the occupants have a hyperextension injury of the neck, there is pain provoked by neck move-ments and all investigations are normal for the age of the patient. The pain and tenderness are situated in the neck and shoulders, often associated with tingling of the fingers. Symptoms may persist for many months, but improvement is usual. The perpetuation of symptoms seems to have much to do with the fact that the injuries often involve compensation claims with protracted legal wrangling that can add to the anxiety of the patients and sometimes predispose to a full-blown compensation neurosis. In the long term, patients who sustain whiplash-associated injury and who pursue litigation are likely to suffer greater levels of pain and poorer function compared with patients who suffer true structural damage and cervical fractures. Patients should be reassured and told to mobilize as normally as possible. Physiotherapists can have a role in their rehabilitation. Careful neurological assessment is mandatory in these cases to exclude more serious structural damage to the vertebral column.

Cervical fractures and the special case of the patient with multiple injuries are discussed in Chapter 11.

MECHANICAL BACK PAIN

Mechanical pain or 'simple back pain' is worse with movement and relieved by rest. It can arise in any aspect of the motion segment – bone, joints, ligaments or discs – and has many possible causes. This type of pain is very common and it is estimated that 80% of people will experience at least one episode of severe back pain during their lives, 80% will resolve spontaneously within 6 weeks and in 80% no clear cause can be identified. However, chronic back pain is considered to limit economic growth in the European Union by 2%. Most causes are trivial and the back pain is self-limiting, usually within 6 weeks. Although the pain can be severe, patients need to be reassured and told to keep active without taking long periods off work and altering their normal life-style. 'The Back Book', written by a multidisciplinary group of experts, can be used to educate patients and those involved in treating them. Expensive investigations are inappropriate and may add to anxiety by revealing 'abnormalities' that are incidental and part of the normal ageing process. Physiotherapists and alternative practitioners provide support, but sound advice and reassurance are crucial.

Investigation by plain radiographs and magnetic resonance imaging (MRI) is usually most helpful in the over 50s, where metastases are possible causes of pain; in the under 20s, e.g. adolescent disc herniation, spondylolysis or benign tumour; or if the history and examination are suggestive of an inflammatory cause for pain, such as ankylosing spondylitis.

Persistent mechanical back pain may be due to degenerative change. Discogenic back pain is made worse by sitting and partial flexion of the lumbar spine. Pain of facet joint origin is aggravated by twisting and extension. Pain-relieving injections and physiotherapy are most commonly employed. Spinal fusion or intervertebral disc replacement is rarely indicated, as results are unpredictable and similar results can be obtained by functional restoration programmes using education, exercise and psychological counselling.

Back pain is often the presenting symptom for litigants in personal injury claims, those with work-related injury, and some with major psychosocial problems. These patients do not need investigation of their back pain as over-investigation and treatment can be counter-productive. Waddell described a number of signs that help to identify abnormal illness behaviour in back pain patients. The signs include apparent limitation of straight leg raising, but no problem sitting upright with extended legs ('flip test') (Fig. 22.5), superficial tenderness to palpation, non-dermatomal numbness, low back pain with skull pressure (simulated axial loading), back pain on simulated rotation of the spine and inappropriate verbalization during examination. Careful interpretation is required, but these non-organic physical signs suggest distress and anxiety.

By contrast, a working party set up by the Royal College of General Practitioners has identified 'red flag' features, which help to select the cases where investigation is required (Table 22.1). Red flag signs and back pain should be investigated by a combination of spinal imaging (MRI and technetium bone scanning) and blood tests including full blood count, inflammatory markers (erythrocyte sedimentation rate (ESR) and C-reactive protein (CRP)), blood cultures, serum biochemistry and plasma protein immuno-electrophoresis. An evaluation of patients for tuberculosis (TB) and tests for HIV may be indicated.

LUMBAR DISC DISEASE

Intervertebral discs start off as spongy structures with a combination of collagen fibres and proteoglycans, but become dehydrated and narrowed with age. Between the ages of 25 and 50 years, discs become susceptible to herniation, i.e. the central nucleus pulposus herniates through a defect in

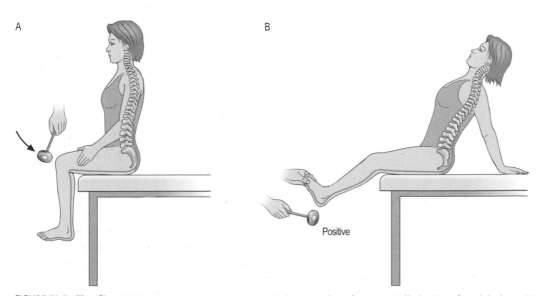

A   B

Positive

FIGURE 22.5   The 'flip test' is a sign of inappropriate pain behaviour; there is apparent limitation of straight leg raising, but no problem sitting upright with extended legs

Table 22.1 Red flag features

Red flag	Reason
Violent trauma, e.g. fall from a height or road traffic accident	Fracture or instability
Constant, progressive non-mechanical pain	Possible tumour or infection
Thoracic pain	Degenerative pain rare. Thoracic spine can be the site of metastases
Presentation under 20 or over 55 years	More serious pathology possible
Previous history of carcinoma	Metastases possible
Systemic steroids	Risk of fracture
Drug abuse, HIV	Risk of infection
Systemically unwell	Extraspinal pathology (aortic aneurysm, pancreatitis, etc.)
Weight loss	Malignancy or infection
Lumbar stiffness	Inflammatory disorder, e.g. ankylosing spondylitis
Widespread neurological signs	Possible intradural tumour or neurological disorder, e.g. demyelination
Structural deformity	Scoliosis, tuberculosis

the annulus fibrosus. Lumbar disc herniation is common and can be asymptomatic.

Pressure of the nucleus upon the posterior longitudinal ligament and dura mater produces acute back pain. Later, the herniation deviates laterally to impinge upon the traversing nerve root. The combination of mechanical pressure and chemical irritation of the nerve causes pain down the leg and may cause alteration of sensation, motor weakness and changes in reflexes. The lowest disc (L5/S1) is most commonly affected and compresses the first sacral nerve (S1), so the symptoms radiate from the buttock to the foot with sensory change on the lateral border of the foot, weakness of the calf muscles and a reduction of the ankle reflex. The second commonest level is L4/5 (Fig. 22.6, position 1) where posterolateral herniation affects the L5 nerve, resulting in pain radiating to the ankle and top of the foot, sensory change on the lateral border of the leg and top of the foot to the big toe (L5 dermatome), and weakness of dorsiflexion of the ankle and toes. The L5 nerve does not supply a reflex, so the ankle and knee reflexes remain intact.

Back and leg pain are made worse by flexion and by sitting as the irritated nerve is stretched over the anteriorly situated disc pathology. Thus, the straight leg raising test (attributed to Lasegue)

produces pain around 40° of hip flexion when the lower limb is raised passively by the examiner. If the knee is flexed, the sciatic nerve tension is released and the pain relieved. Lumbar flexion is impaired, but other movements are normal. The back is not usually tender as the pathology is beyond the reach of the palpating fingers.

Higher lumbar disc herniations are uncommon, but affect upper lumbar nerves, producing a different syndrome with anterior thigh pain (cruralgia) rather than the posterior and lower leg pain of sciatica. The quadriceps muscles are weakened, there is sensory change around the knee and the knee reflex is diminished. The straight leg raise is normal, but the femoral stretch test (knee flexion performed passively on the prone patient) is positive.

About 6% of disc herniations extend laterally rather than posterolaterally and affect the higher, exiting nerve rather than the traversing nerve. Thus, a lateral herniation at L4/5 would affect the L4 nerve producing cruralgia, an anterior thigh syndrome, rather than sciatica associated with the L5 nerve. Lateral disc herniation affects an older age group with severe pain and dysaesthesia because the disc impinges upon the highly sensitive dorsal root ganglion in the exit foramen (see Fig. 22.6, position 3).

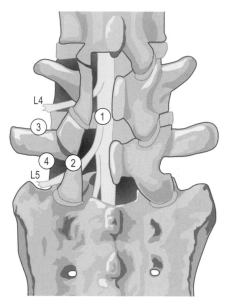

294

FIGURE 22.6   Hemi-laminectomy at L4/5 level with four possible sites of nerve compression:

1. Posterolateral disc compressing L5 nerve as it leaves the theca (common)
2. Overhanging facet joint compressing underlying L5 nerve (common)
3. Far lateral disc compressing the L4 nerve in the exit foramen (rare)
4. Foraminal stenosis compressing L5 nerve at L5/S1 level (rare)

MANAGEMENT OF LUMBAR DISC HERNIATION

Ninety per cent of disc herniations resolve spontaneously by a process of dehydration and resorption of the herniated material. The diagnosis is clinically obvious and there is no benefit in rushing to special investigations. A short period of rest followed by return to activity should be advised. Any improvement in pain levels, tension signs and mobility bodes well for natural healing. For the first 6–12 weeks treatment includes reassurance, analgesics, NSAIDs, physiotherapy and, in some cases, the use of epidural steroid injections for pain relief.

INVESTIGATIONS

When there is no improvement and operative treatment is considered, investigations are needed. Plain radiographs are of little value and involve unnecessary irradiation. MRI is the most valuable investigation and will confirm the presence, level, size and extension of the disc herniation. Water-soluble myelography and computed tomography (CT) were the traditional methods of imaging the disc pathology, but are less accurate and involve irradiation of the spine and pelvis.

OPERATIVE TREATMENT

The best treatment for unresolving disc herniation is microdiscectomy. An operating microscope allows excellent access to the disc through a small incision and window in the laminae and ligamentum flavum. In 90% of cases patients can mobilize rapidly and often return to work within 6 weeks. Complications of this procedure are uncommon, but include nerve damage, dural puncture with cerebrospinal fluid leakage, infection, haemorrhage, recurrent disc herniation and post-discectomy back pain.

CAUDA EQUINA SYNDROME

This is a surgical emergency which arises when many nerves are compressed, usually by a massive central disc herniation. Lower motor neurone dysfunction affects low lumbar and sacral nerves and there is often impaired bladder and bowel function. Alteration of urinary function with difficulty in micturition and any alteration in perianal sensation should suggest the diagnosis. Rapid imaging and surgical decompression are indicated.

SPINAL STENOSIS

Narrowing of the spinal canal can be congenital, but is usually acquired in the over 50 age group with degenerative changes that narrow intervertebral discs and thicken the facet joints with osteophyte formation (Fig. 22.7). In the lateral recesses of the spine, the nerves may be compressed by the overhanging facet joints so the patients present with sciatica fairly similar to that produced by disc herniation. However, there are important differences. Because the thick joints lie posterior to the spinal nerves, the sciatica is worse with standing and walking, but relieved by sitting. Walking is punctuated by periods of rest and flexion. Even lying down in bed can be painful, so the older patient with sciatica may be forced to sleep in a chair or lying in the fetal position. The spinal canal flares at the lumbosacral level, so stenosis is rare

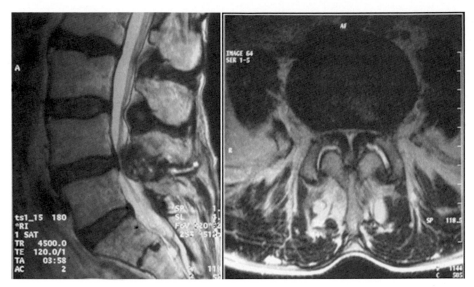

FIGURE 22.7 Magnetic resonance sagittal and axial T2 images showing spinal stenosis at L4/5 level. Note thick posterior facet joints making spinal canal T-shaped

at this level. It most commonly affects L4/5 and L3/4, but can affect all levels of the lumbar spine. The patient usually points to the lateral aspect of the lower leg as the site of the pain (L5 dermatome).

Examination findings are often unimpressive. The straight leg raise is usually normal and lumbar flexion is unimpaired. Extension, however, may provoke the pain. The facet joints may be tender. There are usually few signs of neurological impairment, but occasionally numbness, weakness and even a foot-drop can occur. The pain can resolve, but, because the stenosis persists, the symptoms may recur. Conservative treatment consists of analgesics, NSAIDs, physiotherapy and the use of epidural or perineural steroid injections. Operative treatment involves decompression of the compressed nerves by laminectomy and undercutting of the facet joint(s). The extent of the procedure depends upon the number of levels and whether the stenosis is bilateral or unilateral. The presence of instability, e.g. scoliosis or spondylolisthesis, requires an additional spinal fusion. The results of spinal decompression are very good in the short term, but can deteriorate years later due to continued degeneration.

Central spinal stenosis presents with features akin to those of vascular claudication. It occurs in elderly patients who often have concurrent cardiovascular problems. It may be difficult to distinguish between vascular and spinal claudication and some patients have dual pathology. The pain of vascular claudication is relieved by standing still until the calf muscles recover from the ischaemia, but spinal claudicants often need to bend forward or sit down to relieve their discomfort, as flexion of the spine has the effect of increasing the spinal dimensions and decongesting the contents. The 'spinal claudication' occurs after a set walking distance with tightness or heaviness in the legs and pain radiating from back to buttocks and thighs. Sitting relieves the feeling instantly. Interestingly, patients can often ride a bicycle for miles and can walk uphill more easily than downhill because of the flexed posture involved in these activities. Examination findings are unremarkable and MRI shows central stenosis. Surgical decompression must include central and lateral parts of the canal.

SPONDYLOLYSIS (AKA BROKEN VERTEBRA)

Spondylolysis (see also Chapter 27) is a defect in the isthmus of a vertebra, the part between the superior and inferior facets, the 'pars interarticularis'. It usually affects the 5th lumbar vertebra and is a common incidental finding on radiographs, rarely causing symptoms. It arises as a result of stress fractures and is common in young sportsmen. Symptoms usually settle with rest and bracing, but bone grafting and surgical repair may be necessary.

SPONDYLOLISTHESIS

This is the forward slippage of a vertebra on the one below (see also Chapter 27). It is caused by conditions that induce instability by interfering with the posterior bony elements of the vertebra or with the posterior ligament complexes. The displacement is commonest in the elderly due to degenerative change and in the young with spondylolysis. When it is responsible for continued symptoms a spinal fusion with bone grafting can be curative. Retrolisthesis is the radiological observation of slight posterior displacement of one vertebra on the vertebra below. It comes about because of degeneration and loss of disc height. Apart from the fact that the degenerate level can be the source of some back discomfort, retrolisthesis is a relatively unimportant condition.

THORACIC SPINAL PATHOLOGY

Clinical presentations of thoracic pain are relatively uncommon, but the thoracic spine can contain sinister pathology, such as tumour metastases and infection. Thoracic disc herniation is rare, but can have the serious consequences of thoracic spinal cord compression. Degenerative and inflammatory arthropathies affect the thoracic spine (see Chapter 16). The thoracic spine can be the site of spontaneous ankylosis, where stiffness is induced by ossification of the ligaments, such as the anterior longitudinal ligament, the posterior longitudinal ligament and the ligamenta flava. Forestier described the condition of diffuse idiopathic skeletal hyperostosis (DISH) with bony spurs predominantly on the right side of the lower thoracic spine. The condition is radiographically similar to ankylosing spondylitis, but there is no involvement of the sacroiliac joints in DISH. DISH is common in patients with metabolic diseases, such as diabetes mellitus (see Chapter 14).

FURTHER READING

Benoist M 2003 Natural history of the aging spine. Eur Spine J 12(Suppl 2): S86–S89.

Boden SD, Davis DO, Dina TS et al 1990 Abnormal magnetic-resonance scans of the lumbar spine in asymptomatic subjects. A prospective investigation. J Bone Joint Surg Am 72(3): 403–408.

Boden SD, McCowin PR, Davis DO et al 1990 Abnormal magnetic resonance scans of the cervical spine in asymptomatic subjects. A prospective investigation. J Bone Joint Surg Am 72(8): 1178–1184.

Burton K, Roland M, Waddell G et al 2002 The back book. Stationery Office, London.

Joslin CC, Khan SN, Bannister GC 2004 Long-term disability after neck injury. A comparative study. J Bone Joint Surg Br 86(7): 1032–1034.

Postacchini F 1999 Surgical management of lumbar spinal stenosis. Spine 24(10): 1043–1047.

Postacchini F 2001 Lumbar disc herniation: a new equilibrium is needed between nonoperative and operative treatment. Spine 26(6): 601.

Ranawat CS, O'Leavy P, Pellicci P et al 1979 Cervical spine fusion in rheumatoid arthritis. J Bone and Joint Surg Am 61: 1003–1010.

23

LOWER LIMB

Daniel Porter

Cases relevant to this chapter

15, 23, 69 76, 98

●Essential facts

1. In hip osteoarthritis, early features are exercise-induced groin or anterior thigh pain.

2. Local steroid joint injections in hip osteoarthritis may provide medium-term relief in mild-to-moderate disease.

3. Most hip replacements in the UK are cemented into the bone, although worldwide uncemented components are common; younger patients may be treated with metal-on-metal hip replacements to resurface the joint.

4. About 90% of patients get a pain-free hip once recovery from a hip replacement is complete; risks of surgery are: death (1%), infection (1–2%), dislocation (1–2%) and loosening (1% per annum).

5. The hip is at high risk of avascular necrosis because of its vulnerable blood supply.

6. Spinal pathology from low lumbar spondylosis, nerve roots, sacroiliac disease and spinal stenosis can all radiate to the hip.

7. Meniscal tears result in pain, locking and inability to extend the knee; McMurray's test is positive and a magnetic resonance image can confirm the diagnosis.

8. Osteoarthritis of the knee may affect any of the three compartments, but the medial compartment in most frequently affected and leads to a varus deformity.

9. Assessment of the lower limb includes palpation of the dorsalis pedis and posterior tibial arteries; inability to feel these or identify them on Doppler ultrasound may mean a reduced chance of healing after major surgery on the knee or below.

10. Rheumatoid arthritis often affects the ankle and hindfoot; the destruction of capsule and tendons together with toe subluxation can cause a valgus deformity of the foot.

HIP

Common pathologies around the adult hip are listed below:

- Hip osteoarthritis
- Trochanteric bursitis
- Rectus femoris sprain/avulsion
- Psoas bursa
- Meralgia paraesthetica
- Labral injury
- Avascular necrosis
- Other musculoskeletal pathology
- Non-musculoskeletal pathology.

HIP OSTEOARTHRITIS

This is detailed in Chapter 15.

TROCHANTERIC BURSITIS

A bursa is found deep to the fascia lata tendon sheet over the greater trochanter of the femur. This can be inflamed and produce hip pain on lying and walking. Point tenderness over the greater trochanter is evident, but there is a relatively normal range of hip movement. Ultrasound or magnetic resonance imaging (MRI) can often confirm the diagnosis. Although the condition is self-limiting, it may recur. Steroid injection can be targeted under ultrasound control. Surgery to lengthen the fascia lata or remove a trochanteric spur may be necessary in intractable pain. A common differential diagnosis is gluteus medius tendinopathy, increasingly diagnosed on MRI, which may respond to local injections of steroid into the muscle insertion points onto the ilium, followed by muscle-strengthening exercises.

RECTUS FEMORIS SPRAIN/AVULSION

Young men may present with pain in the groin after sport, frequently first felt when kicking or twisting against resistance. Local tenderness just inferior to the anterior pelvic brim indicates a possible sprain of the rectus femoris origin. Complete avulsion may result in a 'bunching' of the muscle in the upper thigh. Sometimes the avulsed anterior inferior iliac spine is seen on radiographs. In an elite sportsman the fragment and the associated attachment of the short head of rectus may need to be fixed back to the ilium. Other avulsions are the hamstrings from the ischium and the sartorius/tensor fascia lata from the anterior superior iliac spine.

PSOAS BURSA

Sometimes deep hip pain may be associated with swelling. Hip movement may be almost full, but an ultrasound or MRI scan may identify a bursa deep to the psoas over the anterior hip joint or a ganglion emanating from the psoas tendon sheath. Symptoms may improve spontaneously or require surgical decompression.

MERALGIA PARAESTHETICA

The lateral cutaneous nerve of the thigh may be compressed as it perforates the inguinal ligament 1–1.5 cm medial to the anterior superior iliac crest. Symptoms are of pain or dysaesthesia in its distribution. This is most frequent in younger women who are often overweight. Tight trousers have been implicated in some patients. Nerve conduction studies are difficult, but can sometimes confirm the diagnosis. Steroid injection or surgical decompression can be considered in intractable discomfort.

ACETABULAR LABRAL INJURY

The acetabular labrum can be torn in early degenerative hip osteoarthritis and more rarely in sportsmen and women. Pain is elicited with the hip in flexion, adduction and internal rotation. Diagnosis in confirmed on MRI arthrography. In some centres hip arthroscopy and repair is advocated.

AVASCULAR NECROSIS

The hip is at high risk of an avascular insult because of its vulnerable blood supply. Segmental or total collapse is seen as a consequence of osteoarthritis. It also occurs after systemic steroid use, alcohol abuse, fractures, dislocations, in childhood hip disorders, Caisson's (decompression) disease, Gaucher's disease (an inborn error of metabolism) and blood dyscrasias. During the revascularization phase, bone is resorbed and the articular surface collapses resulting in acute pain, effusion and eventual risk of secondary osteoarthritis. In the earliest phase a surgical core decompression of the avascular segment may provide relief and improve the outcome. Rotational osteotomies of the femoral head are undertaken in Japan, but have not gained favour in Europe.

REFERRED PAIN

Spinal pathology from low lumbar spondylosis, nerve roots, sacroiliac disease and spinal stenosis can all radiate to the hip. Apart from a high lumbar disc prolapse, these give symptoms felt more posteriorly.

NON-MUSCULOSKELETAL PATHOLOGY

Inguinal or femoral hernia, appendicitis and pelvic infection should all be considered.

KNEE

SEPTIC ARTHRITIS

Septic arthritis of the knee occurs in children and adults and is an emergency. Within 48 h virulent Gram-positive bacteria can produce proteolytic enzymes that destroy the proteoglycan scaffold of articular cartilage. Infected knees often produce a purulent or watery fluid. If there is a high suspicion of infection urgent lavage should be undertaken without waiting for microbiological confirmation. It is important to discriminate septic arthritis from superficial bursitis, since the latter does not need knee joint aspiration or lavage, which carries the risk of introducing infection into the joint (see Chapter 5). In children knee pain referred from the hip should not be missed (Fig. 23.1).

CYSTS AND BURSAE

Both the pre-patellar and infra-patellar bursae can become inflamed by kneeling. Rest will produce a cure. If chronic, nodular scar tissue may be excised surgically. Infected superficial bursae may need to be incised and drained. It is important to discriminate these from a knee joint infection.

A defect in the knee joint capsule, at the back of the knee in the popliteal fossa, can produce a large ganglion called a Baker's cyst, which is some-times seen in children but is more commonly associated with degenerative disease in adults. This is symptomatic in its formative phase, but usually becomes pain-free. It may be necessary to obtain an ultrasound scan to confirm the diagnosis to exclude a solid tumour. Surgery is rarely necessary. Other ganglion cysts arise from the semi-membranosus tendon sheath and from torn menisci. These may grow to very large proportions.

MENISCI

The semilunar cartilages or menisci act as protective shock absorbers over the lifetime of the knee joint by reducing sheer stresses. Torn menisci were once removed in their entirety through open surgery, but it was found that premature arthritis commonly resulted. In a young patient the menisci are firm and rubbery and require significant twisting force to tear. Sometimes cruciate ligament instability can provide increased sheer stresses which result in meniscal tears. Symptoms are of pain, locking and sometimes an inability to extend the knee. McMurray's test is positive and an MRI scan can confirm the diagnosis. Tears may be described by their site, size and orientation. Menisci are only vascular at their peripheral attachment to the bone and joint capsule. Most tears occur in the avascular part and healing will not occur. Arthroscopic 'keyhole' surgery will allow inspection of the menisci and introduction of small instruments to resect the torn component only (Fig. 23.2). Usually this only consists of 5–20% of the total meniscus, so does not cause arthritis. A large tear of the lateral meniscus (rarer than the medial), however, can result in degenerative change. For these and for tears in the vascular segment, arthroscopically assisted suture repair can be used. In older patients the menisci become more brittle and develop planes of weakness. This may be associated with early arthritis. Unlike this condition in younger patients, no particular injury may be volunteered and symptoms sometimes resolve spontaneously. If not, then arthroscopic surgery can provide relief.

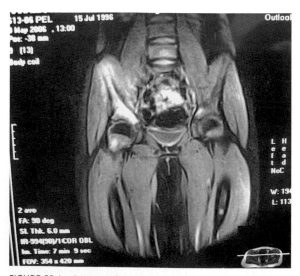

FIGURE 23.1 Osteomyelitis of the right acetabulum causing pain referred to the knee

OSTEOARTHRITIS

See Chapter 15.

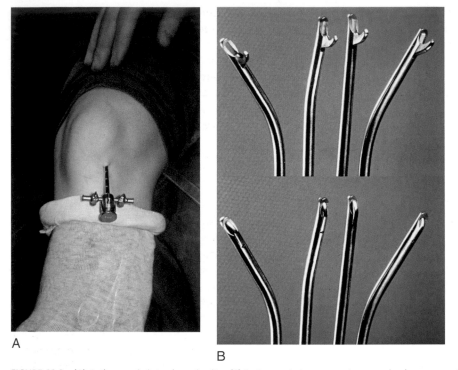

A

B

FIGURE 23.2 (A) Arthroscopic introducer in situ. (B) Instruments to remove torn meniscal component

FOOT AND ANKLE

GENERAL EXAMINATION

When the lower limb is being examined, exposure of the whole limb, including ankle and foot, allows inspection of potential features that identify important co-morbid conditions. There may be a spindle shank, a red shiny hairless foot with poor nail quality and small ulcers, or even dry gangrene of toes. This may indicate peripheral arterial disease and care should be taken to palpate the dorsalis pedis and posterior tibial arteries. Inability to feel these or identify them on Doppler ultrasound may mean a reduced chance of healing after major surgery on the knee or below. The leg may be swollen and oedematous. This may indicate the presence of a deep venous thrombosis – a frequent event after major lower limb surgery and a risk factor for pulmonary embolus. Alternatively, venous incompetence may be the cause, in which case venous ulceration may be identified just proximal to the medial malleolus. Other reasons for pitting oedema include heart failure and hypoproteinaemia. Long-standing diabetes mellitus will cause microvascular disease and peripheral neuropathy. This leads to pressure areas breaking down, and secondary osteomyelitis and amputation of toes may be necessary. Sometimes a frank woody cellulitis affects the whole fore- or hindfoot and necessitates a trans-tibial amputation. A Charcot joint is one that is destroyed rapidly and is usually associated with a peripheral neuropathy; the ankle is typically affected.

ANKLE AND HINDFOOT OSTEOARTHRITIS

The ankle joint is affected by osteoarthritis (OA) less frequently than the hip and knee, but may follow an ankle fracture. Conservative treatment will include shoe-wear modifications to improve shock absorption at heel strike and orthoses to block painful movement at the ankle. Surgery usually involves an ankle fusion as the long-term outcome for an ankle replacement for arthritis is not known. A prerequisite for fusion is a mobile hind- and midfoot. OA of the hindfoot joints may affect the subtalar joint alone or exist in combination with talo-navicular and calcaneo-cuboid joint arthitis. Arthrodesis of these joints is the surgical treatment of choice in intractable pain.

RHEUMATOID ARTHRITIS

Rheumatoid arthritis (RA) often affects the ankle and hindfoot. The destruction of capsule and tendons together with toe subluxations can cause a valgus deformity of the foot. Carefully moulded footwear to diminish contact forces on pressure areas is vital for skin care and to reduce pain. The management of the ankle arthritis may be fusion or joint replacement. Hindfoot arthritis is often treated by fusion of the hind- and midfoot.

FLAT FEET

The medial arch of the foot is maintained by static and dynamic structures. The arch may be viewed as a triangle with the two shorter sides above made of the medial bones of the foot and the hypotenuse base as the long plantar ligament extending from the calcaneus to the base of proximal phalanges. This ligament is the passive structure that keeps the arch from collapsing when standing. Flat foot (pes planus) is a common condition, present in about 5% of the population in school studies (see Chapter 24). Extra-articular extension of rheumatoid disease may cause rupture of the tibialis posterior tendon leading to a painful flat foot.

TOES

A bunion is a prominent first metatarsophalangeal joint (on the little toe side this is a bunionette). Radiographs of the underlying bone may reveal the first metatarsal in varus (metatarsus primus varus) and the great toe in valgus (hallux valgus). Clinical examination may reveal evidence of congenital joint laxity with a somewhat splayed forefoot (laxity of the inter-metatarsal ligaments) with correction of the bunion by gentle compression across the metatarsal heads. This condition is found in many racial groups. The Masai tribe in Africa has hallux valgus, but rarely pain on inflammation and by tradition they do not wear shoes. In contrast, Western fashions may be associated with narrow

shoe wear, which can lead to a painful, inflamed bunion. Management should include education about sensible footwear and often trainers are helpful. A firm moulded insole will elevate the medial arch and help to correct the splaying and reduce pain in about 40%, but compliance is difficult. Surgery to lateralize the 1st metatarsal (1st metatarsal osteotomy) and tighten the medial capsule of the metatarsophalangeal (MTP) joint together with excision of the prominent medial metatarsal head bony spur will correct the bony deformity, at least for a time. In older people with low activity levels an excision hemiarthroplasty (Keller's procedure) may suffice. OA of the first MTP joint causes pain on walking and the joint is stiff in dorsiflexion. An addition of a 'rocker' sole to the shoe allows the foot to roll into the 'toe-off' position of the gait cycle, avoiding the need for painful dorsiflexion of the joint. Surgery is usually arthrodesis.

Together with forefoot splaying, the extensor tendons of the toes can shorten causing hammering (fixed distal interphalangeal joint flexion) or clawing (fixed proximal interphalangeal joint flexion) of the toes. Shoe-wear causes dorsal corns to form over the prominences. Corrective toe surgery may be required. The metatarsal heads may be prominent on the sole of the forefoot when this happens, causing pain over the heads (metatarsalgia) and callosities to form over their plantar surfaces (Fig. 23.3). In RA, subluxation of the MTP joints causes most severe metatarsalgia. Treatment with a metatarsal 'dome' or 'bar' as a shoe insert will give relief by unloading the weight of the foot just proximal to the metatarsal heads. Where the metatarsal heads are abnormal, the interdigital

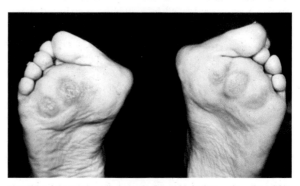

FIGURE 23.3 Hallux valgus and painful callosities associated with metatarsalgia in rheumatoid arthritis

nerves may be subject to abrasion causing a painful traumatic Morton's neuroma. This is most common in the 3rd interspace. The neuroma may be so big as to splay the toes apart when standing. Diagnosis is confirmed on ultrasound or after local anesthetic injection. The neuroma may be treated by cortisone injection or excision.

TOE-NAILS

The toe-nails are important as they may hide important pathology, such as melanoma. This may be amelanotic (pale) and careful examination is necessary to make the diagnosis. Psoriasis leads to nail pitting. In adolescents the nail-fold may become inflamed and infected. Treatment is careful nail care and sometimes antibiotics. Partial or complete nail-bed ablation is reserved for intractable infection.

SPORTS CONDITIONS

In running sports, the plantar ligament may become inflamed at its origin just distal to the plantar surface of the calcaneus – plantar fasciitis. This settles with changes in activity or shoe-wear and a steroid injection may help. The dynamic structure is the tibialis posterior tendon, which inserts onto the navicular and other bones of the medial midfoot to elevate and invert the foot when contracted.

FURTHER READING

Bullough PG, DiCarlo EF 1990 Subchondral avascular necrosis: a common cause of arthritis. Ann Rheum Dis 49: 412–420.

Coughlin MJ 2000 Common causes of pain in the forefoot in adult. Br J Bone Joint Surg 82-B: 781–790.

McNally EG 2002 Magnetic resonance imaging of the knee. BMJ 325: 115–116.

PAEDIATRICS

24

NORMAL VARIANTS IN CHILDREN

David Sherlock

Cases relevant to this chapter

6, 7, 9, 11

●Essential facts

1. In-toe gait becomes evident by age 2 in 14–18% of infants and is usually secondary to persisting femoral anteversion.

2. Children with limb pains and ligament laxity may be diagnosed as having hypermobility syndrome, although most hypermobile children do not suffer such pains.

3. Bow legs (genu vara) are normal till age 2, after which knock-knees (genu valga) become the norm.

4. Painless flat feet that develop normal arches when the child stands on tiptoe require no treatment other than reassurance.

5. Calcaneovalgus is a uterine moulding deformity that usually corrects spontaneously.

Most books cover diseases, yet normal variants and normal developmental stages cause considerable anxiety to parents and doctors. Normal children have a rotational profile to their gait, as shown in Figure 24.1.

GAIT VARIANTS

In-toe gait is seen in 14–18% of infants and is usually noted by age 2. The parents complain that the child in-toes and is clumsy. It is important to eliminate neurological causes (upper motor neurone lesions such as cerebral palsy exhibit increased muscle tone, up-going plantar reflexes and sustained clonus) and to exclude in-toeing due to metatarsus varus of the feet or internal tibial torsion. Usually, in-toeing results from persisting femoral anteversion (PFA), as demonstrated by a greater range of internal than external rotation of the hip. PFA is often associated with generalized ligament laxity, which may explain both the clumsiness and the PFA. Lax ligaments cause inefficient proprioception (clumsiness) and produce less remodelling force on the femoral neck, which is anteverted 40° at birth but only 16° by age 16. Interventions do not alter the natural history; therefore reassurance and explanation are important. These children commonly sit splay-legged in the W shape, but should be dissuaded as this may exacerbate PFA and cause external tibial torsion deformities. Most children improve with age under peer pressure, but all will continue to in-toe with inattention or when tired.

Out-toeing gait is usually noted as the child starts to walk. Fetal moulding from compression by the uterus before birth produces hip flexion and

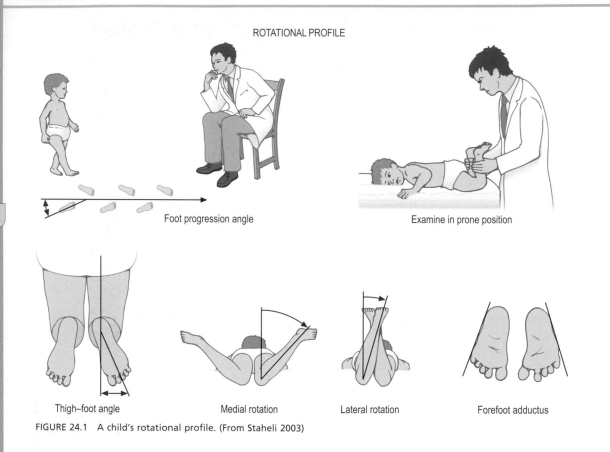

ROTATIONAL PROFILE

Foot progression angle

Examine in prone position

Thigh–foot angle

Medial rotation

Lateral rotation

Forefoot adductus

FIGURE 24.1 A child's rotational profile. (From Staheli 2003)

external rotation contractures, such that all children initially walk out-toed with their hips and knees flexed. These contractures stretch out by age 2, sometimes to reveal an in-toed gait from PFA.

BOW LEGS AND KNOCK-KNEES

All children are bow-legged (genu vara) until age 2 when they become knock-kneed (genu valga). Genu vara appears greater in a child who in-toes. Genu valga is maximal between ages 3 and 4, and may be more marked in children who have ligament laxity or are overweight. The adult alignment of slight valgus is usually achieved by age 9 (Fig. 24.2). Bow legs beyond age 2½ or knock-knees before 18 months are probably pathological, in which case rickets or an inherited skeletal dysplasia that can cause either genu vara or valga should be excluded. Persisting bow legs in a heavy early walker may be due to Blount's disease (medial growth delay or arrest of the proximal tibial

physis). This condition is more common in Afro-Caribbeans. If detected early, it can readily be corrected surgically by a medial periosteal release. If detected late, complex osteotomies are required to correct this tri-planar deformity.

GROWING PAINS

Growth is not painful, but growth plates are weaker during rapid growth. Pain may be nature's way of protecting the growth plate from overuse damage. The pain occurs during the day or in the evening. Children with ligament laxity may be labelled as having hypermobility syndrome, although most hypermobile children do not suffer pain; furthermore, similar pain may occur in children who are not hypermobile. Recent research suggests that children who suffer growing pains have a low pain threshold. Management is by reassurance. Some children wake in the night with severe pain, which is due to cramp. Massage and reassurance will settle this pain within 20–30 min.

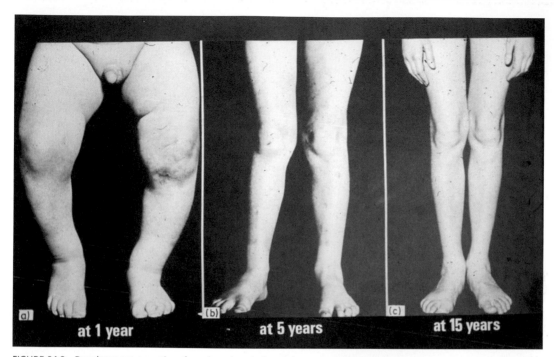

FIGURE 24.2 Development over time from bow legs to knock-knees to normal alignment

ANTERIOR KNEE PAIN

Anterior knee pain arises from the patello-femoral joint, usually after increased activity or prolonged sitting. It affects 19% of girls and 7% of boys during adolescence. There is an association with external tibial torsion. The patella carries up to 12 times body weight and is one of the most heavily loaded joints in the body. During the adolescent growth spurt, the forces on the still immature patella increase markedly. Patello-femoral irritability, sometimes with crepitus, distinguishes anterior knee pain from the tenderness over the tibial tubercle of Osgood–Schlatter's disease (see Chapter 26). Radiographs are normal. Treatment is by regular quadriceps exercises, restriction of activity within the bounds of the discomfort, and avoidance of prolonged kneeling, squatting or sitting with the knee fully flexed. Most outgrow the pain, but a significant minority have anterior knee pain throughout life.

CALCANEOVALGUS

Unless there is an underlying neurological abnormality, calcaneovalgus of the foot results from intrauterine moulding (Fig. 24.3). The deformity

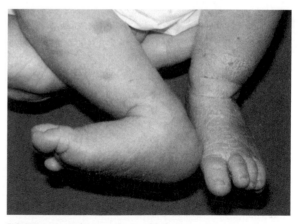

FIGURE 24.3 Calcaneovalgus at birth

corrects with stretching exercises and as the powerful calf muscles gain tone. Correction occurs by 3–6 months of age, so plaster casting is unnecessary.

FLAT FEET

Flat feet, characterized by heel valgus with pronation of the rest of the foot, are classified as postural or structural. In postural flat feet, the arches correct when the child stands on tiptoe. Postural flat feet occur in 97% of children at 18 months but in only

4% of 10-year-olds. Most flat feet resolve spontaneously. Knock-knees make flat feet look worse, which explains why flat feet are most apparent between age 3 and 4. Persisting flat feet are often familial and associated with ligament laxity. Insoles or heel cups do not alter the natural history of postural flat feet, although orthoses can adversely affect the child psychologically. If the foot is painless, treatment with reassurance is appropriate. Bare-foot walking helps the normal development of the foot, but is not always feasible in cold climates. Trainers, often have an in-built arch support which may help if shoe wear is excessive and, unlike orthoses, will not label the child as different from their peers. An older child with aching postural flat feet, particularly in association with ligament laxity, may find an arch support helpful. A very athletic child with flat feet may also benefit in performance and symptoms from a customized arch-supporting insole.

Structural flat feet may be flexible with the primary pathology being tight calf muscles, or rigid. Tight calf muscles are managed by serial plaster casting or surgical release. Rigid flat foot may be overlooked until the child presents with pain. A painful stiff flat foot suggests subtalar pathology such as a tarsal coalition (see Chapter 26), infection, juvenile arthritis, trauma or severe neurological abnormality. In addition to minimal (but usually painful) subtalar movement, there is often associated calf wasting and muscle spasm, causing the foot to evert or, occasionally, to invert. Investigation by magnetic resonance imaging (MRI) or computed tomography (CT) may identify the cause to be tarsal coalition, inflammation or trauma of the subtalar joint, or an infective focus. If performed before the appearance of degenerative change, excision of a calcaneo-navicular bar can successfully restore some subtalar movement and relieve most of the pain. Excision of a talo-calcaneal coalition is less effective, unless the bar occupies less than 30% of the talo-calcaneal joint surface; therefore, in most cases, subtalar fusion is necessary to relieve pain. Where the rigid flat foot is secondary to trauma, chronic inflammation or severe neurological abnormality, it may be difficult to achieve mobility and balance. Some symptoms may be relieved by use of a shoe insert or ankle–foot orthoses combined with appropriately fitted footwear, although great care is necessary if there is impaired sensation in the foot.

SEVER'S DISEASE

This is not a disease, but a type of growing pain that causes posterior heel pain after activity in children, usually between age 9 and 11. At the back of the os calcis is a growth plate capped by a thin plate of bone (apophysis). During rapid growth the growth plate becomes thicker and weaker, providing less support to the apophysis. The Achilles' tendon inserts into one end and the plantar fascia into the other thereby applying traction forces to the apophysis and producing microfractures in it. Unchecked activity risks avulsion of the Achilles' tendon from its insertion, but the pain usually protects against this.

Treatment comprises restricting activity within the bounds of the pain, calf-stretching exercises and possibly wedge-heel trainers (which partially defunction the calf muscles). Once the growth plate closes, the problem disappears.

Similar traction apophysites can occur at the insertion of peroneus brevis into the 5th metatarsal base, at the insertion of the glutei into the greater trochanter, and at the insertion of the medial hamstrings and adductor magnus into the ischium. Osgood–Schlatter's disease and accessory navicular are also examples of traction apophysites.

TOE DEFORMITIES

Curly toes (Fig. 24.4) are common and often familial. The 4th toe is most frequently involved, but the 3rd and occasionally the 5th can be affected. Stretching or strapping the toes is ineffective. Curly toes seldom cause symptoms so intervention is usually not required. Occasionally, pain secondary

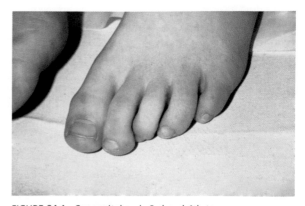

FIGURE 24.4 Congenital curly 3rd and 4th toes

to shoe pressure on the nail or proximal interphalangeal joint warrants surgical division of the flexor tendons. In children with over-riding 5th toes, the 5th toe overlies the 4th. Symptoms are surprisingly rare. If there are symptoms, or cosmetic issues, treatment is surgical. An over-riding 2nd toe is common in the podgy infant foot, but resolves as the foot slims and spreads with weight-bearing. Congenital anomalies such as syndactyly, polydactyly, macrodactyly, delta phalanx and absence of a toe and/or metatarsal often occur in association with other congenital abnormalities. Claw, mallet and hammer toe deformities (see Chapter 26) are usually developmental and become problematic only in later childhood.

FURTHER READING

Do TT 2001 Clinical and radiographic evaluation of bowlegs. Curr Opin Pediatr 13: 42–46.

Gore AI, Spencer JP 2004 The newborn foot. Am Fam Physician 69: 865–872.

Kocher MS, Sucato DJ 2006 What's new in pediatric orthopaedics? Am J Bone Joint Surg 88A: 1412–1421.

Staheli LT 2003 Pediatric orthopaedic secrets, 2nd edn, Hanley and Belfus, Philadelphia.

309

25

UPPER LIMB DISORDERS IN CHILDREN

David Sherlock

●Essential facts

1. Congenital upper limb anomalies may be part of the VACTERL syndrome.

2. Many trigger thumbs recover spontaneously.

3. Syndactyly, polydactyly and, occasionally, trigger thumb are managed surgically.

4. Approximately 400 obstetric brachial plexus palsy (OBPP) cases occur annually in Britain; 50% recover by 2 years, 40% regain useful function, but muscle imbalance may cause shoulder dislocation.

5. Management of OBPP by physiotherapy prevents joint contractures; if the biceps does not recover by 3 months investigation by neurophysiology and X-ray is indicated.

6. Narakas' classification and the speed of biceps recovery are useful guides to outcome.

7. Persisting muscle imbalance and dislocation of the shoulder require surgery.

SPRENGEL'S SHOULDER

This occurs through a failure of the scapula to descend during fetal development. It is often associated with the Klippel–Feil syndrome (congenital fusion of cervical vertebrae and other musculoskeletal and systemic abnormalities). The scapula is tethered to the cervical spine by a bony, cartilaginous or fibrous band.

Clinically the scapula sits high with abnormalities of the muscles. Treatment is surgical, to excise the tether and bring the scapula down to its normal position.

SYNDACTYLY

The commonest congenital hand anomaly, it comprises fusion of two or more fingers. The fusion may be soft tissue only or bony, partial or total. The middle and ring fingers are most commonly affected. It is often familial and may be associated with other conditions. Treatment comprises surgical separation of the digits.

POLYDACTYLY

Polydactyly may be associated with other conditions and is the second commonest hand anomaly. The duplication is either postaxial (of the little finger) or preaxial (of the thumb; Fig. 25.1). The extra digit may be a soft-tissue tag or may comprise partial or complete bony and soft-tissue duplication of the digit. Treatment involves surgical deletion of the extra digit.

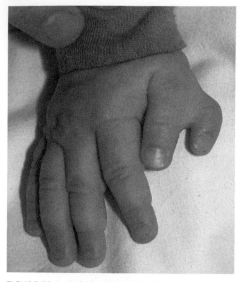

FIGURE 25.1   Polydactyly of the thumb

TRIGGER THUMB

Trigger thumbs may be present at birth or develop later. They result from stenosis of the flexor tendon sheath. Clinically a nodule is palpable at the base of the thumb in the flexor tendon. Often the thumb is fixed in flexion, though early on it can be extended passively. Up to 50% of trigger thumbs resolve spontaneously over 1 year. A persistent trigger thumb is released surgically.

OBSTETRIC BRACHIAL PLEXUS PALSY

Between 0.1% and 4% of live births are complicated by obstetric brachial plexus palsy (OBPP). OBPP includes both Erb's and Klumpke's palsies. Birth weight is the chief etiological factor, not the expertise of the delivery staff. Since birth weights are increasing, OBPP will continue to be a problem.

The injury affects the roots of the brachial plexus, most commonly the upper ones (Fig. 25.2). The outcome depends largely on the severity of the lesion, which is described by the Narakas classification (Table 25.1).

Failure of biceps recovery by 4 months also heralds a poor result.

Treatment initially is physiotherapy to prevent joint contractures due to muscle imbalance. In

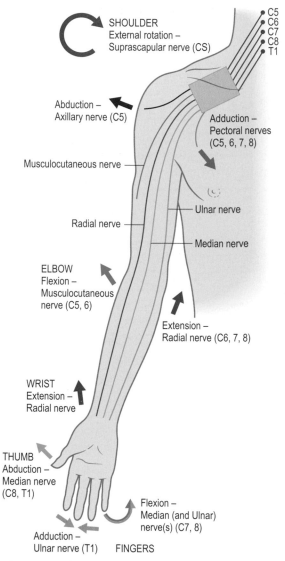

FIGURE 25.2   The anatomy and functions of the brachial plexus (reproduced with permission from *Guidelines for the Scottish National Brachial Plexus Injuries Service* based at the South Glasgow University Hospitals). Courtesy of Medical Illustration Service, Victoria Infirmary, Glasgow

Group 4 cases with no biceps recovery by 4–6 months, nerve repair by grafting or nerve transfers may restore useful, but never good, function. Partial recovery produces muscle imbalance, particularly at the shoulder, which limits function and may cause dislocation of the shoulder. Surgery to weaken the internal rotators or muscle transfers to strengthen the external rotators prevents dislocation and improves function. Muscle transfers can also help residual wrist or hand weakness.

Table 25.1 The Narakas classification

Narakas group	Roots and muscles affected	Outcome
Group 1	C5, 6. Biceps & deltoid	90% recover fully
Group 2	C5, 6, 7. All except long finger flexors	65% recover fully. Rest have permanent deficit
Group 3	C5, 6, 7, 8, T1. All except slight finger flexion	1–2% recover fully. Rest have significant permanent deficit
Group 4	C5, 6, 7, 8, T1 & Horner's. All muscles & sympathetic function	None recovers fully. All have severe permanent deficit

FURTHER READING

Gherman RB, Chauhan S, Ouzounian JG et al 2006 Shoulder dystocia: the unpreventable obstetric emergency with empiric management guidelines. Am J Obstet Gynecol 195(3): 657–672.

Shaw-Smith C 2006 Oesophageal atresia, tracheo-oesophageal fistula, and the VACTERL association: review of genetics and epidemiology. J Med Genet 43(7): 545–554.

LOWER LIMB DISORDERS IN CHILDREN

26

Malcolm F. Macnicol

Cases relevant to this chapter

4, 5, 7–10, 12, 13, 32

●Essential facts

1. Congenital talipes equinovarus is the most common birth deformity of the foot, especially in boys and in identical twins.

2. Pes cavus is produced by four principal patterns of neurological imbalance: soleus and gastrocnemius weakness, with over-action of the long toe flexors; weakness of ankle dorsiflexion resulting in over-action of the long toe extensors; weakness of the intrinsic muscles; and a weak peroneus brevis muscle with an overactive peroneus longus.

3. Tiptoe walking may develop at walking age; most children are neurologically normal.

4. Referred pain from the hip to the knee may be due to Perthes' disease, a slipped upper femoral epiphysis (especially in adolescents) or hip dysplasia.

5. In later childhood and adolescence, ligament tears are more likely than fractures as the skeletal attachments of ligament become stronger.

6. Osteochondritis dissecans can cause clicking, catching and bouts of pain if the affected fragment starts to separate; it is a localized avascular necrosis most commonly affecting the lateral margin of the medial femoral condyle in late childhood and adolescence.

7. In neonates, rapid detection and treatment is required for hip instability and septic arthritis; delay leads to deformity, stiffness, dislocation and osteoarthritis.

8. In mid-childhood, more than 50% of children who present with a limp have a clear diagnosis; a further 40% have transient synovitis of the hip.

9. In the late stage of Perthes' disease, femoral and pelvic reconstruction is indicated if flattening of the femoral head and acetabular deformity have occurred.

PAEDIATRIC FOOT AND ANKLE

DEFINITIONS OF POSITION AND DEFORMITY

The hindfoot (talus and calcaneus) is described as valgus if it deviates laterally, varus if medially. When the tilt is subtalar, involving the heel, the terms eversion and inversion correspond. As with the hand, the midfoot and forefoot are said to pronate when they roll internally, often in conjunction with eversion of the heel, and to supinate when they roll externally with the first metatarsal raised above the 5th and the heel inverted. Similarly, medial deviation of the forefoot (metatarsals and toes) in the horizontal plane is adduction, the opposite being abduction. Dorsiflexion of the foot normally occurs as a total movement, but may be confined to the heel alone, as with the deformity 'calcaneus' seen with a weak calf after poliomyelitis and other neurological conditions including some forms of pes cavus. Equinus describes the toe-down position of the whole foot or the heel, but when only the midfoot and forefoot are plantar-flexed, the term used is 'plantaris'.

The arch of the foot is maintained by the conforming shape of the bones, the ligaments, and the muscles, both intrinsic and from the calf. Maintenance of this medial or longitudinal arch is reliant upon normal muscle action, especially at push-off when walking. A transverse metatarsal arch is also present, although it is less obviously so; in the elderly this arch may be lost along with flattening of the medial arch as the weakening foot pronates.

PRESENTATION OF FOOT DEFORMITIES AT DIFFERENT AGES

Birth

At birth, during infancy and when the child is a toddler, variations from normal may be encountered (see Chapter 24).

Convex pes valgus ('rocker' foot)

This deformity is rare and differentiated from calcaneovalgus by the fact that the heel is in equinus and the deformity relatively rigid. Different grades of severity are recognized, determined by the extent of the underlying dislocation of the talonavicular joint and hindfoot valgus. Surgical treatment is often advised, preferably by the first birthday of the child. A combined procedure, correcting both the hindfoot and midfoot deformities, is now usually preferred and may have to be repeated. Dynamic support for the prolapsing talonavicular joint (hence the term 'vertical talus') is ensured by appropriate re-attachments of the tibialis posterior and sometimes the tibialis anterior tendons.

Metatarsus adductus

This appearance is relatively common and usually benign. Provided the forefoot alignment is correctable and there is no element of supination the condition can be ignored and will lessen during the early years of shoe-wear. Hallux varus or adductus is highly unusual; this congenital condition may require soft-tissue correction later in childhood.

Congenital talipes equinovarus (clubfoot or congenitally inverted foot)

This is the most common significant deformity of the foot encountered at birth (Fig. 26.1). It is more likely to occur in boys. A family history is often identified, reaching its peak with identical twins when the condition is seen in 33% of siblings. Milder forms of the deformity may result from tight uterine 'packaging', including oligohydramnios. The more structurally severe feet have been shown to have neurological, vascular and other soft-tissue abnormalities.

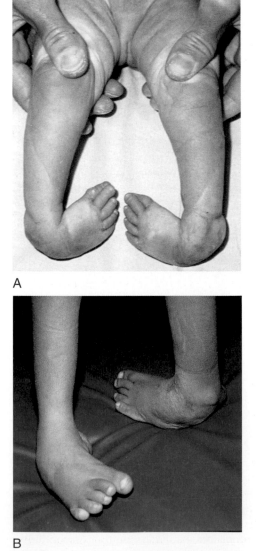

A

B

FIGURE 26.1 Congenital talipes equinovarus (clubfoot). (A) In the infant, (B) as an established deformity in childhood

The prognosis for clubfoot is related to the severity of the presenting deformity, graded from postural to mild, moderate or severe. Atypical syndromic clubfeet are also encountered: the deformities may be very stiff in conditions, such as arthrogryposis, or they may correct more rapidly than the idiopathic forms, potentially leading to over-correction if surgery is undertaken.

A conservative approach should always be tried initially. Dynamic splintage using strapping or more complex devices will correct the postural and milder deformities, and may reduce the moderate deformity. In the severe case dynamic splintage has little to offer, although manual stretching may help to keep the foot in a more supple, partially corrected posture. A programme of carefully defined plaster casting has been advocated by Ponseti. This offers excellent correction of all but the worst deformities, provided it is combined with percutaneous Achilles tendon (and possibly tibialis posterior) release and a subsequent period of Denis Brown boot and bar application.

Surgical release has lost its universal appeal and over-zealous operative intervention may lead to clinical problems as severe as the original deformity, including a fixed valgus of the heel, calcaneo-cavus, gross scarring or irretrievable neurovascular deficit. Correction of late deformity, whether untreated or post-surgical, can be achieved with distraction frames, externally applied. The procedures are demanding for patient and surgeon alike, and may have to be combined with corrective osteotomies and prolonged plaster-cast application.

Childhood

Osteochondritic conditions

These affect the navicular (Kohler's disease) in mid-childhood and the second or occasionally other metatarsal heads (Frieberg's disease) in early adolescence. The former resolves completely, although a strong shoe with an insole, or plaster cast support for a month or two, may be helpful if it is symptomatic. Frieberg's disease leads to pain in the affected metatarsophalangeal (MTP) joint and a tender enlargement of the metatarsal head. An extension osteotomy of the metatarsal neck may relieve metatarsalgia, although the dorsal bony swelling persists. The long-term outcome of this condition, when healed, is poorly recorded.

Pes cavus

A high longitudinal arch is rarely a problem in early childhood, but becomes increasingly symptomatic towards the later stages of skeletal growth. Four principal patterns of neurological imbalance produce these chronic changes in the foot:

1. Weakness of soleus and gastrocnemius, with over-action of the long toe flexors
2. Weakness of ankle dorsiflexion resulting in over-action of the long toe extensors
3. Weakness of the intrinsic muscles
4. A weak peroneus brevis muscle with overactive peroneus longus.

The neurological conditions responsible include cerebral palsy, poliomyelitis, Friedreich's ataxia, myelomeningocele and other abnormalities of the spinal cord, such as spinal dyraphism or syringomyelia, and peripheral neuropathies. The commonest cause of this in the UK is hereditary sensory and motor neuropathy (HSMN) type 1 (Charcot–Marie–Tooth disorder or peroneal muscular atrophy). This autosomal dominant progressive local demyelinating disorder of the lower limbs produces initially a correctible and then a rigid deformity associated with painful calluses. Hammering of the toes and a hindfoot in varus co-exist.

Surgery for clubfoot may also fail to address the cavus deformity, and the persistence of muscle imbalance post-operatively may lead to a high arch and plantaris deformities. Compartment syndromes and damage to one or both of the peroneal tendons may also be causative. Clinical assessment should include neurological examination (loss of light touch, vibration or proprioception; diminished deep reflexes; ataxia and dysarthria; clonus and overt muscle wasting).

When further investigation is warranted, X-rays of the feet and a spinal MR scan are indicated. Imaging of the brain and spinal cord may also be necessary, and both nerve conduction studies and EMG are helpful in ruling out overt nerve deficit. In many cases no cause is uncovered.

Treatment consists of:

1. Soft-tissue surgery (releases and tendon transfers)
2. Osteotomies (first metatarsal, midfoot, calcaneum)
3. Triple arthrodesis of the talus, calcaneum and cuboid.

The toes are often clawed so that flexor tendon releases or tendon transfers may be required. Orthoses will help to reduce local pressure over the metatarsal heads.

Tiptoe walking

This gait pattern may develop at walking age or a little later in childhood. In some cases this is associated with hyper-reflexia and mild, non-progressive diplegia. The majority of children with the condition seem to be neurologically normal, so the term 'tight heel cords' or 'ballerina syndrome' is used. Stretching by physiotherapy or casting is usually effective, but may have to be repeated. Nowadays, lengthening of the Achilles tendon is avoided whenever possible since it is the calf muscle rather than the tendon that is pathologically shortened.

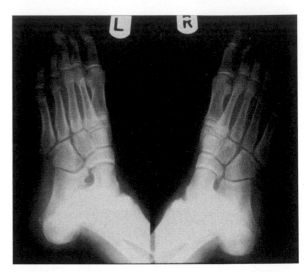

FIGURE 26.2 Radiographic appearance of a calcaneonavicular bar or coalition

Early adolescence

Flat foot, pes cavus and toe deformities

These are common reasons for referral. Surgical intervention is rarely recommended unless the deformity is fixed and progressive. Three conditions should be recognized at this stage of development.

Symptomatic accessory navicular

This forms near the insertion of the tibialis posterior tendon into the midfoot (principally the navicular, but also through slips to all the other tarsal bones). Only rarely is excision of the bony lump required, for example when there is pressure from the shoe or pain at the synchondrosis between the accessory and the parent navicular. More complicated reattachment of the tibialis posterior tendon, attempting to improve the height of the medial arch, is unnecessary. Other bony prominences dorsally, laterally or posteriorly should not be excised.

Tarsal coalition

This produces a rigid structural flat foot. Normally the embryonic mesodermal segments separate to form the different tarsal bones. A coalition represents a failure of complete segmentation, most commonly at the calcaneo-navicular site laterally (Fig. 26.2) and less frequently between the talus and the calcaneum medially. Other coalitions (for example, calcaneocuboid) have been described and they may occur at several sites in the same foot.

The condition is often bilateral and hereditary. Symptoms develop in early adolescence as the cartilaginous bar ossifies and becomes rigid. Excision of the bar is worthwhile if conservative measures fail. Many cases of tarsal coalition remain asymptomatic or cause minimal stiffening.

Hallux valgus

The deviation is one expression of a broad forefoot and the effects of too narrow a shoe upon it. This is not entirely fair to the patient as the deviation may be strongly hereditary, the product of ligament laxity, metatarsus primus varus and a pronating foot. Although many surgical procedures have been described to correct the deformity and its associated first MTP joint bunion, a conservative approach is best, at least until skeletal maturity.

Soft-tissue corrections have been recommended in adolescence, but unless the underlying metatarsus primus varus (medial deviation of the first metatarsal) is corrected, permanent improvement is unlikely. Basal, shaft and distal first metatarsal osteotomies are all effective, particularly the proximal closing wedge or dome osteotomy for more severe cases. A broad forefoot may also produce prominence and a bunion over the 5th metatarsal head (the 'baby bunion' or 'bunionette'). Side-to-side compression from a shoe, especially in the presence of a long toe with slight flexor and extensor muscle imbalance, may also produce mallet, hammer or claw toe (Fig. 26.3).

318

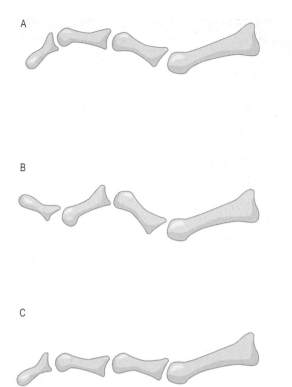

FIGURE 26.3 The different deformities of the lesser toes. (A) Claw toe, (B) hammer toe, (C) mallet toe

Miscellaneous abnormalities

The foot may be the site of inflammatory and primary neoplastic conditions. Infection, pressure ulcers and trauma can produce significant inflammatory responses and chronic dysfunction. Exostoses, including the painful subungual variety, may require excision and 3% of all primary bone tumours affect the foot, including simple and aneurysmal bone cysts, osteochondromata, enchondromata, osteoid osteoma and chondroblastoma. Ankle sprains and fractures are dealt with in Chapter 13.

THE KNEE IN CHILDHOOD

The knee joint is complex, consisting of four compartments if the proximal tibiofibular joint is included. By far the most temperamental component is the patellofemoral, including its anchor points at the quadriceps tendon and the tibial tuberosity.

PRESENTATION AT DIFFERENT AGES

Birth

It is rare to encounter knee deformity or malfunction in the neonate, although patellar clicking may be referred to the hip, confusing the inexperienced. Congenital dislocation (hyperextension) of the knee may be associated with syndromes such as arthrogryposis. Absence of the anterior cruciate ligament (ACL) and shrinkage of the suprapatellar pouch are coexisting abnormalities and the dislocation may be severe or little more than mild subluxation in hyperextension. Valgus deformity may co-exist with fibular deficiency and knee deformity also characterizes tibial hypoplasia or aplasia.

Early childhood

Referred pain

In young children knee pain is a common site for pain that originates from a proximal structure. In the absence of obvious knee pathology it is vital that the clinician should examine the thigh, hip, pelvis and spine to rule out important pathology, such as sepsis, tumour, Perthes' disease or slipped upper femoral epiphysis.

Patellofemoral dysfunction

At this stage patellofemoral dislocations may result in episodes of locking or giving way. Valgus of the knee predisposes to patellar instability and also accentuates the malfunction produced by a discoid lateral meniscus. A snapping knee is produced by tibiofemoral subluxation at an age when many supple children present normally with a positive pivot shift (see Chapter 24).

Mid-childhood

At this age patellofemoral instability persists as a problem with patellar dislocation either in extension or in flexion. Patella alta, valgus alignment, persistent femoral anteversion and poor development of the lower femoral sulcus conspire to produce habitual or intermittent dislocation. Lateral patellar release is rarely sufficient and should be combined with distal, medial realignment of the patellar tendon and possibly a lengthening VY quadricepsplasty, if patella alta is extreme.

Metaphyseal, physeal and avulsion fractures are more common than ligament tears at this age. Fractures may need to be K-wired or screwed into position to preserve ligament function. Ruptures of the medial collateral and anterior cruciate ligaments have been described in young children, but are much more common in adolescence.

The knee, being a large-volume joint, may be the site of rheumatoid synovitis, haemophilic arthropathy with haemarthroses and septic arthritis. Synovitis secondary to viral infection elsewhere in the body (reactive synovitis) and from repeated mild trauma in the sporting child also produces intermittent swelling, pain and stiffness.

Later childhood

Meniscal tears

Meniscal lesions, principally peripheral tears, and ligament injuries become more frequent. An important differential diagnosis is from osteochondritis dissecans (Fig. 26.4), which can cause clicking, catching and bouts of pain if the affected fragment starts to separate. It is vitally important to realize that referred pain from the hip to the knee may catch out the unwary who miss the presence of a slipped upper femoral epiphysis or hip dysplasia. The meniscus functions as a stabilizer of the knee by deepening the tibial plateaux and integrating function with the cruciate and collateral ligaments, capsule and, in the case of the posterior horn of the

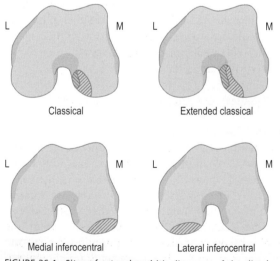

FIGURE 26.4 Sites of osteochondritis dissecans of the distal femur. (From Macnicol 1995)

lateral meniscus, the popliteus muscle. Nutrition and the circulation of synovial fluid are less appreciated roles. In the first half of childhood the meniscus is vascularized from the periphery to its central edge, but this vascular front gradually recedes to the outer third of the meniscus at skeletal maturity. Since peripheral splits are the most common vertical cleavage of the young and vascular meniscus, spontaneous healing is known to occur. If the tear is unstable with abnormal movement of the central part of the meniscus, a small radial tear may develop and the unstable fragment is likely to deform with time. Meniscal suturing is worthwhile if the split is less than half the length of the meniscus and the central portion is not significantly deformed.

A congenital 'discoid' rather than the usual 'horseshoe' shape to the meniscus may lead to intermittent clicking, locking or giving way. MRI will confirm the diagnosis and arthroscopic surgery can recreate the horseshoe shape. Whenever possible, the discoid meniscus should be left intact, or the central torn portion excised to leave some sort of rim. The same principle of preserving meniscal volume characterizes modern treatment of a lateral meniscal cyst, which is almost always caused by a cleavage within the midsubstance of a lateral meniscus. The tear should be 'saucerized' and the cyst drained from within the knee, inserting an arthroscopic instrument through the mouth of the tear and into the cyst. Degenerative change generally follows complete meniscectomy and cyst removal, a practice favoured in the past.

Adolescence

Ligament tears

In later childhood and adolescence these tears are more likely than fractures, as the skeletal attachments of ligament become stronger. However, the ACL may avulse the intercondylar eminence of the proximal tibia where it is attached anteriorly. Varying degrees of osteochondral detachment are described. It is important to reduce and internally fix displaced fragments that fail to reduce by manipulation of the knee and subsequent splintage. If this is not ensured, the avulsed fragment may overlie the anterior meniscal horn and block knee extension. In almost all cases the ACL is also stretched, so some degree of laxity and a long period of recovery are typical, particularly in later adolescence when less corrective bone growth remains. Collateral ligament avulsion should be reduced and internally fixed, particularly fibular head avulsion; interstitial tears can be managed conservatively with partial weight-bearing and maintenance of knee movement and muscle strength.

Posterior cruciate ligament (PCL) avulsion, usually from the upper tibia posteriorly, is only one-tenth as common as ACL injury, but leads to troublesome posterior tibial laxity. Fixation is, therefore, recommended (Fig. 26.5) with a 4-week period of plaster splintage. Knee subluxation or dislocation produces various patterns of ligamentous, meniscal and chondral damage. Neurovascular injury needs to be ruled out and the patellofemoral joint may also have been rendered unstable.

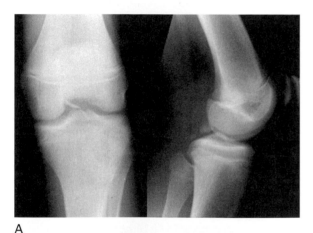

A

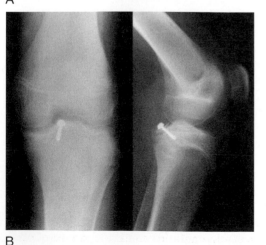

B

FIGURE 26.5 Screw fixation of an avulsed posterior cruciate ligament. (A) Avulsion fragment, (B) reduction

Osteochondritis dissecans

The juvenile knee is prone to separation of an avascular osteochondral fragment, usually from the lateral aspect of the medial femoral condyle – osteochondritis dissecans. Unlike an osteochondral facture, this is an expression of localized avascular necrosis and is, therefore, less likely to heal if separation occurs. It is more common in active children, particularly adolescents, and there is a genetic predisposition. The bones most frequently affected are the lateral femoral condyle and the talus. Pain or discomfort is usually the presenting complaint. If the condition has advanced to involve the cartilage and the fragment detaches, true locking of the knee can occur. The lesion may be less than a centimetre in diameter or may affect as much as half of the condylar surface. Determining whether the fragment is healing or separating can be difficult, but the clinical signs, MR scanning and radiographs offer useful information about the likely prognosis. The fragment may remain attached to the underlying epiphysis by a fibrous bridge and give symptoms of pain and swelling.

The condition can be managed conservatively with avoidance of impact sports if there is no overlying cartilage defect (stage 1), but a loose or detached fragment, fluid around a fragment, or a cyst over 5 mm (stage 2) necessitates arthroscopy. If the fragment is large, drilling into the fragment from the femoral side can occasionally induce healing. Artificial bone anchors have also been used. Smaller separated fragments should be removed arthroscopically, but larger, unstable fragments need to be reduced and fixed in place as their loss hastens osteoarthritis of the knee by a decade or two. Osteochondritis dissecans in adults is more pathological and a large fragment will rarely heal; the consequent articular defect causes premature osteoarthritis. Other sites include the opposite condyle and the patellar articular surface.

Tibial tubercle pain

The older child entering the adolescent growth spurt may experience pain at the front of the knee. This may be bilateral and associated with sporting activity; running, climbing or descending stairs will exacerbate the symptoms. On examination there may be tenderness around the patella or at the tibial tuberosity. If this bony apophysis is enlarged with radiographic evidence of bony fragmentation and sclerosis, the diagnosis is Osgood–Schlatter's condition, an osteochondritis. This is a self-limiting disorder, which only requires reassurance, exercise modification and occasionally physiotherapy.

Jumper's knee (patellar tendinopathy)

'Jumper's knee' is a diagnosis given to young adults who develop pain just below the patella after vigorous leaping activities. It is common in basketball and volleyball players, and in ballet dancers. Tenderness, present on extension, usually disappears on flexion. The diagnosis can be confirmed by MRI; management includes exercise modification, physiotherapy, steroid injection or arthroscopic debridement of the patella.

Joint laxity and patellar instability

Congenital joint laxity may result in patellar dislocation. There may be a history of other family members affected with hypermobility. The patella usually dislocates laterally and often occurs during sport in adolescent girls. It may have spontaneously reduced by the time the first doctor sees the patient and then the only clues are a suspicious history, a large knee joint effusion, and tender, torn quadriceps retinacular fibres supero-medial to the patella. This may be a recurrent problem in the rapidly growing older child and adolescent. Hamstring tension and malalignment are partly to blame. In the inherited collagen disorder, Ehlers–Danlos syndrome, and where there is a bony abnormality, such as a high-riding patella and a shallow intercondylar groove, dislocation may become recurrent or habitual and difficult to treat.

Wherever possible the patellar instability should be managed conservatively with quadriceps exercise, hamstring stretching and possibly patellar taping or bracing during the early stage of convalescence. Occasionally medial reefing and lateral release of the quadriceps retinaculum are required. Inferomedial translation of the tibial tuberosity may be indicated after skeletal maturity.

Haematological and other conditions

The knee may be the site of a haemarthrosis secondary to conditions such as haemophilia, traumatized haemangioma, or a synovial lesion or tear. Reactive and primary synovitis should be considered when there is no history of convincing trauma. Septic arthritis is less common in adolescence but, as with the younger child, high clinical suspicion and speedy diagnosis are paramount if secondary,

possibly permanent, changes are to be avoided. Tumours around the knee (see Chapter 20) are encountered infrequently, apart from osteochondromata, which give trouble in relation to the medial hamstrings, the quadriceps muscle and the proximal tibiofibular joint.

PAEDIATRIC HIP JOINT CONDITIONS
PRESENTATIONS AT DIFFERENT AGES
Birth

Developmental dysplasia of the hip

In the neonatal period, rapid detection and treatment are required for hip instability and septic arthritis. Delay in management of both conditions will lead to severe and sometimes irreversible changes due to deformity, stiffness, dislocation and OA. These severe penalties from late treatment are not seen with rare conditions, such as coxa vara and proximal femoral focal deficiency, although their corrective surgery is still taxing. The golden period for treating hip instability is at birth or in the first 2 weeks of life. Neonatal screening with clinical examination and ultrasound scanning diagnoses most, if not all, cases, with further detection achieved by vigilant examination at 6 weeks and again at 8–9 months of age. The two classical tests are the Barlow test, in which the hips are gently pushed posteriorly to elicit the 'exit clunk' of the dislocatable joint (Fig. 26.6) and then circumducted with forward pressure over the greater trochanters to produce the rarer 'entry clunk' of the dislocated hip (Ortolani's test) (Fig. 26.7). If the hip can be reduced by abducting and flexing the legs, then commercial splints and braces are usually effective (Fig. 26.8). Treated in this way over 95% of unstable hip joints will improve and eventually return to normal.

The natural incidence of developmental dysplasia is 1.5–2.0 cases per 1000 live births. A screening programme should detect over 95% of unstable hips. Unfortunately, risk signs such as female gender, first born, high birth weight, breech presentation, oligohydramnios and the presence of other anomalies do not always identify the likely case. A positive family history is an important indicator.

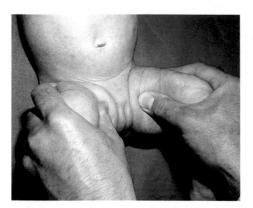

FIGURE 26.6 The Barlow test assesses posterior laxity of the hip joint by eliciting an 'exit clunk'

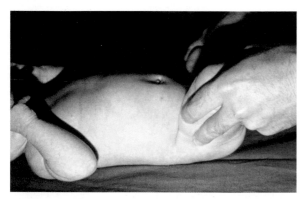

FIGURE 26.7 The Ortolani test checks whether the femoral heads are lying in a posteriorly dislocated position at birth. (When the child starts to walk the femoral head displaces upwards as well as backwards)

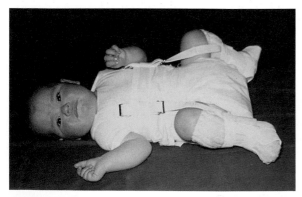

FIGURE 26.8 The Pavlik harness reduces the unstable hip at birth

Racial and cultural differences influence the late diagnosis rate and the birth frequency of the condition. The older the child is at diagnosis, the more necessary surgical intervention becomes, moving progressively from closed reduction (monitored by contrast injected in the joint) after skin traction, to open reduction and then to the use of pelvic or femoral re-directional osteotomies. The longer the femoral head remains dislocated the more likely the child will suffer from residual deformity, stiffness and later OA of the hips. Complications from surgery include further episodes of dislocation, avascular necrosis and residual anteversion of the femur, and infection.

Septic arthritis

This may be multifocal as it often follows septicaemia with bacteria seeding into the metaphyses of long bones and thence into the neighbouring joint (hip, shoulder and knee) since the infective focus is intracapsular (Fig. 26.9). Early drainage rather than aspiration is recommended, with culture and sensitivities of the organism (see Chapter 5) followed by appropriate antibiotics and possible splintage.

Mid-childhood

Irritable hip

In more than 50% of children who present with a limp, a clear diagnosis can be made. In Edinburgh, irritable hip or transient synovitis accounts for a further 40%. By definition, the irritability should be transient: discomfort, muscle spasm round the hip joint and limp disappear within 7–10 days. Most children can be referred back home for bed-rest after clinical examination, routine blood tests and possibly an ultrasound scan of the pelvis and hip joints. Radiographs and MR scanning are not indicated unless the symptoms fail to settle rapidly.

Perthes' disease (Legg–Calve–Perthes' disease)

Perthes' disease is idiopathic osteonecrosis of the proximal femoral epiphysis. It is less than one-tenth as common as transient synovitis, from which it is usually clinically distinct. It affects the proximal epiphysis between the ages of 3 and 10 years (Fig. 26.10), with a median age of 5.5 years, similar to transient synovitis. The male:female ratio is 4:1, 10–20% of cases are bilateral and 8–12% of children have a positive family history. Clinical presentation is usually with a limp, and hip or knee pain. The condition progresses through various radiographic stages, including sclerosis; the formation of a fracture line in some children; fragmentation; and, finally, healing followed by re-ossification.

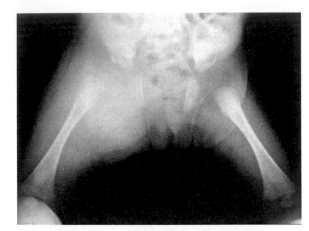

A

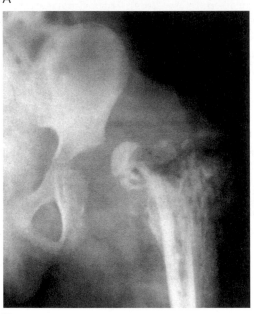

B

FIGURE 26.9   Septic arthritis secondary to a proximal metaphyseal osteomyelitis. (A) Involving the right hip of an infant, (B) producing destructive changes and dislocation in early childhood

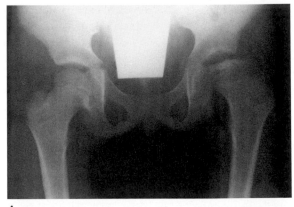

A

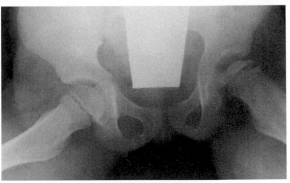

B

FIGURE 26.10   Perthes' disease alters the appearance of the proximal femoral epiphysis. (A) Anteroposterior projection radiographically, (B) 'frog lateral' projection

Children over the age of 7 or 8 years, and girls, recover poorly, although even in younger children (under 5 years) a good outcome is not assured.

Mild disease can be treated with avoidance of high-impact activity, but severe disease requires careful management. The younger the child the better the prognosis, as greater remodelling of the abnormal femoral head can occur. Surgical realignment of the proximal femur and, occasionally, an acetabular procedure to improve femoral head cover are advocated. Intervention of this sort is not without risk so a conservative approach, emphasizing the return of hip movement, is a safe starting point. When the infarction is larger (defined by various radiographic and arthrographic assessments) surgery may be the best option, as it may also be in the child who develops repeated hip spasm.

In the late stage of Perthes' disease further reconstructive femoral and/or pelvic surgery may be indicated if flattening of the femoral head and acetabular deformity have become established. Clearly, it is more successful to prevent deformity as this will lead to the best hip function in adult life. Recent research has suggested that thrombophilia, resultant from an insufficiency of thrombolytic factors (protein S and C), may predispose some children to Perthes' disease. It is also recognized that many of these children are skeletally immature and mildly stunted. Bilateral hip involvement suggests a systemic condition, although the bone age may not be significantly delayed. Hypothyroidism and some skeletal dysplasias may produce similar appearances. Lastly, social deprivation and possible malnutrition have been implicated, all of these factors supporting the concept of the 'at risk' child.

Other causes of limp

Dysplasia

Late hip dysplasia (Fig. 26.11) or even dislocation may present at this age. With better screening and public awareness these 'missed' cases are less likely, but cause considerable consternation. Bilateral developmental dysplasia may produce a symmetrical, waddling gait so that the absence of a unilateral limp may confuse the examiner. The later this hip condition is discovered the worse the prognosis. Acetabular realignment osteotomies and occasional proximal femoral procedures are required to improve the mechanics of the abnormal hip. The guiding principles are that the hip should be mobile and not reduced under compression (Fig. 26.12), and that the best fit between the acetabulum and the femoral head should be achieved by surgical means. The eventual inclination of the socket must be reduced to something like normal and augmentation of the lateral edge of the acetabulum may be needed to ensure a femoral head cover of over 90%.

Infection

Early recognition of septic arthritis or of proximal femoral or periacetabular osteomyelitis should reduce the consequences of hip-joint involvement, which includes acute dislocation and, later, stiffness and long-term deformity or leg shortening. Uncontrolled sepsis may destroy the proximal femur leaving an unstable, adducted and flexed hip with gross femoral shortening. The principles of management of bone and joint infection have already been discussed.

Chronic arthritis

Equally as common as infection (3–4% of the total number of children with limp) is 'reactive arthritis' in association with inflammatory conditions, such as rheumatoid arthritis (RA), ankylosing spondylitis, acute rheumatic fever and viral infection. Haematological abnormalities (leukaemia, haemophilia, sickle cell disease) and a variety of infiltrative and metabolic disorders should also be considered. A team approach is important. The management of neoplasia has already been touched upon and is discussed further in Chapter 20.

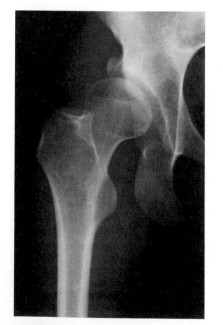

FIGURE 26.11   Late hip dysplasia comprises a sloping acetabulum and femoral head deformity. Note also the 'os acetabuli' and the subchondral sclerosis

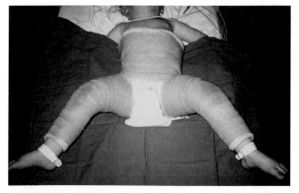

FIGURE 26.12   A plaster cast that controls the reduced hip(s) is applied with the legs abducted and flexed, avoiding extremes of position and compression of the femoral head, as avascular necrosis may otherwise complicate the treatment

Later childhood

In addition to a limp, children may describe referred knee pain as much as any localizing discomfort in the groin or thigh. It is, therefore, very important to examine the hip and spine when assessing the lower limb in childhood conditions such as this.

Limp

Different causes of limp produce changes in gait. A limp may be Trendelenburg in type (articular pathology with inflammation, deformity or weakness), short leg caused by limb discrepancy, or antalgic. When the leg length discrepancy is significant, the child will tend to flex the knee on the longer side, or circumduct that leg, or possibly walk with equinus on the short side.

Miscellaneous

Mechanical, inflammatory, avascular and neoplastic causes of hip disorder have already been considered. Fractures of the proximal femur are either intracapsular (transepiphyseal, transcervical, cervicotrochanteric) or extracapsular (intertrochanteric and subtrochanteric). Complications include avascular necrosis with later deformity and OA, growth arrest and, rarely, non-union. Accurate, early reduction and internal fixation should lessen the risk of these sequelae. Traumatic dislocation of the hip is unusual and is more likely to be posterior. Habitual dislocation may develop. Associated fracture should be carefully excluded. Avascular necrosis is related to the degree of violence producing the dislocation. The condition may be missed, requiring late reduction.

Adolescence

Slipped upper femoral epiphysis

Although relatively rare, this condition may produce catastrophic consequences. The atypical form may occur in mid-childhood, in association with metabolic bone disease, neoplasia and its treatment with chemotherapy or radiotherapy. Various endocrinopathies also predispose to abnormal weakness in the proximal femoral growth plate. The majority of slips, however, occur during the early adolescent growth spurt when the perichondrial ring is relatively weak. The epiphysis slips posteriorly on the neck and also slightly medially, the child with retroversion of the femoral

neck being more at risk. Sudden and major slipping of the epiphysis prevents the patient from weight-bearing or actively straight leg raising, the so-called 'unstable' slip (Fig. 26.13). In many cases the slip is more subtle, however, and may occur gradually over time. In these children, limp and knee pain are crucial presenting features.

Early recognition and treatment will prevent many of the late complications of this condition, including chondrolysis, avascular necrosis and osteoarthritis. Bilateral involvement may be present concurrently or sequentially. Fixation of the contralateral epiphysis is, therefore, advised in younger, more obese patients particularly if there is evidence of metabolic bone disease or an endocrinopathy. In older patients with efficient links to

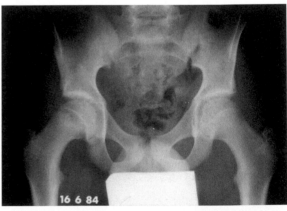

A

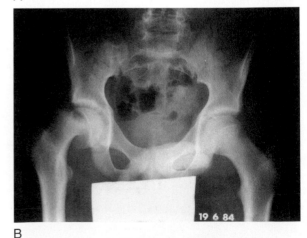

B

FIGURE 26.13 Radiographic changes secondary to slipping of the upper femoral epiphysis. (A) Early displacement of the right epiphysis. (B) The appearance 3 days later after the diagnosis was missed

an orthopaedic clinic, prophylactic fixation of the contralateral epiphysis is probably unnecessary.

Reactive synovitis

Inflammatory disease affecting the hip has already been mentioned and is discussed in greater detail elsewhere (see Chapter 16). Rare conditions such as idiopathic osteoporosis and haemophilia should be considered, in addition to the more common arthropathies. Localized inflammatory processes, such as the snapping hip syndrome (fascia lata rubbing over the greater trochanter), may produce a bursitis in relation to a bony prominence.

Tumour

The hip may be the site of skeletal abnormality in the form of osteoid osteoma, osteochondromata, skeletal dysplasias with bone distortion (including fibrous dysplasia) and leukaemia. Malignant primaries and secondary deposits are rare, but should be considered (see Chapter 20).

Avascular necrosis

Perthes' disease is unlikely to affect the adolescent, but avascular necrosis is still seen. This may be primary (idiopathic) or associated with other conditions including infiltrative disorders and trauma. Steroid treatment for renal conditions such as glomerulonephritis or rheumatoid (juvenile chronic) arthritis may produce iatrogenic avascular necrosis, as may the surgical treatment of developmental dysplasia of the hip and slipped upper femoral epiphysis. Post-fracture avascular necrosis is also encountered.

If the femoral head deforms, and this is more likely when the infarcted area is extensive, movement of the hip will be lost progressively. At first, abduction, internal rotation and extension become limited, before a more generalized stiffness supervenes. A realignment proximal femoral osteotomy with internal fixation can improve function once the extent of the infarction and resultant stiffness is known. Leg-length equalization may also be achieved by this means, but the longer-term results are often disappointing owing to the development of secondary OA.

FURTHER READING

Cassas KJ, Cassettari-Wayhs A 2006 Childhood and adolescent sports-related overuse injuries. Am Fam Physician 73(6): 1014–1022.

De Boeck H, Vorlat P 2003 Limping in childhood. Acta Orthop Belg 69(4): 301–310.

Frick SL 2006 Evaluation of the child who has hip pain. Orthop Clin North Am 37(2): 133–140.

Macnicol MF 1995 The problem knee. Butterworth-Heinemann, London.

THE PAEDIATRIC SPINE AND NEUROMUSCULAR CONDITIONS

27

Athanasios I. Tsirikos and Paul Eunson

Cases relevant to this chapter

3, 7–9, 14, 34

●Essential facts

1. Idiopathic scoliosis is the commonest spinal deformity in children; it is usually painless and affects adolescents most commonly.

2. Congenital scoliosis is due to failure of formation and/or segmentation of the spine.

3. Painful scoliosis needs investigating for an underlying cause.

4. Neuromuscular scoliosis usually produces a long 'C'-shaped collapsing thoracolumbar curve with associated pelvic obliquity.

5. Persistent back pain in children is uncommon and requires further investigation.

6. An infant may be floppy at birth because of a central neurological problem or acute illness, such as infection or hypoxic–ischaemic encephalopathy.

7. Congenital contractures occur in any disorder that limits fetal movement including spina bifida.

8. The commonest single genetic cause of the floppy infant is spinal muscular atrophy; most children have a very poor prognosis.

9. Any boy not walking by 18 months or with global developmental delay or with delayed speech development should have creatine kinase levels checked for a diagnosis of Duchenne's muscular dystrophy.

10. The three main causes of cerebral palsy are abnormalities of brain growth and development, brain damage, and impaired brain function.

11. Spasticity is the commonest tone abnormality in cerebral palsy.

12. To encourage sarcomere growth in a spastic muscle, stretch of the muscle needs to be maintained for about 6 h a day; this can be achieved in calf muscles by using ankle–foot orthoses.

13. With better nutrition, treatment of chest infections and overall care, even children with severe cerebral palsy and profound learning difficulties are likely to survive into adult life.

PAEDIATRIC SPINE

SCOLIOSIS

Scoliosis is a lateral curvature of the spine that measures more than 10°. The deformity may be structural or postural (non-structural). Structural scoliosis can be classified further according to the underlying aetiology into idiopathic, congenital, neuromuscular and syndromic or miscellaneous.

Idiopathic scoliosis

Idiopathic is the most common type of scoliosis in children and adolescents and 2–3% of children have idiopathic scoliosis. The term idiopathic implies that the cause remains unknown. The deformity involves all three planes as the vertebrae at the apex of the curve are rotated towards the convexity of the scoliosis.

Children with idiopathic scoliosis can develop a single thoracic, thoracolumbar or lumbar curvature, or multiple curves along the spine. In the thoracic region, the effect of the rotational deformity of the spine is usually the development of a significant rib prominence, in addition to an elevation of the shoulder line and protrusion of the scapula adjacent to the convex side of the curve, as well as elimination of the normal thoracic kyphosis, which together create most of the cosmetic element of the deformity. Thoracolumbar and lumbar curves produce an asymmetry of the waistline and prominence of the pelvis adjacent to the concavity of the scoliosis, and this is usually the patient's first complaint. In contrast, double thoracic and lumbar curves are often diagnosed late as they are balanced and cosmetically less obvious.

Classification

Idiopathic scoliosis can be classified at diagnosis into infantile (0–3 years), juvenile (3–10 years) and adolescent (AIS) (>10 years up to skeletal maturity).

Aetiology

The cause of this disorder remains elusive, but hereditary or genetic factors are relevant. Studies based on a wide variety of populations have suggested an autosomal dominant, X-linked or multifactorial inheritance pattern and there is a family history of scoliosis in up to 30% of patients with AIS. Connective tissue abnormalities, neuromuscular aberrations, central nervous system asymmetries, hormonal variations and differing growth patterns have been also noted in selected patient populations.

Clinical presentation and prognosis

Infantile idiopathic scoliosis

This has two distinct patterns of development and 80–90% of curves will resolve spontaneously with further growth and do not require treatment other than observation. The remaining 10–20%, however, show rapid progression, are usually resistant to conservative management with a spinal jacket or a brace, and require early surgical treatment. Male and female patients are equally affected. Surgical treatment is indicated in older children with progressive curves or in children with more severe deformities where the use of growing rods can delay spinal fusion for a later age and preserve spinal growth (Fig. 27.1). If left untreated, infantile scoliotic curves will exceed 100° by the age of 10 years and patients can die from cor pulmonale in early adulthood.

Adolescent idiopathic scoliosis

Females are more commonly affected than males and for a curve greater than 20° the ratio is approximately 4:1. The children are born with a straight spine and start developing a scoliosis close to puberty. As they go through their adolescent growth spurt, the deformity progresses more rapidly and becomes clinically apparent. The most frequent pattern of deformity is a right thoracic scoliosis (80–90%). A left thoracic scoliosis is regarded as atypical and other underlying causes, such as spinal dysraphism, should be excluded. Risk factors for curve progression include a younger age or a larger curve magnitude at detection, and are directly related to the amount of remaining growth. Patients who have a rigid thoracic scoliosis often have decreased lung volume, but this is not usually a clinical problem and does not interfere with the level of the patient's activities. In contrast, an adolescent idiopathic thoracic scoliosis that exceeds 90° can cause clinically significant respiratory compromise.

Clinical approach The history of a cosmetically obvious rib asymmetry is highly suggestive of a thoracic scoliosis. Idiopathic scoliosis is not usually

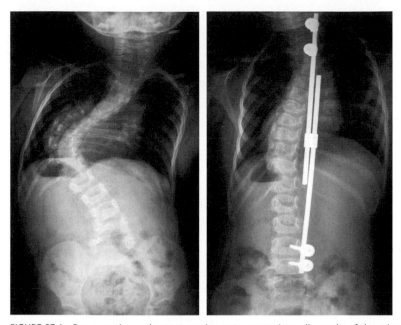

FIGURE 27.1 Pre-operative and post-operative anteroposterior radiographs of the spine show a very severe left thoracic infantile idiopathic scoliosis, which was corrected with the placement of a growing rod with the aim to control the deformity and allow for further growth. At a later stage a definitive spinal fusion will be required to stabilize the spine. The patient's age was 2 years 4 months pre-operatively (2+4). The curve magnitude (°) is indicated on the radiographs

associated with back pain and if children present with spinal pain and/or a stiff back, other causes for the scoliosis, such as an infection, spinal cord tumour, spinal dysraphism, spondylolysis/spondylolisthesis and a herniated intervertebral disc (see 'Red flag symptoms, Chapter 1), should be considered.

Examination Ensure that the patient is appropriately undressed to observe the whole of the trunk. Look at the patient from behind for asymmetry of the shoulder height, a rib prominence, asymmetry of the waistline and stigmata of spinal dysraphism, such as hairy patches, dimples or haemangiomas. There may be flank recession on the concave side and flattening of the waist on the convex side of a thoracolumbar or lumbar scoliosis as well as listing of the trunk towards the convexity of the curve. Perform a forward bend test, ask the patient to lean anteriorly at the waist to 90°, and observe their spine and trunk from behind as they bend forward; this will highlight the flank and ribcage deformity in scoliosis. Assess spinal flexibility and correctibility of the curvature by performing a side-bending test with the patient standing.

Perform a detailed neurological examination evaluating sensation, muscle power and tendon reflexes in the upper and lower limbs, and include abdominal reflexes. Asymmetrically elicited abdominal reflexes may be suggestive of an intraspinal abnormality. Check leg lengths, as a unilateral limb-length discrepancy can cause an obliquity of the pelvis and, as a consequence, a tilt of the spine; this is a good example of a non-structural lumbar scoliosis. Examine the feet, as a cavovarus deformity may suggest an underlying neuromuscular condition (e.g. Charcot–Marie–Tooth disease; see above). Neurological examination should be normal in idiopathic scoliosis and abnormal neurological findings are an indication to perform an MRI of the whole spine and a possible referral to a neurologist.

Radiographic evaluation Obtain anteroposterior (AP) and lateral radiographs of the spine with the patient standing to document the type and location of the scoliosis. The magnitude of the curve can be measured using the Cobb method in both the coronal (frontal) and the sagittal (lateral) planes of the spine (Fig. 27.2).

The Cobb angle and the amount of remaining spinal growth are essential guides to treatment and scoliosis progression during follow-up. A preoperative MRI of the whole spine extending from the

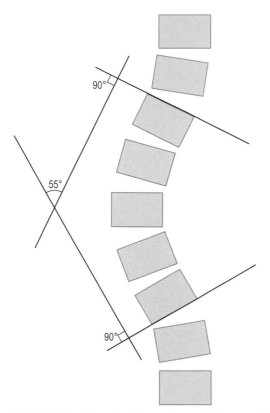

FIGURE 27.2 Cobb angle. The vertebrae at either end of the curvature are located and lines drawn from the superior surface of the uppermost vertebral body and the inferior surface of the lowermost vertebral body. The perpendicular lines to the superior and the inferior end-plates of the two end vertebrae included in the curve are used to form the Cobb angle

Table 27.1 Guidelines for treatment for patients with an adolescent idiopathic scoliosis

Curve magnitude (°)	Treatment
<20–25	Observation
25–40	Bracing
>40–50	Surgical correction and fusion with instrumentation and bone graft

20–25°, a minimal cosmetic deformity and an otherwise normal clinical examination.

Bracing with a lightweight, detachable, custom-moulded, underarm orthosis can be used in a growing child who has a moderate curve ranging from 20–25° up to 40° and whose apex lies below the level of the 6th thoracic vertebra. The aim of a brace (see Chapter 6) is to modify spinal growth and stop curve progression. Brace management cannot lead to resolution of the scoliosis and, at best, will maintain the size of deformity seen at the initiation of bracing. Therefore, the indication for bracing is for small-to-moderate curves that are cosmetically acceptable at the time of initial diagnosis. The child is asked to wear the brace for approximately 20 h a day until skeletal maturity. Compliance can be a significant problem.

Surgical correction should be considered if the curve is greater than 40° and likely to deteriorate with remaining spinal growth, or if there is an established scoliosis greater than 50°. The aim of surgery is to prevent further deterioration by stabilizing the spine and to correct all the components of the deformity (spinal curvature, rib prominence, shoulder or waistline asymmetry, thoracic translocation and listing of the trunk). This can be achieved with the use of spinal instrumentation and bone graft to produce a solid bony arthrodesis (fusion) across the instrumented levels (Fig. 27.3). The general principle when selecting the extent of the fusion is to try to maintain as many mobile segments as possible in order to preserve spinal flexibility.

Post-operatively children are mobilized as soon as possible and bracing is not usually necessary. A small percentage of patients may have to wear an underarm spinal jacket or brace if the fixation of the spine is not secure enough.

foramen magnum proximally to the sacrum distally is required for patients with an abnormal neurological examination, an atypical curve pattern, those children with abnormalities of the skin or subcutaneous tissues overlying the spine or for patients with an infantile or juvenile scoliosis.

Young children with infantile scoliosis or patients with very severe curves, and especially those who will require a combined anterior and posterior spinal fusion, may also necessitate a pre-operative cardiopulmonary assessment.

Treatment The aim of the management of scoliosis is to ensure that a child does not enter adulthood with a significant curve (Table 27.1). Observation is indicated for growing patients with small adolescent idiopathic scoliotic curvatures of up to

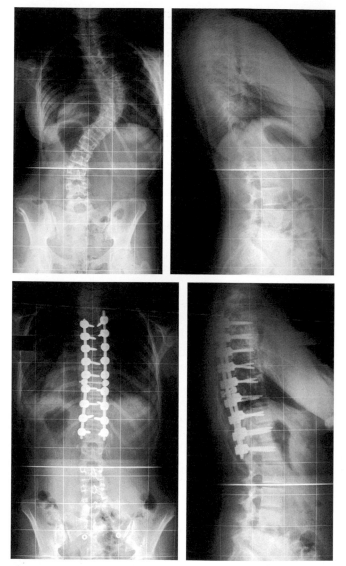

FIGURE 27.3   Pre-operative and post-operative anteroposterior and lateral radiographs of the spine showing a severe right thoracic adolescent idiopathic scoliosis, which was corrected with a posterior spinal fusion

Congenital scoliosis

Congenital scoliosis is caused by developmental vertebral anomalies that occur in the mesenchymal period, during the first 6 weeks of intrauterine life, and produce a lateral longitudinal imbalance in the growth of the spine. Although the vertebral anomalies are present at birth, the clinical deformity may not become evident until later childhood. The anomalies can affect any part of the spine and are classified as defects of vertebral formation or vertebral segmentation, and mixed anomalies (Fig. 27.4). These malformations often cause a structural deformity in one or two planes

and a progressive curvature as the spine grows. As the child grows, a structural compensatory scoliosis often develops above or below the congenital scoliosis, and creates a more significant imbalance of the spine.

Congenital scoliosis may also be associated with congenital malformations affecting the intraspinal neural structures (up to 40%), genitourinary (25%) and cardiac (10%) systems, cervical spine (Klippel–Feil syndrome – 25%) and shoulder (Sprengel's deformity – 7%).

Congenital scoliosis is usually progressive and does not respond to conservative management. It is impossible to create growth on the concavity of

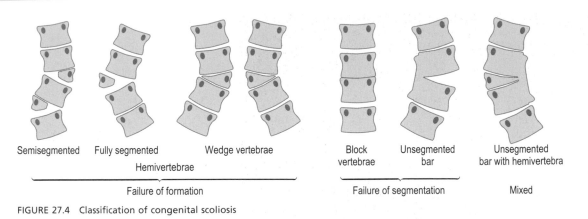

| Semisegmented | Fully segmented | Wedge vertebrae | | Block vertebrae | Unsegmented bar | Unsegmented bar with hemivertebra |

Hemivertebrae

Failure of formation

Failure of segmentation

Mixed

334

FIGURE 27.4   Classification of congenital scoliosis

the scoliosis where it is either retarded or non-existent due to malformation, and the aim of surgery is to balance spinal growth by stopping the accelerated growth on the convexity of the curve. The key to successful treatment is early diagnosis while the curve is still small and there is an opportunity to balance the growth of the spine prophylactically (Fig. 27.5). If the patient presents with a more severe deformity at a later stage, salvage surgery will be required and usually involves an extensive spinal arthrodesis with a suboptimal outcome.

Spina bifida (myelomeningocele)

Spina bifida is a malformation of the development of the vertebral arches of the spine and is often associated with abnormalities of the spinal cord (spinal dysraphism; see above).

There is a spectrum of spinal abnormalities that may include any of the following:

- Defects of the neural arch
- Widened distance between the pedicles with deficient posterior bony elements
- Congenital vertebral abnormalities (see above).

These anomalies may produce a kyphosis (paralytic or congenital), a lordosis (secondary to hip flexion contractures), a scoliosis (usually paralytic but also as a result of mixed paralytic and congenital curves) or a combination of deformities affecting both the coronal and the sagittal planes of the spine. Bracing is not effective in controlling paralytic curves and is also hampered by insensate

skin, as the cord abnormality produces a lower motor neurone lesion. Spinal fusion is indicated where there is increasing spinal deformity to produce a stable posture for sitting and standing, to relieve bony prominences that may cause skin-pressure problems and to improve respiratory function.

Neuromuscular scoliosis

Neuromuscular scoliosis occurs in patients with upper or lower motor neurone lesions, and in muscular conditions (Table 27.2). The spinal deformity is the consequence of a generalized muscle weakness affecting the trunk, with or without associated spasticity, and the effect of gravity. This type of scoliosis is typically characterized by an early onset with rapid progression and a poor response to orthotic management, particularly during the adolescent growth spurt. The scoliosis that develops is a long 'C'-shaped curve with the apex most frequently located in the thoracolumbar spine and can occasionally be associated with an increased kyphosis or lordosis. The curve commonly extends to the pelvis causing marked pelvic obliquity.

The deformity of the trunk and the pelvis may add to the child's functional loss from their underlying disorder. The spinal malalignment and trunk decompensation can affect standing balance in ambulatory patients and limit their ability to walk. In non-walkers the imbalance can lead to sitting intolerance and cause a child to become a hand-dependent sitter. It can also produce pain from

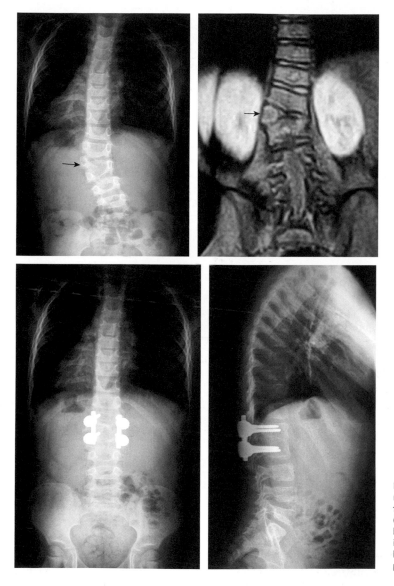

FIGURE 27.5 Pre-operative anteroposterior radiograph and magnetic resonance image of the spine showing a left L1 hemivertebra (black arrow). Posterior resection of the hemivertebra and segmental fusion with instrumentation resulted in a normal spinal balance in both the coronal and the sagittal planes

Table 27.2 Incidence (%) of neuromuscular conditions associated with scoliosis

Condition	Incidence (%)
Cerebral palsy	25
Myelomeningocele	60
Spinal muscular atrophy	67
Freidrich's ataxia	80
Duchenne muscular dystrophy	90
Spinal cord injury in children (before age 10 years)	100

impingement of the ribs against the iliac crest on the concavity of the scoliosis as the spine collapses and the pelvic obliquity progresses. Scoliosis in this group of severely disabled children may create cardiopulmonary complications and deteriorate pre-existing feeding disorders.

The management of neuromuscular scoliosis is directed at maintaining or improving functional abilities and the quality of life. Bracing may provide trunk support and improve posture, but does not prevent curve progression. Seating can be adapted to accommodate the spinal deformity, but also does not correct the deformity. Trunk support and seating modifications can be used as a temporizing measure to maintain function in young children with flexible deformities, to allow further spinal growth and delay surgery. Spinal fusion is the only treatment that is effective in these patients and involves an extensive spinal arthrodesis with instrumentation and allograft bone. It is indicated to improve seating stability, maintain function, improve the quality of life and prevent cardiorespiratory compromise (Fig. 27.6). A multidisciplinary approach is essential when surgical treatment is anticipated to reduce the significant risks of potentially life-threatening complications that can occur in the peri-operative period.

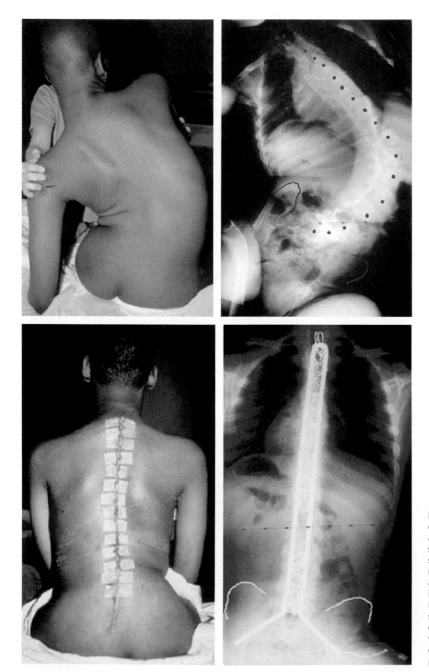

FIGURE 27.6 Pre-operative and post-operative clinical photographs and anteroposterior radiographs of the spine show a typical severe long C-shaped right thoracolumbar neuromuscular scoliosis with significant associated pelvic obliquity causing impingement of the ribs against the iliac crest on the concavity of the scoliosis in a patient with quadriplegic cerebral palsy. A posterior spinal fusion was performed and resulted in correction of the scoliosis and a level pelvis

KYPHOSIS AND LORDOSIS

In the lateral (sagittal) plane, kyphosis is a forward bend of the spine and lordosis is a backward bend of the spine. The spine has a physiological kyphosis in the thoracic and a lordosis in the cervical and lumbar spines (Box 27.1). The normal thoracic kyphosis should not exceed 40–50° and the normal lumbar lordosis should be up to 60°.

Congenital kyphosis, like congenital scoliosis, can occur as the result of an anterior failure of vertebral segmentation (anterior unsegmented bar) or failure of vertebral formation (anterior hemi-

vertebra). Congenital kyphosis is often associated with neurological compromise as the cord is stretched over the angular deformity and early surgical treatment is required.

A kyphotic deformity can develop following spondylodiscitis where there is infection of contiguous vertebral end-plates, after irradiation to the spine to treat a neoplastic lesion or steroid therapy causing generalized osteopenia, and following spinal trauma that involves the anterior column of the spine and produces foreshortening of the anterior aspect of the vertebral body (anterior wedge or compression fracture). Kyphosis can occasionally be seen in patients with rheumatological disorders.

Scheuermann's disease (juvenile kyphosis) is characterized by at least three contiguous anteriorly wedged vertebrae and affects boys more than girls. The cause of the condition is largely unknown and should be differentiated from a postural (roundback) kyphosis where there are no structural abnormalities. If the Scheuermann's deformity is severe and creates back pain that is refractory to conservative measures, surgery to straighten and fuse the spine may be indicated (Fig. 27.7).

An increased lumbar lordosis is most commonly seen in association with a flexion contracture of the hips that causes an anterior pelvic tilt.

Box 27.1
Aetiology for an increased kyphosis

- Congenital
- Neuromuscular
- Post-traumatic
- Postural
- Scheuermann's disease
- Juvenile rheumatoid arthritis and ankylosing spondylitis
- Post-infection, e.g. TB

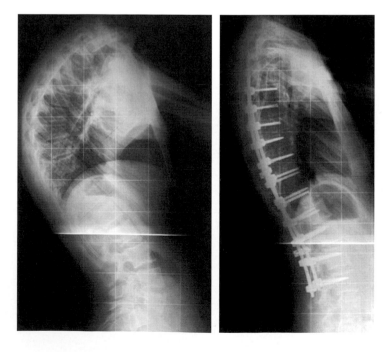

FIGURE 27.7 Scheuermann's kyphosis and anterior wedging of three consecutive thoracic vertebrae in an adolescent male who underwent a posterior spinal fusion combined with multi-level posterior wedge osteotomies. This resulted in restoration of a normal sagittal balance of the spine

337

BACK PAIN IN CHILDREN

Severe back pain occurring during childhood and adolescence is relatively uncommon, but persisting pain often has a serious underlying cause and should be investigated thoroughly (Table 27.3; see also Chapter 1, 'Red flags').

Clinical approach

The history should attempt to differentiate mechanical from non-mechanical sources of spinal pain. Mechanical pain is aggravated by physical activities and alleviated by rest or change of body position. In contrast, non-mechanical pain is more constant and remains unaltered by activity. Is there a history of preceding trauma or infection? A recent urinary tract infection or otitis media may point towards a discitis or vertebral osteomyelitis. Are there any general symptoms, such as high temperature, lethargy, malaise, pallor, anorexia, weight loss, bowel or bladder function change, which may implicate malignancy or infection? About 6% of children with acute lymphocytic leukaemia present initially with back pain. Did the pain appear acutely or was there a gradual onset of symptoms? How long did the pain last? Mild pain that has been present for a short period following intense athletic activities can be attributed to muscle sprain or overuse, but spinal pain that has persisted without improvement over weeks or months requires further investigation. Which factors provoke or worsen the pain? Spondylolysis and spondylolisthesis frequently arise in children participating in sports that involve repetitive hyperextension of the spine.

Enquire about location, radiation, severity, frequency and nature of the pain, and its effect on activities. Back pain can be localized to a small area of the spine – a typical example being pain associated with spondylolysis/spondylolisthesis or spinal neoplasms. In contrast, generalized thoracic discomfort in adolescents is commonly seen in Scheuermann's kyphosis. Radiation of the pain to the buttocks or the lower limbs, with or without associated neurological findings such as numbness, tingling or muscle weakness, may indicate a disc herniation or a space-occupying intraspinal lesion. Bowel or bladder incontinence, loss of balance or coordination, and change in the gait may be related to spinal cord pathology, including spinal dysraphism or neoplasm. Mild changes in gait and loss of previous motor skills suggest subtle neurological changes.

Persistent night pain, unrelated to physical activities and unresponsive to rest, may be the initial complaint in a tumour, infection or inflammatory condition involving the vertebral column or the spinal cord. Immediate relief of the pain (including night pain) with the use of aspirin or

Table 27.3 Differential diagnosis of back pain in children and adolescents

Developmental	Infection	Traumatic	Neoplasms		Visceral
Scheuermann's kyphosis	Discitis	Spondylolysis/ Spondylolisthesis	*Benign*		Abdominal neoplasms, pyelonephritis, appendicitis, retroperitoneal abscess
			Posterior	Anterior	
			Osteoid osteoma Osteoblastoma Aneurysmal bone cyst	Histiocystosis (eosinophilic granuloma)	
Painful scoliosis	Vertebral osteomyelitis	Herniated disc	*Malignant*		Gynaecological problems
			Leukaemia, lymphoma, sarcoma		
	Tuberculous spondylitis	Slipped vertebral apophysis			
		Vertebral fractures			
		Muscle strain			

non-steroidal anti-inflammatory drugs (NSAIDs) is suggestive of an osteoid osteoma. Patients with back pain and other joint symptoms relieved by NSAIDs may have juvenile rheumatoid arthritis or ankylosing spondylitis.

Enquire about the family history as conditions such as idiopathic scoliosis, disc herniations, and inflammatory joint or hereditary neurological diseases may have a familial pattern of inheritance. Psychological causes of back pain do exist in children, but have a much lower prevalence than in the adults. Children can also mimic the symptoms of their parents, siblings, grandparents or friends. Children with complaints of spinal pain often report other unassociated sources of pain, such as recurrent headaches and abdominal discomfort. Conversion and psychosomatic conditions are a diagnosis of exclusion, but should always be considered.

The age of the child may also assist in differentiating between conditions. In children of less than 10 years of age, infection (especially discitis) and tumour are the most frequent causes of back pain. In children older than 10 years the conditions that are most commonly encountered are more benign and include overuse syndromes, spondylolysis, spondylolisthesis and Scheuermann's kyphosis. In general, young children are unlikely to exaggerate their symptoms.

Inflammatory conditions, such as juvenile ankylosing spondylitis, can be seen occasionally in children and adolescents. Often the complaints are of vague spinal pain, symptoms in other joints, mainly the hips, and systemic manifestations, such as stiffness, fatigue and decreased stamina.

Examination and investigations

The child should then be examined using the principles detailed above. An AP and lateral radiograph of the spine localized to the symptomatic area comprise the initial radiological investigation. Disc narrowing, irregularity of the vertebral endplates, Schmorl's nodes, destructive radiolucent or radiodense lesions, vertebral scalloping, congenital vertebral anomalies, evidence of a fracture or a pars interarticularis defect and osteopenia, are some of the abnormal findings detectable on plain radiography. Anterior or posterior wedging of vertebral bodies suggestive of vertebral fractures will be evident on lateral views. Irregularity of vertebral end-plates usually points towards infection, and if

that involves multiple levels mycobacterial infection must be excluded. Absence of a pedicle or the spinous process may indicate the presence of a tumour, while increased interpedicular distance across one or more levels suggests the presence of an intraspinal pathology, such as spinal dysraphism or neoplasm. If spinal instability is suspected, an AP and standing lateral flexion–extension views should be obtained. Adequate visualization of the pelvis is necessary, as pelvic pathology may manifest as low back pain.

Further imaging may be required (see Chapter 4). A technetium bone scan can delineate discitis, vertebral neoplasms, occult or stress fractures. CT is helpful for bony pathology and MRI is the optimal study to assess the spinal cord and exclude the presence of intraspinal dysraphic lesions, neoplasms, herniated discs, slipped vertebral apophysis, discitis and cord damage after spinal trauma. Routine laboratory tests are not generally indicated in the evaluation of paediatric back pain, but can be invaluable when an infection, neoplasia or inflammatory aetiology is suspected.

Spondylolysis and spondylolisthesis

Spondylolysis is a unilateral or bilateral defect in the pars interarticularis and can occur in children and adolescents who undertake physical activities that include repetitive hyperextension of the trunk (gymnasts, swimmers, dancers). Spondylolysis most commonly affects the 5th lumbar vertebra. Spondylolisthesis occurs when one vertebral body moves anteriorly in relation to the adjacent inferior vertebral body or the sacrum. The most common location for a spondylolisthesis is the lumbosacral joint with the body of L5 displacing forward in relation to the sacrum. The classification is shown in Table 27.4. Dysplastic and isthmic spondylolisthesis may occur in children and adolescents.

Children usually present in early adolescence complaining of mechanical midline low lumbar pain precipitated by strenuous activities and protracted standing. Hamstring tightness and the Phalen–Dickson sign (walking with the hips and knees flexed) may be evident. The pars defect is best shown on localized CT scans at the level of the spondylolysis/listhesis.

Management is usually conservative and involves activity modification, pain relief and physiotherapy to reduce extension stresses on the spine. NSAIDs should be avoided in patients with an acute unilateral spondylolysis because they can inhibit ossification and healing of the pars defect. Some children may benefit from a short underarm brace, which can be successful in relieving the symptoms in up to 80% of patients with grade 0 or 1 spondylolisthesis. Posterolateral spinal fusion in situ with the use of autologous bone graft across

Table 27.4 Newman classification of spondylolisthesis

Type of spondylolisthesis	Cause of spondylolisthesis
Lytic	Stress fracture of pars interarticularis separating posterior elements from vertebral body
Degenerative	Arthritic changes in the posterior facet joints leading to joint subluxation and instability
Traumatic	Fractures and ligament injuries leading to instability and vertebral displacement
Dysplastic	Congenital abnormalities of posterior facet joints which allow severe displacement due to lack of the normal restraints
Pathological	Instability due to primary bone tumours, metastases or generalized pathology

the affected motion segment is usually effective for persisting symptoms. In the presence of a severe spondylolisthesis, the use of instrumentation with bone graft can restore the lateral balance of the lumbosacral junction (Fig. 27.8). In general, surgical treatment should be considered in growing children with a spondylolisthesis of greater than 50% due to the high risk of further progression, where there is evidence of progressive slippage radiologically and for persisting pain in spondylolysis.

Spinal infection

This includes infection affecting the disc in isolation (discitis) and a vertebral osteomyelitis; the latter may progress to soft-tissue involvement and abscess formation. It usually results from haematogenous seeding of bacteria originating from other sources of infection, such as otitis media, urinary or upper respiratory tract infections.

Back pain is the presenting symptom in 50% of children with discitis. Children younger than 3 years of age are less likely to complain of back pain, but will present with a limp or difficulty weight-bearing, not wanting to be moved very much. They may also present with generalized malaise and fever. The older child (between 3 and 8 years of age) may present with less specific symptoms, including vague abdominal or back pain, mild fever, elevated blood white cell count and decreased activity. Adolescents will complain mostly of back pain, which is usually well localized in the lower

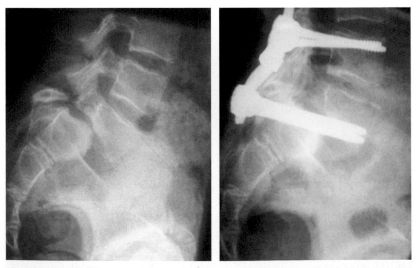

FIGURE 27.8 Adolescent patient with bilateral spondylolysis and a severe isthmic spondylolisthesis at L5–S1 who underwent a posterior spinal fusion extending from L4 to S1, which restored the sagittal balance of the spine across the lumbosacral joint

thoracic, thoracolumbar or lumbar spine and may have developed an abnormal antalgic posture, which is more evident with flexion (painful scoliosis). They may also report radicular pain affecting the buttock and leg due to nerve root irritation.

Vertebral osteomyelitis occurs as bacteria spread from the intervertebral disc to the vertebral body. Children with vertebral osteomyelitis usually have more significant systemic symptoms than those with a discitis. The symptoms include an elevated temperature, back pain, abdominal, chest, neck or flank pain, gait abnormalities with a noticeable limp and increased tenderness on the spine with stiffness on examination.

Clinical approach

A low-grade fever may be present and younger children may refuse to crawl or walk. Usually there will be localized tenderness on palpation at the site of infection. There may be signs of an irritable hip, paravertebral muscle spasm, limitation of spinal motion and hamstring tightness. Limitation of straight leg raising may be present, but other abnormal neurological findings are usually absent. A complete neurological examination should be performed.

Investigations

Full blood count with white cell differentials, erythrocyte sedimentation rate (ESR), C-reactive protein (CRP) and blood cultures are required. The white blood cell count is often within normal limits or slightly elevated with mild leucocytosis. An AP and lateral plain radiograph of the spine can be normal at the early stages of the infection. When the symptoms have been present for at least 1 week, the plain radiographs may reveal intervertebral disc space narrowing and involvement of the vertebral body. MRI is best for further imaging as it shows the affected disc space, neural structures and surrounding soft tissues, and can differentiate between isolated disc involvement and vertebral osteomyelitis, epidural or paraspinal abscesses. Needle biopsy of the disc space or the vertebral body is not usually required if a spinal infection is suspected; however, this will be necessary if there is suspicion of a tumour.

Treatment

Staphylococcus aureus is the organism most commonly identified and the patients are initially treated with intravenous anti-staphylococcal antibiotics until the symptoms subside followed by a course of oral antibiotics for 3–6 weeks. The development of an epidural abscess or neurological compromise is a surgical emergency. The development of a post-infection spinal deformity may also require surgical reconstruction.

Tuberculous spondylitis (see Chapter 29)

Intervertebral disc herniation

The incidence is much less common than in adults and accounts for only 1–4% of all disc herniations. The most commonly affected segments are L4/L5 and L5/S1. The incidence of a herniated disc in males is greater than in females by a ratio of 2:1 or 3:1, but as girls mature faster than boys they are more likely to develop disc herniations at an earlier age.

Clinical presentation

Symptoms are often intermittent and there is often a delay in diagnosis. Children commonly present with back pain and trunk stiffness, with or without sciatica. Symptoms may be aggravated with prolonged sitting and standing or by coughing and sneezing. A history of trauma is given as a precipitating factor in about 50% of the patients. Children tend to have a paucity of abnormal neurological findings. However, straight and crossed leg raising tests are usually positive. Motor weakness and bowel or bladder dysfunction are uncommon. The back is rigid with marked limitation of spinal mobility, especially in the lumbar spine during flexion. There is also localized tenderness on palpation in the lower lumbar region adjacent to the disc pathology with associated elimination of normal lumbar lordosis. Scoliosis may be present with a significant trunk shift due to paraspinal muscle spasm, but no evidence of vertebral rotation. Plain radiographs may show a coronal or sagittal plane deformity due to asymmetrical muscle spasm. MRI is the most useful imaging test to illustrate the pathology.

Treatment

Initially children should be managed conservatively; this includes bed-rest, NSAIDs and muscle relaxants, followed by gradual mobilization. The symptoms will persist in about 40% of cases and indications for surgery include failure of conservative measures and a significant or progressive neurological deficit. Approximately 90% of patients report good or excellent short-term results after disc excision.

Neoplasms

A benign or malignant tumour should always be considered in the differential diagnosis for back pain in children and adolescents. Malignant primary tumours of the spine are rare in children. Non-mechanical pain and red flag features are the predominant presenting symptom of a tumour, but occasionally the symptoms can be non-specific and cause a delay in diagnosis. The presence of a painful scoliosis (antalgic scoliosis), localized tenderness on examination or a palpable mass are important physical signs to guide the diagnosis.

Benign tumours include an osteoid osteoma, osteoblastoma, aneurysmal bone cyst and eosinophilic granuloma. A Ewing's sarcoma and an osteosarcoma are the most common examples of primary malignant bone tumours affecting the spine. Spinal involvement causing persistent back pain may be the first presentation of an acute lymphocytic leukaemia.

DISORDERS OF UPPER MOTOR NEURONE, SPINAL CORD, PERIPHERAL NERVES AND MUSCLE IN CHILDREN

The majority of children with a disorder of motor pathways from cortex to muscle will present with delayed motor milestones. This may be from birth with a child who is weak and floppy. Some experienced mothers may have been aware that their child moved less than usual in utero. Other children may present with delayed sitting, crawling or walking (Table 27.5). Such motor delay is found in children with global developmental delay, but the problems in development of language or hand skills may not be apparent until the child is older.

An infant may be floppy at birth because of a central neurological problem or acute illness, such as neonatal infection or hypoxic–ischaemic encephalopathy. The presence of contractures at

Table 27.5 Usual age of achieving major motor milestones for term infants

Skill	Age	Comments
Sitting	6 months	
Crawling	9 months	10% of children bottom-shuffle rather than crawl
Standing	10 months	
Walking	12–14 months	97% walk 6 steps unaided by 18 months
Reaching for toy	6 months	Manipulates toy by 14 months

birth – arthrogryposis – points to a peripheral neuromuscular disorder, such as congenital muscular dystrophy. Congenital contractures may be seen in any disorder that limits fetal movement, including spina bifida. There may be associated brain and eye malformations in congenital muscular dystrophy and these children require detailed investigations including neuroimaging and genetic studies. The congenital myopathies may also present with weakness and low tone at birth, and are differentiated by muscle biopsy and gene analysis. Although individually rare, it is important to make a diagnosis as some are associated with malignant hyperpyrexia.

In all the neuromuscular conditions that present at birth, close attention must be paid to respiratory function as the child grows. Kyphoscoliosis may progress rapidly as part of the condition, further impairing lung function. Nocturnal ventilation or airways pressure support may be required from early childhood.

SPINAL MUSCULAR ATROPHY

The commonest single genetic cause of the floppy infant is spinal muscular atrophy (SMA). The clinical phenotype can vary considerably with children with mild forms being able to walk eventually, but the majority of children with SMA have a very poor prognosis. Mothers may be aware of reduced fetal movements, and children are weak and floppy from or soon after birth (Fig. 27.9). Weakness is progressive, sparing facial muscles initially. Respi-

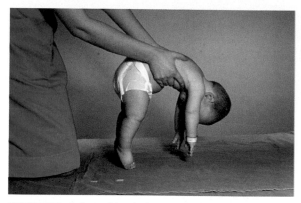

FIGURE 27.9 Infant with spinal muscular atrophy type 1 showing truncal hypotonia (Courtesy of Dr J K Brown)

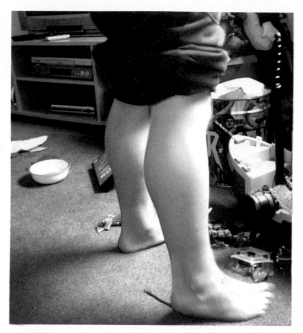

FIGURE 27.10 Pseudohypertrophy of muscles in muscular dystrophy

343

ratory failure devolops and the children often have a bell-shaped chest. Survival beyond the age of 18 months is rare, although with the use of home ventilation some children will survive much longer. Intellect is normal. It is not clear whether this prolonged survival is accompanied by an acceptable quality of life.

DUCHENNE MUSCULAR DYSTROPHY

Delay in gross motor skills in a boy is the usual presentation of Duchenne muscular dystrophy (DMD). Occasionally, the presenting symptom may be delayed language skills. Dystrophin, the protein missing in DMD, is also expressed in the brain, and the mean IQ of boys with DMD is lower than that of their peer group. Creatine kinase (CK) blood levels can be used as a screening test for DMD and levels are usually many times above normal.

Any boy not walking by 18 months, with global developmental delay or with delayed speech development should have CK levels checked. If the level is very high, the family should be offered gene analysis for their son. Genetic testing can identify the gene abnormality – deletion in Xp21 gene – in 60–70% of boys and thus avoids the need for muscle biopsy. Determining the genetic defect gives the family a definitive diagnosis and also allows for genetic counselling of family members and prenatal diagnosis in subsequent pregnancies.

Clinical features include weakness, hypotonia and muscle hypertrophy (Fig. 27.10) early in the disease, followed by muscle atrophy. The boys may develop a foot drop because of muscle weakness

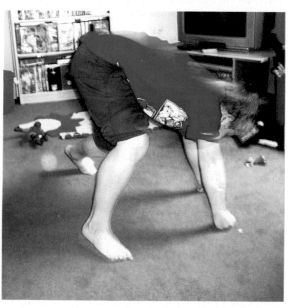

FIGURE 27.11 Boy demonstrating Gower's sign, which may be found in any cause of lower limb weakness

and occasionally present as a toe-walker. Once the boy becomes significantly weak, he rises from the floor in a typical fashion, pushing himself up with his hands. This is known as Gower's sign, but may be found in other causes of lower limb weakness (Fig. 27.11).

There is not yet a specific treatment for DMD. The boys will slowly lose motor skills in later childhood and the majority stop walking by early teenage years. Encouraging the boys to remain mobile on their feet for as long as possible should be tempered by the need to allow social mobility within their peer group. Interacting with friends is far easier in a powered wheelchair than in a walking frame with an adult supervisor hovering in the background.

Respiratory failure often develops in teenage years and the first symptoms may be morning headaches due to hypercarbia during sleep causing raised intracranial pressure. Nocturnal continuous positive airway pressure through a mask may relieve these symptoms and is usually well tolerated. Meticulous attention should be paid to treatment of intercurrent chest infections and it would be appropriate to offer the boys immunization against influenza and pneumococcus. Spinal deformity may also develop as in other childhood neuromuscular conditions once the boys stop walking and standing. If surgery to stabilize the spine is to be offered, it should be done early whilst the boy still has reasonable cardiorespiratory function. Although cardiac muscle is also involved in DMD, symptomatic cardiomyopathy is unusual, unlike in other neuromuscular conditions, such as Becker muscular dystrophy and Friedreich's ataxia.

Steroid therapy has been advocated in DMD to slow down the rate at which the boys lose motor skills. The mechanism by which steroids work at the cellular level is unclear. If therapy is used before the weakness has progressed to loss of walking, some boys will benefit significantly, although the side effects of weight gain, osteoporosis, fractures and cataracts may outweigh the benefits.

Survival is improving in DMD due to better management of chest infections and respiratory failure. At last, there are some possibilities of gene therapy for DMD, through techniques such as gene patching for gene deletions and drug therapy to bypass stop codon mutations. These may be available within the next 10 years. Hence it is essential to delay the secondary complications of DMD in boys being diagnosed now.

BECKER MUSCULAR DYSTROPHY

Becker muscular dystrophy (BMD) is caused by a mutation in the dystrophin gene that permits some dystrophin expression, hence BMD is a much less severe clinical phenotype than DMD. The boys retain community mobility into adult life, survive into middle age, at least, but are at risk of cardiomyopathy. There are rare autosomal genetic muscular dystrophies with phenotypes similar to DMD that usually require a muscle biopsy to reach the specific diagnosis.

HEREDITARY MOTOR AND SENSORY NEUROPATHY (CHARCOT–MARIE–TOOTH DISEASE)

Disorders of peripheral nerves such as hereditary motor and sensory neuropathy are rare in early childhood, and usually present in the older child with footdrop, abnormal walking pattern and clawing of the toes. Deterioration is slow, the sensory component is minimal until late in life and there is often a family history. Examination will reveal signs of a lower motor neurone lesion – wasting, weakness and diminished reflexes. The different types are clinically very similar and are distinguished by different patterns of inheritance and nerve conduction studies.

MYOTONIC DYSTROPHY

Myotonic dystrophy in childhood presents in one of two ways. The congenital variety may present as a floppy baby with arthrogryposis, feeding and respiratory difficulties. The child will be slow in all aspects of development. This disorder may also present in the older child with fatigue, expressionless face, articulation difficulties and, eventually, difficulty in relaxing grip.

CEREBRAL PALSY

Cerebral palsy is the motor symptoms caused by a non-progressive insult to the developing brain. There are three broad causes of cerebral palsy: abnormalities of brain growth and development, brain damage and impaired brain function. Depending on the timing, the extent and the distribution of the brain insult, the child may have problems in other areas of development – vision, language, learning or epilepsy – and these may be more disabling than the motor insult itself.

Cerebral palsy can be classified by:

1. Geographical distribution of the motor impairment
   a. hemiplegia
   b. diplegia
   c. quadriplegia
2. Abnormalities of tone and movement
   a. spastic – an increase of tone on passive stretch of muscle
   b. dystonic – an increase in tone on voluntary movement, change of position or posture
   c. dyskinetic – combination of above with involuntary movements
   d. ataxic – poor balance, often with low trunk muscle tone
3. Timing of insult
   a. antenatal
   b. perinatal
   c. postnatal
4. Gestation at birth
   a. premature
   b. term
5. If any additional impairments are present, this can be added to the diagnostic label, thus enabling communication between health professionals about that child's particular problems, e.g. a 2-year-old child with spastic quadriplegia of perinatal onset at term with associated learning difficulties and epilepsy.

The neurological examination of a child with cerebral palsy and spasticity will reveal signs of an upper motor neurone lesion:

- Weakness
- Poor control of fine movements
- Increased tone
- Brisk deep tendon reflexes.

Hemiplegic cerebral palsy is frequently caused by haemorrhage and/or ischaemia in the territory of the middle cerebral artery (Fig. 27.12). Diplegic cerebral palsy is usually caused by damage to the periventricular white matter (Fig. 27.13). There are many risk factors for diplegic cerebral palsy including prematurity and the causes of prematurity. Damage to developing white matter by cytokines is a common feature of pathogenic mechanisms. Quadriplegic cerebral palsy usually involves widespread damage in watershed areas between vascular territories, and in severe cases

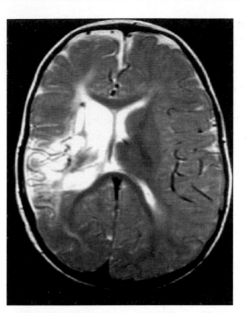

FIGURE 27.12 Magnetic resonance image of child with hemiplegic cerebral palsy demonstrating a middle cerebral artery infarct

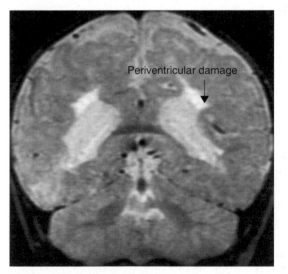

Periventricular damage

FIGURE 27.13 Periventricular damage typically seen in diplegic cerebral palsy

may result in severe atrophy of the brain with cystic changes. Dyskinetic cerebral palsy in its pure form is associated with damage to basal ganglia.

An affected limb may be short and in the severely affected child growth may be poor. Motor control of eye movements, facial muscles, and the muscles of chewing and swallowing may also be affected. Problems in the bulbar muscles – again with weakness, poor motor control, increased tone and exaggerated reflexes – will affect speech and feeding, and put the child at risk of aspiration pneumonia.

There are many recognized risk factors for cerebral palsy, some maternal, some antenatal and some perinatal. Placental dysfunction probably predisposes some fetuses to impaired brain blood supply, which can be exacerbated during labour. Only a small percentage (<10%) of cerebral palsy is due to brain damage acquired during labour and delivery.

The mode and age of presentation of cerebral palsy varies considerably from child to child. If a child has developed a severe neonatal encephalopathy from hypoxic–ischaemic encephalopathy or neonatal septicaemia, their development may never be normal. The child will go through a stage of altered conscious level, poor feeding, impaired spontaneous movements and low tone. It may be some months before the child starts to develop abnormally increased tone, appear microcephalic or show delay in acquisition of visual skills. Such a child is likely to develop a severe quadriplegic cerebral palsy with global developmental delay and will not be able to walk. Many, but not all, have learning difficulties and it is important to encourage language including non-verbal communication.

The child who subsequently develops a hemiplegia may not present until 6 months or older when it is apparent that one hand is not being used as much as the other. A mild hemiplegia may only be apparent when the child runs with poor reciprocal arm movement on the affected side or on performing intricate bimanual tasks. Virtually all children with hemiplegia walk well and it is associated epilepsy (present in up to 40%) or learning problems that impair quality of life as older children and adults (Fig. 27.14).

Children with diplegic cerebral palsy have motor skills that range from excellent with some sporting abilities to limited household mobility or even transfer ability only. The child may present with delayed gross motor skills, increased tone in the legs or toe-walking (Fig. 27.15). The majority will either have been born prematurely or their mothers will have had problems during pregnancy between 20 and 32 weeks, such as premature labour or antepartum haemorrhage.

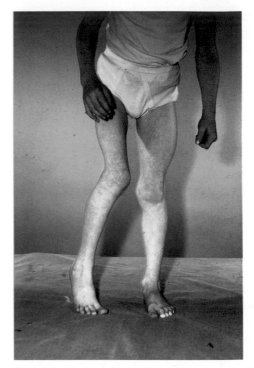

FIGURE 27.14 Boy with right hemiplegic cerebral palsy demonstrating wasting and contractures in the right leg

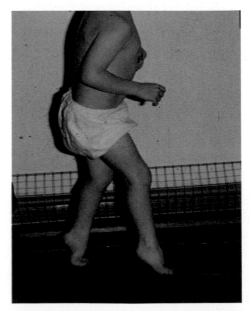

FIGURE 27.15 Child with diplegic cerebral palsy showing equinus position at ankle with foot contact by the forefoot only

The commonest tone abnormality in cerebral palsy is spasticity, measured as an increase in tone related to the velocity at which you stretch the child's muscle. Severe spasticity may be painful, interfere with function and may dislocate joints due to uneven pull of muscles. The hip joint is most vulnerable to dislocation in children with cerebral palsy, and appropriate positioning in sitting and lying of the child with severe spasticity from an early age may retard lateral migration of the hip joint. Therapies that reduce spasticity (predominantly drug therapy such as muscle relaxants, botulinus toxin injections and intrathecal baclofen) may prevent hip joint dislocation if used early, although the evidence for this is not yet strong. Spinal deformity is also commonly seen in total body involvement cerebral palsy.

Any child with reduced mobility is at risk of osteoporosis and the non-mobile child with cerebral palsy is no exception. It is unusual for the osteoporosis to be severe enough to lead to frequent or spontaneous fractures, but it may exacerbate the torsional effects of spasticity on bones. The use of a standing frame daily can encourage bone mineralization and is also an effective way of stretching hamstrings and hip flexors. Children with poor hip-joint development are at risk of developing painful arthritis of the hip in young adult life.

However, to encourage sarcomere growth in a spastic muscle, stretch of the muscle needs to be maintained for about 6 h a day. This can be achieved in the calf muscles by the use of well fitting ankle foot orthoses, which may also improve the gait pattern of the child with mobility. It is difficult to maintain stretch on other muscles during waking hours, hence the development of sleep systems that encourage good positioning at night.

The role of the physiotherapist is crucial in the management of the child with cerebral palsy. Ideally, they should be involved from the time the child is identified as at risk of developing cerebral palsy, e.g. at discharge from neonatal intensive care unit. The physiotherapist's role will change as the child's skills and difficulties develop. There are many different philosophies of physiotherapy with no good evidence that any of the mainstream types are better than others. An experienced physiotherapist will use a range of techniques adapted to meet the needs of the individual child with the judicious use of aids, such as orthoses, good seating techniques, and education of parents and other carers in a daily pattern of exercises. However, it is important that the therapy does not take over the child's or family's life, and the family should be given realistic goals as to what therapy should achieve.

The child with severe cerebral palsy in previous years was at risk of hip dislocation, multiple contractures, severe spinal deformity and cardiorespiratory failure (Fig. 27.16). With better nutrition, treatment of chest infections and overall care, even children with severe cerebral palsy and profound learning difficulties are likely to survive into adult life. However, it is important that quality of life is maintained as well as length of life. In the less severely affected child with cerebral palsy, there is more to life than walking, and social mobility and independence for the teenager and young adult with severe diplegic cerebral palsy may be better in a powered chair than in a walking frame or with sticks.

There is a small group of children described as having hypotonic cerebral palsy. Some may have an unidentified disorder of spinal cord, anterior horn cell, muscle or nerve, which may have a genetic origin. A few subsequently develop an ataxic cerebral palsy, with learning difficulties and perhaps epilepsy. Hypotonic children are also at risk of hip dislocation and kyphoscoliosis, not through spasticity, but through laxity of soft tissues and weakness. They may also be prone to the joint pains seen in children with hypermobility syndromes.

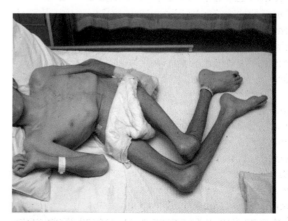

FIGURE 27.16 Boy with severe quadriplegic cerebral palsy, wasting and windswept posture with fixed contractures

FURTHER READING

Angevine PD, Lenke LG 2006 Thoracic and thoracolumbar idiopathic deformity. Neurosurg Clin N Am 17(3): 289–298.

Cassar-Pullicino VN, Eisenstein SM 2002 Imaging in scoliosis: what, why and how? Clin Radiol 57(7): 543–562.

Cutts S 2006 Managing scoliosis in adolescents. Practitioner 250(1685): 40–41, 43–44.

Steinbok P 2006 Selection of treatment modalities in children with spastic cerebral palsy. Neurosurg Focus 21(2): e4.

Straub V, Bushby K 2006 The childhood limb-girdle muscular dystrophies. Semin Pediatr Neurol 13(2): 104–114.

ARTHRITIS IN CHILDREN

28

Sally Edmonds

Cases relevant to this chapter

91, 94

●Essential facts

1. Juvenile idiopathic arthritis (JIA) affects 0.1% of the population.

2. The onset of JIA can be: polyarticular (five or more joints at presentation), oligoarticular (fewer than five joints at presentation) or systemic (features such as fever and rash at presentation).

3. Twenty per cent of children with anti-nuclear antibody (ANA)-positive oligoarticular JIA develop asymptomatic anterior uveitis, which can cause blindness if untreated.

4. Most children with polyarticular JIA do not have rheumatoid factor.

5. Polyarticular JIA may cause short stature and local growth impairment, such as micrognathia and retrognathia, brachydactyly and small hands and feet.

6. Typical features of systemic-onset JIA include high spiking fever, a transient episodic erythematous rash, lymphadenopathy, hepatosplenomegaly and pericarditis.

7. The differential diagnosis for systemic JIA includes infection, inflammatory bowel disease and malignancy (especially leukaemia and neuroblastoma).

8. Enthesitis-related arthritis is associated with HLA-B27 and usually presents with an enthesitis or a peripheral oligoarthritis.

9. In juvenile psoriatic arthritis most children present with an oligoarthritis of the knees or ankles, or the interphalangeal joints of the fingers and toes.

10. Persistent inflammation in a lower limb joint may lead to leg length discrepancy due to a longer affected limb.

11. Non-steroidal anti-inflammatory drugs (NSAIDs) are the first-line treatment for most children with JIA, and cause less gastrointestinal toxicity than in adults.

12. Intra-articular steroid injections are a safe, effective treatment in JIA.

13. Children with persistent joint inflammation despite treatment with NSAIDs and intra-articular steroids should be offered disease-modifying anti-rheumatic drugs (DMARDs), usually methotrexate; if they fail to respond, anti-TNF treatment should be given.

14. Multidisciplinary management of JIA includes rheumatologists, paediatricians, orthopaedic surgeons, ophthalmologists, clinical nurse specialists, physiotherapists, occupational therapists, podiatrists, orthotists, dieticians and clinical psychologists.

Arthritis is commonly thought of as a disease of older people and it may be surprising to learn that children, sometimes less than 1 year old, may also be affected. Whilst children obviously do not suffer from the degenerative arthritis that is becoming such a burden in the ever ageing population, they are susceptible to a number of different inflammatory arthritides. Juvenile idiopathic arthritis (JIA) affects approximately 0.1% of the population, although prevalence rates vary between countries and races. The childhood arthritides, just as in adulthood, are a heterogeneous group of diseases, but most are different from adult rheumatoid arthritis (RA).

CLASSIFICATION

It is difficult to classify diseases where the precise aetiology is unknown, and JIA is no exception. For arthritis to be classified as 'juvenile' rather than 'adult' the age of onset must be before 16 years. The duration of the arthritis must be a minimum of 6 weeks in at least one joint, and other causes of arthritis, such as infection, must have been excluded. Broadly, JIA is classified as having three types of onset: polyarticular (five or more joints at presentation), oligoarticular (fewer than five joints at presentation) and systemic (features such as fever and rash at presentation). Presentation in this context means the first 6 months of disease. The most recent classification of idiopathic arthritis in childhood is shown in Box 28.1.

Box 28.1
Classification of juvenile idiopathic arthritis

- Systemic onset
- Polyarthritis (rheumatoid factor negative)
- Polyarthritis (rheumatoid factor positive)
- Oligoarthritis (persistent)
- Oligoarthritis (extended)
- Enthesitis-related arthritis
- Psoriatic arthritis
- Other (not meeting above criteria, or meeting more than one criterion)

OLIGOARTICULAR JUVENILE IDIOPATHIC ARTHRITIS

Oligoarthritis is by far the most common subgroup of JIA, accounting for approximately 50% of cases. This type of arthritis may persist with fewer than five joints being affected, or, if more joints become affected after the first 6 months of disease, then it is said to have become 'extended' oligoarticular JIA and, not surprisingly, has a worse prognosis than those that have persistent oligoarticular disease. This type of juvenile arthritis most commonly affects young girls, usually in the 4–6 years age group. The knee is the most common joint to be affected, with wrists and ankles also likely to be involved (Fig. 28.1).

Eye disease in oligoarticular juvenile idiopathic arthritis

Children with oligoarticular JIA are susceptible to inflammatory eye disease (anterior uveitis/iridocyclitis), especially if they are anti-nuclear antibody (ANA) positive. The overall incidence of uveitis in children with arthritis is in the order of 20%. It is essential to remember that this type of eye disease is asymptomatic and must, therefore, be screened for as soon as the joint disease is diagnosed. Unfortunately, eye disease may pre-date joint disease, and irreversible damage may have occurred before anyone is aware that the problem exists. Screening for uveitis is a simple, rapid process, performed by an ophthalmologist using a standard slit-lamp ophthalmoscope. If uveitis is detected, most cases respond very well to topical steroid therapy. By contrast, undetected uveitis in childhood can lead to blindness.

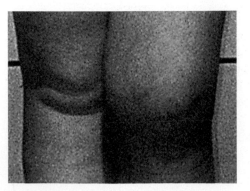

FIGURE 28.1 Oligoarticular juvenile idiopathic arthritis

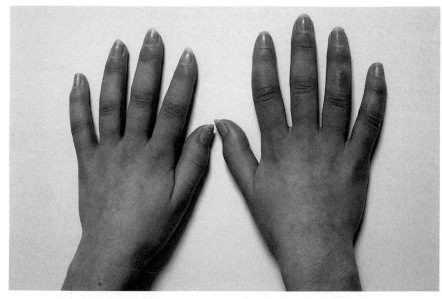

FIGURE 28.2 Polyarticular juvenile idiopathic arthritis

POLYARTICULAR JUVENILE IDIOPATHIC ARTHRITIS

Arthritis affecting five or more joints at presentation may be rheumatoid factor (RF) negative or positive (Fig. 28.2). The latter is much less common in children than in adults, and usually affects teenage girls. When it does occur, it behaves very much like adult RA and responds to the same drugs. RF-negative polyarticular disease, like RF-positive arthritis, tends to be symmetrical, but differs in that it may affect the distal interphalangeal joints, which RF-positive disease never does (one of the few 'nevers' in medicine!).

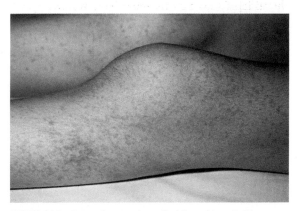

FIGURE 28.3 Systemic-onset juvenile idiopathic arthritis

SYSTEMIC-ONSET JUVENILE IDIOPATHIC ARTHRITIS

As the name implies, this is chronic arthritis in childhood that is associated with systemic features including: high spiking fever, with one or two daily spikes, often in the afternoon or early evening; transient episodic erythematous rash, often described as 'salmon pink'; lymphadenopathy; hepatosplenomegaly; and pericarditis in about 30% of cases. The systemic features may, and often do, precede the arthritis (Fig. 28.3). Girls are only slightly more commonly affected than boys, and onset is usually between 3 and 4 years of age.

ENTHESITIS-RELATED ARTHRITIS

As with the adult forms of the disease – principally adult ankylosing spondylitis (AS) – this type of juvenile arthritis is strongly associated with HLA-B27. However, unlike adult AS, children rarely present with sacroiliitis, and much more commonly present with an enthesitis (inflammation at a site where ligament, tendon or fascia attaches to bone) or a peripheral oligoarthritis, usually in the lower limb. Enthesitis is common in the foot, particularly at the calcaneal enthesis.

JUVENILE-ONSET PSORIATIC ARTHRITIS

Juvenile psoriatic arthritis is defined as the association, but not necessarily the coincidence, of arthritis and psoriasis. The child himself/herself may not have the typical psoriatic rash at the time of diagnosis, but may have a family history of psoriasis, or other features such as nail pitting or dactylitis. Approximately 70% of children will have an oligoarthritis at presentation, either of the knees or ankles, or the interphalangeal joints of the fingers and toes. Again, girls are more commonly affected than boys.

DIFFERENTIAL DIAGNOSIS

The differential diagnosis of systemic-onset JIA may be particularly difficult, not only because the systemic features may pre-date the arthritis, but also because many conditions may present with fever and rash. The three conditions most frequently mistaken for systemic JIA are infection, inflammatory bowel disease and malignancy. Of the malignancies, leukaemia and neuroblastoma most commonly present with arthralgia.

Arthritis where only one or two joints are affected may also pose problems with diagnosis. Septic arthritis, although uncommon, must always be excluded. There are usually clues, such as a high C-reactive protein (CRP) level, which would usually be normal or only slightly elevated if the diagnosis was oligoarticular JIA. Reactive arthritis, seen in association with an extra-articular infection, both viral and bacterial, is common, and taking a careful history is essential. Reactive arthritis is most commonly seen following gastrointestinal infections such as *Salmonella* and *Shigella*, but post-streptococcal arthritis is not uncommon in children, although true rheumatic fever is rare.

Hip disease is unusual at the onset of JIA, and if a child presents with hip pain other causes must be excluded. Whilst straightforward 'irritable hip' is common, more serious diagnoses, such as infection, congenital dislocation, slipped upper femoral epiphysis and malignancy, should not be forgotten.

COMPLICATIONS OF JUVENILE ARTHRITIS

Extra-articular complications, other than those seen in association with systemic disease, are rare. Eye disease in association with oligoarticular JIA has already been discussed. Enthesitis-related arthritis is also associated with eye disease, but, like the adult HLA-B27-associated diseases, this tends to be symptomatic uveitis, where the eye is red and painful, and screening is, therefore, unnecessary.

Disturbances of growth, both local and generalized, may occur in JIA. Polyarticular disease itself may cause inhibition of growth, not only in terms of short stature, but also more specific growth abnormalities, including micrognathia and retrognathia secondary to temporo-mandibular joint involvement, brachydactyly and small hands and feet. Steroids given systemically may further inhibit growth and also cause generalized osteoporosis. However, ongoing active disease is also detrimental to growth and bone density, and it is achieving the right balance between amount of steroid given and disease activity that is crucial.

Local growth disturbances can also occur. In a growing child, persistent inflammation in a joint may lead to overgrowth of that joint. If this occurs at the knee, leg-length discrepancy occurs (Fig. 28.4).

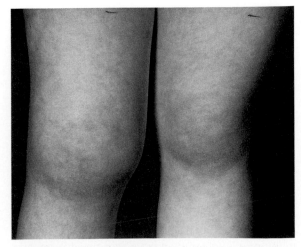

FIGURE 28.4 Leg-length discrepancy due to overgrowth of inflamed knee

As with any chronic inflammatory disease, AA amyloid may occur in JIA, especially in the systemic-onset subgroup (see section on amyloidosis in Chapter 18). However, amyloidosis is less common these days, probably because of improved treatments.

INVESTIGATIONS

Initial investigations may not be particularly helpful in making a diagnosis of JIA, as they are often normal, particularly in oligoarticular disease, but may be useful for differentiating JIA from other conditions such malignancy. A full blood count (FBC) and inflammatory markers in the form of erythrocyte sedimentation rate (ESR) and CRP should be performed in most children. Blood should also be sent to look for ANAs, because of their significance in relation to eye disease. RF is almost always negative, and needs to be looked for only in older children or teenagers who present with polyarticular disease. Other investigations, such as viral titres, serum ferritin (raised in systemic-onset JIA) and antistreptolysin O titres, may be appropriate, depending on individual circumstances. Plain X-rays are also often unhelpful initially, but may need to be done, for example in a child presenting with hip pain where the diagnosis may be 'orthopaedic' rather than 'rheumatological'. Other, more specialized investigations, such as ultrasound and magnetic resonance imaging, have their place, but clearly need to be used discriminatingly.

MANAGEMENT OF JUVENILE IDIOPATHIC ARTHRITIS

The approach to the management of children with arthritis is often different to that of adults, not only because the childhood arthritides are, on the whole, different diseases to the adult forms, but also because factors such as growth must be taken into consideration. Children may be more resistant to drug toxicity than adults, particularly with respect to the non-steroidal anti-inflammatory drugs (NSAIDs). However, other drugs, for example glucocorticoids, may have adverse effects on children, such as inhibition of growth, that would not be a problem in adults.

DRUG THERAPY

NSAIDs remain the first-line treatment for most children with JIA, and cause less gastrointestinal toxicity than they do in adults. Ibuprofen, naproxen and diclofenac are the most commonly used anti-inflammatories in children. The doses given may be quite high; for example, ibuprofen may be given at doses of 20–40 mg/kg/day. Some NSAIDs, including ibuprofen, come in liquid or dispersible forms, which are of great value in treating children.

Children should be reviewed after 1 or 2 months on NSAIDs, and if there has been no improvement additional treatment should be considered. Intra-articular steroid injections are a safe and effective way of reducing swelling and inflammation in individual joints and several joints may be injected at one time. In younger children, this needs to be done under general anaesthetic, but older children will usually tolerate the procedure under sedation or local anaesthetic.

Children who have persistent joint inflammation in spite of treatment with NSAIDs and intra-articular steroids will need disease-modifying anti-rheumatic drugs (DMARDs). Methotrexate is by far the most commonly used DMARD, but sulfasalazine, hydroxychloroquine and ciclosporin are also used. Methotrexate may be given orally, although some children do not absorb it very well, in which case it may be given as a subcutaneous injection. The starting dose for methotrexate is usually 10 mg/m^2 of body surface area as a weekly dose, building up to 20 or 25 mg (and sometimes more) as necessary. More recently, the biologic agents, in particular, the anti-TNFα drug etanercept, are being used in children who have particularly resistant disease.

Systemic glucocorticoids will need to be employed if a child has life-threatening complications of systemic disease or, less commonly, if there has been a general deterioration in the child's health or a more serious joint problem, the aim being to enable the child to function more normally. The starting dose would be in the region of 1–2 mg/kg of prednisolone, but should be kept to a minimum and an alternate-day regimen used whenever possible.

NON-DRUG THERAPY

The key to the successful management of a child with chronic arthritis is a team approach. In addition to rheumatologists, paediatricians, orthopaedic surgeons and ophthalmologists, the team includes clinical nurse specialists, physiotherapists, occupational therapists, podiatrists, orthotists, dieticians and clinical psychologists.

The clinical nurse specialist has a vital role to play in helping the child and their family in coming to terms with the diagnosis. He or she can give general advice and answer many of the questions that are bound to arise and, specifically, give information about the drugs that will be prescribed. These nurses are often the main link between the child and their family and the doctors.

Physiotherapy is vital for maintaining joint mobility, increasing muscle strength and preventing deformity. Exercise also helps to stimulate skeletal growth and prevent osteoporosis, and an exercise programme, tailored to the individual child, should be part of the daily routine. Hydrotherapy is particularly useful for treating children with arthritis, as the warmth and buoyancy of the water enable the child to move more freely and achieve more than they would on dry land. Children should be encouraged to go swimming, and cycling is also an excellent form of exercise.

The role of the occupational therapist is to assess functional skills and provide training in independence, to adapt equipment and provide aids, to assess hand function, to encourage activities to improve dexterity, muscle power and joint range, and to provide splints. Splinting is essential in maintaining joint position and function, although children often do not like wearing them! Great care must be taken over the making and fitting of splints so that the child will co-operate with wearing them. So-called 'night resting' splints for the knee and wrist are the most commonly employed splints.

It should never be forgotten that the child with JIA may well grow up into the adolescent, and then the adult, with JIA. This transition needs to be managed carefully, preferably by a physician who has a particular interest and expertise in this area, in order that this particularly difficult time is eased both for the patient and their family.

FURTHER READING

1. Hull RG 2001 Guidelines for the management of childhood arthritis. Rheumatology 40(11): 1309–1312.
2. Sathananthan R, David J 1997 The adolescent with rheumatic disease. Arch Dis Child 77: 355–358.
3. Southwood TR 1997 Classifying childhood arthritis. Ann Rheum Dis 56: 79–81.

DEVELOPING WORLD

355

29

MUSCULOSKELETAL PROBLEMS IN THE DEVELOPING WORLD

Benjamin Joseph

Cases relevant to this chapter

33

●Essential facts

1. There are differences in disease patterns in the developing world due to the following: diseases unique to tropical areas; poverty resulting in poor hygiene and malnutrition; genetic effects; social customs.

2. Over 70% of patients with human immunodeficiency virus (HIV) infection have musculoskeletal problems including myopathies, bone and joint infections, neoplasia, inflammatory arthritides and avascular necrosis of bone.

3. Reiter's syndrome is 100 to 200 times more frequent in HIV-infected patients than in the general population; up to 10% of HIV-infected

patients develop Reiter's syndrome with severe symptoms that do not respond well to anti-inflammatory drugs.

4. HIV-associated arthritis is a sub-acute oligoarthritis, which responds well to intra-articular steroid injections.

5. Tuberculosis of the spine accounts for 40–60% of all cases of skeletal tuberculosis.

6. Skeletal manifestations of sickle cell disease are due to blockage of the small vessels within bone by sickled red blood cells, resulting in thrombosis and infarction of bone; the necrotic bone is susceptible to infection.

Diseases of the musculoskeletal system seen in the developing world differ from those seen in the UK (Table 29.1) for four reasons: many patients live in tropical areas with diseases unique to these environments; poverty contributes through poor hygiene and malnutrition; there are differences in genetic predisposition to disease; and different social customs influence the pattern of disease. It is important to be aware of these differences while either working in the developing world or dealing with immigrants from the developing world.

MUSCULOSKELETAL PROBLEMS ASSOCIATED WITH HUMAN IMMUNODEFICIENCY VIRUS INFECTION

The musculoskeletal system may be affected in over 70% of patients with human immunodeficiency virus (HIV) infection by inflammatory, infective

Table 29.1 Factors contributing to differences in prevalence of various diseases of the musculoskeletal system in the UK and in the developing world

Condition	Prevalence in the UK	Prevalence in the developing world	Reasons for the difference in prevalence
Developmental dysplasia of the hip	High	Low	Genetic and racial factors (the condition is distinctly uncommon in African races)
Primary osteoarthrosis of the hip	High	Very low	Genetic and racial factors
Nutritional rickets	Very rare	High	Poverty and malnutrition are common in the developing world
Chronic osteomyelitis	Rare	Common	Early diagnosis and treatment of acute osteomyelitis often not possible due to poverty
Symptomatic hallux valgus	High	Very rare	Social customs (footwear is often not used in the developing world and those who use footwear seldom use closed-toe shoes)

Table 29.2 Musculoskeletal manifestations of HIV infection and AIDS

Myopathies	Pyomyositis
	Polymyositis
	AZT myopathy
Skeletal infections	Tuberculous osteomyelitis
	Bacillary angiomatosis
Neoplasia	Non-Hodgkin's lymphoma
	Kaposi's sarcoma*
Inflammatory arthropathies	Reiter's syndrome
	Psoriatic arthritis**
	HIV-associated arthritis
	Painful articular syndrome*
	Hypertrophic osteoarthropathy
Osteonecrosis	Osteonecrosis of the femoral head

Note:
* Seen in patients with AIDS
** May precede full-blown AIDS
The other conditions listed in the table are seen in patients with HIV infection and they usually appear before the onset of full-blown AIDS

or neoplastic processes that are either unique to HIV infection or secondary to immunocompromise. Musculoskeletal involvement includes myopathies, bone and joint infections, neoplasia, inflammatory arthritides and avascular necrosis of bone (Table 29.2).

MYOPATHIES

Myopathies may be caused by bacterial infection (pyomyositis), non-infective inflammation (polymyositis) or by drugs used in the treatment of HIV infection (AZT myopathy). In the early stage of pyomyositis the symptoms include cramp-like pain localized to a single muscle group (most frequently the quadriceps) and low-grade fever. The affected muscle is indurated and feels like wood. The second, suppurative, stage is characterized by increasing pain, high-grade fever and abscess formation. In the final stage the patient is toxic, the muscles are necrotic and septic shock may ensue. The mortality rate may be as high as 20%. Blood cultures are positive in only 5% of cases. Early diagnosis and management with parenteral antibiotics combined with surgical drainage is essential. Polymyositis may be one of the first manifestations of HIV. Bilateral symmetrical progressive proximal muscle weakness with elevated creatine kinase (CK) levels occurs. EMG demonstrates myopathic potentials, and on histological examination perivascular lymphocytic infiltration and muscle necrosis are seen. Treatment with anti-inflammatory drugs and oral prednisone in doses of up to 60 mg per day is very effective. Toxic mitochondrial myopathy that is reversible can occur after prolonged use of AZT (AZT myopathy). The clinical manifestations are similar to those of polymyositis. Antiviral therapy with alternative drugs is needed in these patients.

TUBERCULOSIS

Tuberculosis has re-emerged as a major public health problem after the HIV epidemic. The prevalence of tuberculosis is 500 times greater in HIV-infected persons than in the general population. The duration of anti-tuberculous therapy should be longer in HIV-infected patients. TB is discussed in more detail in Chapter 5.

BACILLARY ANGIOMATOSIS

Bacillary angiomatosis caused by *Bartonella henselae* is a multi-system infection that only occurs in immunocompromised individuals. One-third of patients develop lytic skeletal lesions characterized by cortical destruction and periosteal reaction. The overlying skin may be inflamed, giving the appearance of cellulitis. Biopsy of the lesion and Warthin–Starry staining helps to identify the organism. Bacillary angiomatous osteomyelitis responds favourably to erythromycin. A delay in the diagnosis should be avoided as disseminated angiomatosis involving several organs can be fatal.

NEOPLASIA

Non-Hodgkin's lymphoma occurs with a frequency that is 60 times greater in patients with AIDS than in the general population. Involvement of bone may occur either primarily or secondarily in up to 30% of patients. The radiological appearance may be similar to that of osteomyelitis and hence a confirmatory biopsy is mandatory. Treatment entails chemotherapy and radiation.

About 20% of patients with AIDS develop Kaposi's sarcoma. However, skeletal involvement is rare.

ARTHROPATHIES

About one-third of HIV-infected patients have some form of arthralgia during the course of the disease. Reiter's syndrome, psoriatic arthritis, HIV-associated arthritis, painful articular syndrome, acute symmetrical polyarthritis and hypertrophic osteoarthropathy are all more prevalent or unique

to these patients. Interestingly, immune-mediated arthritis of systemic lupus erythematosus (SLE) and rheumatoid arthritis (RA) improves as the immune system deteriorates.

REACTIVE ARTHRITIS IN HUMAN IMMUNODEFICIENCY VIRUS INFECTION

Reactive arthritis (see Chapter 16) is 100 to 200 times more frequent in HIV-infected patients than in the general population. Up to 10% of HIV-infected patients develop reactive arthritis with severe symptoms that do not respond well to anti-inflammatory drugs. In the foot, enthesopathy may involve any of the tendons around the ankle or the plantar fascia and the pain may be very disabling. Methotrexate is contra-indicated since it may induce full-blown AIDS and Kaposi's sarcoma.

PSORIATIC ARTHRITIS

This is 10 to 40 times more frequent in HIV-infected patients than in the general population. These patients usually have severe skin disease and the arthritis may precede development of full-blown AIDS.

HUMAN IMMUNODEFICIENCY VIRUS-ASSOCIATED ARTHRITIS

HIV-associated arthritis is a sub-acute oligoarthritis unique to HIV-infected patients. The symptoms that develop over a few weeks include severe incapacitating pain, often of the ankle or knee. The synovial fluid has less than 2500 cells/mm^3 and the synovium shows features of chronic inflammation with mononuclear cell infiltration. Intra-articular steroid injections dramatically relieve symptoms in these patients.

PAINFUL ARTICULAR SYNDROME

This is seen in about 10% of patients with AIDS. Severe pain in the knee, shoulder or elbow may mimic septic arthritis. There is no effusion in the affected joint. The pain is self-limiting; it usually resolves in a day and responds well to anti-inflammatory drugs.

HYPERTROPHIC OSTEOARTHROPATHY

HIV patients with *Pneumocystis jiroveci* pneumonia may develop hypertrophic osteoarthropathy, which resolves if the pneumonia is treated.

AVASCULAR NECROSIS OF THE FEMORAL HEAD

Avascular necrosis of the femoral head may occur in a proportion of HIV-infected patients and should be considered as a possible diagnosis of hip pain in these patients.

BONE AND JOINT TUBERCULOSIS

SPINAL TUBERCULOSIS

Tuberculosis of the spine accounts for 40–60% of all cases of skeletal tuberculosis. The thoracolumbar spine is most frequently involved and the disease most commonly starts adjacent to the intervertebral disc. The first plain radiographic finding may be a reduction in the disc space. The disc and the contiguous vertebral end-plates are soon destroyed. As the disease progresses the vertebral body gets destroyed and a kyphotic deformity develops. A cold abscess forms and is most commonly seen in the paravertebral region. Granulation tissue, disc material and pus may produce cord compression. The neurological compromise is aggravated by increasing kyphosis. A diagnosis must be made before onset of neurological signs from the plain radiographic appearances. A CT-guided needle biopsy should confirm the diagnosis when in doubt. If diagnosed early, ambulatory short-course (6–9 months) therapy with rifampicin, isoniazid and ethambutol is effective in curing the disease. If more advanced destruction of the vertebrae has occurred and neurological signs are present, surgical debridement, cord decompression and spinal fusion hasten healing and minimize the risk of progression of the neurological deficit and the spinal deformity.

OSTEOARTICULAR TUBERCULOSIS

Although any synovial joint may be affected by tuberculosis, the hip and knee are the most com-

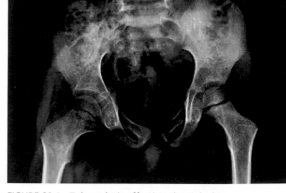

FIGURE 29.1 Tuberculosis affecting the right hip

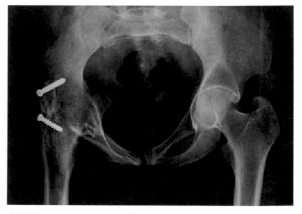

FIGURE 29.2 Arthrodesis of late-stage tuberculosis of right hip

monly affected and the ankle, elbow and wrist joints are less frequently involved (Fig. 29.1). The disease passes through stages of synovitis, early arthritis and late arthritis. In the stage of synovitis an effusion is present and pain is present only in the terminal ranges of movement. In the later stages articular cartilage destruction is associated with increasing pain, muscle spasm and fixed deformities. Diagnosis can seldom be confirmed by culturing the synovial fluid, but the chance of confirmation increases if synovial tissue is cultured. Treatment with antituberculous drugs and rest of the joint is effective in the stage of synovitis and the early arthritis stage. However, in the later stage of arthritis, joint function may not be restored even after eradicating the infection. In such instances arthrodesis (Fig. 29.2) or excision arthroplasty may be needed to improve function and to relieve pain.

HAEMOGLOBINOPATHIES

SICKLE CELL DISEASE

The skeletal manifestations of sickle cell disease are largely related to blockage of the small vessels within the bone by sickled red blood cells, resulting in thrombosis and infarction of bone. The necrotic bone in the region of infarction is susceptible to infection. The symptoms may be on account of the initial thrombotic episode, which is referred to as a crisis, or related to the effects of the infarcted bone or on account of the infection of the infarcted bone.

VASO-OCCLUSIVE CRISIS

The crisis is characterized by pain, fever and leucocytosis and, hence, the clinical picture may be indistinguishable from acute haematogenous osteomyelitis. Bilateral symmetrical involvement of the hands and feet can occur. Treatment with anti-inflammatory analgesics, oxygen and intravenous fluids is usually effective. Some authors suggest that since the propensity of infection is high in these patients it is wise to cover each crisis with a suitable antibiotic to prevent secondary infection. Joint effusion may occur during the crisis. This is characteristically non-inflammatory and tends to subside within 14 days with rest and analgesics.

AVASCULAR NECROSIS OF BONE

Avascular necrosis (AVN) of bone occurs anywhere in the skeleton where significant vaso-occlusion occurs. However, avascular necrosis in certain sites, such as the femoral head, produces progressive symptoms with long-term morbidity and disability. AVN of the femoral head may occur in less than 20% of patients with sickle cell anaemia, slightly more frequently in patients with sickle cell haemoglobin C disease, and to a variable extent in patients with sickle cell thalassaemia or sickle cell trait. If AVN of the femoral head occurs in a young patient, collapse of the epiphysis occurs and the changes are similar to those seen in Perthes' disease. More commonly, AVN of the femoral head occurs after puberty. In these older patients, segmental collapse of the epiphysis occurs with very little

remodelling. Secondary degenerative arthritis ensues in these patients. In the young child with Perthes'-like changes, treatment using a varus osteotomy of the proximal femur may help in preventing the femoral head from becoming deformed. In the adult with degenerative arthritis, a total hip replacement may be considered. However, it needs to be emphasized that complications following total hip replacement in patients with sickle cell disease are very common and that the chance of 5-year survival of the prosthesis may be as low as 50% (see Chapters 2 and 19 for more information on AVN).

OSTEOARTICULAR INFECTION

In patients with sickle cell disease, bacteria commonly colonize infarcted bone following an episode of bacteraemia. Osteomyelitis is not restricted to the metaphysis of long bones, but can involve any part of the diaphysis of long or short bones, and several bones may be affected simultaneously on account of the multiplicity of infarcts. These patients are particularly prone to develop salmonella osteomyelitis. Diaphyseal sequestration with formation of a prominent involucrum is noted in patients with sickle cell osteomyelitis. Osteomyelitis can be differentiated from vaso-occlusive crisis by the presence of positive cultures and characteristic bone lesions. Patients presenting with pyrexia, bone pain, leucocytosis and radiological changes in the bone should be treated immediately with intravenous broad-spectrum antibiotics (to cover salmonella species as well) after specimens for bacteriological examination have been obtained.

FURTHER READING

Bennett OM, Namnyak SS 1990 Bone and joint manifestations of sickle cell anaemia. J Bone Joint Surg Br 72-B: 494–499.

Biviji AA, Paiement GD, Steinbach LS 2002 Musculoskeletal manifestations of human immunodeficiency virus infection. J Am Acad Orthop Surg 10: 312–320.

Hanker GJ, Nuys V, Amstutz HC 1988 Osteonecrosis of the hip in the sickle-cell diseases. Treatment and complications. J Bone Joint Surg Am 70-A: 499–506.

Rajasekaran S, Shanmugasundaram TK 2002 Spinal tuberculosis. In: Bulstrode C,

Buckwalter J, Carr A et al (eds) Oxford textbook of orthopaedics and trauma. Oxford University Press, Oxford, p 1545–1561.

Small PM, Selcer UM 2000 Tuberculosis. In: Strickland TG (ed.) Hunter's tropical medicine and emerging infectious diseases, 8th edn. Saunders, Philadelphia, p 491–512.

Theis J-C, Joseph B 2000 Orthopaedics. In: Strickland TG (ed.) Hunter's tropical medicine and emerging infectious diseases, 8th edn. Saunders, Philadelphia, p 117–124.

PROBLEM-ORIENTATED SECTION

CASES

The following section contains 100 cases followed by the answers. For each case we have listed the relevant chapters that you may want to review before or after you look at the case or answer.

CASE 1

4, 20

A 12-year-old boy presents with a painful right knee and a limp. His mother says he strained his knee playing football a few weeks before, and he has been struggling to run since. His family has noticed a swelling over the inner aspect of his shin below the knee. He is not sleeping well.

His knee X-ray is shown.

1. What are the critical features in the history and examination?

2. What do the X-rays show?

3. What is the treatment?

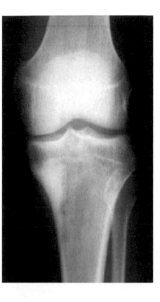

CASE 2

4, 6, 7

An 82-year-old man had a right hip replacement performed 17 years earlier. He now complains that his right hip feels unreliable and has started to click when he gets up out of a chair.

When he walks you notice that he hesitates slightly to put full weight on the right foot. He has a negative Trendelenburg test and has excellent movement in the right hip and no pain. He has about 1 cm of true shortening in the right femur. There are no signs of inflammation or infection clinically.

His hip X-ray is shown.

1. What is the likely cause of his symptoms?

2. What other investigations might be helpful?

3. How should he be managed?

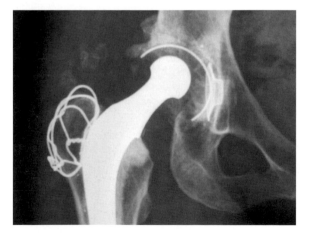

CASE 3

4, 6, 27

A 13-year-old girl has noticed that one of her shoulders seemed a bit higher than the other. When she was swimming with her family, her mother thought that her daughter had a twisted back. There was no history of back pain or spinal trauma.

Her back X-ray is shown.

1. What does the X-ray show?
2. How should this be managed?

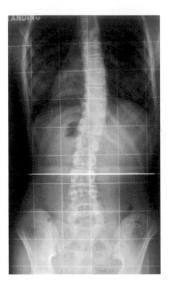

CASE 4

6, 26

A 5-year-old boy is brought to his general practitioner because his mother has observed that he has developed a limp. There is no history of trauma and he is a healthy boy who is active. He has complained recently of some pain in the left knee. When you observe him walking you notice that he has a left-sided limp and the left leg seems a bit stiff when he walks. You examine his left knee and find that it is normal. You correctly think you should examine his left hip because you have remembered about referred pain. You find that there is a restriction of internal rotation and extension. Leg lengths appear equal.

The boy's X-ray is shown.

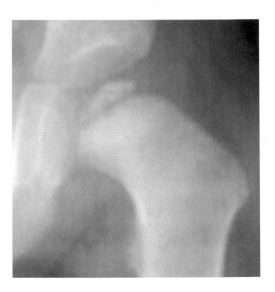

1. What is the likely diagnosis?
2. What factors affect the prognosis?

CASE 5

26

A 13-year-old boy complains of intermittent pain in the right knee which has been troubling him for 3 months. He is not particularly sporty but recalls a knock on the knee whilst playing football around the time the problem began. His general health is otherwise normal. You observe that when he walks he has a slight limp on the affected side and his right foot is more externally rotated than the left. There is no abnormality in the knee when you examine the joint. You examine the hip and find that as it flexes it goes into external rotation.

1. What is the diagnosis?
2. What is the next step?
3. What is the likelihood of him developing the same condition on the opposite side?

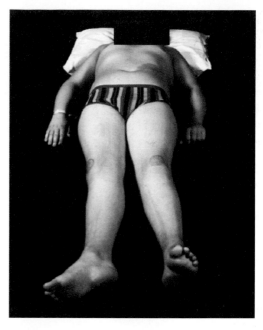

CASE 6

1, 24

The parents of an 18-month-old toddler are concerned that she has bandy legs. She has a normal birth history and subsequent milestones. Her parents say she eats a balanced diet and there is no history of skeletal dysplasia. Her clinical photograph is shown.

1. What should you examine?
2. What is the diagnosis?
3. What is the prognosis?
4. What do you advise the parents?

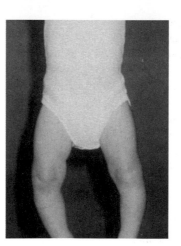

CASE 7

24, 26, 27

A 4-year-old boy is brought to you because he walks on tiptoe. His parents report that he has always done so since he started to walk at 24 months of age. They say his shoes are wearing out quickly and they find this expensive. He was born at 32 weeks of gestation by normal delivery. Parents feel that he is a bright lad but seems a bit unsteady on his feet and they say his upper limb function is fine. You observe him walking and he walks on tiptoe when in shoe wear and when walking barefoot. You look at his shoes and they are worn out at the toes. When you examine him you find that his feet are a normal shape but his legs seem a bit stiff, although you do not find any restriction of movement at the hips, knees or ankles. He has brisk but symmetrical knee and ankle reflexes.

1. What is the differential diagnosis?

2. Which parts of the brain control movement?

3. What is the most likely cause for his tiptoe walking pattern?

CASE 8

26, 27

The parents of a 3-year-old boy have noticed that he has become a bit clumsy when standing up and walking. He has started to walk on tiptoe. His general health is normal; he was born at term and walked at 15 months. There is no family history of walking difficulties.

1. What is the likely cause of this boy's walking difficulty?

2. How can this be diagnosed?

3. What is the likely outcome?

CASE 9

6, 24, 26, 27

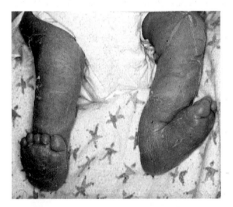

You are called to the neonatal unit as the midwife who delivered this newborn baby is concerned about the shape of the baby's feet. The baby was born at term and the delivery was uncomplicated.

1. How would you describe the shape of the left foot?

2. Suggest two causes for the appearance of the baby's left foot.

3. What else should you examine?

CASE 10

6, 26

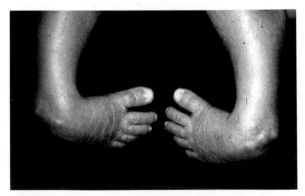

This is the clinical photograph of a neonate. There are bilateral foot deformities.

1. What is this condition?

2. What else in the child should you examine?

3. What is the next step?

4. In a unilateral case will the child have symmetrical calf muscle bulk and foot size?

CASE 11

1, 24

The mother and grandmother of a healthy 3-year-old boy report that he wakes up at night about once a week crying and pointing to his legs saying that they are sore. His mother says that she has to console him, rub his legs and occasionally give him some paracetamol elixir before he settles down. You enquire further and his mother says that as far as she is concerned he is a healthy but very active boy who is 'on the go' all the time. The boy's grandmother states that she thinks that he has growing pains because her daughter, the boy's mother, had them when she was his age.

1. What is the problem?
2. What should be considered when examining the child?
3. What is the outcome?

CASE 12

4, 5, 26

A 3-year-old girl is brought to the Accident & Emergency Department because she has suddenly stopped walking and will not take weight on her right leg. The parents say that she has not been unwell and, as far as they know, she has not fallen over. You examine her and find that she seems well but holds her right thigh slightly flexed at the hip and dislikes her hip being rotated or abducted. She has normal movements in the right knee and the left hip and knee. She does not appear to have a fracture in the lower limb clinically.

1. What else should you examine?
2. What is the differential diagnosis?
3. What investigations should be done?

CASE 13

1, 4, 26

A 6-year-old girl has been noted to have a short left leg. The illustration shows a 2.5 cm discrepancy between her legs.

1. What is true and apparent leg length discrepancy?

2. What other investigations are helpful?

3. The child has a predicted 3.5 cm discrepancy at skeletal maturity. How should this be managed?

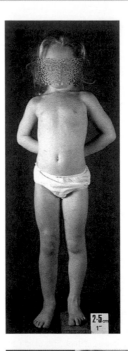

CASE 14

6, 21, 27

This man has a right-sided hemiplegia. He has a flexed wrist which cannot be straightened.

1. What functional difficulties might this cause the patient?

2. How might the wrist posture be improved?

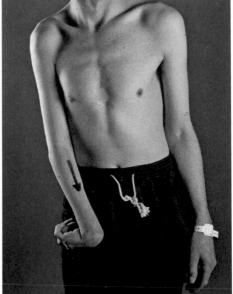

CASE 15

6, 23

A 60-year-old woman has increasing pain in her left forefoot. She cannot get into high-heeled shoes.

1. What is the diagnosis?

2. What are the treatment options?

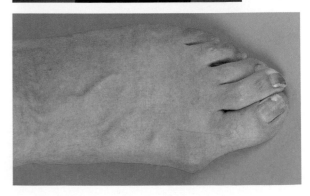

CASE 16

1, 6, 7, 16

This 70-year-old farmer has difficulty getting his left Wellington boot on. He is slower around the farm and his wife says he wakes often during the night with leg pain. He denies much discomfort.

1. What are the cardinal features shown here?

2. How would a walking stick be held?

3. Is the lack of pain critical to decision-making about treatment?

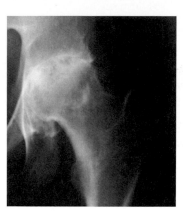

CASE 17

1, 6, 22

A 47-year-old builder's labourer presents with chronic back pain, which has prevented him from working for 3 years. Repeated investigations have all proven negative. He has recently attended a medical examination at the request of the Department of Work and Pensions and has been told that his Incapacity Benefit is to be withdrawn as he is thought to be fit and capable of work. He is distressed and states that his pain is as bad as it has ever been and that there is no way he can possibly return to work. He requests stronger analgesics and an MRI to determine the cause of his symptoms. There are no 'red flags' on taking a full history. You examine him and find that when the chest is examined on the couch he can do a full 'long sit' but that his straight leg raising is only 20° on the right and 30° on the left. There are no neurological signs.

1. What other 'inappropriate' back pain signs would you expect to find?

2. What investigations would you order?

3. What treatment might be considered?

CASE 18

1, 4, 22

A 70-year-old man has great difficulty walking out. He experiences pain in his right leg after a few yards, and this is relieved by rest. He has intermittent back pain. He is a moderate smoker (10 cigarettes per day), but his foot pulses are normal. A line drawing of an axial cross-section of one of his lumbar vertebrae is shown.

1. What is abnormal about this?

2. How does this abnormality cause his symptoms?

3. How can the diagnosis be confirmed?

4. What are the treatment options?

CASE 19

1, 5, 6, 21

A woman cleaner attends the clinic with a painful elbow. Examination confirms tenderness over the lateral epicondyle of the humerus.

1. What is the likely diagnosis?

2. What muscles attach to the common extensor origin?

Supracondylar ridge

Common extensor origin

CASE 20

1, 5, 6, 21

A 52-year-old secretary complains of a sore wrist after using a computer keyboard, particularly when pressing the spacebar. She can accurately locate the pain to the lateral aspect of the distal radius and thinks the wrist is more swollen.

1. What is the most likely diagnosis?

2. Is there a test for this condition?

3. What is the differential diagnosis?

4. What are the options for treatment?

CASE 21

1, 6, 14, 16, 21

A 23-year-old pregnant woman is regularly woken at night with discomfort and numbness in both hands, which she relieves by getting up and walking about, shaking the hands.

1. What is the most likely diagnosis?

2. Why does it occur?

3. What is the likely prognosis?

4. What is the best form of treatment?

CASE 22

21

A 60-year-old gravedigger with a known high alcohol intake has developed gradually progressive contractures of the small fingers that are now interfering with his ability to grip a spade.

1. What is the condition?

2. What is the significance of the high alcohol intake?

3. What other conditions are associated with this disorder?

4. What treatments are available?

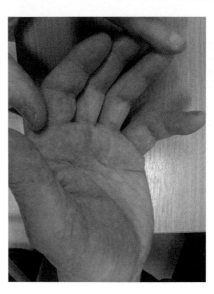

CASE 23

4, 5, 23

A 14-year-old boy complains of pain, redness and swelling of his left great toe. He says that the toe has been discharging from one of the nail-folds. There is no history of injury and he feels well.

1. What is this condition?

2. What should be done?

CASE 24

1, 4, 20, 22

A 55-year-old woman had a breast carcinoma treated by lumpectomy and radiotherapy, but 10 years later presented with thoracic back pain, a nagging discomfort which interfered with her sleep. She had cutaneous discoloration from prolonged use of a hot water bottle to relieve her back pain ('erythema ab igne').

Initially she tried chiropractic treatment, but had increasing back pain and then numbness in her lower limbs with a feeling of 'heavy legs' and walking difficulty. She had MRC grade 4 power in all muscle groups of the lower limbs and a sensory level detectable at T9 level. She had slight impairment of proprioception, brisk reflexes and an extensor plantar response on the right side. She could walk with a frame, but her impaired proprioception and weakness prevented her from walking unaided. She had control of her bladder and bowel function.

1. How many red flag signs did she manifest?

2. What is the most likely diagnosis?

3. Was it safe for her to have chiropractic treatment?

4. What tests are required to reach a diagnosis?

5. What treatment is required for pain and for her spinal cord dysfunction?

374

CASE 25

3, 4, 20

A16-year-old boy has discovered a swelling on the inside of his left knee. He is well and there is no pain; there is no history of significant injury. You examine the knee and there seems to be a bony lump at the medial side of the distal end of the femur. It is not tender. An X-ray is shown.

1. What is the diagnosis?

2. What other assessment is necessary?

3. What is the treatment?

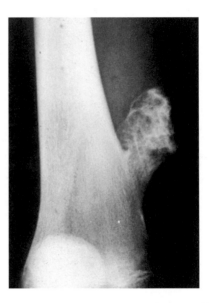

CASE 26

4, 5, 6, 7

An 85-year-old man complains of increasing pain in his left thigh and reduced walking distance 15 years after a left total hip replacement.

An X-ray of a Charnley total hip replacement is shown.

1. What does this X-ray show?
2. What is the natural history of this problem?
3. How can this problem be managed?

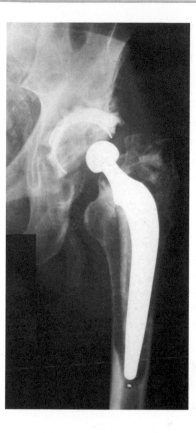

CASE 27

4, 5, 6, 7

A patient who received a total knee replacement 6 months ago says her knee has 'never been right' since. It took several weeks to heal and has produced increased pain and a red hot swelling adjacent to the knee recently.

1. What is the likely diagnosis?
2. How can the diagnosis be confirmed?
3. What is the treatment?

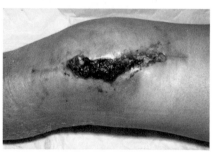

CASE 28

1, 4, 22

A patient who underwent a spinal decompression for neurogenic claudication 12 h previously has experienced increased back and leg pain in the recovery ward with progressive weakness of the legs.

Shown is a copy of the nursing observation chart.

1. What is the purpose of the nursing chart?

2. At what point should the doctor be informed of a significant change?

3. What is the likely diagnosis and management?

		returned theatre									
		12.00	13.00	14.00	15.00	16.00	18.00	20.00	22.00	23.00	23.15
left leg sensation		N	N	N	N	reduced	reduced	reduced	reduced	absent	absent
right leg sensation		N	N	N	N	N	reduced	reduced	reduced	reduced	reduced
left leg power		5	5	5	4	4	4	4	3	3	2
right leg power		5	5	5	5	4	4	4	3	3	3

CASE 29

1, 4, 22

A 75-year-old man with type 2 diabetes mellitus had been in good general health, but presented with a history of falls and unsteadiness which had come on over a period of 8 months and seemed to be increasing in severity. He had no pain anywhere. Until 8 months earlier he had been able to walk distances of several miles, but by the time of presentation he could only manage 20 yards with an awkward, scissoring gait. He had strong upper limbs, but had noticed some loss of fine hand control with difficulty fastening buttons. He described his hands as feeling slightly numb – 'a woolly feeling'.

Examination revealed normal blood pressure and pulse and normal cranial nerve function. He had normal sensation in his upper limbs apart from slight numbness in the middle, ring and little fingers. Power seemed normal in all muscle groups of the upper limbs. Jaw, deltoid, biceps and brachioradialis reflexes were normal, but both triceps reflexes were brisk.

Lower limb sensation was altered in a stocking distribution, tone was increased and power seemed only slightly reduced in all four limbs. Knee reflexes were brisk but ankle reflexes were absent and plantar responses were equivocal. He had ankle clonus bilaterally. He walked with a scissoring gait and had a positive Romberg's test.

1. What is the reason for his gait disturbance and falling?

2. What is the significance of his tendon reflex findings and at what level of his nervous system would you expect to find any pathology?

3. The sagittal MRI is shown. What is the pathology and does it explain his neurological picture?

4. What is the natural history of his condition and can it be modified? How?

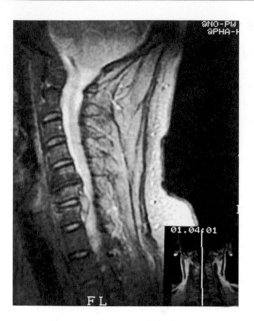

CASE 30

1, 4, 20, 22

A 50-year-old man presented with pain in the neck and left arm with paraesthesiae and numbness in the thumb and index finger. He had lost 20 kg of weight and had a general malaise. He was unaware of any lower disturbance, but neurological assessment revealed a brisk set of reflexes in the left lower limb. Routine blood tests yielded a mild anaemia (Hb 10.1 g/dl) and a very high erythrocyte sedimentation rate (ESR) (110 mm/h). Plasma proteins were raised and immuno-electrophoresis showed a monoclonal gammopathy with a raised IgM.

1. What is the likely diagnosis?
2. Why does he have evidence of a radiculopathy of C6 and also a mild myelopathy of the upper limbs?
3. What tests are indicated to clarify the diagnosis?
4. What treatment is required:
   a. for the neurological condition?
   b. for the underlying condition?

CASE 31

1, 4, 6, 22

A 48-year-old-man presented with a 1-year history of neck pain followed by pain radiating down the right arm with some tingling in the thumb. The pain intensified on lateral cervical rotation to the right and was worse on vertical compression of the head. The pain had also been disturbing his sleep at night.

There was subtle sensory change in the thumb and index finger, but no detectable weakness. The reflexes were all present, but the right biceps reflex was sluggish in comparison to the left. The lower limb neurological examination was normal. Gait was normal. The plain radiographs of the neck showed multi-level cervical spondylosis.

Physiotherapy, cervical traction and acupuncture had been tried, but without any improvement in pain levels.

1. At which level is the pertinent pathology and how can you best determine this?
2. What treatment is indicated?
3. Is operative treatment ever required?
4. How would any operation be performed?

CASE 32

4, 5, 26

A 19-month-old girl was noted by her mother to be unwilling to walk and apparently unable to take her weight on her left leg. She became miserable and refused to eat. Her mother took her to a paediatric emergency department where it was established that she had previously been healthy apart from a cough and runny nose 2 days before.

Examination at that time showed a listless girl who had a fever of 38.5°C and a tachycardia. She lay still, held her left hip abducted and externally rotated, and resented attempts to move her leg.

Radiographs of her hip and lower limb were normal. Her white cell count was $18.9 \times 10^9/l$, ESR 32 mm/h and C-reactive protein (CRP) 94 mg/l.

1. What is the differential diagnosis?

2. What further investigations may help to determine the diagnosis?

3. What is the appropriate management?

CASE 33

1, 4, 22, 29

A 34-year-old Asian man presented with a long history of low back pain and a 3-week history of severe sciatica and dysaesthesia in the right leg. He looked ill and had lost weight over a 6-month period. He had a productive cough and night sweats. His pain was relentless in all positions except in extreme flexion of hip and knee on the right side. He had an absent right ankle reflex, hyperaesthesia of the right foot and was reluctant to move his back. He had severe sciatica during attempted raising of the straight leg.

1. What baseline investigations help to differentiate between mechanical causes of sciatica and more serious pathology?

2. What spinal investigations are indicated?

3. What treatment is indicated?

CASE 34

1, 4, 22, 27

A 15-year-old girl presented with back pain of 1 year's duration associated with a 3-month history of pain radiating from her back via the buttock to the upper thigh into the lateral aspect of the right leg and dorsum of the right foot. She also complained of occasional tingling in the sole of the right foot. Symptoms were made worse by any vigorous activity and relieved by lying down on her back. There were no sphincter disturbances. She is a very keen gymnast and ballet dancer but has had to stop this because of her symptoms. On examination she was of slim build and in excellent health. There was no scoliosis, forward flexion of the lumbar spine was restricted and she was tender over the lower lumbar spine and sacrum. There were no root irritation or compression signs in the legs, but straight leg raising was limited by short hamstrings. A lateral radiograph of the lumbar spine is shown below.

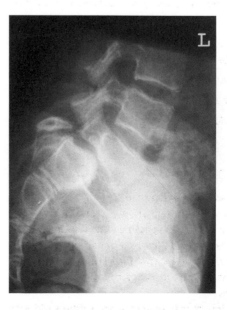

1. What is the abnormality shown on the lateral radiograph?
2. What is the underlying cause of the abnormality in this patient?
3. What treatment is required?

CASE 35

8, 9, 13

A 35-year-old cyclist commuting to work was knocked off his bicycle and landed heavily onto his left shoulder. His presenting radiograph is shown in figure A.

1. What fracture is visible and what is the treatment of choice?
2. A radiograph at 12 weeks is shown in figure B. What complication has occurred?
3. What is the treatment?

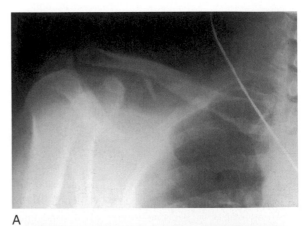

A

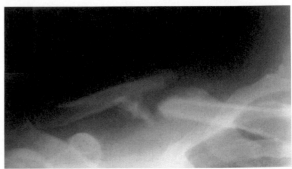

B

CASE 36

9, 13

A 22-year-old man falls on extended outstretched hand during a football match. He presented with a painful swollen left shoulder. On physical examination the humeral head was palpable in a subcoracoid position. The radiograph is shown.

1. In what directions can the shoulder dislocate?
2. What are the most well recognized associated injuries?
3. What is the appropriate treatment for this injury?

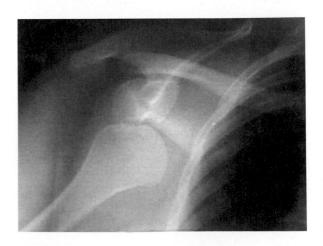

CASE 37

8, 9, 13

A 61-year-old woman fell down some steps and landed heavily onto her left arm. She sustained a shoulder injury.

1. What injury has she sustained?
2. Where is the humeral head situated?
3. What aspects of clinical examination are important?
4. What are the options for treatment?

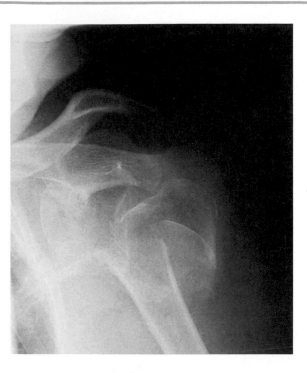

CASE 38

8, 9, 13

A 21-year-old man crashed his motorcycle and sustained the fracture of the humerus, shown in the figure. He was unable to actively dorsiflex his wrist.

1. What is the associated soft-tissue injury likely to be?
2. What are the typical physical findings?
3. What is the usual treatment of humeral shaft fractures?
4. What are the indications for operative treatment?
5. What type of fixation implant is preferred?

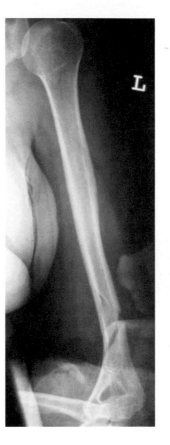

CASE 39

9, 12, 13

A 6-year-old falls off a swing and lands awkwardly onto the right arm and complains of pain in the elbow and tingling in the index and middle fingers. When you examine the child you find that they have a thready radial pulse and have altered perception to light touch on the volar (anterior) surface of the thumb.

The radiograph is shown.

1. What type of fracture is this?
2. What accounts for the physical signs observed?
3. What is the initial management?
4. What is the preferred treatment?

CASE 40

8, 9, 13

A 54-year-old woman fell heavily onto her outstretched right arm and presented complaining of elbow pain. Physical examination revealed a swollen bruised elbow. There was no distal neurovascular deficit.

The radiograph is shown.

1. What injuries can be detected on the plain radiographs?
2. What is the preferred treatment?
3. What complications can be expected?

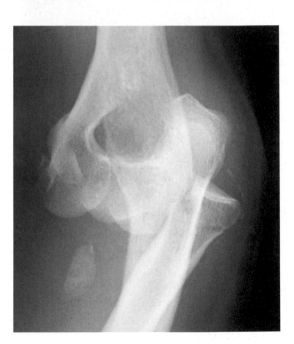

CASE 41

8, 9, 13

An 81-year-old woman fell heavily onto the point of her left elbow and sustained the injury shown in the figure.

1. What fracture can be seen?
2. Apart from the fall, what may contribute to causation of this injury?
3. What is the source of the main deforming force?
4. What is the usual treatment?

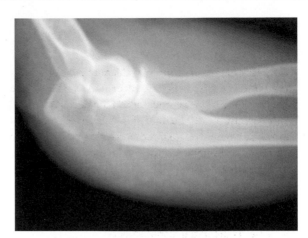

CASE 42

8, 9, 13

A 34-year-old man crashed his motorcycle and was admitted with a painful swollen forearm with obvious deformity. Pain gradually increased in the 6 h after admission despite splintage and adequate analgesia.
    The radiograph is shown.

1. What complication should be considered?
2. How can the diagnosis be confirmed?
3. Describe the pathophysiology and the long-term sequela if not recognized and treated appropriately.
4. What is the correct management of this injury?

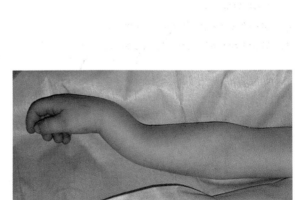

CASE 43

8, 9, 12, 13

A 5-year-old boy fell off a swing and landed on his outstretched hand. There is an obvious deformity of the right forearm.
    The appearance of the arm (A) and a lateral radiograph of the forearm (B) are shown.

1. What is the diagnosis?
2. What specifically would you examine in the child's arm?
3. The injury is treated by closed reduction, application of a full-arm plaster under general anaesthesia and elevation of the arm afterwards. You are called to the ward 6 h later and are told that the child has intolerable pain in the affected arm that has not improved with elevation or

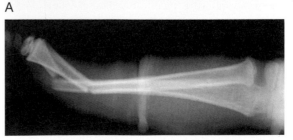

A

B

analgesia. When you examine him he has pink fingers which are a little swollen, the radial pulse is concealed by the plaster and he appears to have intact sensation. He is very reluctant to move his fingers himself and cries when you try to extend his fingers passively. What might the problem be?

CASE 44

12, 13

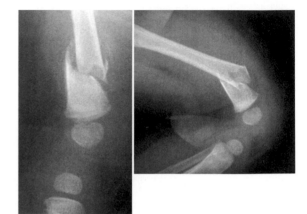

An 8-week-old baby is brought by her parents to the Accident & Emergency Department with a swollen left thigh. She had seen the general practitioner (GP) on the previous day, for her routine child health check. The GP had performed a test for congenital dislocation of the hips, following which the baby was reported to be 'crying all the time' and 'hasn't moved her leg since'.

On examination, the baby is well nourished and well cared for. The left thigh is swollen with an area of red-blue bruising on the anterior aspect, just above the knee.

She lives at home with her parents, and is the younger of two children. The older brother (aged 2 years) is reported to be in good health. She was a full-term normal delivery, and required no resuscitation or special care. The father is unemployed.

The X-rays of her left femur are shown.

1. What is the most likely explanation for the diagnosis?

2. What other features in the history would you seek? From whom?

3. What other investigations would you consider?

4. Which other agencies would you involve, and what do you expect of them?

5. What are the issues for the 2-year-old brother?

CASE 45

8, 9, 13

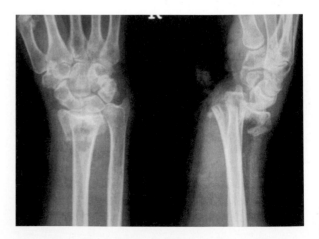

A 74-year-old woman slipped on ice and sustained the injury shown in the figure. On clinical examination the wrist was deformed and there was impaired sensation with paraesthesia in the thumb, index, middle and radial side of the ring finger.

1. What is the term used to describe the clinical deformity shown?

2. What eponymous terms are commonly used to describe fractures in this location?

3. What is the significance of the sensory symptoms?

4. What is the appropriate management of the fracture?

5. What are the most common complications?

CASE 46

8, 12, 13

A 12-year-old boy sustained an injury to his right wrist after a fall off a skateboard.

A radiograph at presentation is shown.

1. What fracture is visible?

2. What reduction manouevre is usually employed?

3. What is the usual treatment?

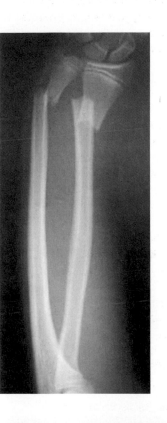

CASE 47

8, 9, 13

A 34-year-old man fell heavily while playing football and landed on his outstretched hand. He presented with wrist pain.

The radiographs are shown.

1. What fracture is visible?

2. What is the most common clinical finding?

3. What is the usual treatment?

4. What are the well recognized complications of this injury and why do they occur?

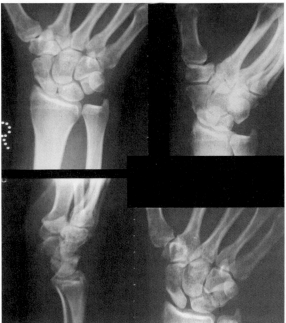

CASE 48

8, 9, 13

A 21-year-old boy was involved in a fight. He sustained a laceration over the 5th metacarpophalangeal (MCP) joint. He presented 5 days later with increasing pain and swelling. There was a pyrexia of 38.5°C.

The radiograph is shown.

1. What fracture is visible?

2. What is the likely associated complication?

3. What is the appropriate treatment?

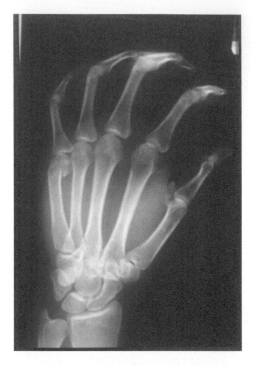

CASE 49

1, 13

A 15-year-old boy finds a piece of broken glass on the beach and cuts the volar aspect of his right fifth finger at the level of the proximal phalanx. On presentation his hand had the position shown.

1. What is the likely diagnosis?

2. What other associated injury might be present?

3. What is the relevant anatomy and surgical management?

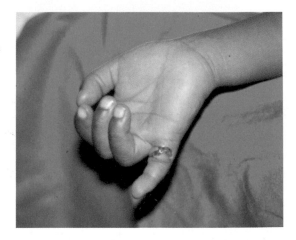

CASE 50

8, 22

A 30-year-old woman fell from a first-floor balcony and injured her back at the thoraco-lumbar junction. She was brought to hospital on a rigid stretcher. She was unable to move her legs and had no sensation below the umbilicus. No other injuries had been sustained. There was a palpable step in her back at the thoraco-lumbar junction with localized tenderness overlying it. There was an unusually wide gap between two of the spinous processes corresponding to the site of tenderness. She had paralysis of all muscle groups in the lower limbs with no detectable reflexes in her legs. She also had perineal numbness and a sensory level at the umbilicus. There was no abdominal tenderness and palpation did not reveal an enlarged bladder.

1. What is the diagnosis?
2. What investigations are required?
3. What early management is needed?
4. What are the later treatment options?

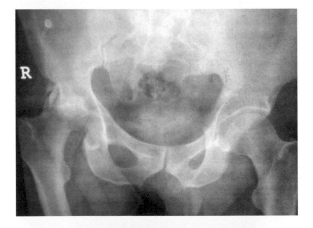

CASE 51

1, 8, 9, 13

A 44-year-old man driving a car was involved in a head-on collision with another vehicle. He presented with pain in his right hip.
   A radiograph of the hip is shown.

1. What is the injury shown?
2. What is the typical position of the leg in this situation?
3. What are the most common associated injuries?
4. What is the appropriate management?

CASE 52

12, 13

A 12-year-old slips on wet grass and twists their ankle. When you examine them they are unable to bear weight on the affected limb and the ankle is very swollen.
   The radiographs are shown.

1. What types of physeal injury are there and what type is this?
2. What are the principles of management of a physeal injury?
3. What are the possible long-term problems associated with a physeal injury?

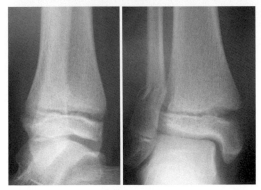

CASE 53

8, 9, 13

An 85-year-old woman slipped on a supermarket floor and presented with a painful right hip. The leg was shortened and externally rotated on examination.

A radiograph of the hip is shown.

1. What is the injury shown and how would you classify this fracture?
2. What are the complications associated with this injury?
3. What is the relevant anatomy of the blood supply?
4. What treatment options are commonly used and why?

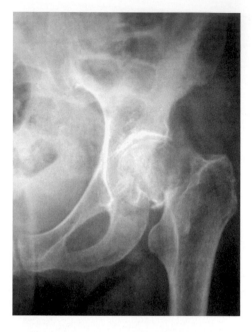

CASE 54

8, 9, 10, 11, 13

A 23-year-old man was involved in a collision with a car and sustained a femoral shaft fracture shown in figure. There was an ipsilateral tibial shaft fracture. At the time of presentation the patient was tachycardic with a pulse of 110/min. The BP was 110/60 mmHg.

1. What is the most appropriate system of assessment for this patient?
2. What are the key elements of this approach?
3. What are the risks associated with these long-bone fractures in a young patient?
4. What are the treatment options usually considered and what are the advantages and disadvantages?

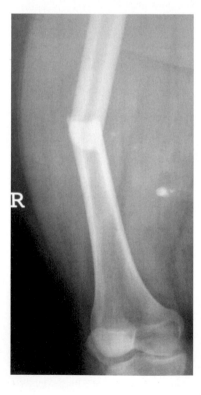

CASE 55

1, 7

A 25-year-old man was playing football on a wet pitch. He changed direction to chase the ball and his studs caught on the pitch surface twisting his right knee, which gave way. He described a 'popping' sensation in the knee. He was unable to play on. The knee swelled and became very painful within 4 h and he attended the casualty department. Aspiration of the knee yielded 80 ml blood (see figure). The radiographs were normal.

1. What is the differential diagnosis?
2. What physical signs are helpful to differentiate?
3. What additional investigation is most useful?
4. What is the likely treatment?

CASE 56

1, 7

A 24-year-old man was playing American football. He landed heavily on his left knee. The knee was stiff after the injury. He was able to play on for part of the game but eventually had to discontinue due to pain over the medial side of the joint. Some swelling occurred over the next 48 h and he was unable to straighten the knee. He consulted his general practitioner who referred him to a knee clinic. The radiographs were normal.

1. What is the differential diagnosis?
2. What physical signs are helpful to differentiate?
3. What additional investigation is most useful?
4. What is the likely treatment?

CASE 57

1, 8, 9, 13

A 42-year-old woman riding pillion passenger on a motor cycle was involved in a crash when the driver lost control on a wet surface and was involved in a collision with a car. She was complaining of right leg pain when seen in casualty. There was a large wound over the lower third of her right leg (shown).

1. What fracture is visible?
2. How is this injury classified?
3. What are the important steps in the early management?
4. What is the definitive management?

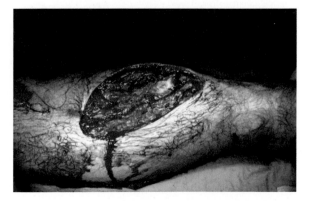

CASE 58

8, 9, 13

A 58-year-old woman slipped on ice and presented complaining of right ankle pain. On clinical examination there was marked ankle swelling, with deformity and generalized tenderness.

A radiograph is shown.

1. What fracture is visible?
2. How is this injury produced?
3. What is the appropriate treatment of this injury?

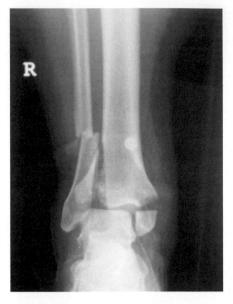

CASE 59

8, 9, 13

A 26-year-old male rock climber fell 20 feet and landed heavily on his right foot. He presented complaining of severe pain in the right hindfoot region.

A CT scan with a reconstruction image of his hindfoot is shown.

1. What fracture is visible?
2. What is the most well recognized complication of this injury and what is the anatomical explanation?
3. What is the appropriate treatment of this injury?

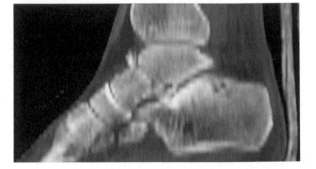

CASE 60

8, 9, 13

A 64-year-old woman fell and sustained a right distal radial fracture treated by reduction and cast immobilization. The fracture united. The cast was removed 6 weeks after injury. The wrist was noted to be rather stiff and the patient was reviewed again 4 weeks after cast removal. At this stage she was complaining of constant pain in the right hand and wrist with stiffness and swelling. The fingers and hand were swollen with a red, shiny appearance and were hypersensitive.

1. What complication has arisen?
2. What is the postulated cause?
3. What treatment is available?

CASE 61

8, 9, 13

A 43-year-old man with epilepsy presented to an Accident & Emergency Department after a fit. He was in a drowsy post-ictal state at the time of presentation but complained of shoulder pain. Radiographs were taken which were considered to show no major abnormality (shown). He was discharged when alert and referred to a fracture clinic for a further opinion. He was seen 1 week later still complaining of shoulder pain.

1. What abnormality is shown on the initial radiographs?
2. What is the characteristic feature in the history that should alert the doctor to this possibility and what is the most useful clinical sign?
3. What additional investigations would be helpful?
4. What is the treatment of choice?

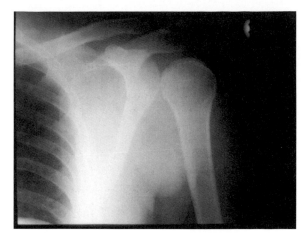

CASE 62

8, 9, 10, 11, 13

A 26-year-old male motorcyclist was involved in a head-on collision with a car. He was admitted in hypotensive shock.

The pelvic radiograph is shown.

1. What pattern of pelvic injury is shown?
2. What are the likely associated injuries?
3. What are the priorities in the early management?
4. What options are there for definitive treatment of the orthopaedic injury?

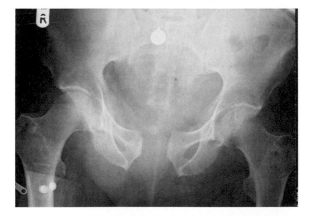

CASE 63

8, 9, 10, 13, 19

A 77-year-old woman was blown over by the wind while out shopping. She was admitted complaining of right hip pain.

The presenting radiograph is shown.

1. What fracture is visible and how can it be classified?
2. What is the best choice of treatment for this injury?
3. What are the possible complications?

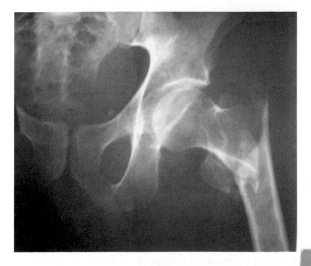

CASE 64

8, 9, 10, 13

A 68-year-old woman fell while playing golf and landed heavily on her left side. She presented complaining of severe pain in the left hip. There was no shortening or external rotation of the left leg, but the left hip was painful to move.

Radiographs of the hip are shown.

1. Is there a fracture clearly visible?
2. What additional investigations would help?
3. What is the treatment of choice?

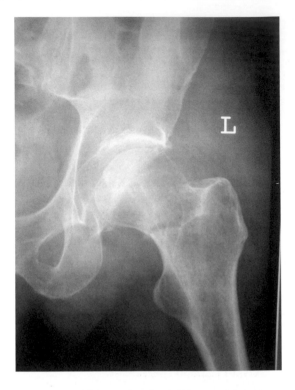

CASE 65

8, 9, 10, 12

A 3-year-old boy was at a funfair and fell off a merry-go-round ride twisting his right leg. Radiographs demonstrated a spiral fracture of the femur.

1. What is the initial management of this injury?
2. What are the advantages and disadvantages of the treatment methods generally used for this fracture?

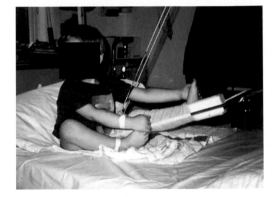

CASE 66

1

A 44-year-old woman was participating in Scottish country dancing at a wedding. She landed on her left leg and developed severe pain over the posterior aspect of the heel. She initially attended a physiotherapist and was treated for a calf muscle sprain. The pain persisted and she subsequently saw her general practitioner who referred her to the local Accident & Emergency Department. When she presented it was 2 weeks after the initial injury. She was limping and had diffuse swelling and resolving bruising over the posterior aspect of her heel above the level of the calcaneus.

1. What is the most likely diagnosis and what are the other common activities associated with this injury?

2. What clinical signs are helpful in making the diagnosis?

3. Are there any investigations that may help in doubtful cases?

4. What are the options for treatment at this stage?

CASE 67

8, 9, 13

A 21-year-old male soccer player sustained an inversion injury of his left foot and presented complaining of foot and ankle pain. On examination there was swelling and bruising along the lateral aspect of his foot and ankle. Tenderness was maximal along the lateral border of his foot.

Radiographs of the foot are shown.

1. What fracture is visible?

2. What other injury should be considered?

3. What is the appropriate treatment?

4. What is the most common complication?

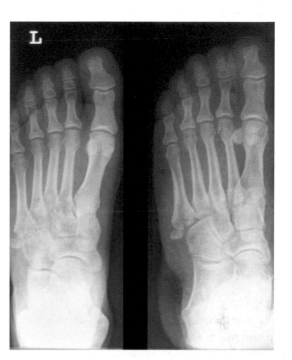

CASE 68

1, 4, 5, 6, 15, 16

A 21-year-old man returned from a holiday in Ibiza 10 days before presenting to the Accident & Emergency Department with a 1-day history of a hot, swollen right ankle, pyrexia of 39.5°C, rigors and general malaise. It emerges that whilst away on holiday he suffered from some nausea and vomiting for 24 h, followed by diarrhoea for about 1 week associated with some blood in the stool. He also became aware of some discomfort on micturition and noticed an offensive discharge on his underwear which he is sure is from his penis. He had a sore right eye for a few days but this has cleared up now. Examination reveals that his right ankle is warm, very swollen and tender, and slightly red. All other joints are normal, and there are no abnormalities in the chest, cardiovascular system and abdomen.

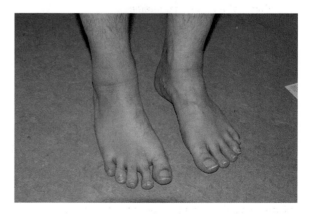

1. What is the differential diagnosis?

2. What are the most appropriate investigations?

3. How should he be managed?

CASE 69

1, 3, 23

A 50-year-old woman presents with sore knees for the last 4 years. She has no evidence of swelling, and her pains are relieved by simple analgesia. On examination the only abnormality is shown in the photograph.

1. What is the abnormality?

2. What is the diagnosis?

3. What is the most appropriate treatment?

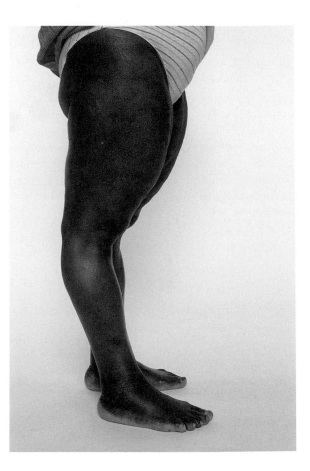

CASE 70

5, 15, 16

A 70-year-old man presents with joint pains for 3 years. The condition has affected his hands, wrists, feet and ankles. Four months ago he was commenced on a new treatment, and although his joints are improving he has developed lumps on his hands. He has widespread changes of joint swelling in small- and medium-sized joints and firm lumps on his fingers as shown in the picture.

1. What are the lumps?

2. What is the diagnosis?

3. What is the most likely drug to have caused these lumps to appear?

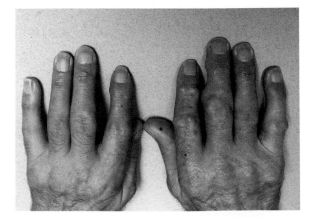

CASE 71

1, 5, 15, 16

A 43-year-old joiner (carpenter) presents to you with a 2-day history of a hot painful left knee, fever, nausea, vomiting and rigors.

1. What are the features in the history that you would consider relevant?

2. You examine him and discover that he has a red hot swollen left knee. All his other joints are normal and there is no relevant other history except that he injured his left foot approximately 3 days previously and has a small puncture wound between the fourth and fifth toes. The knee is aspirated and you obtain 45 ml of thick, purulent material. What is your next step?

3. How long would you continue treatment for?

4. What is the likely outcome?

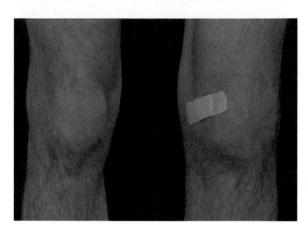

CASE 72

4, 5, 16, 17

A 25-year-old woman is 16 weeks' pregnant with her first baby. She presents with a 6-week history of swelling, stiffness and pain in her knuckles and wrists, associated with tiredness and a rash. Her blood pressure has been rising over the last 4 weeks, and is currently 145/97 mmHg. She has routine blood tests which show a normal haemoglobin, but reduced white cell count (neutrophil count 1.7×10^9/l) and platelets (66×10^9/l).

1. What is the differential diagnosis?

2. What investigations would you recommend?

3. How would you manage this patient?

CASE 73

1, 5, 13, 19, 20

A 69-year-old man presents with a 1-month history of left shin pain, which is gradually getting worse. He has had some night disturbances. He is generally tired and in the last 2 weeks has become breathless on minimal exertion. He smokes 35 cigarettes per day and admits to a regular productive cough in winter, more recently flecked with blood. On examination you find that he is tender over the shin. He has not lost any height but has lost 5 kg in weight in the last 2 months. He is otherwise well. Systems enquiry is negative. His haemoglobin result is 7.8 g/dl with a microcytic hypochromic picture.

1. What does the X-ray show?
2. What is the differential diagnosis?
3. What should be done for his pain?

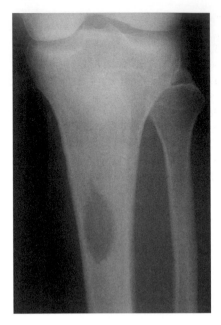

CASE 74

1, 3, 4, 5, 6, 22

A 40-year-old bricklayer was lifting a pile of bricks and experienced sudden, severe back pain. He was unable to continue working and was taken home for a period of rest. A few hours later he had mild bilateral sciatica and progressive numbness around the buttocks, genitalia and soles of both feet. Over the next 3 days his pain increased. He was unable to stand with his back straight and his walking distance was reduced to a few yards due to a combination of pain and weakness. He could not pass urine, but had no discomfort in the suprapubic region. He had experienced faecal soiling of his underwear. There was sacral dermatomal numbness, absent ankle reflexes and weak plantar flexion of both feet. The straight leg raising test was restricted to 45° on both sides. A full bladder could be detected with overflow incontinence. Rectal examination revealed a patulous anus due to reduced anal sphincter tone.

1. What is the likely diagnosis?
2. What are the pathognomonic clinical features?
3. What tests should be done?
4. What treatment is required?

CASE 75

1, 5, 6, 16

A 17-year-old girl presents with a 5-day history of acute onset of swelling, pain and redness affecting the right knee and right ankle. She had been in good health previously. She admits to having had sexual intercourse with four new partners in the last 3 weeks. One week ago she recalls having a little soreness in the right eye, but no loss of vision or blurring, and the eye cleared up within the last 24 h. On examination, she has a large effusion in the right knee and synovitis of the right tibiotalar joint. Her temperature is 38.9°C.

1. What is the most important test?
2. What is the differential diagnosis?
3. What is the most appropriate treatment?

CASE 76

1, 4, 5, 6, 7, 15, 23

A 76-year-old man presents to clinic with a 5-year history of progressive pain and stiffness affecting his left knee. He has a past history of myocardial infarction within the last 6 months, and has also suffered from angina since then. Over the past 2 years he has been unable to walk to the local shops without stopping at least four times (approximately 1 mile away); however, most of the time this is due to his angina and not to his knee pain. The pain is all around the left knee, and can be associated with occasional swelling. Driving has been unaffected since he has an automatic car. Examination reveals a slight bowing of his left knee at rest, and on standing he has a marked valgus deformity. The joint line is swollen with what feels like a bony enlargement of the distal end of the femur and the proximal tibia. The knee has 30° of fixed flexion at rest and flexes to 120° before there is pain.

1. What is the most likely diagnosis?
2. What medical treatments should be considered?
3. If he fails to improve with medication, what else can be done?

CASE 77

4, 5, 16

A 57-year-old woman with rheumatoid arthritis for the past 3 years attends the routine follow-up clinic. Her diagnosis was based on the onset of a widespread inflammatory arthritis of small- and medium-sized joints, an elevated CRP and a positive rheumatoid factor. After failing to respond to non-steroidal anti-inflammatory drugs, she was established on sulfasalazine 2 g per day with good effect. Unfortunately after 18 months she had a flare of disease and was switched to methotrexate, increasing the dose to 20 mg per week in the last 8 months to establish good control. She feels well but her general practitioner has sent a note with the latest blood results (see table) from the last 3 months which have caused some concern.

1. What do the results show?
2. What action should you take immediately?
3. What is the next stage in her treatment?

	01/02/2006	01/03/2006	05/04/2006
Haemoglobin (13–17 g/dl)	10.1	10.3	10.2
White cell count (4–11 × 10^9/l)	4.6	7.2	5.1
Neutrophil count (2–7 × 10^9/l)	3.1	4.6	3.8
Platelets (150–400 × 10^9/l)	345	236	431
ESR (mm/h)	12	15	7
Albumin (35–50 g/l)	38	41	39
Bilirubin (3–17 μmol/l)	7	11	8
Aspartate transaminase (15–42 IU/l)	86	36	190
Alkaline phosphatase (80–250 IU/l)	510	189	1130

CASE 78

16, 18, 22

A 78-year-old woman with rheumatoid arthritis is admitted from home as an emergency. She has had rheumatoid arthritis for the past 34 years starting in hands, feet, knees, wrists and elbows. She was originally treated with penicillamine tablets with modest improvement, until she developed increasing nausea and eventually stopped the drug. She was switched to gold injections with partial response, supplemented by prednisolone at increasing doses, currently 15 mg per day for the past 5 years. Her gold treatment was switched to methotrexate 3 years ago but she can only tolerate 10 mg per week due to diarrhoea. Her general practitioner was called to see her at home yesterday with a history that she is not able to get out of bed and has admitted her with a presumed flare of her arthritis causing the immobility. On re-taking the history, there is no mention of worsening arthritis; in fact she feels that her current medication is actually keeping the arthritis under good control for the first time in years. However, she cannot move properly and feels stiff especially in her legs. Examination of her joints shows a considerable amount of accumulated damage with typical forefoot deformities of rheumatoid arthritis in her feet, bilateral ankle valgus and pes planus; her knees have crepitus and small effusions but are non-tender. Hips (both replaced in the past 10 years) move well and are pain free. In the upper arms there are signs of ulnar drift, volar subluxation of the wrists, fixed flexion contractures of the right elbow to 30°, and very restricted glenohumeral movement bilaterally. Her ESR is 35 mm/h, which is similar to her usual results over the past 12 months; the CRP is 15 mg/l (normal value <2 mg/l).

1. What further examination should you perform?

2. What tests would you undertake?

3. How should the patient be managed?

CASE 79

1, 5, 6, 16

A 50-year-old woman with known psoriasis for the previous 25 years presents with a 3-month history of a swollen 4th right toe, and some pain in her knees. Over the past 15 years she has noticed a gradual onset of spine stiffness which is associated with occasional bilateral buttock pain. The stiffness is usually gone by lunchtime, and these symptoms were only elicited on direct questioning.

On examination, she has a diffusely swollen 4th toe of the right foot, bilateral knee swelling and tenderness, and widespread small plaque psoriasis.

1. What is the diagnosis?

2. What investigations are of help?

3. What is the best treatment for this patient?

CASE 80

5, 6, 16

A 25-year-old man presents to his general practitioner with back pain that has developed over the last couple of months. The general practitioner takes a history and finds that there was no obvious precipitant to this, and that the patient complains of significant early morning stiffness. The doctor suspects that the patient may have ankylosing spondylitis and orders an X-ray and a test for HLA-B27.

1. What is the likelihood of ankylosing spondylitis if the X-ray is negative?

2. What is the likelihood of ankylosing spondylitis if the X-ray is negative but the HLA-B27 test is positive?

3. If the X-ray is negative, in what circumstances would an MRI scan be useful?

CASE 81

5, 16

A 49-year-old woman with a 6-year history of rheumatoid arthritis presents to clinic. She has failed to respond to sulfasalazine given for at least 6 months; she was switched to methotrexate and improved on 15 mg per week for 18 months. After this time her joint disease became more active and failed to improve on increasing the dose of methotrexate to 20 mg per week, even switching to the subcutaneous route. Additional hydroxychloroquine did not improve her arthritis. She was prescribed leflunomide 10 mg per day, but this caused severe diarrhoea, and she stopped after 1 week. Attempting to restart caused the diarrhoea to return. She came off the drug 2 weeks ago. On examination today she has widespread inflammatory arthritis involving most of her MCP and PIP joints, wrists, elbows, shoulders and ankles. Her CRP is 46 mg/l (normal value <2 mg/l). Her disease activity score (DAS) is shown in the table. These figures represent a high level of disease activity (good control would be a score of <3.2).

1. What treatment plan do you have for this patient?

2. What precautions are required?

3. How will you monitor her response to new treatment?

Tender joints	Right	Left	Swollen joints	Right	Left
Shoulders		X	Shoulders		
Elbows	X				X
Wrists	X		Wrists	X	
MCP1	X		MCP1	X	
MCP2	X	X	MCP2	X	X
MCP3	X	X	MCP3	X	X
MCP4	X		MCP4	X	X
MCP5	X		MCP5	X	
PIP1	X	X	PIP1	X	
PIP2		X	PIP2		X
PIP3	X		PIP3	X	
PIP4			PIP4		
PIP5	X		PIP5		
Knees			Knees		
Tender joint count (0–28)					15
Swollen joint count (0–28)					13
CRP (normal value <2 mg/l)					46
Visual analogue scale of general health of patient (0–100 mm)					31
DAS 28 CRP*					5.96

* Calculated as follows: $0.56 \times \sqrt{(\text{tender joint count})} + 0.28 \times \sqrt{(\text{swollen joint count})} + 0.36 \times \ln(\text{CRP} + 1) + 0.014 \times \text{VAS} + 0.96$

CASE 82

1, 5, 7, 13, 16, 19

A 59-year-old woman presents to the clinic with a history of established rheumatoid arthritis for the previous 14 years. She has been troubled day and night for the last week with pain in her left shoulder. She is being treated with etanercept injections 50 mg per week, methotrexate 15 mg per week and some analgesia.

On examination she has rheumatoid hand deformities and nodules at both elbows. The left shoulder is very stiff with almost no movement in any direction. The deltoid and trapezius muscles are wasted. Passive movement of the shoulder is limited by pain and there is a lot of crepitus on attempted abduction. By contrast the right shoulder has a better range of movement, but is still limited in abduction, although not painful.

1. What is the likely cause of the left shoulder problem?

2. What tests should be done?

3. What treatment could be offered?

CASE 83

1, 4, 5, 6, 14

A 24-year-old woman presents with a 6-month history of generalized ill health, following a series of 'flu-like' illnesses. She complains of joint and muscle pain, being tired all the time, having abdominal bloating with constipation and poor concentration. She has gained a stone in weight in the 6 months 'because I am too tired to exercise'. There is no significant past or family history. Physical examination reveals an essentially fit woman, with a flat affect.

1. What is the differential diagnosis?

2. What investigations are appropriate?

3. The investigations are all normal. What would be your final diagnosis?

4. How would you manage this patient?

CASE 84

1, 5, 17

A 68-year-old man presents with a 1-week history of new, unaccustomed headache, affecting both temples. His general health has been poor for the last month, with increasing pain and stiffness in his shoulders and hips. He has struggled to get out of bed in the morning and describes this as most unusual. His appetite has been poor and he has lost 4 kg in weight during this period. Three days ago he noticed some blurring of vision in his right eye, and was seen urgently in the eye department. An ophthalmologist has diagnosed anterior ischaemic optic neuropathy and referred him to you for an urgent opinion.

1. What is/are the most likely diagnosis(es)?

2. What is the most important investigation?

3. What treatment would you suggest and when would you start it?

CASE 85

1, 5, 14, 16, 17, 20

A 68-year-old woman is referred for an urgent appointment because of weight loss, stiffness and weakness for the previous 8 weeks. She has been going gradually downhill during this time, losing 6 kg in weight, and feeling less able to get out of bed in the mornings. She gets a little better by lunchtime and has taken to staying up later at night. She finds it difficult to dress in the mornings and sometimes gets stuck in a chair in the evenings, if she has rested too long in one place. She complains of pain in the shoulders and lower back. Her general practitioner has undertaken some tests including a rheumatoid factor which is positive at 20 IU/l and an anti-nuclear antibody, which is positive at 1/40; her ESR is 75 mm/h and the CRP is 60 mg/dl. On examination she is stiff with no evidence of muscle wasting or weakness; her joints are normal apart from mild changes of osteoarthritis in both hands.

1. What is the differential diagnosis?

2. What is the most likely diagnosis?

3. How are you going to manage her?

CASE 86

5, 15, 16

A 78-year-old man is referred to the clinic with a problem of lumps on his hands that have been coming on slowly over the past 6 years. They are not painful normally, but 1 week ago he cut his hand whilst peeling potatoes. The cut sliced into one of the lumps, which has been oozing white chalky material ever since. He has multiple medical problems mainly due to heart failure. He remains a heavy smoker and had a myocardial infarction 10 years earlier. He has longstanding angina and progressive breathlessness on exertion due to a combination of emphysema and heart failure. His long list of medication includes aspirin, diuretics, ACE inhibitors and digoxin. He lives alone. He still smokes 20 cigarettes per day but drinks only in moderation (up to 3 units per day). Examination reveals some swelling of his MCP and PIP joints and he admits to some stiffness in his hands in the mornings. There are numerous firm subcutaneous lumps on the fingers of both hands and similar lumps at the elbows.

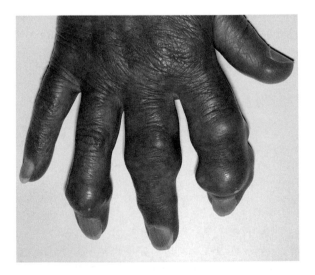

1. What is the most likely diagnosis?

2. What investigations should you perform?

3. How can you manage his problem?

CASE 87

1, 4, 5, 17

A 38-year-old woman presents with a 1-month history of increasing lethargy and malaise and low-grade fever. In the past month she has also noticed pain and swelling in the small joints of her hands with morning stiffness of 2 h. Her hair has been falling out and it often blocks the plughole of her shower. In the last 3 days she has also experienced pain on the right lower side of her chest, which is worse on deep inspiration. Her past history is unremarkable apart from Raynaud's phenomenon for the past two winters. She is currently taking no medication and has no known allergies. The patient is aware that one of her maternal aunts has been on dialysis for the past 5 years. On clinical examination her temperature is 37.8°C and she has palpable lymph nodes in her neck and axillae. She has three small oral ulcers on her buccal mucosa and there is erythema and scaling on her scalp with broken hairs present. She has swelling and tenderness of 20 small joints in her hands and feet. There is also a pleural rub audible at her right base. You make a provisional clinical diagnosis of a connective tissue disease.

1. Describe the range of investigations required at this stage.

2. Which serological tests (including autoantibodies) might help to inform the clinical features described or observed?

3. Will her hair loss be permanent?

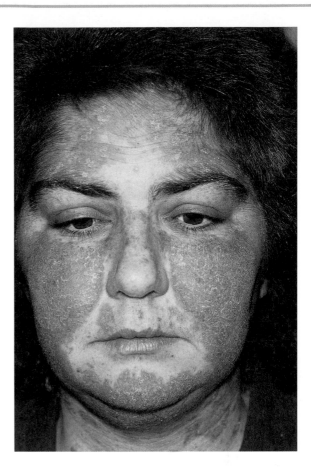

CASE 88

1, 4, 17

An anxious 47-year-old woman is referred urgently to clinic with a history of back pain for 4 years, shoulder pain intermittently for the previous 18 months, treated with physiotherapy with good effect; she has developed hand and wrist pains for the past 2 months and her general practitioner has checked an ESR (90 mm/h) and a rheumatoid factor (475 IU/l). She is very concerned that she has developed rheumatoid arthritis. On examination, you find that her hands are normal at present but she tells you that they are swollen first thing in the morning. No other joints bother her, except her spine, where she has limited forward flexion due to pain, but normal movement in all other directions. She denies any skin or hair problems. Her eyes have been gritty feeling in the last 4 years. She has difficulty swallowing foods without a drink of water. She has no history to suggest lupus. Her blood pressure and urinalysis are normal. You check her CRP level, which is normal, and start her on an anti-inflammatory agent and review her 4 months later. She is still complaining of pain in her hands, but again you cannot find any signs of joint swelling, and she has a normal range of movements in all her peripheral joints. You repeat her ESR and it is still high (89 mm/h) and her rheumatoid factor is still positive (530 IU/l), but her CRP remains normal.

1. What is the likely diagnosis?
2. What investigations would help you confirm the diagnosis?
3. How might you manage this patient?

CASE 89

4, 17, 18

A 23-year-old woman presents to the clinic with abnormal blood results. She has not had any clinical symptoms. Her obstetrician has referred her because she has had four miscarriages in the past 3 years, all in the first or second trimester. Following the second miscarriage she had a deep vein thrombosis. The blood results (see table) alarmed her obstetrician – hence the referral.

1. What do the blood results show?
2. What is the diagnosis and what other features might you expect?
3. How should she be managed?

Haemoglobin (12–15 g/dl)	11.1
White cell count (4–11 × 10⁹/l)	4.5
Neutrophil count (2–7 × 10⁹/l)	3.1
Platelets (150–400 × 10⁹/l)	45
ESR (mm/h)	132
CRP (<2 mg/l)	<2
Anti-nuclear antibody (normal <1/160)	1/80
Anti-ds DNA (normal 0–20 IU/l)	11
C3 (65–190 mg/dl)	110
C4 (14–40 mg/dl)	35
Prothrombin time (10–14 s)	12
APTT (22–34 s)	72

CASE 90

4, 5, 17, 18

A 33-year-old woman presents with a history of painful, cold hands for the past 4 months. They turn white, then dusky blue, then bright red before going back to normal again. The episodes started in January and have improved a little since the start of May with the warmer weather. Both index fingers and the right ring finger are predominantly affected, but the episodes sometimes affect the left little finger as well. The attacks are happening about three times per week at present, having been on most days in January. They do seem to relate to a change in temperature and she has started wearing gloves all the time. She noticed a very painful sore on the right index fingertip 2 months ago, and the skin cracked and then healed but has left a pitted scar. On further questioning she admits to an acid taste in her mouth when she wakes in the morning and occasional bouts of indigestion. On examination, she has cold hands with some whitening of the index fingers; peripheral pulses are all normal. You notice discrete small (2 mm) red blanching marks on her face and neck. The joints of her hands look normal, but she is unable to make a full fist with either hand. Her feet are also cold, although the peripheral pulses are all present. You notice that the 4th toe of the left foot and 3rd toe of the right foot are pale.

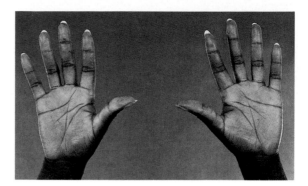

1. What is the most likely diagnosis?
2. What tests would you recommend?
3. What treatment and advice would you offer?

CASE 91

1, 5, 6, 18, 28

A 9-year-old girl is taken to Accident & Emegency by her parents who have noticed that she is limping. She is normally a very active child but has stopped running around, although can still ride her bike. Her parents think that her left knee is a little swollen. There is a history of a sore throat a few weeks previously, but no history of trauma. There is no significant past medical history. On examination, she is a well child, with a moderately swollen, non-tender right knee. She cannot fully straighten the knee and her quadriceps are wasted. The remainder of the examination is unremarkable.

1. What is the differential diagnosis?
2. What investigations would you do?
3. How would you manage her?

CASE 92

15, 19, 20

A 78-year-old man is referred to the clinic with a long history of back pain for the past 14 years. He has been investigated previously and found to have degenerative disc disease and managed quite well with exercise and simple painkillers. His general practitioner (GP) has referred him back because of new onset of pain in the right buttock and stiffness of the right leg, which stops him doing his back exercises. His GP ordered an X-ray of the hips, which is shown. You examine the patient and find that his hip movement appears to be full but it is painful when he walks, and he has a pronounced limp. He feels well in himself and has not lost any weight. His back is a little stiff but no different from before. His GP has ordered some blood tests as follows: ESR 5 mm/h, CRP 8 mg/l, routine blood count normal, routine biochemistry normal apart from the alkaline phosphatase, which is 1200 IU/l (normal range up to 500 IU/l).

1. What does the X-ray show?

2. What is the diagnosis?

3. How should he be managed?

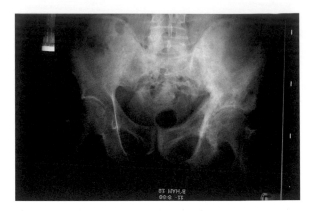

CASE 93

1, 4, 5, 17

A 76-year-old man has noted a 3-week history of fatigue, 4 kg weight loss, and joint pains in his hands and ankles. He has noticed some nasal crusting and bleeding, with severe tenderness over the cheeks. One week ago he started coughing up blood, and a chest X-ray was performed, showing infiltrates in both lung fields at mid-zone, and some nodules in the right lower lobe. Examination reveals swollen, tender and warm MCP joints. The ankles are also swollen and tender without any sign of pitting oedema. His CRP is 158 mg/l. The creatinine has risen from 150 µmol/l on admission 1 week ago to 250 µmol/l today. His urine contains 15 red cells per high power field, and occasional red cell casts.

1. What is the most likely diagnosis?

2. What tests would be most helpful?

3. How would you treat him?

CASE 94

4, 5, 17, 18, 20, 28

A 32-year-old man attends the clinic. His disease started at the age of 9 with a 6-week history of a swollen left knee and right ankle. Investigations fail to reveal any sign of infection, but he has a raised ESR and a very high CRP. Initial treatment with anti-inflammatory drugs was unhelpful, and he had the joints injected with steroid. Within 8 months, he had a recurrence of swelling in the same joints, and also further spread of swelling and pain in both his wrists, some toes and finger MCP joints. A diagnosis was made and he was started on methotrexate. After 2 years he stopped taking treatment even though it helped him. He refused to take any more, mainly because he did not want to have blood tests. After a further 3 years, he would not attend clinic. He moved away from the area and did not seek any more help. His parents supported his decision. Eventually, he was referred to the adult service, but did not attend many of the appointments and always politely declined any offer of help or blood tests, until, eventually, he stopped attending altogether.

On every visit his joint disease was getting progressively worse with significant swelling and restriction in range of movement. He was also noted to have poor spine posture with a significant stoop, and very limited back movements. Finally he has been referred back to clinic because his legs have become much more swollen than before, and his current general practitioner (GP) has noticed that he has some protein in his urine (see table), and a blood pressure of 172/97 mmHg. He allowed his GP to do a blood test showing a haemoglobin of 9.8 g/dl (normochromic, normocytic picture) and a significantly elevated CRP (150 mg/l).

1. What was the original diagnosis?
2. What is the most likely explanation for his recent leg swelling and proteinuria?
3. What is the connection between the two problems?

Blood test	Result	Units	Normal range
Sodium	136	mmol/l	135–145
Potassium	3.4	mmol/l	3.5–5.0
Urea	4.5	mmol/l	2.5–6.7
Creatinine	69	µmol/l	70–150
CRP	150	mg/l	<2
Bilirubin	13	µmol/l	3–17
ALT	34	IU/l	10–45
Alkaline phosphatase	116	IU/l	95–320
Albumin	21	g/l	35–50

Urine test	Result	Units
Urine protein	2598	mg/l
24-h protein	4468.6	mg/24 h
Collection time	24	h
24-h volume	1.72	litres

CASE 95

13, 19, 20

A 68-year-old woman presents with an osteoporotic vertebral fracture. She complains that she should not have developed the condition, because she has exercised regularly, particularly since reaching the menopause, and drinks over a litre of milk per day in addition to taking calcium and vitamin D supplements. She knows that her father had a hip fracture in his 60s, but her mother and female relatives have not had any fractures that she is aware of.

1. Is the patient correct regarding the interpretation of her family history?

2. What would be the correct advice to her regarding the effectiveness of exercise and calcium and/or vitamin D supplementation in osteoporosis prevention and treatment?

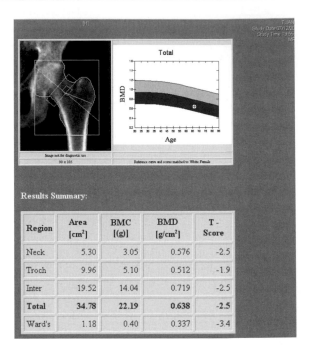

Results Summary:

Region	Area [cm²]	BMC [(g)]	BMD [g/cm²]	T-Score
Neck	5.30	3.05	0.576	-2.5
Troch	9.96	5.10	0.512	-1.9
Inter	19.52	14.04	0.719	-2.5
Total	34.78	22.19	0.638	-2.5
Ward's	1.18	0.40	0.337	-3.4

CASE 96

1, 5, 6, 21

A 21-year-old young man presents to clinic with a 1-month history of a sore right elbow. He works as a cook in a chip shop and has had to go off sick for the last week as his arm is too sore to lift the chips out of the fryer. He is in good health otherwise. On examination he has tenderness over the lateral aspect of the right elbow, but no swelling or redness. The left elbow is normal; all other joint areas are pain-free.

1. What is the most likely problem?

2. If he also complained of heel pain and had a history of acute iritis in the past, what diagnosis would you consider?

3. How would you manage this problem?

CASE 97

1, 5, 6, 7, 21

A 54-year-old woman presents to clinic with a sore right shoulder for the past 2 months. The pain came on gradually over this time and is stopping her from writing comfortably, and makes driving a little difficult. On examination, she has a good range of shoulder rotation, flexion and extension. Shoulder abduction is a little awkward but she manages it quite well. However, if her scapula is fixed, she struggles to abduct the arm beyond 30°.

1. What is the clinical syndrome?
2. What is the differential diagnosis?
3. How would you manage this patient?

CASE 98

14, 15, 19, 20, 23

A 21-year-old Pakistani woman is referred to the clinic with pain in her hips and shoulders. The problem has been present for about 3 months and is gradually getting worse. She finds it difficult to get out of a chair at home and is struggling to look after her 2-year-old son, as she cannot lift him. You are unable to get any further history and the examination is refused; she wears traditional dress and is covered from head to foot; her husband explains that she always dresses this way. The patient agrees to a blood test (see table).

1. What do the blood tests show?
2. What is the most likely diagnosis?
3. What treatment would you recommend?

Blood test	Result	Units	Normal range
ALT	33	IU/l	10–45
Sodium	139	mmol/l	135–145
Potassium	3.5	mmol/l	3.5–5.0
Urea	3.5	mmol/l	2.5–6.7
Creatinine	82	µmol/l	70–150
Calcium	1.92	mmol/l	2.12–2.62
Albumin	43	g/l	35–50
Total bilirubin	9	µmol/l	3–17
Alkaline phosphatase	956	IU/l	75–250
CRP	<8	mg/l	<2

CASE 99

4, 14, 17, 20

A 32-year-old man presents with a 6-month history of increasing fatigue and generalized weakness. He is usually a very keen sportsman but had to give up both weight training and jogging 4 months ago. In the last 4–5 weeks he has noticed increasing difficulty dressing in the morning, climbing stairs and getting up out of bed. He does not describe any joint pain or swelling, but he is generally stiff in his hips and shoulders for 2–3 h in the morning. In the past 6 months he has also noted some scaly erythematous lesions over the dorsum of both hands and he has developed photosensitivity. In the past 2 months he has had a persistent dry cough and exertional dyspnoea.

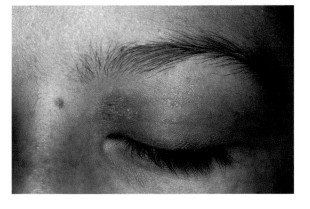

On examination there are erythematous scaly lesions over the dorsum of both hands and facial erythema. The proximal muscles of his upper and lower limbs show some evidence of wasting and he has grade 4 weakness on formal testing. He is also unable to rise from a squat position and his neck flexors are weak. He has bi-basal end-inspiratory crackles on chest examination.

1. What is the diagnosis?
2. What investigations are appropriate?
3. What treatment is indicated at this stage?

CASE 100

13, 16, 18, 21

A 67-year-old woman with rheumatoid arthritis for the past 15 years has suddenly started to drop her knives and forks. She is well controlled on methotrexate 12.5 mg per week and simple analgesia. She has not had any pain or swelling in her hands for 6 months. Examination shows that she has changes of longstanding rheumatoid arthritis with ulnar deviation, some swan neck deformities, but no active synovitis. The right 5th finger is not painful. You can extend it at the MCP joint without any pain but the patient cannot do this herself.

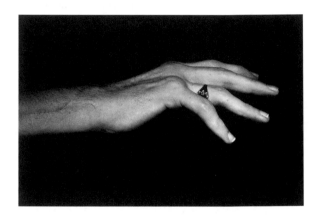

1. What does the picture demonstrate?
2. What complication of her disease has arisen?
3. How should this complication be managed?

ANSWERS

CASE 1 ANSWERS

4, 20

1. The critical feature is the asymmetric visible swelling below the joint. A 'swollen knee' and limp could indicate one of several common inflammatory or traumatic diagnoses. The earlier football injury is a 'red herring', which should not mislead, as parents often ascribe the onset of tumour symptoms to a knock sustained in sport.

2. The X-ray shows a sclerotic tibial lesion with calcification extending into the soft tissues. This lesion arises from the tibial metaphysis and on biopsy is shown to represent an osteosarcoma.

3. Treatment for osteosarcoma was revolutionized by the advent of effective chemotherapy in the 1980s. Many children and adolescents will receive 'neoadjuvant' chemotherapy, often including the drug methotrexate. Neoadjuvant treatment involves chemotherapy both before and after definitive surgery. Increasingly 'limb salvage' surgery will allow an affected limb to be saved, although amputation is still performed in about 20% of patients.

CASE 2 ANSWERS

4, 6, 7

1. The X-rays show a Charnley hip replacement. A trans-trochanteric approach to the hip was made at the original surgery and wires inserted to reattach the greater trochanter to the femur. There is wear of the high-density polyethylene cup as the prosthetic femoral head should lie in the centre of the cup, but it has migrated proximally. The joint is becoming unstable as a result of the wear.

2. Exclude infection and check his erythrocyte sedimentation rate (ESR), C-reactive protein (CRP) and white count. An aspiration arthrogram will also help to exclude infection within the hip joint and can also demarcate prosthetic loosening.

3. Revision of the hip replacement is indicated if his symptoms are troublesome and he is fit for surgery.

CASE 3 ANSWERS

4, 6, 27

1. The postero-anterior X-ray shows an adolescent idiopathic scoliosis. Note that the film has been taken as the patient stands and is shown with heart on the left so that one is looking at the spinal deviation from behind. The direction to which the convexity of the curve points indicates the side of the curve; right thoracic and left lumbar curves are a common combination.

2. The child should be examined from behind to observe her shoulders for asymmetry of height, scapular protrusion that may suggest an underlying rib hump, and the pelvis for symmetry of height of the iliac crests. A forward bending test is then performed as the rotational component of the scoliosis increases with spinal flexion. A 'postural' curve will disappear whereas a significant 'structural' curve, such as occurs in adolescent idiopathic scoliosis, will highlight rib cage elevation, deformity and asymmetry. The child should be assessed neurologically and this should be normal in adolescent idiopathic scoliosis. Curve magnitude and location of the apical vertebra are obtained from X-rays using Cobb's angle (see text on spinal deformity, Chapter 27). In general, for angles of less than 20° curves are kept under observation, bracing is used for those between 20° and 45° and surgery for curves greater than 45°. An MRI examination of the thoracolumbar spine is an essential preoperative requisite to exclude any co-existing spinal skeletal or neurological anomaly.

CASE 4 ANSWERS

6, 26

1. This is Perthes' disease – perhaps better termed a 'condition' – which represents an avascular necrosis of the capital (upper femoral) epiphysis and the X-ray shows collapse of the capital epiphysis.

2. The prognosis will depend on the extent of involvement of the head, the child's age at presentation and the sex of the child. The younger the child is at presentation, the better the outlook, and boys have a better prognosis than girls. A 5-year-old boy presenting for the first time with whole head involvement would be expected to have a better outcome in terms of sphericity of the femoral head at maturity than a 9-year-old girl presenting for the first time with a similar extent of necrosis.

CASE 5 ANSWERS

26

1. This is a slipped upper (capital) femoral epiphysis (see X-ray). This affects children usually between the ages of 10 and 15 years. It may be classified according to

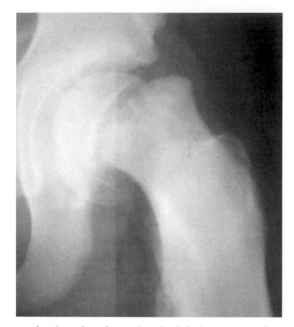

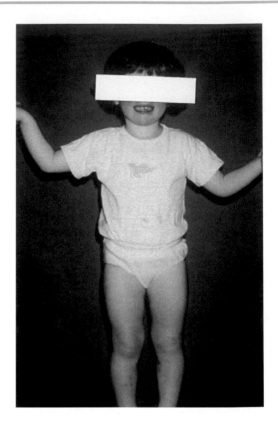

the time that the patient had their symptoms (acute, chronic, acute on chronic), the severity of the slip (mild, moderate and severe) or whether the patient could bear weight on the affected leg with or without walking aids or not (stable or unstable).

2. He should be admitted to hospital, placed on bed-rest and have the slip stabilized on the next convenient operating list.

3. The likelihood of developing a slip in the contralateral hip is about 30% and the boy and his parents should be made aware of this. There is some controversy as to whether or not the opposite side should be stabilized prophylactically at the time of fixation of the symptomatic side. This will depend on the surgeon's, patient's and family's views.

CASE 6 ANSWERS

1, 24

1. Assess limb alignment with the child standing. Check limb length and the child's torsional profile (see Chapter 1 on Physical examination) as external femoral torsion and internal tibial torsion can exacerbate the appearances of bow legs

2. The toddler has physiological bow legs (genu varum).

3. This is a physiological condition often seen in toddlers and normally resolves by about the age of 2 years. It is important to ensure that the deformity is symmetrical as a unilateral bowing may be an indication of a structural abnormality in the lower limb, which would require further investigations.

4. Take the parents' concerns seriously and allow time to discuss the condition with them. If the lower limbs are symmetrical in alignment and length, it is highly likely that the appearances are physiological and there is no underlying structural reason for the appearances. Thus further imaging is not required and the parents can be reassured that the appearances can be expected to improve over the next 12 months or so (see figure). No treatment is required; special shoe wear and exercises are of no proven benefit.

CASE 7 ANSWERS

24, 26, 27

1. The differential should include habitual toe walking, congenitally short gastrocnemei and diplegic cerebral palsy.

2. In broad terms the motor cortex, cerebellum and basal ganglia. A lesion of the motor cortex will produce spasticity, a lesion of the cerebellum results in ataxia and that of the basal ganglia will produce dyskinesia.

3. This boy has diplegic cerebral palsy as he was born prematurely, had a delay in walking, walks on tiptoes, and has increased tone and brisk reflexes in the lower

limbs. If he were a habitual toe walker he would have normal muscle tone and calf muscle length, and if he had congenitally short gastrocnemei he would have normal tone but a restriction in ankle dorsiflexion.

CASE 8 ANSWERS

26, 27

1. Duchenne's muscular dystrophy (DMD). This is the commonest inherited disease of muscle and is an X-linked recessive condition that can also arise spontaneously in about 15% of cases. Other conditions to consider are spinal muscle atrophy and other muscle dystrophies.

2. Plasma creatinine kinase is often grossly elevated in DMD. DNA analysis of peripheral blood can also show deletion of the dystrophin gene on the X chromosome.

3. The muscle weakness is progressive and many children lose the ability to walk between the ages of 8 and 12 years. As they become wheelchair dependent they often develop contractures at the hips, knees and ankles and a neuromuscular scoliosis. Pulmonary function deteriorates in their second decade; this is often made worse by the scoliosis and patients have difficulty in clearing secretions. Patients usually succumb to respiratory failure or infection at around 20 years of age.

CASE 9 ANSWERS

6, 24, 26, 27

1. Calcaneovalgus. The foot is deviated away from the midline (valgus) and the heel is excessively dorsiflexed (calcaneus; the opposite is equinus).

2. The calcaneovalgus may be an example of a 'packaging disorder' where the foot has been moulded into its shape by the pressure from the uterus. The foot will respond readily to passive stretching and there should be an excellent outcome. The foot posture may also result from a neurological disorder affecting the baby.

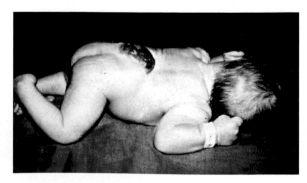

3. You must examine the baby's hips for stability and their spine. The photograph shows the baby's back and there is a myelomeningocele. This is an example of spina bifida, which produces a lower motor neurone lesion. The tibialis anterior (L4) is working and is dorsiflexing the ankle. The excessive dorsiflexion (calcaneus) has arisen because the posterior calf muscles (L5, S1, 2) are paralysed and there is an unopposed action of tibialis anterior.

CASE 10 ANSWERS

6, 26

1. This is clubfoot or talipes equinovarus. Equinus indicates a plantarflexed position at the ankle, and varus a deviation towards the midline.

2. As a matter of routine you should examine the hips to exclude instability, and the spine to exclude spinal dysraphism as a cause of a neurological clubfoot. In the latter case there may be a hairy patch or sacral dimple overlying the lower spine.

3. The feet should be examined to assess their stiffness. A programme of passive stretching of the feet begins shortly after birth and plaster casts or strapping are used to hold the position of the feet. In the past about 50% of feet might be operated on because of a deformity resistant to stretching, but recently a more conservative approach has become more widespread.

4. There will be permanent thinning of the calf muscles on the affected side and a difference in shoe size because the foot on the affected side is usually smaller. If treatment is successful in producing a plantargrade and reasonably flexible foot, these features are not likely to affect function greatly.

CASE 11 ANSWERS

1, 24

1. The grandmother is right, although growing pains do not have any connection with growth itself, but do occur in young growing children. The cause is unknown, but the above history is typical. The peak incidence is between 4 and 8 years of age and is thought to be muscle fatigue in the thighs and calves.

2. Observe the child's gait and examine their legs and spine carefully and include a neurological assessment. The diagnosis is made from the history and the absence of any objective abnormal physical findings. Remember referred pain, though. Only obtain X-rays

if there is loss of movement at a joint or tenderness in a specific area. A bone scan might be indicated to exclude an osteoid osteoma, a benign bone-forming tumour that can produce bone pain, but this is likely to affect one limb only whereas 'growing pains' are usually symmetrical.

3. The condition resolves spontaneously and the frequency and intensity of the pains abate. Inform the parents and child that the condition is self-limiting, but that the child should be reviewed if pains persist, particularly at night, and/or affect one limb only. Bone tumours are rare and musculoskeletal infection is not as common as it was, but worsening night pain affecting one limb or limb segment should be considered as a 'red flag' symptom.

CASE 12 ANSWERS

4, 5, 26

1. Examine her abdomen and spine; remember referred pain.

2. Irritable hip, septic arthritis of the hip, osteomyelitis of the proximal femur or pelvis, and Perthes' condition.

3. Check her temperature. X-ray the right hip and femur to exclude a fracture. If there is no fracture or hip pathology such as Perthes' condition on the plain X-ray, obtain an ultrasound of the hip. Take blood for a CRP or ESR and white cell count to exclude infection. Obtain urine for culture. If the investigations show that she is afebrile, has a normal or only slightly raised CRP or ESR and white cell count, but that she has an effusion of the right hip demonstrated on ultrasound, the diagnosis is an irritable hip. It is not necessary to admit her to hospital as in most cases the pain settles over 48–72 h and the child starts to walk again. Irritable hip may be associated with a recent viral infection or be an early sign of Perthes' condition. The parents should be told that if she becomes unwell or starts to develop a fever they should return to hospital promptly. This is to re-evaluate her, as missed septic arthritis of the hip can have a disastrous outcome.

CASE 13 ANSWERS

1, 4, 26

1. True leg length discrepancy is the difference in overall length when measured from the anterior superior iliac spine to the medial malleolus when the legs are placed symmetrically. Apparent leg length discrepancy is the difference in leg length when measured from the xiphisternum or umbilicus to the medial malleoli.

2. The discrepancy can also be assessed clinically by placing blocks under the short leg and assessing when the pelvis is level. Radiological imaging is obtained from a CT scanogram of the lower limbs. The image can be digitized to give lengths of the thigh and shin segments. An X-ray of the left wrist is taken to assess the child's bone age, which may be different from their chronological age.

3. A discrepancy predicted to be 3.5 cm at skeletal maturity is best managed by an epiphyseodesis (surgical destruction of a growth plate) of the long leg. This may involve the distal femoral or proximal tibial growth plates, or both, depending on the discrepancy and the amount of residual skeletal growth left. The distal femoral plate grows at about 3/8" (1 cm) and the proximal tibial plate at 2/8" (0.7 cm) per year. Girls stop growing at about 14 years of age and boys at about 16 years of age. Knowing the child's bone age helps to predict when skeletal maturity will occur and one can then calculate when the growth arrest at a physis should be made.

CASE 14 ANSWERS

6, 21, 27

1. Access for skin hygiene can be hampered by the flexed position of the fingers, thumb and wrist, and the skin can become macerated in the wrist and palm creases. The posture of the hand is not functional for putting on and removing clothing, and the hand cannot rest on a flat surface. The patient may also feel self-conscious about the posture of his hand.

2. If there is excessive muscle tone from the upper motor neurone lesion, but adequate muscle length, an injection of botulinum toxin into the wrist and finger flexors may help. Botulinum toxin inhibits the action of acetylcholine at the neuromuscular junction. The pharmacological effect wears off after about 3 months. If there is shortening of the flexors and a fixed contracture of the wrist, surgical lengthening of the flexors and a wrist fusion are likely to improve posture, hygiene and cosmesis, but not necessarily hand function. Hand orthoses are poorly tolerated.

CASE 15 ANSWERS

6, 23

1. A painful red bunion occurs when the forefoot is chronically forced into shoes too tight for the

forefoot. There is usually evidence of 'hallux valgus' deformity on X-ray. Hallux valgus is a common condition that is most evident in people with evidence of joint or soft-tissue laxity. This is not pathological, and may affect up to 10% of the population, women more than men. The intermetatarsal ligaments stretch and the forefoot splays outwards on standing. This makes the condition painful on compressing the forefoot within tight fashion shoes, but is often not painless when barefoot or in trainers.

2. If correctible passively, there is a good chance of improvement with footwear advice. Sometimes a moulded instep orthosis can also help by allowing the forefoot to take its original shape within the shoe. If pain persists, excision of the bunion with an osteotomy to correct the underlying 'metatarsus primus varus' (first metatarsal in varus) is performed in younger people. Older patients with low demand may have an excision arthroplasty with excision of the base of the proximal phalanx (Keller's procedure). Osteoarthritis of the first metatarsophalangeal joint may also respond to this operation, or to an arthrodesis.

CASE 16 ANSWERS

1, 6, 7, 16

1. Cardinal radiographic features of osteoarthritis are:
   a. joint space narrowing
   b. peri-articular osteosclerosis (whiteness on an X-ray 'negative' as shown here)
   c. marginal osteophytes
   d. subchondral cysts.

2. Non-surgical treatments include analgesia and use of a stick. In most patients, the stick should be held in the opposite hand to off-load the painful hip when weight-bearing on the painful side. Very occasionally a patient with a waddling-type gait may find relief by holding the stick in the hand on the affected side hard against the affected leg during stance.

3. In many patients without a significant inflammatory component, and in whom there is no joint collapse, pain may not be a major complaint. Instead it may be possible to identify a gradual deterioration in walking distance and a gradual reduction in work-related and recreational activities. Inability to tie or put on shoes reflects stiffness of the hip joint. Capsular contracture is part of the pathology of osteoarthritis.

   Although total hip replacement is most reliable in its ability to reduce pain from arthritis, in the pain-free but very stiff patient there may be a marked increase in activity level after the operation and a concurrent increase in quality of life. Dislocation is a risk of total hip replacement and individuals who require to squat or twist as part of their work are at special risk. Strategies to reduce this risk include careful mobilization in the first 6 weeks after surgery.

CASE 17 ANSWERS

1, 6, 22

1. Waddell's inappropriate back pain signs include, as well as the positive 'long sit', pain in the low back on applying pressure to the top of the head (crown pressure sign), pain in the low back when the patient is asked to place their hands flat against their upper thighs and the pelvis is rotated on the hips, without any back movement (trunk rotation sign), back pain when the knee and hip are flexed together, and exaggeration of pain on attempted straight leg raise.

2. Further investigations should be resisted. Plain X-rays will show some degenerative changes, which are normal in middle age. An MRI will either be normal or show minor abnormalities of doubtful significance. It is highly unlikely that an operable lesion will be identified or that a reputable surgeon would consider surgery. It is important not to overmedicalize such patients.

3. The first task of management is to explain that there is no pathological or anatomical abnormality that requires or will respond to invasive intervention. The patient has to be told that the pain is mechanical in origin and that the first line of management is physical rehabilitation, coupled with education about the nature and origin of the pain. Emphasis should be placed on regaining physical fitness and avoidance of activities that are likely to aggravate the pain. It is important to refer the patient to a physiotherapist or other therapist who regularly deals with patients with back pain and who is prepared to be involved over a significant period of time. Often a fitness trainer with an interest in this type of client is an alternative approach. If these approaches do not succeed formal pain management, including cognitive behavioural therapy, should be considered.

CASE 18 ANSWERS

1, 4, 22

1. The abnormality in the patient's spinal canal produces a 'trefoil' outline. This is usually due to an arthritic

(spondylitic in the spine) process which produces osteophytic overgrowth impinging on the canal, known as spinal stenosis.

2. This tends to pinch the spinal nerves. Below the cord (L1/L2), the cauda equina is compressed. Sometimes individual nerve roots are also compressed as they pass through their own exit foramina. It is thought a 'double' compression, occurring at two levels, may be required to block microvascular blood supply to the nerve roots, leading to pain in the muscle supplied by one or more affected nerve roots. The symptoms are known as 'claudication' after the Roman emperor Claudius who walked with a limp.

3. The diagnosis can be confirmed by excluding the other major cause of claudication – 'intermittent' or vascular claudication. This may require a vascular referral. A CT or MRI scan of the lumbo-sacral spine will confirm spinal stenosis. The side and level of maximum stenosis can often be identified and this ought to correlate with the symptoms.

4. Sometimes caudal epidural steroid injections may help, but to be curative treatment is usually surgical. Decompression of the posterior elements (laminectomy) together with nerve root foraminal decompression is the commonest procedure.

CASE 19 ANSWERS

1, 5, 6, 21

1. Tennis elbow (lateral epicondylitis) is a painful overuse condition in which the common extensor tendon origin becomes inflamed and painful. The diagnosis is made by a suitable history of overuse (e.g. in tennis) of the extensor muscles of the forearm. The common extensor origin is tender and forced extension of the wrist and digits against resistance increases the discomfort. This is usually self-limiting, and a period of rest and perhaps anti-inflammatory medication is all that is required to allow the symptoms to settle. Occasionally the condition becomes chronic. Ultrasound treatment, steroid injection and common extensor surgical release have been tried. A similar condition affects the common flexor origin (golfer's elbow). The diagnosis is made in the same way.

2. Extensor digitorum communis, extensor digiti minimi, extensor carpi ulnaris, extensor carpi radialis brevis. (Brachioradialis and extensor carpi radialis longus originate from the supracondylar ridge.)

CASE 20 ANSWERS

1, 5, 6, 21

1. The most likely diagnosis is de Quervain's disease. In this condition there is a pathological thickening within the wall of the sheath through which the tendons of extensor pollicis brevis and abductor pollicis longus pass to the thumb. This constricts the sheath causing pain when the thumb is moved. The thickening may be visible and palpable. Although this condition is often called stenosing tendovaginitis, it is not due to inflammation of the lining of the sheath. Anatomical variations such as subcompartments of the sheath and multiple tendons are common and may be predisposing factors. The condition is most often seen in perimenopausal women and sometimes in the postpartum period, indicating that hormonal factors may be involved. It is not thought to be caused by work or repetitive movements, but when the condition is present such activities may provoke pain.

2. In Finkelstein's test the thumb is passively adducted across the palm and then the wrist is deviated in an ulnar direction. When the test is positive the discomfort that it provokes is accurately localized to the first dorsal compartment of extensor retinaculum of the wrist, which lies just proximal to the tip of the styloid process.

3. The main differential diagnosis is osteoarthritis at the base of the thumb metacarpal, which is common in women in the same age group. The joints that are affected are the trapeziometacarpal or scapho-trapeziotrapezoid joints (see Anatomy section, Chapter 1). When both joints are involved the condition is called pantrapezial osteoarthritis. Osteoarthritis can be distinguished from de Quervain's disease by physical examination. In osteoarthritis the discomfort is located distal to the radial styloid process. The pain is aggravated by compressing the joint by gripping the thumb ray and then twisting it (the grinding test, which should be done gently). X-rays will confirm the diagnosis.

4. Splinting the thumb will give temporary relief. It is important to note that a simple wrist splint is ineffective because it still allows the painful movements of the thumb. Most patients find that a splint is cumbersome and limits the ability to do daily tasks. The uncomfortable area may be infiltrated with a mixture of steroid and local anaesthetic, injected around the tendons. Surgical treatment

involves releasing the tendons in the first dorsal compartment. Care must be taken to release all subcompartments and it is particularly important that the incision does not damage the terminal branches of the radial nerve. The symptoms from the resultant neuroma may be considerably more disabling than the original condition.

CASE 21 ANSWERS

1, 6, 14, 16, 21

1. Carpal tunnel syndrome. This is a fairly common condition in the later stages of pregnancy. The symptoms result from increased pressure on the median nerve in the carpal tunnel, beneath the flexor retinaculum at the wrist. Although unpleasant tingling (paraesthesia) usually occurs in the median nerve distribution, this is not invariable and the whole hand may be affected. Symptoms are characteristically worse during the night or when holding the hands elevated, for example holding a phone or newspaper. Physical signs are usually absent. Wasting of the thenar muscles is not usually seen in this particular group, although it may occur in older women with carpal tunnel syndrome. Before wasting develops there may be weakness of abduction of the thumb. Phalen's test involves holding the wrists flexed for 60 s. It is positive if the tingling is reproduced. Tapping on the median nerve at the base of the palm may again cause tingling (Tinel's test). These tests are not particularly sensitive or specific and the diagnosis should not be based solely on their presence or absence. Motor and sensory nerve conduction tests are more reliable and will usually demonstrate slowed conduction in both motor and sensory fibres of the median nerve in the wrist.

2. When it occurs during pregnancy the condition is believed to be associated with increased fluid retention. Similar symptoms can occur when there is a space-occupying lesion within the carpal tunnel, for example a ganglion or proliferative synovium associated with rheumatoid arthritis. Most cases occur in middle-aged women without a clear cause and in these cases the condition is termed idiopathic carpal tunnel syndrome. Carpal tunnel syndrome may occur in endocrine disorders such as diabetes mellitus and hypothyroidism.

3. In most cases the symptoms resolve within a few weeks of childbirth.

4. Since the condition is likely to resolve, conservative treatment is preferred in pregnant patients. Wearing a splint on the wrist prevents the wrist going into flexion, which can trigger symptoms. An injection of steroid and local anaesthetic into the carpal tunnel may be helpful in resistant cases. Surgical release of the flexor retinaculum is rarely needed in this group, although it is usually the treatment of choice in older women with idiopathic carpal tunnel syndrome.

CASE 22 ANSWERS

21

1. This is the typical appearance of Dupuytren's disease, a proliferative disorder of the palmar and digital fascia of unknown cause. It is equally common in those who do not do heavy manual labour. There is often, but not always, a strong family history of the condition. It occurs in those of Northern European origin and is quite rare in other racial groups. It is more common in men and becomes more common with age. In many cases the condition is mild, with slight nodularity in the fascia that does not interfere with function.

2. Dupuytren's disease has been shown to be more common in people with a heavy alcohol intake and particularly in those with alcoholic liver disease. However, it is a very common condition and its presence does not indicate that the person is a heavy drinker.

3. Dupuytren's disease is very common in both type 1 and type 2 diabetics. The contractures tend to be milder in diabetics and the condition is more diffuse. There is a less clear association with epilepsy, which has not been clearly confirmed in all studies. Associated fibrotic conditions should be identified, such as Garrod's pads (swellings over the proximal interphalangeal (PIP) joints of the fingers), Ledderhose's disease (involvement of the plantar fascia) and Peyronie's disease (fibrosis of the corpus cavernosum of the penis).

4. In many cases without significant contractures, simple advice is all that is required. It is important to realize that excision of early nodules in an attempt to prevent later contractures may have exactly the opposite effect by causing an increase in proliferative activity in the area of the scar. No regimens of splintage or exercise have been shown to be effective. Surgery is reserved for contractures that are interfering with function but no operation cures the patient of

Dupuytren's disease, as it is programmed into that patient to form proliferative tissue in the fascia, either in the area of previous excision (recurrent disease) or elsewhere (extension of the disease). A strong family history, extensive palmar involvement and evidence of fibrotic disease elsewhere indicate a high likelihood of recurrence.

CASE 23 ANSWERS

4, 5, 23

1. This is an ingrowing toenail. Infection of the lateral nail-fold has caused granulation tissue to form over the nail-plate.

2. Antibiotics on their own are not likely to resolve the condition and usually are only indicated if there is a surrounding cellulitis or lymphangitis. A wedge of the lateral nail-plate can be removed under local analgesia and this gives an opportunity for the granulation tissue to resolve. The nail-plate will regrow after wedge excision and is associated with about a 30% likelihood of the infection and granulation tissue recurring. Definitive treatment is ablation of the lateral part of the germinal matrix of the nail-bed using liquefied phenol BP or surgical excision of the nail-bed. The advantage of phenol over surgical excision is that it can be done in the presence of infection as phenol is an antiseptic.

CASE 24 ANSWERS

1, 4, 20, 22

1. Her red flag features included: age, thoracic back pain, previous cancer history, non-mechanical pain and neurological picture, i.e. five relevant red flags.

2. There is a high chance of her clinical features being due to a metastatic cancer deposit, even though her breast cancer was diagnosed and treated 10 years earlier. After breast cancer, metastases can appear even later.

3. Because back pain in cancer patients may signify a pathological fracture of a vertebra, manipulative treatment of the back pain is strongly contra-indicated as it may lead to spinal cord damage.

4. Plain radiographs may show vertebral body collapse, but MRI and CT scanning show much more detail, especially helping to differentiate between extradural soft-tissue metastasis and cord compression due to vertebral body fracture with collapse, i.e. a mechanical problem demanding a mechanical solution.

A tissue diagnosis is needed and a sample is obtained through needle biopsy under X-ray or even CT guidance.

5. Initially, systemic steroids (dexamethasone) may be used to reduce oedema of the cord. If the spinal cord dysfunction is mild and the cord compression is due to extradural soft-tissue tumour, radiotherapy and chemotherapy may suffice. If there is mechanical bony compression of the cord, surgical decompression is best with instrumentation to stabilize the pathological fracture. The surgical procedure will be planned according to the position of the pathology; in this case it is mostly anterior so, ideally, the surgical procedure would be anterior thoracotomy with removal of the diseased vertebral body and interbody fusion using instrumentation and bone grafting. In cases with a poorer prognosis the decompression can be carried out posteriorly with supporting instrumentation. Radiotherapy would be used as an adjunct. Treatment is palliative rather than curative with rehabilitation according to the degree of disability. Bone pain can be controlled by bisphosphonates. Diamorphine may be required.

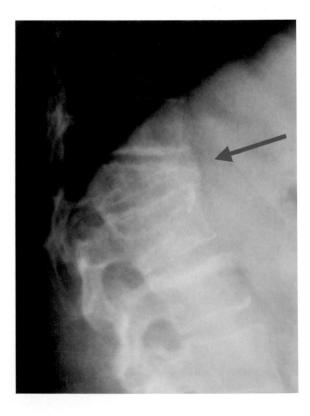

CASE 25 ANSWERS

3, 4, 20

1. The X-ray shows an osteochondroma, so called because it has a bony base (osteo-), a cartilage cap (-chondro-) and is a benign tumour (-oma). About 1% of children will develop a noticeable osteochondroma. The diagnosis is made on clinical examination and X-ray. Most are asymptomatic, but sometimes they can cause discomfort when muscle or tendon rubs over the surface of one. An osteochondroma will usually grow up to skeletal maturity and then stop, although occasionally one may continue to grow into adulthood. It is thought to arise from the perichondrial ring which surrounds the childhood growth plate, since the histology of the cartilage cap is quite similar to the columnar architecture of the growth plate.

2. It is important to check for other osteochondromas. If they occur, then the condition may be hereditary multiple exostoses (HME), an autosomal dominant inherited condition affecting about 1 in 50 000 people in which many osteochondromas are found. In this condition there is often short stature, deformity of forearms and legs, and occasionally malignant change in an osteochondroma to form a chondrosarcoma in adulthood (less than 5% of HME).

3. Treatment mostly depends upon symptoms. Many painful osteochondromas will settle with observation, but sometimes excision is warranted. In HME removal of osteochondromas is quite common, and correction of long-bone deformity may also be required.

CASE 26 ANSWERS

4, 5, 6, 7

1. This X-ray shows a cemented total hip replacement. The implant is loose at both the acetabular and femoral sides of the joint since there is a clear surrounding lucency at the bone–cement interface. Proof of this would be gained by performing a hip arthrogram in which radio-opaque contrast is injected into the artificial hip joint under aseptic conditions and X-ray control. Contrast leaking into the bone–cement interface indicates loosening. Loosening can be either septic or aseptic. An aspiration sample taken at the same time as the arthrogram can be sent for microbiology, but a negative result does not exclude infection entirely. Loosening at 15 years after primary surgery, however, is much more likely to represent an aseptic process.

2. All non-biological implants will eventually fail under load. The natural history of aseptic loosening at the bone–cement interface is one of progressive symptoms, with progressive cortical and medullary osteolysis through bone phagocytosis. Eventually the femur may fracture, or the acetabular component may spin or even perforate into the pelvis.

3. Treatment depends upon the patient's general condition, but if an improvement in mobility is anticipated in a resilient patient then revision total hip replacement could be undertaken. Outcome overall is often satisfactory, but this is a much more extensive procedure than the primary operation with a higher general complication rate, and a lower implant survival rate.

CASE 27 ANSWERS

4, 5, 6, 7

1. The likely diagnosis is infection within the total knee replacement. The clinical picture of pain, redness, swelling and heat is one of acute inflammation, possibly with a pointing abscess.

2. Temperature and inflammatory markers (white cell count, ESR, CRP) may be elevated. A knee arthrogram could be performed. Here radio-opaque contrast is injected into the artificial knee joint under aseptic conditions and X-ray control. Contrast leaking into the bone–cement interface indicates loosening. An aspiration sample taken at the same time as the arthrogram can be sent for microbiology, but a negative result does not exclude infection entirely.

3. If there is a clinical abscess, then surgery to drain and debride the knee replacement is indicated. Septic loosening of the prosthesis means that a simple 'washout' will not suffice, and revision of the prosthesis should be undertaken. Early debridement of a possibly infected joint replacement is preferable to late debridement, and hence careful clinical observation in the immediate post-operative phase is vital. This may be performed as a single-stage procedure, in which the implants are replaced with new ones during the same operative procedure. Alternatively a two-stage procedure can be undertaken in which the new prosthesis is implanted several weeks after removal of the infected components. In the intervening period a 'cement spacer' is often interposed between the femur and tibia, and appropriate antibiotics given. The advantage of a two-stage revision is that the re-infection rate is low, but patient morbidity may be higher.

CASE 28 ANSWERS

1, 4, 22

1. The nursing chart is a record of post-operative patient observations; here a selection is recorded. Both pulse and blood pressure are rising, supporting evidence for an increasing level of pain. Leg sensation and power are recorded because of spine surgery adjacent to nerve roots supplying the lower limbs. Any life- or limb-threatening deterioration should be detected early by this chart.

2. The doctor should be informed when pain is not controlled by prescribed medications, and certainly when a deterioration in neurology is first detected (by 16.00 hours).

3. The likely diagnosis is a compressive lesion affecting the nerve roots. This is usually due to an acute haematoma. An emergency MRI scan should be undertaken to confirm the diagnosis, followed by immediate surgical evacuation of the haematoma.

CASE 29 ANSWERS

1, 4, 22

1. The picture described is of a myelopathy that is affecting the lower limbs, but also certain parts of the upper limbs. If the upper limbs were normal there could be a problem in the thoracic cord, but with the upper limb involvement the lesion must be in the cervical spine. The lack of pain is typical and is partly responsible for the fact that myelopathy does not present until the condition is well advanced.

2. The jaw reflex is normal, so placing the lesion below brain level. The biceps and brachioradialis reflexes are normal, but the abnormal triceps reflexes means that there is cord pathology at a level between the 6th and 7th cervical vertebrae (C6/7). The knee reflexes are brisk as one would expect, but the ankle reflexes and plantar responses are inhibited by the presence of a diabetic peripheral neuropathy.

3. The MRI shows a minor abnormality at C5/6, but a more significant stenosis at C6/7 due to a combination of disc and osteophyte narrowing the spinal canal and compressing the spinal cord. The level of this pathology would exactly explain the neurological picture.

4. Cervical myelopathy carries a variable prognosis and sometimes remains static for long periods of time. However, when there is evidence of a quadriparesis and a rapidly deteriorating myelopathy, there is an inevitable progression to severe disability with loss of all useful function in the hands and legs. No conservative treatment is helpful, but operative decompression can halt the progression of the condition. Modest improvement of function is possible, but complete recovery is unlikely except in early and mild cases.

CASE 30 A3NSWERS

1, 4, 20, 22

1. The high ESR and general malaise suggest more serious pathology including neoplasia and infection. An ESR of over 100 mm/h raises the possibility of myeloma in middle-aged patients. The plasma proteinaemia and monoclonal gammopathy are in keeping with the diagnosis of multiple myeloma.

2. The C6 radiculopathy and myelopathy suggest a condition at the C5/6 level with compromise of the 6th cervical nerve and spinal cord itself. This could mean a reduced biceps reflex, but increased triceps and lower limb reflexes.

3. Besides the blood tests mentioned above, Bence Jones protein may be found in the urine. Plain radiographs of the neck show loss of density of the C5 vertebra with collapse of the vertebral body. MRI shows collapse of the vertebral body and axial slices show a major soft-tissue abnormality extending on the left side of the midline, impinging upon the spinal cord and encompassing the 6th cervical nerve. A needle biopsy under X-ray guidance should be carried out and the tissue samples examined histologically and by tissue culture for the possibility of infection.

    In this case the diagnosis of multiple myeloma was confirmed.

4. The neurological problems – radiculopathy and myelopathy – were treated by anterior vertebrectomy of the diseased 5th cervical vertebra with anterior cervical fusion using bone-graft and plate fixation. Decompression rapidly improved the pain and neurological deficit, but was clearly not the answer to the neoplastic process. Therefore, radiotherapy to the cervical spine was indicated together with the appropriate chemotherapy to control the myeloma.

    The patient in question survived for 3 years before dying from the multiple myeloma, but had no brachialgia or neurological problems after his operation. The operative treatment, therefore, provided useful palliation.

CASE 31 ANSWERS

1, 4, 6, 22

1. The most likely problematic level is at C5/6 because the clinical features suggest a C6 nerve deficit (weak biceps). MRI or CT of the cervical spine is indicated.

2. Treatment should be conservative as the natural history of disc disease usually results in complete resolution of the symptoms. Physiotherapy with traction and manipulation can help, as can other techniques, such as acupuncture and transcutaneous nerve stimulation. As they had not helped this patient, treatment might extend to nerve root or epidural injections of steroid. The changes seen on this scan would be equivalent to those on scans of asymptomatic subjects so caution should be exercised to avoid over-treatment of the changes that may simply reflect benign degenerative changes associated with ageing.

3. If symptoms persisted and were troublesome enough, an operation could offer definitive treatment.

4. This is usually carried out anteriorly and after discectomy an anterior cervical fusion is performed. It is possible to perform cervical discectomy without fusion, but there is an incidence of significant cervical pain afterwards.

CASE 32 ANSWERS

4, 5, 26

1. The differential lies between acute septic arthritis of the hip and acute osteomyelitis of the femur. Both may present in a similar manner and the posture of the child is characteristic. In a larger child it may be possible to demonstrate discrete swelling and tenderness overlying the femur in osteomyelitis, but such distinction may be difficult in the younger child. The history of preceding upper respiratory tract infection raises the possibility of transient synovitis or 'irritable hip', but this would be unlikely to result in such high levels of the inflammatory markers.

2. Ultrasound scan is simple, safe and non-invasive, but should be interpreted with care. An effusion in the hip joint does not exclude a proximal femoral osteomyelitis, as there may be a sympathetic effusion in the adjacent joint. However, absence of an effusion would point towards osteomyelitis as the cause, and detection of a subperiosteal pus collection would confirm the diagnosis. Aspiration of any effusion under ultrasound control may help distinguish between infected and sympathetic collections.

Isotope bone scanning may be used on occasion to localize the site of infection, but it may not be readily available as an emergency and there are concerns about radiation. MRI scan will clearly distinguish between a primary septic arthritis and acute osteomyelitis, but this may not be available as an emergency investigation.

3. If septic arthritis is suspected, blood cultures should be taken. The joint must be opened to obtain infected material for culture, to wash it out thoroughly and to establish adequate drainage. Appropriate antibiotic therapy should then be started and given intravenously initially. If acute osteomyelitis is suspected, intravenous antibiotics prescribed on a 'best guess' basis should be started and the progress closely monitored by the child's temperature and serial estimation of inflammatory markers. Ultrasound evidence of a subperiosteal collection that fails to resolve may be an indication for surgical drainage of pus. In both scenarios, supportive measures such as pain control, nutritional support and close watch on fluid balance are important.

CASE 33 ANSWERS

1, 4, 22, 29

1. An Asian with a generalized illness and spinal trouble demands early investigation for a possible diagnosis of tuberculosis (TB) of the spine.

A full blood count may reveal a chronic anaemia and a lymphocytosis. The ESR and CRP are usually very high.

A chest radiograph may show hilar lymph node enlargement of features of pulmonary TB. Mantoux or Heaf skin tests are usually positive. Sputum culture may yield acid-fast bacilli.

2. Plain radiographs of the spine show loss of definition of the disc space and may show erosion of the end-plates (see figure).

An X-ray-guided aspiration and needle biopsy is required. Samples need standard bacterial culture and specific TB culture using Lowenstein–Jensen culture medium. Histological examination of the tissue biopsy requires Gram and Ziehl–Nielsen staining. This patient's sample was positive for TB culture and acid-fast bacilli could be seen on histological examination as well as granulomata with caseation.

3. Treatment: rest in an orthosis and anti-tuberculous chemotherapy may suffice, even in the presence of an epidural abscess, but if there is no clinical improvement, surgical drainage and instrumented

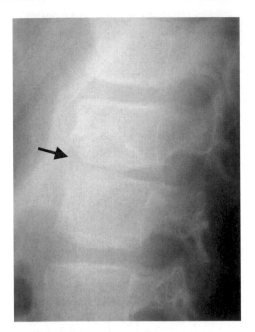

spinal fusion may be required. This patient improved on chemotherapy alone. Therapy with two or three anti-tuberculous drugs continues for at least 6 months. It is important to monitor treatment progress by weekly measurement of inflammatory markers. Serial radiographs and MR scans can also be helpful in assessing resolution of the infection. The natural history of a tuberculous spondylodiscitis is to heal by a process of ankylosis with bony bridges forming to immobilize the affected motion segment.

CASE 34 ANSWERS

1, 4, 22, 27

1. There is a spondylolisthesis of the 5th lumbar vertebra on the sacrum. Spondylolisthesis is classified according to the degree of slip of the AP diameter of the vertebral body upon the vertebra below. Grade I is a 0–25% slip, grade II 25–50%, grade III 50–75%, grade IV 75–100%, and grade V ('spondyloptosis') is where the vertebra has slipped right off the vertebra below.

2. Bilateral pars interarticularis defect. The slip often develops gradually and there may be adaptation of the tissues with few deleterious effects. Whilst the spondylolisthesis can present in childhood with back pain, a spinal deformity, tight hamstrings and even neurological deficit (numbness, weakness and sphincter disturbance), it is just as likely to be picked up in adulthood in the course of investigation for chronic back pain and it can turn up as an incidental finding during investigation of other conditions.

3. Treatment of spondylolisthesis depends upon the cause, the degree and the severity of symptoms. Most forms of spondylolisthesis can be managed conservatively with only a small proportion needing spinal fusion. By the time a patient reaches the age of 30 years the spondylolisthesis usually stabilizes spontaneously and any back pain is just as likely to have a completely separate cause. The young patient with severe symptoms and an unstable slip is different and there is good evidence that a spinal fusion with bone grafting in situ will suffice. Pain is relieved and the relief of hamstring muscle spasm improves the posture and sagittal balance. This girl underwent surgery.

CASE 35 ANSWERS

8, 9, 13

1. The patient has sustained a fracture of the midshaft of the clavicle. This is a very common injury and the treatment of choice is non-operative. Patients are provided with a sling and analgesia. Regular follow-up is required to ensure the fracture progresses to union, which normally occurs in adults within 2–3 months of injury.

2. The radiographs at 12 weeks indicate there has been no progression to union. Non-union is a well recognized complication of clavicular fractures in adults and occurs in 10% of cases. It is more common in fractures with more than 1 cm of displacement between the bone fragments or in those with comminution.

3. The most appropriate treatment is plating, occasionally with bone grafting. This is successful in obtaining union in more than 90% of cases. The radiograph below shows the bony union progressing after plating.

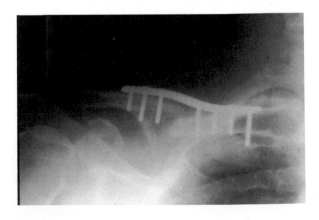

CASE 36 ANSWERS

9, 13

1. The patient has sustained an anterior dislocation of the shoulder. The humeral head has come to lie in a subcoracoid position. Anterior dislocations account for 95% of shoulder dislocations. The other directions encountered in clinical practice are posterior and the very rare 'luxatio erecta' when the humeral head dislocates in an inferior direction.

2. Anterior dislocations may be complicated by traction nerve injuries, most commonly involving the axillary nerve. However, in older patients, brachial plexus palsies are not unusual. Rotator cuff tears are also frequent in patients over the age of 40 years who sustain a shoulder dislocation. These are difficult to diagnose at the time of the dislocation. They should be suspected in patients who fail to mobilize the shoulder in the weeks following injury.

3. A closed reduction under sedation is the most appropriate treatment for the acute case. A period of immobilization in a sling for a period of 4–6 weeks is usually recommended for younger patients to minimize the risk of recurrent dislocation. In patients over the age of 40 years the risk of recurrent dislocation is small and early mobilization can be safely attempted once the initial pain and swelling have settled.

CASE 37 ANSWERS

8, 9, 13

1. The patient has sustained a fracture dislocation of the shoulder.

2. The humeral head is visible in a dislocated position. Note that the head is separated from the humeral shaft and the greater tuberosity. The lesser tuberosity is not visible as a separate fragment and is probably still attached to the humeral head.

3. This is a high-energy injury and there is a significant risk of an associated axillary nerve neuropraxia or even a brachial plexus injury. There is also a risk of fractures elsewhere. Clinical examination should, therefore, be conducted with these possibilities in mind. The neurological status was actually normal. However, there was a painful deformed wrist and radiographs confirmed a comminuted intra-articular distal radial fracture.

4. Options for treatment: non-operative treatment is not feasible in this situation. A closed reduction of the dislocated head is impossible because it is separated from the humeral shaft. The choices are either open

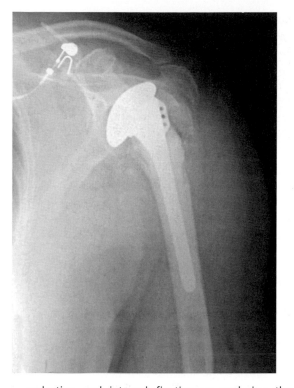

reduction and internal fixation or replacing the humeral head with a shoulder hemiarthroplasty. Internal fixation is feasible if the bone is of good quality and the humeral head has an adequate soft-tissue attachment to provide a blood supply. Surgical exploration was carried out. This revealed that the bone was very osteoporotic and the lesser tuberosity was also detached from the humeral head. The humeral head, therefore, had no soft-tissue attachments and in this situation (a four-part fracture dislocation) shoulder joint replacement (see figure) was a better option. This was performed and the patient made a satisfactory post-operative recovery. The distal radial fracture was considered unstable as it was very comminuted and it was treated with external fixation.

CASE 38 ANSWERS

8, 9, 13

1. Fractures of the humerus are associated with injury to the radial nerve in 10–15% of cases. If the patient lacks active dorsiflexion of wrist then it is likely there is a radial nerve palsy present.

2. Physical examination is rendered difficult in the presence of a humeral shaft fracture. The radial nerve supplies all the muscles involved in extension of the arm, forearm and wrist. It supplies triceps,

brachioradialis, supinator, extensor carpi radialis brevis and longus, extensor carpi ulnaris, extensor digitorum communis, extensor pollicis longus, and abductor pollicis longus. In patients with humeral shaft fractures it is usually possible to test the wrist, finger and thumb extensors. If a radial nerve palsy is present, there is an area of numbness also present involving the dorsal aspect of the first web space.

3. The treatment of choice for an isolated closed humeral shaft fracture is non-operative. A plaster U-slab is applied. This can be changed to a functional brace at 3–4 weeks. Union will occur in more than 95% of cases between 8 and 12 weeks.

4. Operative treatment is indicated in patients whose fractures fail to heal or show signs of progression to union with the 8–12-week time-frame. Some fractures cannot be maintained in a satisfactory position in a cast and this is also an indication for internal fixation. However, modest degrees of malunion are well tolerated in the humerus and up to 20° of angulation or rotation can be tolerated without functional limitation. Fixation is also generally indicated in patients with multiple long bone fractures, open humeral fractures and humeral fractures with a vascular injury. An isolated radial nerve palsy in itself is not an indication for fixation.

5. Plating is the preferred method of fixation for humeral shaft fractures. The other main alternative is intramedullary nailing. This has been associated with a higher complication rate in clinical practice than plating. Intramedullary nails are inserted at the shoulder or the elbow. If inserted at the shoulder they are often associated with pain due to penetration of the rotator cuff. The elbow entry point is at a relatively weak bony point and iatrogenic fracture may occur. Non-union has also been more common with intramedullary nailing. The humerus is subject to a lot of torsional force during normal use. Plates are good at resisting this type of force. Nails, by comparison, are less suited to resisting torsional motion. This excess motion at the fracture site contributes to a higher risk of non-union. Nails may be preferable for segmental fractures where the bone is fractured at two locations. Nails are also more suitable for treatment of pathological fractures.

CASE 39 ANSWERS

9, 12, 13

1. This is a humeral supracondylar fracture and is a common elbow injury in children.

2. The brachial artery and median nerve have been contused by the injury or the fracture haematoma has caused some local pressure on these two structures.

3. X-ray the limb and apply temporary splintage. Provide intravenous or intranasal analgesia. The child should be admitted to the ward prepared for theatre and have their pulse and sensation checked regularly. Loss of the pulse and an ischaemic hand is a surgical emergency.

4. The fracture is reduced under general anaesthesia and pinned using percutaneous wires. The fracture will heal rapidly and the wires can be removed at 3 weeks as an outpatient procedure without the need for general anaesthesia.

CASE 40 ANSWERS

8, 9, 13

1. The patient has sustained a fracture dislocation of the elbow. There is a dislocation with an associated fracture of the coronoid process of the ulna and a radial head fracture. This combination of injuries is often referred to as the 'unhappy triad' of the elbow, signifying that it is a well recognized injury pattern commonly associated with a poor outcome. It is often the result of high-energy trauma and a careful clinical evaluation should be part of the initial work-up to detect any associated neurovascular problems or signs of fractures elsewhere in the upper limb.

2. This injury is not amenable to non-operative treatment. The presence of the coronoid process fracture and the radial head fracture greatly increases the instability of the elbow and an adquate closed reduction cannot be maintained. These injuries require internal fixation of the coronoid process to restore ulnohumeral stability. The fracture is exposed through a posterior approach. The proximal ulnar shaft and coronoid fracture is reduced and fixed with a plate. The options for the radial head fracture are either reduction and fixation with screws, if there are no more than three main fragments, or, if there is more comminution than this, a radial head replacement is preferred.

3. The most common complication following an injury of this severity is elbow stiffness. Heterotopic ossification of the elbow is not unusual following injuries of this type and the extensive surgery required. If this occurs the stiffness may be severe and disabling. The functional range of motion required for normal elbow activities is 30–120°. If the range of motion is

less than this then normal activities of daily living may be interfered with. Elbow stiffness can be minimized if the internal fixation has secured a good-quality stable reduction that allows early motion and avoids the need for prolonged immobilization. Physiotherapy to supervise rehabilitation is helpful. If stiffness occurs and causes significant disability then further surgery to carry out a soft-tissue release can be performed, usually 4–6 months after the initial injury.

CASE 41 ANSWERS

8, 9, 13

1. The patient has sustained an olecranon fracture of the elbow.

2. This injury is more common in elderly women. It is associated with the presence of osteoporosis, which should be considered as a possibility, particularly if there are any other risk factors.

3. The triceps muscle inserts onto the olecranon and applies a deforming force, which tends to distract the fracture.

4. Non-operative treatment is difficult since there is no practical way with closed methods of treatment to overcome the triceps force distracting the fracture. Internal fixation is, therefore, the method of choice. In most patients, the method selected is termed 'tension band wiring'. This system comprises K-wires applied parallel across the fracture and a figure of eight loop of flexible wire (see Chapter 13). When the triceps contracts or the elbow flexes, tension in the wire increases and it applies compressive force across the fracture, hence the name.

CASE 42 ANSWERS

8, 9, 13

1. The patient has sustained a fracture of the mid-shaft of the radius and ulna as a consequence of a high-energy injury. The appropriate initial management is temporary immobilization of the fracture in a plaster backslab with provision of adequate analgesia. If the patient is still complaining of severe pain despite these steps, then the diagnosis of compartment syndrome should be considered. This condition occurs most commonly in the leg and forearm. It is uncommon in older patients with low-energy trauma, but is not unusual in young adults with high-energy forearm fractures.

2. There are no pathognomonic clinical findings and the diagnosis is often difficult to make on clinical grounds alone, particularly since most fracture patients are in pain anyway. However, most patients experience some degree of relief of pain with splintage of the fracture and analgesia. If pain persists or increases, this should alert the clinician to the possibility that the patient is developing a compartment syndrome. The most useful clinical finding is the presence of increased pain on passive flexion and extension of the fingers. Signs of distal vascular impairment or neurological compromise develop late in the evolution of the condition, often after there has been muscle necrosis. Earlier diagnosis can made with the aid of compartment pressure monitoring. A compartment pressure of less than 30 mmHg can be considered normal. Pressures of greater than 40 mmHg are generally considered too high, but there is a relationship with the diastolic pressure that has to be taken into account. There should be a pressure differential of more than 30 mmHg between the diastolic pressure and compartment pressure. Pressure differentials of less than this value indicate muscle perfusion is likely to be inadequate, irrespective of the absolute compartment pressure.

3. Compartment syndromes are characterized by the development of muscle ischaemia after trauma. Skeletal muscle is enveloped by a fascial layer that has limited capacity to expand. Following fracture or muscle injury there is typically a combination of muscle contusion and bleeding from bone ends and damaged muscle in addition to an acute inflammatory response. This results in soft-tissue swelling. In the case of muscle, particularly in the leg and forearm, the muscle swells in well defined fascial compartments. Once the elastic limit of the fascia is reached, then further bleeding and inflammation cannot be accommodated by an increase in compartment size. This results in pressure being transmitted directly to the compartment contents. Initially, this causes occlusion of veins, but not of arterioles. This results in a rapid increase in compartment pressure, which eventually occludes the arterioles. Once this occurs, then muscle ischaemia follows and, in a short period of time, ischaemic muscle necrosis. In the acute phase of the condition the breakdown of muscle results in the release of myoglobin into the systemic circulation. This is toxic to the renal tubule and acute renal failure may occur due to acute tubular necrosis. In the longer term, the dead muscle is replaced with fibrous tissue and a contracture termed 'Volkmann's ischaemic contracture'.

4. The correct management of the condition involves early recognition of the compartment syndrome before muscle necrosis has supervened. A prompt surgical fasciotomy is carried out to allow for muscle swelling to occur safely without any vascular compromise to its blood supply.

CASE 43 ANSWERS

8, 9, 12, 13

1. There are fractures of both bones of the forearm. The ulnar fracture is complete and the radial fracture is a greenstick (as seen on the lateral film).

2. At presentation you should check that the radial pulse is present, the fingers are well perfused and there is no neurological deficit. Check also that there is not a second injury in the arm by examining gently the child's shoulder, elbow and wrist. Do not palpate the fracture as the injury is obvious. Although the clinical signs of a fracture are pain, swelling, deformity, loss of function and crepitus you should never test for crepitus in a conscious patient.

3. The forearm may have started to swell at the site of the fracture and despite post-operative elevation of the arm the plaster will constrict the swollen arm. An early compartment syndrome may also be developing. Have no hesitation in splitting the cast on its medial and lateral aspects down to skin. It is not vital if the position of the fracture is lost as a result – this can always be retrieved, but irreversible muscle necrosis is a functional disaster.

CASE 44 ANSWERS

12, 13

1. There is a displaced spiral fracture of the distal end of the femur. The texture of the bones looks normal, excluding the possibility of osteogenesis imperfecta or metabolic bone disease. This fracture in a non-mobile child is highly suggestive of non-accidental injury. In the absence of any bone disease, it is highly unlikely that a Barlow or Ortolani procedure would cause the fracture.

2. See text on Assessment (Chapter 26). The general practitioner (GP) records show that 3 weeks prior to the current presentation the baby had been seen at the same hospital Accident & Emergency department with a sub-conjunctival haemorrhage and was assessed by the paediatric registrar who attributed the haemorrhage to 'sneezing'. Two weeks later, her father brought her back to hospital, with a history that she had a 'breath-holding attack'. During an overnight admission, the baby was noted to be well with no signs or symptoms of illness. The father has learning difficulties and is receiving therapy for 'anger management'. This background information suggests that father was the constant person present whenever the baby presented for medical attention and should alert you to the possibility of the baby's problems being fabricated or induced by the father.

3. See text on Differential diagnosis and investigations (Chapter 4). The chest X-ray from the skeletal survey showed a healing fracture at the posterior end of the left 12th rib.

4. See text on Inter-agency working (Chapter 12).

5. You should consider, with social services and the police, whether the 2-year-old brother is safe to remain at home while the inquiry continues (multi-agency risk assessment). He will need a medical examination to look for signs of neglect or abuse. Discuss with a radiologist whether he needs a skeletal survey to exclude occult fractures.

CASE 45 ANSWERS

8, 9, 13

1. The patient has sustained a distal radial fracture with dorsal displacement and angulation of the distal fragment. This produces a typical clinical appearance of the wrist termed a 'dinner-fork' deformity.

2. Three eponymous terms are used to describe fractures involving the distal radius. The most common type is the Colles fracture, characterized by a fracture of the distal radius with dorsal displacement, dorsal angulation radial displacement and impaction of the distal fragment. The Smith fracture is a fracture with volar displacement of the distal fragment. A Barton's fracture is a partial articular injury. The most common pattern is characterized by a volar fracture fragment of the distal radius allowing volar displacement of the carpus.

3. The patient has sensory disturbance in the distribution of the median nerve. Median nerve dysfunction occurs in 10% of patients with distal radial fractures. It is due to a combination of the trauma sustained at the time of injury and the tension on the nerve produced by the deformity.

4. The most common initial management is a closed reduction and cast application. This will relieve tension on the nerve and the neurological symptoms may resolve. If this fails to occur then a carpal tunnel decompression and some form of fixation will be required. Cast treatment alone is sufficient in the

majority of Colles' fractures. However, approximately 30% of these injuries are unstable and a satisfactory reduction cannot be maintained in a plaster cast. Instability is more common if there is fracture comminution and in older patients. If the reduction cannot be maintained, then operative treatment is usually considered, generally with some form of external fixation. Internal fixation is often used in younger patients if there are any intra-articular extensions that are displaced.

5. Malunion and carpal tunnel syndrome are common complications. Malunion can affect up to 30% of cases. Rates are lower with active intervention when loss of reduction is recognized at an early stage and appropriate treatment is undertaken. Carpal tunnel syndrome is encountered in 10% of cases. Symptoms resolve in 50% of cases after a satisfactory reduction. In 5% of cases symptoms persist. Treatment is a carpal tunnel decompression, but it may be necessary to address any malunion contributing to nerve compression. Rupture of the extensor pollicis longus tendon occurs in 2% of cases, usually several weeks after injury. It is thought to be due to attrition rupture of the tendon. If there is sufficient disability then a tendon transfer can be carried out (extensor indicis to extensor pollicis).

CASE 46 ANSWERS

8, 12, 13

1. The patient has sustained a completely off-ended distal radial fracture of his right wrist.

2. These injuries may be difficult to reduce by closed manipulation. The usual technique is initially to increase the deformity to hitch the dorsal cortex of the distal fragment back on to the dorsal cortex of the proximal radial shaft. Traction and plantarflexion are then used to complete the reduction.

3. Occasionally soft-tissue interposition may prevent a satisfactory closed reduction. In these circumstances an open reduction may be required and internal fixation of the fracture is often used. In younger children a Kirschner wire may be used but in teenagers some of these fractures can be treated by a plate.

CASE 47 ANSWERS

8, 9, 13

1. The patient has sustained a fracture of the waist of the scaphoid.

2. There may be very little to find on clinical examination – the wrist is not deformed and there may be very

little swelling. Typically the patient has well localized tenderness in the 'anatomical snuffbox'. This is an area on the radial side of the wrist delineated by the tip of the radial styloid and the tendons of extensor pollicis longus and abductor pollicis. It is the surface marking closest to the body of the scaphoid bone. Tenderness well localized to this area should alert the examiner to the possibilty of a scaphoid fracture.

3. The usual treatment is a period of immobilization in a scaphoid cast. This is a forearm cast that extends to the level of metacarpophalangeal (MCP) joints. It differs from a standard distal radial fracture cast by having an extension up to the interphalangeal joint of the thumb. The thumb should be positioned in opposition to the other fingers to avoid stiffness due to adduction contracture. Surgical treatment of the scaphoid is most commonly indicated if it fails to unite in a cast. However, internal fixation may be indicated at the outset if the fracture is very displaced or if it is associated with an adjacent fracture (often a radial styloid fracture) or a carpal dislocation (usually a perilunate dislocation).

4. Non-union and avascular necrosis are well recognized complications of scaphoid fractures. Non-union is more likely to occur with high-energy fractures with displacement. Avascular necrosis occurs because of the blood supply of the bone. The vascular supply enters the distal pole mainly from the dorsal side and supplies the bone in a distal-to-proximal direction. Fractures through the waist of the bone may disrupt this blood supply with avascular necrosis developing. The risk of the complication is greater with more proximal fractures and a shorter proximal pole fragment. Treatment of either non-union or avascular necrosis or non-union is by internal fixation, usually with bone grafting. In late cases, secondary osteoarthritis may have developed and fixation is no longer an option. A limited or total wrist fusion is often considered in this situation.

CASE 48 ANSWERS

8, 9, 13

1. The patient has sustained a fracture of the neck of the 5th metacarpal. This injury is commonly sustained in fights when the assailant lands a punch against their opponent.

2. There is a laceration with associated cellulitis and swelling. The source of the laceration is almost always due to contact with a tooth. There is a very high incidence of infection of these lacerations.

Furthermore there may have been penetration of the MCP joint, which can result in a septic arthritis.

3. Taking into account the risk of septic arthritis, the most appropriate management is early exploration of the wound. In this case it confirmed there had been penetration of the joint with introduction of bacteria into the joint cavity and development of septic arthritis. Drainage of pus was required with copious lavage of the joint cavity. The fracture of the 5th metacarpal is of less consequence. Usually these injuries heal with non-operative treatment with minimal functional impairment despite some degree of angular malunion. In this case the fracture was stabilized with wires at the time of surgery. These wires can be removed at 4 weeks.

CASE 49 ANSWERS

1, 13

1. The patient is most likely to have a flexor tendon injury. The extended posture of the little finger is not normal – when the hand is fully relaxed a position of slight flexion of all fingers is usual. The completely extended posture of the finger as shown suggests that the tendons of both flexor digitorum superficialis and profundus have been severed.

2. It is quite common to injure one or both digital nerves in association with flexor tendon injury. The digital nerves run along the radial and ulnar border of each finger. The sensation should be checked carefully at presentation since the nerve will need to be repaired if severed.

3. The flexor tendons have a complex anatomical arrangement as they run into the finger, characterized by a series of pulleys that allow tendons to glide without bowstringing. The tendon is divided into five zones (see hand section in Chapter 13). This injury has occurred in zone 2 where the tendon has a poorer blood supply, and repair is often complicated by stiffness. However, early surgical repair of both tendons is considered the best choice of treatment. Modern suture techniques are designed to allow early mobilization to minimize the risk of stiffness.

CASE 50 ANSWERS

8, 22

1. Spinal injury with spinal cord damage at T10 level. Some cases with injury of the conus medullaris can have sparing of sacral nerve function, but the presence of perineal numbness means that there is a higher

cord lesion. Great care is required in moving the patient.

2. Plain radiographs of the spine showed vertebral fracture and loss of alignment. A CT scan allows assessment of the full extent and severity of the injury. MRI allows soft-tissue assessment so ligamentous damage can be seen as well as haemorrhage and oedema of the spinal cord.

3. The patient needs insertion of a urinary catheter and management of an acute spinal injury is commenced – regular log-rolling to avoid pressure sores, horizontal posture and intravenous fluids to prevent hypotension, which can damage the cord through ischaemia. This is particularly important in injuries above T6 where there is major autonomic nervous system disturbance and spinal shock. Haemorrhage and oedema can cause an extension of the level of cord damage so high-dose methylprednisolone administered intravenously within 8 h of injury has been tried as a means of reducing this secondary damage. There is heated debate about the scientific basis for routine use of high-dose steroids. Neurological recovery depends upon the degree of damage to the cord itself. There was recovery in this patient so the early paralysis was mainly due to swelling and contusion of the cord.

4. Early transfer to a specialist spinal injuries rehabilitation unit is essential. Skin care, bladder care, manual evacuation of the rectum, anti-coagulation to reduce the risk of thromboembolic disease, physiotherapy, occupational therapy and psychological support are required.

   The spine may be internally fixed with pedicle screws to prevent deformity and restore stability. The unstable spine would carry the risk of further spinal cord damage.

CASE 51 ANSWERS

1, 8, 9, 13

1. The patient has sustained a dislocation of the hip. There is an associated posterior wall acetabular fracture. The dislocation is posterior, which accounts for 90% of hip dislocations.

2. The patient typically holds the leg in a flexed, adducted, internally rotated position with some shortening of the leg.

3. In this situation the patient was involved in a head-on collision. The hip dislocation occurs as a consequence of force delivered along the femoral shaft. As a result,

fractures of the patella or femur are not unusual. A posterior force delivered to the proximal tibia may result in a fracture or a rupture of the posterior cruciate ligament. Posterior wall acetabular fractures and fractures of the femoral head itself may also occur. Finally, the sciatic nerve runs close to the posterior aspect of the hip joint and sciatic nerve injury occurs in approximately 15% of hip dislocations. Careful neurological assessment is necessary to detect this complication. The hip dislocation will make a standard neurological examination difficult. However, the diagnosis is likely if the patient has weakness of plantarflexion and dorsiflexion with sensory disturbance below the knee.

An urgent closed reduction of the hip is required. There is a risk of avascular necrosis and this is minimized by reducing the dislocation as soon as possible. Additional oblique views of the acetabulum (Judet views) will usually identify the presence of a posterior wall fracture. A CT scan will also confirm the diagnosis. Most posterior wall fractures are best treated by open reduction and internal fixation unless they are very small.

CASE 52 ANSWERS

12, 13

1. There are five types according to the Salter–Harris classification. The radiographs show a type I physeal injury of the distal tibial growth plate.

2. The principles of management are the same as for any other fracture – accurate reduction and immobilization until union. The type II injury is the commonest and generally has a good outlook.

3. There are two main potential problems after a growth plate injury – premature growth arrest and when the injury involves that articular surface of the joint (types III and IV). A premature growth arrest may result in an angular deformity subsequently, because of asymmetrical growth at the physis. A limb-length discrepancy may also result. This will depend not only on the extent of the damage to the growth plate, but also its location. For example about three-quarters of femoral length originates from the distal femoral growth plate and only one-quarter from the proximal one. Thus, damage to the distal femoral growth plate is likely to have a greater effect on growth of the femur than an injury to the proximal growth plate. The type III and IV injuries involve the joint surface as well as the growth plate and it is important that the articular surface and the physis are reduced

accurately; this usually means an open (surgical) reduction and fixation. Failure to obtain an accurate reduction of the joint surface under these circumstances may predispose the child to post-traumatic osteoarthritis.

CASE 53 ANSWERS

8, 9, 13

1. The patient has sustained a displaced subcapital hip fracture. Fractures of the hip are common injuries and classified based on location. They may be intracapsular (subcapital or transcervical) or extracapsular (basal cervical, intertrochanteric or subtrochateric). Intracapsular fractures are usually sub-classified as displaced (80%) or undisplaced (20%).

2. In displaced subcapital fractures the blood supply to the femoral head may be damaged. This may interfere with fracture healing. If the fracture is treated with reduction and fixation the main risks are non-union, failure of fixation and avascular necrosis at a later stage even if healing has occurred.

3. The blood supply of the adult femoral head is derived from three sources. A limited degree of perfusion reaches the femoral head via the intramedullary circulation and there is an additional supply that enters the head through the insertion of the ligamentum teres. However, the majority of the blood supply is derived from capsular vessels. These are formed from the anastomosis of the medial and lateral femoral circumflex vessels at the base of the femoral neck. These vessels are branches of the profunda femoris artery. This anastomosis gives rise to capsular vessels, which reach the femoral head by travelling along the inner layer of the hip capsule and which enter the femoral head just below the level of the articular surface. They may be torn in subcapital fractures with displacement of the femoral head.

4. The main options for treatment are reduction and fixation or alternatively some form of hip arthroplasty. Reduction and fixation is the usual treatment of choice in younger patients (i.e. most patients under 60 years). In older patients this treatment is associated with a 40% rate of reoperation due to fixation failure, non-union and avascular necrosis. It is, therefore, not commonly used in most patients with this injury who are over the age of 70 years. Replacement of the hip by either a hemiarthroplasty or total hip arthroplasty is the preferred option for most patients. Hemiarthroplasty may be cemented

or uncemented. In patients with very low functional demands (demented patients or patients with very limited mobility) a simple uncemented hemiarthroplasty is often chosen. In fit older patients a cemented hemiarthropl.asty or total arthroplasty is a better choice.

CASE 54 ANSWERS

8, 9, 10, 11, 13

1. This patient has been involved in a high-speed motor vehicle accident. The femoral and tibial shaft fractures are obvious and may distract attention from other potentially life-threatening injuries that may not be apparent. The slightly low blood pressure and tachycardia in a patient of this age suggest that significant blood loss has occurred. A systematic approach to clinical assessment and initial management is required that will identify all injuries and allow prioritization of management. This system is referred to as the ATLS (advanced trauma life support).

2. The ATLS system is designed for a rapid and effective evaluation and initial management of a patient with multiple injuries. The initial step is a primary survey (ABC=airway, breathing and circulation) to detect and rectify immediately life-threatening injury (airway obstruction, major thoracic trauma causing serious respiratory compromise and hypovolaemic shock). This is followed by a secondary survey, which is a head-to-toe examination to detect other potentially important, but not immediately life-threatening, injuries. A limited history is obtained from the patient, relatives or paramedical staff and includes basic details about the victim's allergies, medication, past medical history, last meal and the accident environment (AMPLE). Lateral cervical spine, chest and pelvic radiographs are obtained in all patients. Fluid resuscitation and airway protection are an integral part of the early assessment and management.

3. Multiple long-bone fractures are associated with a number of potential complications in the early stages of treatment. Important general complications include hypovolaemic shock and fat embolism syndrome (see Chapter 10). Other general complications include DVT and pulmonary embolus, although these usually occur later than 72 h in most cases. Early local complications can also occur particularly in the leg, where compartment syndrome may develop. It also occurs in the thigh, but is rare. Open fractures of the tibia have a risk of deep

infection, which can be minimized by thorough debridement, early stabilization and prompt soft-tissue cover. Nerve and vessel injury may also occur, but are, fortunately, rare.

4. In general, the evidence in the literature favours early skeletal stabilization of long-bone fractures in multiple-trauma patients. This has been shown in numerous studies to be associated with a lower risk of pulmonary complications and other general fracture complications. Stable skeletal fixation also reduces local complications, including malunion and non-union. For most long-bone fractures of the tibia and femur in adults, an interlocking intramedullary nail is the treatment of choice. Plating is technically more demanding and is associated with a higher complication rate. There is still a role for external skeletal fixation, particularly in the unstable multiple-trauma patient who may have other injuries requiring surgical intervention. In this situation a prolonged orthopaedic procedure may be undesirable. External fixation can be used as a temporary measure and more definitive fixation can be carried out subsequently if indicated at a later stage when the patient is fit.

CASE 55 ANSWERS

1, 7

1. This patient has developed a haemarthrosis after a twisting injury to the knee. In 70% of cases this is due to a tear of the anterior cruciate ligament (ACL). The history of a 'popping' sensation is commonly reported. There are other causes of a haemarthrosis that should be considered. Fractures of the tibial plateau or osteochondral fractures of the femoral condyle are less common causes but do occur and are the indication for obtaining plain radiographs in this situation. Dislocation of the patella may be associated with a haemarthrosis, but there is usually a clear description of the patella being dislocated and the subsequent reduction. Meniscal tears do not typically cause a haemarthrosis unless there is a peripheral detachment. A rupture of the patellar or quadriceps tendon will cause a lot of bleeding, but as the capsule is disrupted there is no contained haemarthrosis in these injuries. They are very uncommon in younger patients.

2. The acutely injured knee is difficult to examine due to pain and apprehension on the part of the patient. Aspiration of the haemarthrosis relieves pain and facilitates examination. Nevertheless, many of the

more provocative knee tests (e.g. McMurray test, pivot shift test) will be impossible to perform reliably in the early stages after injury. The Lachman test is the most useful method of assessing the ACL acutely. Gentle varus or valgus testing with the knee in slight flexion can be used to test collateral ligaments. Meniscal tears are uncommon in this clinical setting, but clinical diagnosis is not reliable in the early stages. Many of these patients are misdiagnosed as having meniscal tears. This is because the tense haemarthrosis prevents full extension of the knee and there is frequently some degree of medial collateral ligament (MCL) and medial capsular injury. The injury, therefore, simulates a locked knee. A careful history of the injury with particular reference to the rapid onset of generalized knee swelling should alert the clinician to the correct diagnosis.

3. The MRI scan is the most useful additional diagnostic investigation. This will accurately visualize the ligaments and menisci in doubtful cases.

4. The management of most ligament injuries in the acute setting is non-operative. ACL tears or the combination of an ACL and MCL tear are often associated with marked swelling and stiffness of the knee in the weeks after injury. This is not an ideal time to carry out surgical reconstruction since the risk of severe post-operative stiffness is increased. A programme of physiotherapy is the more appropriate initial management to allow time for swelling and stiffness to resolve. In patients with ACL tears surgical reconstruction can be carried out at a later stage if required. In many younger patients who are athletically active, symptomatic instability is very common following this injury and a reconstruction of the ligament within the first year of injury is preferable.

CASE 56 ANSWERS

1, 7

1. This patient has developed an effusion following a knee injury. The swelling developed over a period of 48 h and was not particularly marked. It is, therefore, more likely to be a synovial effusion rather than a haemarthrosis. This makes the diagnosis of a mensical tear more likely than an ACL tear, which is typically associated with a tense haemarthrosis. Isolated MCL sprains often develop a synovial effusion and there is always medial joint tenderness. However, meniscal tears are associated with well localized joint margin tenderness. MCL sprains tend to have

tenderness more diffusely, although it is frequently maximal at the femoral insertion, which is superior to the joint line.

2. Meniscal tears are characterized by the presence of a small effusion and well localized joint margin tenderness. The meniscus is avascular and, therefore, meniscal tears are only associated with a haemarthrosis when there is a peripheral detachment, which is uncommon. In this case the patient was unable to extend the knee fully. This raises the possibility of a displaced bucket-handle tear of the meniscus. Remember, however, that a tense haemarthrosis will also prevent full knee extension. Provocative tests including the McMurray test and the Apley grinding test are neither sensitive nor specific. The acutely injured knee is difficult to examine due to pain and apprehension on the part of the patient. Aspiration of the haemarthrosis relieves pain and facilitates examination. Nevertheless, many of the more provocative knee tests (e.g. McMurray test, pivot shift test) will be impossible to perform reliably in the early stages after injury. The Lachman test is the most useful method of assessing the ACL acutely. Gentle varus or valgus testing with the knee in slight flexion can be used to test collateral ligaments. Meniscal tears are uncommon in this clinical setting, but clinical diagnosis is not reliable in the early stages. Many of these patients are misdiagnosed as having meniscal tears. This is because the tense haemarthrosis prevents full extension of the knee and there is frequently some degree of MCL and medial capsular injury. The injury, therefore, simulates a locked knee. A careful history of the injury with particular reference to the rapid onset of generalized knee swelling should alert the clinician to the correct diagnosis.

3. The MRI scan is the most useful additional diagnostic investigation. This will accurately visualize the ligaments and menisci in doubtful cases.

4. The options for meniscal tears are arthroscopic partial meniscectomy or repair. Surgical repair is mainly considered in peripheral tears in younger patients whose tears are diagnosed and treated within 2 weeks of injury. Tears in the non-vascularized area of the meniscus do not heal reliably. Similarly, tears which are diagnosed late or in older patients are not usually considered suitable for repair. The alternative of arthroscopic meniscectomy is a simple and effective means of treating meniscal pathology. The disadvantage is that it involves removal of a portion of the meniscus, which may increase the risk of

osteoarthritis developing in the longer term. This is less of a consideration in older patients.

CASE 57 ANSWERS

1, 8, 9, 13

1. The patient has sustained a fracture of the midshaft of the tibia and fibula. This is an open fracture with a larger wound in communication with the fracture site.

2. Open long-bone fractures are classified using the Gustilo classification. A puncture wound of less than 1 cm with a low-energy injury is a Grade I open fracture. A wound of between 1 cm and 10 cm with no deep soft-tissue contamination is a Grade II open fracture. A Grade IIIA injury is a wound of more than 10 cm with some deep soft-tissue contamination. A Grade IIIB injury is similar, but there is periosteal stripping of bone and usually a local or free flap is required to cover the soft-tissue defect after debridement. A Grade IIIC open fracture is one with an associated vascular injury that requires repair. Although based to some extent on wound size and contamination, a high-energy fracture is always rated as at least a Grade IIIA injury, irrespective of wound size.

3. The initial steps should be to cover the wound with a sterile dressing and splint the fracture. The patient should be assessed for other injuries. Assuming the tibial fracture is the only fracture, the most important step is an adequate debridement of the wound. This involves excision of the wound edges, removal of any devitalized soft tissue or bone fragments and copious lavage. As a routine all patients should also be given anti-tetanus toxoid. Broad-spectrum antibiotics are also given, but the wound debridement is the most important element of the acute management.

4. Once the wound has been debrided the fracture should be stabilized. In high-energy open fractures, external or internal fixation is the usual method considered. In lower-limb diaphyseal fractures intramedullary nails are usually chosen. In the upper limb, plating of diaphyseal fractures is the method of choice. For articular or metaphyseal injuries either internal or external fixation may be used. External fixation is often chosen if there is extensive soft-tissue damage or swelling. If there is a large open wound, split skin grafting, a local flap or free flap may be required. Ideally, the wound should be closed or covered within the first week to minimize the risk of infection.

CASE 58 ANSWERS

8, 9, 13

1. The patient has sustained a displaced ankle fracture with a fracture of the medial and lateral malleolus. There is talar shift with lateral and posterior displacement of the talus in relation to the distal tibia.

2. These injuries are the result of rotation of the talus within the ankle mortice. Typically the patient goes over on the foot. This imparts a torsional force to the talus. The talus rotates externally. Initially, there is rupture of the talofibular component of the lateral ligament complex. Continued rotation then results in a lateral malleolar fracture. With further rotation there may be a fracture of the posterior lip of the distal tibia (posterior malleolus). As rotation progresses the medial side structures are stressed by the rotating talus resulting in either a medial malleolar fracture or tear of the medial deltoid ligament.

3. A closed reduction should be carried out as soon as possible, usually with sedation and analgesia. Although anatomical reduction is not often achieved, the reduction is generally adequate to produce a significant improvement in the position and reduce pressure on the overlying skin. This will reduce the degree of soft-tissue swelling and minimize the risk of blistering, which may interfere with surgical treatment. Once reduction is achieved, the ankle should be splinted in position with application of a plaster backslab. These injuries are best treated by open reduction and internal fixation to restore perfect anatomical alignment in order to minimize the risk of late osteoarthritis.

CASE 59 ANSWERS

8, 9, 13

1. The patient has sustained a displaced talar neck fracture. Fractures of the talar neck are classified based on the degree of displacement of the fracture, but also the loss of ankle and subtalar joint conguency. A Hawkins I fracture is undisplaced with no ankle or subtalar incongruency. A Hawkins II fracture has some displacement with loss of subtalar congruency. A Hawkins III fracture is displaced with dislocation of the talar body – there is total loss of ankle and subtalar joint congruency.

2. The most well recognized complication of this injury is avascular necrosis. The blood supply of the talus is mainly derived from the artery of the tarsal

sinus (formed by branches of the dorsalis pedis and peroneal arteries) and the artery of the tarsal canal (a branch of the posterior tibial artery). These form an anastomosis in the tarsal canal that provides the blood supply of the talus, via branches entering the inferior surface of the talar neck. The blood supply of the body is, therefore, supplied from distal to proximal and is at risk when there is a fracture of the talar neck, particularly if the fracture displaces.

3. Prompt reduction of the fracture is required if displaced. Most injuries are best treated by internal fixation unless the initial fracture is completely undisplaced. The usual method of fixation is with screws. Following this the patient is mobilized in a plaster cast. Non-weight-bearing or touch weight-bearing is recommended for the first 6 weeks after injury. Once the fracture has healed (usually between 6 and 12 weeks), the patient can progress to full weight-bearing. Patients require to be followed up for 2 years after injury as avascular necrosis may develop at any stage during this time interval.

CASE 60 ANSWERS

8, 9, 13

1. The patient has developed a complex regional pain syndrome. The condition has also been described using other terms reflecting the location or possible pathophysiology. These terms include 'hand–shoulder syndrome', 'reflex sympathetic dystrophy' and 'causalgia'.

2. The exact cause is not known. However, the condition typically occurs following injury and is most commonly encountered in the hand and wrist in clinical practice. It is characterized by development of considerable swelling and stiffness of the hand and wrist. This is accompanied by changes in the skin, which in florid cases is characterized by a shiny red or purple appearance with loss of the normal skin crease markings. The term 'reflex sympathetic dystrophy' implicates a disorder of the autonomic nerve supply after injury. This may well be part of the patho-physiology, but is probably not the actual cause. It appears to be an exaggerated and persistent manifestation of the normal inflammatory response to injury. It is now more commonly referred to as complex regional pain syndrome.

3. There is no specific treatment for the condition. A prolonged supervised course of physiotherapy to minimize stiffness is advisable. There is often a psychological component to the patient's complaints

and continued encouragement with the rehabilitation programme is important. Other treatments including pharmacological alteration of pain perception (e.g. with gabapentin) and local sympathetic nerve blocks (with guanethidine) can be tried as an adjunct to treatment.

CASE 61 ANSWERS

8, 9, 13

1. The patient has sustained a posterior dislocation of the shoulder. Unlike anterior dislocation the radiographic signs on the AP radiograph are more subtle and the diagnosis is commonly missed.

2. Patients who present with shoulder pain after an epileptic fit or an electric shock, or who have sustained a high-energy injury, should be suspected of having a posterior dislocation. In this case the history of epilepsy and related seizures should increase suspicion that a posterior dislocation has occurred. On clinical examination, patients with a posterior dislocation have the shoulder fixed in internal rotation. If the elbow is flexed to 90°, it will be apparent that the shoulder is internally rotated and no external rotation is possible. In this situation posterior dislocation must be excluded before the patient can be discharged.

3. An axillary or modified axial view of the shoulder will identify the posterior position of the humeral head. The former view can be difficult to obtain in the acute setting when there is a lot of pain. The modified axial view is easier to obtain. A CT scan is the most useful form of imaging. This allows confirmation of the diagnosis. In addition it will accurately identify impaction fractures of the humeral head, which may influence the choice of treatment. These fractures are referred to as Hill–Sachs lesions in anterior dislocations and reverse Hill–Sachs lesions in posterior dislocations. In the case of posterior dislocations, the humeral head is closely applied to the sharp posterior border of the glenoid fossa and if the diagnosis is not made quickly a large impaction defect may occur.

4. The treatment of choice is an early closed reduction. This is often not possible if the diagnosis is delayed. Under these circumstances an open reduction may be necessary. If there is a large humeral head impaction fracture then bone grafting of the defect may be necessary to stabilize the shoulder. If the defect occupies more than 40% of the humeral head, then a shoulder replacement may be required.

CASE 62 ANSWERS

8, 9, 10, 11, 13

1. This pattern of pelvic disruption is often referred to as an 'open book' injury. External rotational forces are applied to the hemipelvis on one or both sides resulting in a pubic symphyseal disruption. As the hemipelvis is externally rotated, there is disruption of the sacrospinous and sacrotuberous ligaments and eventual disruption of the anterior sacroiliac ligaments with opening up of the sacroiliac joints.

2. This pattern of pelvic disruption is often associated with disruption of pelvic vessels, particularly pelvic veins. There is a large increase in pelvic volume and patients are frequently hypotensive at presentation. The bladder and urethra are susceptible to injury. The presence of blood at the external urinary meatus, a scrotal haematoma and a high-riding prostate on rectal examination are often present when there is urethral disruption.

3. The initial priorities are to save the patient's life and to identify injuries that may not be life-threatening, but will require treatment. An ATLS system of examination is required to do this. In this case the presence of hypotensive shock was the immediate threat to survival and reversal of this is the first step. A fluid challenge with crystalloid solutions (normal saline usually) is carried out. Blood can be cross-matched for transfusion. In critical cases O-negative blood can be given without cross-matching. Reduction in the pelvic volume will tamponade bleeding and may help. This can be achieved by application of a pelvic binder in the acute resuscitation phase or later by external fixation of the pelvis. A CT scan can be obtained in patients who are sufficiently stable to identify additional abdominal injury. A retrograde urethrogram and cystogram is necessary before catheterization. Urinary drainage must be obtained. Patients with a bladder rupture require laparotomy and repair. Urethral ruptures are very difficult to treat surgically in the acute situation. One option is to establish suprapubic catheter bladder drainage and carry out delayed urethral reconstruction several months after injury.

4. Open-book fractures can be treated by external fixation alone. However, the device is cumbersome and pin-track infection is almost invariable. Mobilization is difficult. Plating is often chosen if the patient's condition can be adequately stabilized. This results in a more rigid anatomical reduction, which allows earlier mobilization.

434

CASE 63 ANSWERS

8, 9, 10, 13, 19

1. The patient has sustained a displaced intertrochanteric hip fracture. Classification of hip fractures is based on the location and fracture morphology. The most important aspect in location of the hip fracture is whether it is extracapsular or intracapsular. Fractures in the pertrochanteric region (basal cervical, inter-trochanteric, subtrochanteric) are extracapsular and the blood supply is excellent. Non-union is, therefore, uncommon. The morphology of the fracture may be classified as unstable or stable. Two-part fractures are generally stable after reduction. However, three-part fractures with a large posteromedial fragment (containing the lesser trochanter) or those with greater degrees of comminution are unstable. These are more likely to be complicated by fixation failure.

2. Internal fixation is the treatment of choice for this fracture. The most commonly used implant is a sliding hip-screw device consisting of a side-plate and hip screw. The hip screw can subside into a barrel at the upper end of the plate to minimize the risk of the hip screw cutting out of the osteoporotic femoral head. Fractures with subtrochanteric extensions are more easily treated with an intramedullary rod with a hip screw. Consideration should be given to treating patients for osteoporosis. Younger patients under the age of 70 years should have a DEXA scan and can be treated with bisphosphonates if indicated. Patients over this age can be commenced empirically on vitamin D and calcium supplements and bisphosphonates without the need for additional investigations.

3. Patients are susceptible to local or general complications following fixation of these fractures. Local complications include wound haematoma, wound infection and failure of fracture fixation. If the hip screw is well placed in the femoral head then fixation failure is rare. However, fixation failure is more common in unstable fractures or comminuted fractures with a subtrochanteric extension. General complications are frequent in the elderly female patients who sustain this injury. These include deep vein thrombosis and pulmonary embolus, pressure sores, and urinary tract infection. The incidence of stroke and myocardial infarction is increased in the post-operative period, particularly in patients with arterial disease.

CASE 64 ANSWERS

8, 9, 10, 13

1. There is an undisplaced subcapital hip present, but it is difficult to identify on the anteroposterior (AP) view. Approximately 2% of hip fractures are not easily seen on plain radiographs. The other possibility is that there may be a pubic ramus fracture. These may be easily overlooked particularly if undisplaced.

2. All patients should have a lateral view of the hip in addition to the AP view. This may confirm the diagnosis. The drawback is that a good-quality lateral view is often difficult to obtain in a painful hip. Bone scans will confirm increased uptake in the hip, but are not absolutely specific. An MRI scan in this situation is a good option as it is a very sensitive investigation for diagnosis of fractures that may not be visible on a plain radiograph. In addition, it is highly specific. Other less common causes of hip pain, such as pathological lesions, will also be detected. It is the investigation of choice in doubtful cases.

3. This fracture is undisplaced. Many of these fractures are quite stable and will remain undisplaced while they heal. However, the risk of displacement is 15% with non-operative treatment. If the fracture displaces the treatment is more difficult and will often require some form of hip arthroplasty. For this reason, most surgeons opt to treat these injuries by fixation with hip screws. These devices can be inserted with minimally invasive surgery and the procedure carries a low morbidity.

CASE 65 ANSWERS

8, 9, 10, 12

1. A femoral nerve block gives excellent analgesia and a Thomas splint can be applied while the block is working. If there is a strong clinical suspicion of a femoral fracture the block can be inserted before the child has X-rays taken. After this there is a choice of management.

2. The child can continue to be managed in the splint until the fracture unites, or she could be placed in a spica plaster cast. This would require a general anaesthetic, but does not need to be done as an emergency and can be done on the next convenient theatre list. In the meantime the limb should be splinted. Children can also be looked after at home either in a spica or on a Thomas splint. It will take about 5 weeks for this fracture to heal (see Chapter 12 for the 'Rule of thumb' for fracture healing).

CASE 66 ANSWERS

1

1. This patient has sustained an Achilles tendon (TA) rupture. This is a well recognized injury associated with a dorsiflexing force suddenly applied to the forefoot that is resisted by powerful plantarflexion of the gastrocnemius soleus complex. This occurs in sports with explosive lower-limb muscle action. The most common sport associated with TA rupture is squash. However, the injury is also observed in soccer players, sprinters and certain types of dancing, as in this case. The injury is most common in patients aged between 30 and 50 years who have developed age-related degenerative changes in the tendon. More rarely, patients on steroid medication for other reasons sustain this injury.

2. The diagnosis is frequently missed, mainly through lack of awareness. The patient often gives a very clear-cut description of a sudden pain in the heel with an audible or palpable tearing sensation. Patients commonly state they feel as if they 'had been kicked in the back of the heel'. This latter description is so characteristic of the injury that it could be considered almost pathognomonic of the condition. If the patient presents acutely there is usually a palpable gap in the tendon on clinical examination. With later presentation the gap is filled with organized haematoma and is more difficult to discern. The Simmonds test is a useful method of confirming the diagnosis. The patient is placed prone with both feet extending just below the examination couch. With the calf completely relaxed, manual compression of the gastrocnemius muscles with the hand of the examiner is associated with passive plantarflexion of the foot if the Achilles tendon is *intact*. If the tendon is ruptured this motion does not occur.

3. The diagnosis can usually be made on the basis of history and examination in most patients. However, in patients who have a partial injury or who present late, the degree of disruption may be more uncertain. In these situations either an ultrasound scan or an MRI scan can be useful in confirming the diagnosis. The ultrasound scan has the advantage in partial rupture that the extent of tendon disrupted can be estimated as a percentage of the normal diameter, which may be helpful in deciding on what treatment to choose.

4. Achilles tendon rupture may be treated non-operatively or operatively. If non-operative treatment

is chosen the usual method is a period of below-knee cast immobilization for 10 weeks, with 4 weeks in full equinus, 4 weeks in semi-equinus and 2 weeks in a neutral cast. Acute ruptures may be treated surgically with an open or percutaneous technique. The main risk of treatment is re-rupture, which is just below 5% in operatively treated cases and between 8% and 10% for non-operative cases (although there is wide variation in the figures reported in the literature). Although the risk of re-rupture is higher with non-operative treatment, there is no risk of wound infection or breakdown, which can occur with operative repair and can be very difficult to manage. Non-operative treatment is safer in older patients and those with risk factors for wound problems, including smoking, diabetes and steroids. Operative treatment is often offered to younger athletically active patients or patients who present late, as in this case. Non-operative treatment is less likely to be successful in patients who present late since tendon apposition will not be achieved due to retraction of the proximal end and formation of scar tissue. This patient presented at 2 weeks and is probably at high risk of a poor result with non-operative treatment and should be treated by surgery unless there are contraindications.

CASE 67 ANSWERS

8, 9, 13

1. The patient has sustained a fracture of the base of the 5th metatarsal.

2. Taking into account the inversion injury that caused the fracture, care should be taken to exclude an associated ankle fracture or ligament injury. There may be a disruption of some of the components of the lateral ligament complex or a fracture of the lateral malleolus. If there is any doubt, a radiograph of the ankle should also be obtained.

3. The majority of these injuries can be treated non-operatively. A below-knee plaster for 3–4 weeks can be used, but is not absolutely necessary. It is usually required in patients with a lot of pain or in older patients who find crutches and partial weight-bearing difficult. Occasionally, the fracture fragment formed by the base of the metatarsal is significantly displaced by the pull of the peroneus brevis (inserted on the base) and in these cases screw fixation may be considered.

4. Non-union is an uncommon but well recognized complication of this injury. Fractures of the shaft of the 5th metatarsal at the junction of the proximal

with middle third (Jones fracture) are more commonly associated with non-union.

CASE 68 ANSWERS

1, 4, 5, 6, 15, 16

1. The differential diagnosis of an acute monoarthritis in this young man includes, in approximate order of probability:

   a. reactive arthritis, secondary to enteric or *Chlamydia* infection

   b. post-infectious arthritis, secondary to gonococcal infection

   c. arthritis associated with inflammatory bowel disease

   d. septic arthritis

   e. gout

Considering these in turn, there is strong evidence to support reactive arthritis since he has an acute inflammatory arthritis with preceding gastroenteritis, urethritis and probable conjunctivitis. The triggering infection cannot be ascertained with certainty; he may have had infection with an organism, such as *Salmonella*, *Campylobacter* or *Shigella*, and have developed a 'reactive' sterile urethritis in association with his arthritis. Alternatively, he could have acquired *Chlamydia* infection with subsequent reactive arthritis; gastrointestinal symptoms might be unrelated or due to sexually acquired proctitis – chlamydial or gonococcal, or both since dual infection is common. If he has contracted gonoccal, his arthritis may be a post-infectious one rather than the classical reactive arthritis that follows *Chlamydia* infection. Conjunctivitis is not a feature of post-gonococcal arthritis, but incidental conjunctivitis is not uncommon in Ibiza clubbers. Lastly, his gastrointestinal symptoms may be the first presentation of inflammatory disease and the arthritis associated with this; this would not explain any of his genitourinary symptoms and is, therefore, a less attractive option.

Any febrile man with a history of rigors and a single hot joint must be assumed to have septic arthritis, unless there is definite evidence to the contrary, and this must be included in the differential despite the other features that make reactive arthritis more likely. Lastly, gout needs to be considered in a patient who may have consumed considerable quantities of alcohol during his holiday and, thus, increased his chance of developing gout.

2. Synovial fluid should be aspirated and sent for microscopy and culture. This will help to exclude septic arthritis and gout, whilst sterile, cellular fluid will confirm an inflammatory arthritis. Blood cultures should also be taken, and ESR, CRP and white blood cell count measured to indicate the extent of the inflammatory response. To identify any organism that could trigger reactive arthritis, a stool sample should be cultured and a urethral swab or first-pass urine tested for *Chlamydia*, preferably using a sensitive nucleic acid amplification technique. Rectal and throat swabs may also be required. Radiographs are not useful diagnostically; autoantibodies are not likely to be present. HLA-B27 measurement may be useful since reactive arthritis in this group is more severe and long-lasting.

3. Acute management consists of symptom control with adequate doses of a non-steroidal anti-inflammatory drug (NSAID), unless there is a contra-indication, such as aspirin-sensitive asthma or an ulcer history (unlikely at this age). Additional analgesics may be required. Aspiration will improve symptoms and, when septic arthritis has been excluded, intra-articular depot steroids are indicated and can be repeated a few days later if there is only a partial response to the first injection. If a diagnosis of reactive arthritis is established, patient education is of great importance emphasizing that, whilst resolution of symptoms may take more than 1 year, there is a 90% chance of full recovery. This is essential to manage expectations in someone who has probably not had more than a few days' illness before. Gastrointestinal infection does not require antibiotics, but *Chlamydia* or gonococcal infection must be treated conventionally. Prolonged antibiotics are not indicated since they do not alter the course of arthritis. In cases of severe persistent symptoms a disease-modifying drug, usually sulfasalazine, may be introduced, but this is rarely required in the first 6–12 weeks of management.

CASE 69 ANSWERS

1, 3, 23

1. The photograph shows that both knees are hyperextended at rest (genu recurvatum). There is no swelling in these joints.

2. This patient has hypermobility of her knees and probably also has hypermobility at a number of other sites. Typically you can expect patients to complain of creaking or clicking noises in their joints. They may suffer pain and occasional swelling in the joints, but not necessarily directly after overstretching or injury.

Formal assessment of hypermobility includes looking for hyperextension of the little finger MCP joints, extending the thumb parallel to each wrist, hyperextending the elbows and knees, and demonstrating excessive forward flexion of the lumbar spine.

3. Explain the diagnosis and reassure the patient that they do not have arthritis. Exercise is the most important treatment, encouraging aerobic exercise especially. Patients may need some encouragement, but formal physiotherapy is not usually required; information and advice about exercise should suffice, supported by simple analgesia.

CASE 70 ANSWERS

5, 15, 16

1. In this patient, the long history of joint problems, together with the photograph showing swelling of the MCP and PIP joints in a symmetrical fashion, suggests that the patient has rheumatoid arthritis.

2. The differential diagnosis would include gout, especially with the appearance of lumps that might be tophi. Chronic tophaceous gout may develop after long-term diuretic use, especially in elderly females. In younger patients, especially women, consider the possibility of systemic lupus erythematosus (SLE) causing the arthritis, and occasionally also causing nodules. In the absence of the lumps, psoriatic arthritis might produce the same clinical appearance. If you look closely at the picture, however, you can also see some small dark lesions, which represent small-vessel vasculitis. The combination of arthritis, lumps and vasculitis strongly supports a diagnosis of seropositive nodular rheumatoid arthritis.

3. Typically, nodules are brought on by the use of methotrexate in patients with rheumatoid arthritis. This may sound like a reason not to use methotrexate, but in fact most patients prefer the appearance of nodules to the pain of inflammatory joint disease and are willing to accept the appearance of nodules as an acceptable side effect. The nodules can be removed surgically, but there is a significant risk that they will recur. In pathological terms, rheumatoid nodules are non-caseating chronic granulomata with pallisading histiocytes and lymphocytes around a central area.

CASE 71 ANSWERS

1, 5, 15, 16

1. In this case, a septic arthritis has to be very high on the differential diagnosis list, as does acute crystal arthri-

tis. You are, therefore, going to be interested in knowing whether there has been any direct trauma to the joint as part of his job, such as a nail or wood splinter, or whether he has received trauma elsewhere in the body, since most cases of septic arthritis arise from bacteraemic spread. If this is not the first presentation of his condition it is worth enquiring about whether he has had similar previous episodes and what they were like. This would be making you think more about acute crystal arthritis, such as gout and pseudogout, and, therefore, you would want to enquire about his alcohol intake (relevant to gout). Ask about a family history of this type of condition (relevant for both gout and pseudogout). Ask about the presence of other co-morbid conditions, such as hypertension, that might require the patient to take diuretic therapy (a potent cause of hyperuricaemia) or the presence of diabetes or other endocrine and metabolic disorders, many of which predispose to pseudogout. If there is a family history of recurrent joint swellings then that might also support the idea of this being gout or pseudogout. Occasionally, patients with reactive arthritis (see Chapter 16, p 224) can present in this way and, therefore, a gentle enquiry into recent changes in dietary habits with associated diarrhoea or foreign travel, and an even more gentle inquiry into any change in sexual partners and/or the presence of urethral discharge, are the relevant questions to ask.

2. You would also need to take blood cultures to enhance your likelihood of achieving a diagnosis, and on the basis of the pus in the joint you would probably want to start him on intravenous antibiotics and fluids. The antibiotic choice would obviously depend on his possible drug allergies, but, in the circumstances, *Staphylococcus aureus* is a highly likely candidate as is *Streptococcus*. On these grounds you would probably start him on intravenous flucloxacillin and benzyl penicillin or amoxicillin. You would continue to aspirate the joint daily, until the effusion settles, and then start some physiotherapy to try to regain joint range of movement.

3. The current suggestion is a minimum of 2 weeks of intravenous antibiotic therapy followed by a further 4 weeks of oral antibiotic therapy. You would be guided by the blood and synovial fluid culture results with regard to the choice of antibiotic. If it was a staphylococcal infection you might elect to stop benzyl penicillin and introduce fusidic acid instead so that you had two drugs working against that organism (flucloxacillin and fusidic acid).

4. Most patients respond well to antibiotic treatment initiated early, but there are some possible sequelae. About 30% of patients would be expected to have residual loss of joint range of movement as a result of the infection. There is a small risk of bacteraemic spread with liver abscesses or lung abscesses.

CASE 72 ANSWERS

4, 5, 16, 17

1. Pregnancy usually has an immunosuppressive effect on joint disease, so many patients with rheumatoid arthritis or psoriatic arthritis experience remission or significant improvement during pregnancy. It is unusual for joint inflammation to occur during pregnancy. In the post-partum period, however, it is possible to see flares of arthritis, or new presentation of arthritis. Characteristically, SLE may present during pregnancy or worsen during pregnancy. However, you should also consider the possibility of infection, especially viral infections, such as parvovirus B19, which may be damaging to the fetus. In the case of this particular patient, however, the combination of arthritis with neutropenia and thrombocytopenia should make you think about SLE.

2. Helpful investigations would certainly include an anti-nuclear antibody (ANA), double-stranded DNA and complement levels looking for consumption of complement. It may be necessary to consider a bone marrow aspirate or biopsy to ensure that the cytopenias are not due to marrow failure. If the marrow stores are plentiful, you would be reassured.

3. Treatment in this patient would probably be with systemic corticosteroids and low-dose aspirin. Use of steroids at significant doses increases the risk of congenital cleft lip and cleft palate especially if given in the first trimester. In patients with established SLE, pregnancy may be attempted as long as disease is in remission, on or off treatment with drugs such as low-dose corticosteroid, hydroxychloroquine and even azathioprine. In SLE it is preferable to keep patients under control rather than risk a flare during pregnancy. Combined management between rheumatologists and obstetricians would be very important for this patient.

CASE 73 ANSWERS

1, 5, 13, 19, 20

1. Metastatic cancer in the shaft of the left tibia; there is a large lucent area representing bony destruction.

2. Disseminated malignancy must be the most likely problem, and with the finding of an iron-deficient picture of anaemia, and the cough, with occasional haemoptysis and weight loss you have to consider the likelihood of a primary tumour in the lung, which is likely to have spread to cause the widespread metastases in bone. The typical tumours that metastasize to bone are lung, prostate, thyroid, adrenal, kidney and breast, but other common tumours also spread to bone. A differential diagnosis would include sepsis and polymyalgia rheumatica. A search for the primary tumour is important, but occasionally in the absence of an obvious primary, a bone biopsy may be considered. This may be hazardous, however, since the procedure may result in local seeding of the tumour.

3. It is most likely that the tumour is widespread and, therefore, palliative measures should be considered to manage the pain, including local radiotherapy if the tumour is radiosensitive, along with appropriate pain relief. The prognosis is likely to be poor.

CASE 74 ANSWERS

1, 3, 4, 5, 6, 22

1. Central disc herniation with cauda equina syndrome because of the rapid onset of bilateral neurological trouble and probable urinary retention. The picture is one of a profound lower motor neurone lesion affecting many of the sacral nerves. Central disc herniation is uncommon (1–2% of all disc herniations) and frequently misdiagnosed.

2. The case described here is florid with a full house of clinical features due to sacral nerve dysfunction, but there is a whole spectrum of different presentations. There may be very little pain and profound sphincter disturbance or severe sciatica, bilateral lower-limb neurological deficit and relative sparing of sacral roots 2, 3 and 4.

   The key sign is perineal numbness, the presence of which demands urgent investigation. Because the normal bladder sensation is lost, the patient may be oblivious of their urinary retention, so it is important to be mindful of the possibility and seek bladder distension by palpation and percussion of the lower abdomen.

3. An urgent MRI proves the diagnosis. The MRI T2 sagittal (A) and axial (B) images show that an L5/S1 disc herniation extends into the canal and upwards behind the body of L5. On the axial view the theca and nerves (lighter colour) are displaced and

compressed by the disc material (dark). Water-soluble myelography and computed tomography can be used in the absence of MRI. If the admitting hospital does not have the facility to arrange an MRI within 12 h of presentation, a transfer to another centre is indicated.

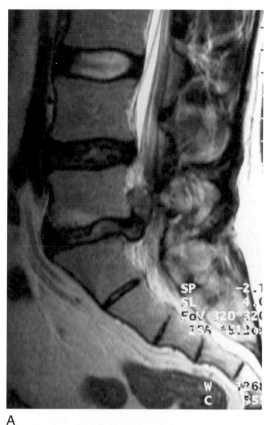

A

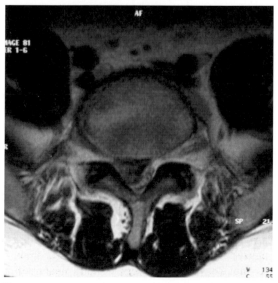

B

4. Immediate urinary catheterization is necessary to decompress the bladder and prevent over-distension, which would damage the detrusor muscle. Discectomy and cauda equina decompression must be carried out as an emergency – ideally within 24 h. The disc material is often sequestrated within the spinal canal, i.e. separated from the intervertebral disc itself, so special care must be taken to clear all the disc fragments. A large meta-analysis has shown that prompt treatment can produce good results, but treatment later than 48 h after presentation is associated with poorer outcome due to permanent bladder and bowel dysfunction. In both sexes sexual dysfunction can be a problem.

The real problem is that patients often present many days after the onset of their cauda equina compression and delay is compounded by failure of doctors to detect the more subtle variations of presentation. The patient is taught self-catheterization to stimulate bladder recovery.

If the 5th lumbar nerves are affected, the patient may be left with unilateral or bilateral foot-drop and walking can be assisted by provision of a custom-made orthosis to splint the ankle at a right angle.

CASE 75 ANSWERS

1, 5, 6, 16

1. This patient presents with an acute oligoarthritis, which reduces the risk of septic arthritis, but does not eliminate it. Therefore, the most important test is to aspirate the knee and ask for an urgent Gram stain, and to culture the fluid as well as taking blood cultures, given the pyrexia.

2. The history of recent change in sexual partner, sore eye and oligoarthritis should make a sexually acquired reactive arthritis the most likely diagnosis even though the patient does not describe any urethral discharge – this is often unnoticed in women compared to men. *Chlamydia trachomatis* is the most common organism, but others are possible including *Neisseria gonorrhoeae*, which may cause either septic arthritis or reactive arthritis or both. The patient should be referred to a sexual medicine clinic for appropriate swabs to be taken. Other potential causes are septic arthritis or inflammatory oligoarthritis related to psoriasis or inflammatory bowel disease, but these are much less likely given the clinical presentation.

3. She will probably need admitting to observe the temperature and to rest affected joints. Once the knee aspirate has been sent, you may consider introducing intravenous antibiotics if you suspect sepsis, especially if the aspirate is purulent, or if the patient has previously received any antibiotic treatment in the last few days. Once sepsis has been ruled out, you may consider injecting the affected joints with steroid, adding a regular anti-inflammatory agent and analgesic to her treatment. She will need physiotherapy to help mobilize again and may even require crutches for a time. Explain the diagnosis to the patient. If she does have an ongoing genital infection, this should be treated, although it will not affect the outcome of the arthritis, which is complete resolution in most patients within 3–6 months.

CASE 76 ANSWERS

1, 4, 5, 6, 7, 15, 23

1. The most likely diagnosis is osteoarthritis of the left knee. If his clinical symptoms were of pain in the knee but without any clinical signs in the knee you should consider hip disease, and routinely examine the hip. The clinical findings in this case are very typical of knee pathology (see figure). Arterial insufficiency may cause leg pain due to ischaemia and, given his

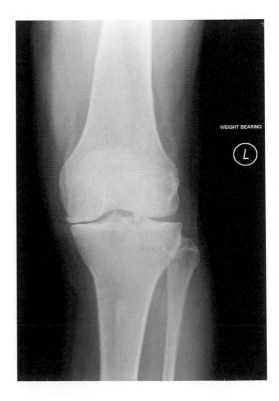

history of myocardial disease, it would be important to examine his pulses and consider a diagnosis of intermittent claudication as a cause of his leg pain, especially if his knee looked normal on examination.

2. The presence of a flexion deformity and limited knee range, accompanied by a valgus deformity, suggests that surgical intervention might be required. However, in terms of medical management, it is important to determine how much movement and strength can be regained from exercise and analgesia. NSAIDs would be relatively contra-indicated given his age and cardiovascular problems. Corticosteroid injections do not have role in this case.

3. The failure of medical management might suggest that surgical intervention should be considered, but this is a major operation and his peri-operative mortality risk will be very high, unless his cardiovascular disease can be improved. You may want to refer him to a cardiologist to improve this and possibly consider him for a revascularization procedure (e.g. CABG, angioplasty) if appropriate. Once his heart has improved, he may then be reconsidered for knee replacement. Make sure you check peripheral pulses just in case he also has peripheral vascular disease.

CASE 77 ANSWERS

4, 5, 16

1. This woman with rheumatoid arthritis has developed liver function abnormalities on taking methotrexate. The results indicate elevation of the aspartate transaminase and the alkaline phosphatase. They are more than four times the upper limit for the laboratory. The bilirubin is normal. Looking back over the previous results you note that on one occasion, the liver function tests had risen to two times the upper limit of normal, but settled spontaneously.

2. Immediate action must be to stop the methotrexate until the results return to normal. You should enquire about the use of any new concomitant therapy or change in alcohol intake as other potential causes of liver dysfunction. Diclofenac as well as other NSAIDs can cause liver function abnormalities. If there was a clinical history to suggest it, you might need to investigate for other causes of abnormal liver function, such as obstructive liver diseases, hepatitis caused by viruses, etc., but in most cases, when you stop the methotrexate, you would expect the results to return to normal rapidly, demonstrating that the drug is almost certainly the cause.

3. You would probably re-establish the patient on methotrexate when the liver function returned to normal, but typically at a lower dose – perhaps 17.5 mg or 15 mg per week. You may need to add another agent to her treatment, in case her disease does become more active on the lower dose, but this may not become apparent for a few weeks. Hydroxy-chloroquine, leflunomide or even sulfasalazine (despite it losing efficacy previously) could be given together with the new lower dose of methotrexate. If these measures fail, you will need to stop methotrexate and consider other agents, including leflunomide alone or anti-tumour necrosis factor (TNF) therapy.

CASE 78 ANSWERS

16, 18, 22

1. The patient presents with immobility as her main complaint. It is not unusual for the GP to assume that this represents a flare of her arthritis. However, the history and physical findings as well as the laboratory results are against this conclusion. In this setting, you need to consider the possibility that she has developed a complication of the arthritis or its treatment. If pain had been a significant feature in the history, then you should consider the possibility of a fracture. Elderly patients with rheumatoid arthritis and steroid therapy are at high risk of osteoporotic fractures. If there is an obvious site of pain and limited movement due to pain, this may be the site of fracture (e.g. neck of femur); if pain is diffusely around the pelvic area, then an insufficiency fracture of the sacrum or pelvis should be considered. The presence of prosthetic joints in the hips raises the possibility of mechanical failure of the prosthetic joints, or infection (even with an apyrexial patient, because steroids may mask signs of infection), or loosening of the prosthesis. However, the absence of pain makes these problems less likely and you need to think about a neurological cause for her immobility. Rheumatoid arthritis commonly affects the cervical spine, with production of pannus in the atlanto-axial area, and erosive changes in the odontoid peg. Atlanto-axial subluxation, vertebral subluxation and sub-axial subluxation are all feared complications of rheumatoid arthritis, which may lead to cord compression and eventually to paraly-sis of the limbs. You need to perform a careful examination of her neck and a neurological examination looking for evidence of cord compression at the neck, typically producing upper motor neurone

442

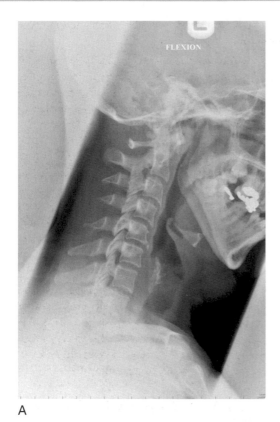

A

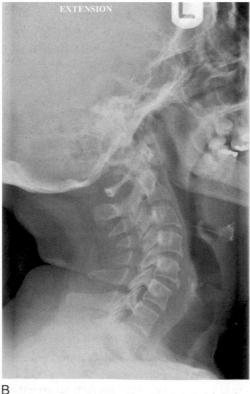

B

signs in the legs, sometimes with lower motor neurone signs in the arms.

2. A simple lateral radiograph of the cervical spine taken in flexion (A), and repeated in extension (B), will demonstrate the presence of atlanto-axial instability (see figures). The most effective investigation is an MRI scan of the neck to demonstrate the presence of pannus and look at the cord signal for signs of cord oedema or compression.

3. Management depends on the degree of neurological deficit present. If there is none, a conservative approach may be used, but with neurological weakness, it is important to fix the neck in a stable position with a firm and extensive collar, and to consider the role of decompression, or internal fixation of the cervical spine, to prevent further neurological damage.

CASE 79 ANSWERS

1, 5, 6, 16

1. The combination of peripheral joint involvement and axial involvement with psoriasis would make the diagnosis of psoriatic spondyloarthritis most likely. The swollen digit is characteristic of dactylitis, which is not seen in rheumatoid arthritis, whereas it is very typical of psoriasis-related arthritis. Spinal examination shows very limited lumbar spine movement in all directions and chest wall expansion restricted to 2 cm.

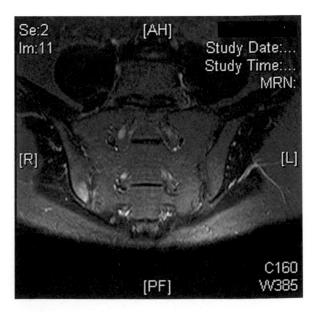

2. Blood should be taken for CRP and baseline blood tests prior to commencing disease-modifying anti-rheumatic therapy. Imaging of the sacroiliac joints with plain X-ray or MRI (see figure) would help to confirm the presence of sacroiliac inflammation; typically in psoriatic spondyloarthritis, the lesions may be asymmetrical.

3. Management includes anti-inflammatory agents, analgesics and a disease-modifying agent. Use of leflunomide or methotrexate should be considered. Physiotherapy is important to mobilize the joints and spine; you may want to consider injecting steroid locally into the swollen finger if it is very painful.

CASE 80 ANSWERS

5, 6, 16

1. In this difficult situation the two most likely diagnoses are either a mechanical cause of low back pain or seronegative arthritis, most likely ankylosing spondylitis (AS). Whilst neither condition is rare, the former is far more common as a presentation to general practitioners. The utility of diagnostic tests is determined by Bayesian analysis, which takes into account the prior likelihood of an outcome in addition to the sensitivity and specificity of a test, in determining the posterior probability/ultimate likelihood of the condition in that setting. The post-test probability of AS in the event of a negative X-ray is difficult to determine with accuracy due to the

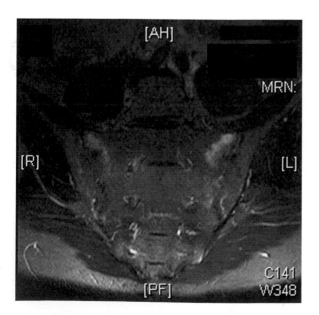

limited information available from longitudinal inception cohort studies.

2. In most Caucasian populations the prevalence of carriage of HLA-B27 is 6–9%, but only 1–5% of carriers develop ankylosing spondylitis. Thus, in the absence of any knowledge of the person's clinical history, the probability of ankylosing spondylitis in a carrier of HLA-B27, called the prior probability, is 1–5%. However, it has been estimated that if a patient presents to a general practitioner with inflammatory pattern low back pain, then the probability of ankylosing spondylitis is 14%. Bayesian analysis then shows that if the patient tests positive for HLA-B27, the probability of the disease increases to 59%. If the HLA-B27 test is negative then the diagnosis can be excluded.

3. When the patient then goes on to have an MRI scan (see figure), if this is positive then the probability of AS is 93% and if negative 14%. These calculations need to be considered with caution due to the paucity of data, particularly regarding the specificity of MRI in pre-radiographic ankylosing spondylitis.

CASE 81 ANSWERS

5, 16

1. The patient has failed at least two disease-modifying drugs and continues to have active disease. She would, therefore, be eligible to receive anti-TNF therapy; current choices include adalimumab, etanercept and infliximab.

2. A careful history to rule out current infection; a check for a current or previous history of tuberculosis is particularly important – with a chest radiograph at baseline. Patients should not have had any premalignant conditions or malignancy within the past 10 years (or any malignancy with a low risk of cure), except basal cell skin cancers. Patients with multiple sclerosis and also patients with heart failure are excluded. The patient needs counselling on the advantages and disadvantages of this type of therapy, and may require practical advice on self-administration of subcutaneous injections (for adalimumab and etanercept). Alternatively the patient must be able to attend hospital on a regular basis to receive intravenous infusions of infliximab.

3. It is important to explain to each patient that the treatment is given under careful supervision. Regular monitoring is required, especially early on, to ensure that the treatment is not causing side effects and,

perhaps more importantly, to ensure that the treatment is working. Patients should be reviewed at 3 months to reassess their disease status; if there has not been a significant fall in disease activity (a DAS score falling by at least 1.2 or falling to below 3.2) the treatment should be either discontinued or supplemented with a previously tolerated dose of a conventional disease-modifying drug. In this case you might restart methotrexate at 15 mg per week and reassess in a further 3 months.

CASE 82 ANSWERS

1, 5, 7, 13, 16, 19

1. The clinical features suggest that she may have developed end-stage disease in her left shoulder (secondary osteoarthritis) as well as rotator cuff damage. It does sound as if there are problems developing in the opposite shoulder as well, probably with rotator cuff disease.

2. An X-ray of the shoulder may be diagnostic (see figure) showing loss of glenohumeral joint space and upward subluxation of the humeral head in relation to the glenoid cavity, secondary to rotator cuff injury. If she had been on long-term steroid treatment, another consideration would be avascular necrosis of the humeral head, which may give a flattened appearance on plain X-ray. If the X-ray was normal, but suspicion was high for avascular necrosis, an MRI scan would indicate the presence of bone oedema in the humeral head, which is diagnostic.

3. Shoulder joint replacement may be the best long-term solution for her pain, but may not restore much

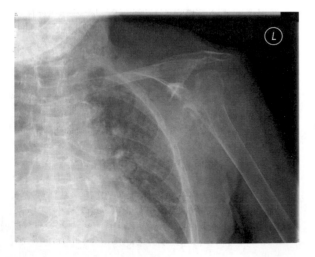

function if the rotator cuff is severely damaged and cannot be reattached. Conservative therapy would be with analgesia, physiotherapy and, possibly, the use of suprascapular nerve blocks for pain relief. The role of intra-articular steroids would have been earlier in the disease course when there was active synovitis. You may want to consider further assessment of the opposite shoulder perhaps with more careful follow-up and ask the patient to report back early if she develops more symptoms, since she may require repair of her rotator cuff, possibly with a decompression of the acromion to preserve its function.

CASE 83 ANSWERS

1, 4, 5, 6, 14

1. This young woman presents with a number of relatively non-specific symptoms. With the flat affect, clinical depression should be considered. Weight gain, with constipation, might suggest hypothyroidism, but the patient is young and there is no past history to suggest an autoimmune thyroiditis previously. Change in bowel habit and ill-health might be due to coeliac disease. Joint pain with no evidence of synovitis could suggest systemic lupus erythematosus. Other disorders, such as hepatitis, could be responsible, but the possibility of chronic fatigue syndrome should be considered.

2. Simple screening investigations should be undertaken, including a full blood count, inflammatory markers, liver, renal and thyroid function, and an autoantibody profile, including antiendomysial antibodies to screen for coeliac disease. Specific questions relating to depression, including suicidal ideation, should be asked and if in doubt a psychiatric opinion should be sought.

3. If screening is normal, then a positive diagnosis of a fatigue syndrome can be made.

4. Management should include a full discussion of the condition, its likely causation, natural history, prognosis and principles of treatment. Care should be taken to explain the need for paced activity and the avoidance of prolonged rest, which can cause physiological deconditioning. It is important to explain that all chronic, disabling disorders are accompanied by psychological distress and help may be required to relieve this. The help of a multi-disciplinary team with experience of dealing with chronic fatigue should be sought.

CASE 84 ANSWERS

1, 5, 17

1. The patient presents with classical symptoms of generalized pain and then sudden onset of a new headache, followed by rapid visual loss. Polymyalgia and giant cell arteritis (GCA) (temporal arteritis) must be the most likely combination of problems. There is considerable overlap between the two diseases. The weight loss and general unwellness may sometimes suggest an underlying malignancy or sepsis in the differential diagnosis, but the headache and visual symptoms strongly point to GCA, in this case with polymyalgia rheumatica. The combination occurs in around 30% of cases. The headache is usually more like head pain, often with localized scalp tenderness. It is useful, although unusual, to get a history of jaw claudication (pain on chewing) or tongue claudication (pain on speaking). The visual loss in these patients is usually irreversible and may occur in around 10% of patients at presentation. The fear is that it may become bilateral, making the condition an ophthalmological emergency.

2. The most useful investigation is a biopsy of the temporal artery (see figure) from the affected side, although the yield of positive results is higher if both sides are sampled. The lesions can be patchy in the course of the artery (skip lesions), suggesting that the longer the sample of artery the better.

3. In most conditions, it is important to undertake investigations before starting patients on definitive treatment. However, in this case it is essential to start treatment on clinical suspicion of the disease in order to try to prevent further visual loss as a result of ciliary artery occlusion, resulting in the typical

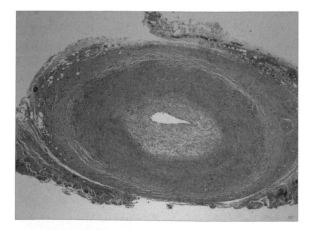

ischaemic lesion in the retina (anterior ischaemic optic neuropathy). Start patients on 60 mg prednisolone per day and taper slowly over the next 18–24 months.

CASE 85 ANSWERS

1, 5, 14, 16, 17, 20

1. The new presentation of generalized stiffness and weight loss in an elderly patient should make you think about malignancy with metastatic bone deposits causing the pain. Hyperthyroidism might be a cause of weight loss, but hypothyroidism is more likely to result in the stiffness and slowing down, so it does not quite fit; neither would cause the ESR and CRP to increase. Depression in the elderly can present in this way, but would not cause the ESR and CRP to increase. Muscle inflammation (polymyositis, dermatomyositis or inclusion body myositis) would be associated with considerable muscle pain and weakness, usually with wasting after this length of time. Chronic infections may sometimes present like this. Rheumatoid arthritis can start with generalized stiffness and pain, but you would expect some evidence of joint swelling especially in small- and medium-sized joints. The low levels of rheumatoid factor and ANA are likely to be irrelevant in someone of this age.

2. The most likely diagnosis is polymyalgia rheumatica.

3. Treatment is with a low dose of corticosteroids. Typically patients respond well to 15 mg per day for 1 month, reducing by 1 mg per month to discontinue. Higher starting doses are seldom justified, although if patients also develop giant cell arteritis, you must use more, typically 40–60 mg per day starting dose. In the elderly, bone protection against steroid-induced osteoporosis would be justified, using a bisphosphonate or vitamin D3 or both.

CASE 86 ANSWERS

5, 15, 16

1. The presence of numerous lumps on the fingers and active joint swelling should raise the possibility of rheumatoid arthritis; however, the fact that the patient is on diuretics and aspirin, and that one of the lesions is leaking white chalky material, is very suggestive of chronic tophaceous gout. Many of these patients have not experienced attacks of acute gout. Urate clearance is chronically inhibited by the diuretic and aspirin. Other causes of lumps and arthritis include SLE, although these are unusual on

the hands, and the age and gender would be unusual. Occasional patients may present with Gottron's papules, which are subcutaneous thickening of skin over the dorsum of the PIP and occasionally MCP joints. Tendon xanthomata are usually asymptomatic, but would be associated with other features of dyslipidaemia.

2. The most useful test would be to send the white material for examination under polarized light microscopy, which would reveal the presence of large numbers of weakly negative birefringent crystals. The material should also be sent for culture since the patient is at risk of developing a superadded infection. A blood sample should be tested for uric acid levels and for creatinine, since poor renal function may contribute to impaired urate clearance. A creatinine clearance measurement or estimation should be performed, in anticipation of starting allopurinol.

3. Initial management of the wound with sterile dressings is important. The culture result should be obtained to determine if there is any infection. The presence of multiple tophi indicates excess urate and is an indication to start allopurinol therapy. It is unlikely that the patient will be able to stop the diuretic treatment for their heart disease; therefore, long-term allopurinol is going to be required. The dose of allopurinol is adjusted according to renal clearance. It is unlikely that the patient will experience acute gout, but as a preventative measure it may be appropriate to use prophylactic colchicine 500 μg twice a day for the first month of allopurinol therapy.

CASE 87 ANSWERS

1, 4, 5, 17

1. This woman presents with a complex medical history and a combination of clinical symptoms and features that suggest SLE. In particular, her history of recurrent oral ulceration, inflammatory arthritis and pleuritic type chest pain would all be in keeping with SLE. Her constitutional upset, hair loss and recent history of Raynaud's phenomenon would also support the diagnosis. Her maternal aunt, who is having dialysis therapy, suggests that there may be a family history.

Simple investigation can be extremely informative and a full blood count may demonstrate additional abnormalities, such as haemolytic anaemia, leuco-penia or thrombocytopenia. A urine dipstick is essential to exclude any early renal involvement. An estimate of the degree of any proteinuria as well as her glomerular filtration rate would also be important at baseline. Blood should be sent for serological testing and in particular the presence of antinuclear antibodies and/or antibodies to double-stranded DNA would help confirm the diagnosis. Additional serological testing is considered in answer 2 below.

Patients with SLE are at increased risk of infection, which can often coincide with their initial presentation. As a result, it should not be assumed that the fever is due to active inflammation and thorough investigation to exclude infection should be undertaken. In this specific case a chest X-ray, cultures of any sputum as well as urine and blood cultures should be sent.

The pleuritic chest pain may reflect serositis of a primary inflammatory aetiology. As mentioned above it can also reflect infection. The third possibility is that she may have suffered a pulmonary embolism and, therefore, a ventilation perfusion scan should be undertaken to exclude this diagnosis.

Once these investigations are complete if there remains any residual doubt as to the underlying diagnosis then a tissue biopsy can sometimes be necessary. In this particular case a lymph node biopsy would exclude any chronic infection or an underlying neoplastic disorder. Also, if any urine abnormalities were detected then a renal biopsy would be indicated.

2. More than 90% of patients with SLE will have a positive ANA and about 60% will also have antibodies to double-stranded DNA. Hypergammaglobulinaemia is also common. The ANA is useful to support the diagnosis; however, antibodies to dsDNA and Sm are more specific for SLE. With regard to disease activity high titres of double-stranded DNA and/or hypocomplementaemia may reflect the underlying inflammatory process and in about one-third of patients changes in the serological tests over time will reflect inflammatory disease activity. Persistent profound abnormalities of these tests should alert the physician to the possibility of underlying nephritis and in such cases the renal function should be observed carefully.

In this case, the presence of antiphospholipid (APL) antibodies and/or the lupus anticoagulant (LAC) is important to detect. These tests are associated with an increased risk of thrombotic complications. The combination of a positive test along with pleuritic chest pain would raise further the possibility of venous thromboembolism. In the context of having a thrombosis, APL or LAC positivity has major prognostic significance, as it would suggest that life-long anticoagulation would be indicated.

3. Alopecia in SLE can be subdivided into cases of scarring and non-scarring alopecia. The majority of patients with acute lupus eruptions can show evidence of scalp erythema and mild scaling associated with diffuse or more localized hair loss. In these cases, as inflammatory disease activity comes under control then hair growth will return.

Less commonly, alopecia can occur in the context of discoid lupus. This usually presents as discrete erythematous papules with dense overlying scaling, which cause complete destruction of skin appendages including hair follicles. Areas of depigmentation can also occur. As a result, the alopecia may be permanent and cosmetically quite disfiguring.

CASE 88 ANSWERS

1, 4, 17

1. The patient presents with some features to suggest rheumatoid arthritis. The pattern of joint pain and the presence of rheumatoid factor are suggestive, as is the raised ESR. But if all this was joint inflammation, you would really expect to see something on joint examination. It is possible that the clinical features might vary a little, but on repeat clinical evaluation some months later there is still no joint inflammation to show. The back and shoulder problems are unlikely to be connected since the shoulder problems have resolved, and the back examination findings strongly suggest mechanical back problems. To confound the problem, the CRP is normal. With such a high ESR, why is the CRP normal? This may provide one clue towards the answer in this case. In many patients with active SLE, the ESR may be high whilst the CRP is normal, but there are no pointers to SLE in this patient. The strongly positive rheumatoid factor should make you think of causes of a strongly positive rheumatoid factor. Apart from rheumatoid arthritis, think about primary Sjögren's syndrome, where rheumatoid factor is commonly found. Ask about a typical history of dry gritty eyes, possible recurrent conjunctivitis, and dry mouth.

2. Further confirmation may be achieved by testing for anti-Ro and anti-La antibodies. You can check her tear production with a simple test (Schirmer tear test) or check salivary flow rates. Many patients do develop arthralgia as part of the condition.

3. The main treatment is education and support. Explain that this is not rheumatoid arthritis; provide artificial tears or suggest possible use of stimulants to encourage better salivary and lachrymal flow. Liaison with ophthalmology and oral medicine colleagues for advice and help on eye and dental hygiene is very useful. Most patients with long-standing Sjögren's read about the risk of lymphoma development, but recent studies show that this is around 10%; it is important to explain this risk to patients and ask them to return for assessment urgently if they develop persistent gland swelling. If the patient had been of child-bearing years, you would also need to counsel her on the risk of fetal heart block if she has anti-Ro and anti-La antibodies (the risk is about 1%).

CASE 89 ANSWERS

4, 17, 18

1. The blood tests show a mild anaemia, normal ANA and dsDNA, normal complement levels, low platelets, normal prothrombin time, but a prolonged APTT.

2. The results suggest the presence of a lupus anticoagulant, and further testing should be performed to confirm this – a typical test would be the dilute Russell viper venom test. In addition, blood should be tested for the presence of antiphospholipid antibodies. The combination of recurrent miscarriages, clotting abnormalities, low platelets and a pulmonary embolus would be diagnostic of the antiphospholipid antibody syndrome. The syndrome may be primary, as in this case, or secondary to SLE, in which case you would expect the presence of some other systemic features, typically a butterfly rash, photosensitivity, mouth ulcers, joint pains, etc.

3. The fact that she has had a pulmonary embolus would suggest that lifelong anticoagulation will be required. Aspirin and heparin should be given throughout any future pregnancies (this will improve, but not ensure, the outcome of future pregnancies) and thereafter she should be given warfarin. The INR should be maintained at between 2.5 and 3.5 (higher than for uncomplicated pulmonary emboli).

CASE 90 ANSWERS

4, 5, 17, 18

1. The patient has presented with classical features of Raynaud's phenomenon, of recent onset and affecting

fingers and toes in an asymmetrical distribution. Clinical features that make you think this must be secondary Raynaud's are the tissue injury to the right fingertip, and the presence of the red blanching lesions of telangiectasia. Add to that the fact that she has indigestion, and the picture is very suggestive of limited cutaneous scleroderma. Your next step would be a careful examination of the skin especially on the dorsum of the hands and feet looking for skin tightness or tethering, especially since you have noted that she is unable to clench her fingers into a fist despite the fact that the joints all look normal.

2. ANA testing and specifically testing for anti-centromere antibody is a useful test, although not all patients will be positive. You might consider a barium swallow or upper GI endoscopy to investigate the indigestion, which may be due to oesophageal involvement by the scleroderma. A monitoring programme of echocardiography and lung function testing should be considered because these patients may develop pulmonary hypertension in future.

3. The most important advice to give her is to stop smoking. She should take extra care to wrap up well a few minutes before going out, and to stay wrapped up for a few minutes after arriving anywhere, in order to avoid experiencing a large temperature gradient. If these measures fail, you can consider the use of calcium channel blockers or other vasodilators, such as prazosin or losartan. For severe Raynaud's features, there is an important role for intravenous prostacyclin given as a continuous infusion, typically over 3–5 days. The benefit may last for 4–6 weeks and the procedure can be repeated. If she is developing worsening indigestion, a proton pump inhibitor should be considered. She should be told about her disease and the need for regular monitoring of blood pressure (if hypertension develops it should be treated with an ACE inhibitor). Currently there are no known effective treatments to alter the underlying disease process.

CASE 91 ANSWERS

1, 5, 6, 18, 28

1. Septic arthritis should always be considered, although this is unlikely in a well child with no other medical problems. The main differential is between a reactive arthritis, possibly related to the sore throat, or oligoarticular JIA. Rarer causes, such as malignancy, should not be forgotten, but again this is less likely in a well child, and investigations should help to exclude this.

2. Unless there is a high suspicion that this is septic arthritis, there is no need to aspirate the knee acutely. The child should have blood taken for a full blood count, ESR and CRP, all of which are likely to be normal. It is probably too late to do a throat swab, but serum should be sent to look for rising antistreptolysin O titres. Blood should also be sent to look for anti-nuclear antibodies.

3. This child should be started on an anti-inflammatory drug such as ibuprofen. A dose of 20 mg/kg/day in divided doses would be reasonable. She needs to be seen by the physiotherapist for quadriceps strengthening exercises and to encourage the knee to straighten. The occupational therapist will need to make her a resting splint to wear at night, also to encourage the joint to fully extend. If the knee does not settle with these measures after 1–2 months, intra-articular steroid injection should be considered, probably under general anaesthetic in a child so young. Once the swelling has settled and the knee is straight, she should be encouraged to return to full activity as soon as possible. If the diagnosis is felt to be oligoarticular JIA, she should be referred to the ophthalmologists for screening under slit-lamp examination, and be kept under review by the paediatric rheumatologist.

CASE 92 ANSWERS

15, 19, 20

1. The left hemi-pelvis shows extensive changes of coarsening of trabeculae and thickening of cortex.

2. The differential diagnosis is of metastatic bone tumour; sclerotic lesions are often seen in patients with primary tumours – of the prostate in men or of the breast in women. Osteosarcoma should be considered, but the patient is quite well. The most likely diagnosis is Paget's disease of bone, a common disorder affecting approximately 3–4% of the adult population. Pathological phases include early excessive resorption of bone trabeculae followed by intense osteoblastic repair. Complications that may develop include sarcomatous transformation (in approximately 1%), neurological deficits (usually from bony encroachment on the nerve), pathological fracture and arthropathy.

3. Use analgesia with NSAIDs for symptom relief. If pain is not controlled and there is clear evidence of active disease (as evidenced by the elevated alkaline phosphatase) then it would be justifiable to treat with a bisphosphonate.

CASE 93 ANSWERS

1, 4, 5, 17

1. This patient presents with a multisystem illness, involving the joints, the kidneys, the lungs and the upper airways, along with systemic features. The more systems that are affected at the same time, the narrower the differential diagnosis becomes, because there are fewer and fewer diseases that can be responsible. The triad of upper and lower airways inflammation together with renal inflammation is characteristic of the small-vessel vasculitis called Wegener's granulomatosis. Conceivably, a systemic infection with bacteria or fungi could cause the airway disease, but you should be able to culture organisms easily in someone who is this unwell and producing sputum.

2. The most important test to perform is a renal biopsy to determine the nature of the kidney involvement, and help to decide appropriate treatment. An ANCA test for cytoplasmic ANCA and a specific ELISA test for PR3 antibodies would be further evidence in favour of a diagnosis of Wegener's granulomatosis.

3. Treatment depends on the extent and severity of organ involvement. In this patient, if a renal biopsy demonstrates the presence of focal segmental glomerulonephritis, then cyclophosphamide and prednisolone are the recommended treatments to induce remission, followed by maintenance therapy with either azathioprine or methotrexate combined with lower doses of steroids. These patients require careful follow-up, since around 50% may experience a relapse of disease requiring more intense immunosuppression again.

CASE 94 ANSWERS

4, 5, 17, 18, 20, 28

1. The original presentation is of childhood-onset joint inflammation with no detectable cause, such as infection. The diagnosis is most likely to be juvenile-onset idiopathic arthritis (JIA). Young boys are less likely than young girls to develop JIA, and you should wonder about this being a form of juvenile spondyloarthritis. It is very important to examine his spine now and in future, since some of these children may progress to ankylosing spondylitis and benefit from treatment of the spinal disease. From the later history it does sound like this is the case in him.

2. If he had been taking any medication, it would be important to document the drug history. NSAIDs can cause leg swelling through renal effects, and this is reversible on stopping the drug.

3. Unfortunately, long-standing inflammation of this type can lead to excess formation and deposition of amyloid (secondary amyloidosis) due to excess production of serum amyloid A protein, one of the acute-phase proteins. Amyloid is typically deposited in the kidney causing tubular damage, leading to excess protein leak, and eventually to renal failure and death if untreated. It is essential to limit further deposition of amyloid fibres by controlling systemic inflammation, usually with potent immunosuppressive or cytotoxic drugs to slow down this process. Amyloid is not completely reversible, but the large bulk that accumulates before causing clinical symptoms means that, in practice, it is very difficult to control once established. Biochemistry testing shows low serum albumin and excess urine protein. Amyloid deposits may occur in all large organs, such as the liver, spleen and the heart, as well as the gut, leading to many problems.

CASE 95 ANSWERS

13, 19, 20

1. In polygenic diseases, such as osteoporosis, the condition is typically inherited from both sides of the family. Indeed, it is thought that where a heritable condition is more prevalent in one gender then affected individuals of the opposite gender must have greater genetic risk factors to develop the condition and, therefore, have greater risk of passing the condition on to their children. This has been shown to be true in some conditions, such as ankylosing spondylitis, where, although men are affected considerably more often than women, children of affected women are more likely to develop the condition than children of affected men. In osteoporosis, with regard to BMD there is good evidence that children of affected men and women are at increased risk of the condition. There are few data regarding fracture, but it is unlikely that this is any different to the inheritance of BMD. Therefore, this woman was mistaken in her belief that she was unlikely to inherit the condition because her father rather than her mother was affected.

2. There is considerable controversy regarding the efficacy of either calcium/vitamin D intake or exercise in

the prevention or treatment of osteoporosis. There is good evidence that in the growing skeleton weight-bearing exercise increases bone density significantly, whereas in later life the beneficial effect appears to be much less. Extreme lack of exercise such as bed-rest or weightlessness does lead to marked bone loss. Similarly, evidence for beneficial effects of calcium and vitamin D is greatest during growth and the evidence that it is effective in preventing or treating osteoporosis in later life is weaker. There are good data indicating that in people who are vitamin D deficient, vitamin D replacement is effective, but limited data that it is effective when used in normal or institutionalized individuals not known to be vitamin D deficient. Thus, whilst there are epidemiological links between these environmental factors and disease, this finding has not yet translated into robustly effective preventative or treatment regimens.

CASE 96 ANSWERS

1, 5, 6, 21

1. The clinical features are those of acute lateral epicondylitis (tennis elbow). Most sufferers do not play tennis. The problem is of acute inflammation around the insertion point of the common extensor tendons of the forearm (the site of insertion of tendon into bone is called an enthesis, hence the term enthesitis).

2. Enthesitis at a number of sites, coupled with a history of iritis, should immediately make you consider the diagnosis of ankylosing spondylitis and it would be important to examine his back carefully looking for restriction of spinal movement in all directions. In most patients who eventually have a diagnosis of ankylosing spondylitis made, the symptoms have been present for years, despite the fact that careful clinical examination may reveal the spinal stiffness. In retrospect, patients may recall back problems for long periods of time, but may have ignored them thinking they are just normal.

3. Rest, ice, compression and elevation may be effective for acute episodes, but after 1 month it is likely that more help may be required. Analgesics and limited use of NSAIDs may help. Physiotherapy to restore muscle strength and movement is important. For acutely tender elbows, a local steroid injection (usually with hydrocortisone 25 mg) may provide short-term relief, but long-term outcome is inferior to physiotherapy, or no intervention. The use of

longer-acting steroid preparations may be more effective, but carries a risk of local skin atrophy and depigmentation, which, although harmless, may be unsightly and permanent.

CASE 97 ANSWERS

1, 5, 6, 7, 21

1. The patient has developed a classical painful arc syndrome, with limited abduction beyond 30°. The supraspinatus muscle is responsible for the initial movement, but then the rotator cuff muscles take over, especially the deltoid. Impingement or damage to the rotator cuff may result in this syndrome.

2. Partial- or full-thickness tears of the rotator cuff, subacromial bursitis, acromioclavicular joint arthritis, calcified coracoacromial ligament, and structural abnormalities of the acromion.

3. In most patients, exercise and analgesia are the most effective treatments. In resistant cases, a local steroid injection may be helpful; however, in patients who have a full-thickness tear, reconstructive surgery may be necessary.

CASE 98 ANSWERS

14, 15, 19, 20, 23

1. The biochemistry results are of a raised alkaline phosphatase and a low calcium.

2. The findings are indicative of osteomalacia. This can be confirmed by measuring her vitamin D levels. Her diet may be deficient in vitamin D and her lack of sunlight exposure would prevent her from making vitamin D from the cholesterol pathway. Other cases of a low vitamin D include malabsorption, as seen in patients with coeliac disease.

3. The patient will need regular calcium and vitamin D. It is unlikely that the patient would be willing to increase her exposure to sunlight, but this would help if it can be encouraged.

CASE 99 ANSWERS

4, 14, 17, 20

1. The clinical history is strongly suggestive of dermatomyositis. This connective tissue disease presents with skin rashes and an inflammatory myositis. The rash observed on his hands is typical of Gottron's papules and photosensitivity is also recognized in this condition. He has had a gradual onset of increasing proximal muscle weakness over the past 6 months

evidenced by his deteriorating functional status. On objective testing his muscles are weak in a pattern suggestive of proximal myopathic process. His shortness of breath may relate to respiratory muscle weakness, but in view of the clinical finding of inspiratory crackles this suggests that he has an underlying interstitial lung disease.

2. The key investigations for this man are:

a. Measurement of muscle enzyme particularly creatinine kinase (CK). This is usually significantly elevated in the context of myositis. His renal function should be checked and if his CK is grossly elevated then myoglobinuria should be considered. An EMG and muscle biopsy are important in evaluation as these will confirm the inflammatory nature of his muscle disease and exclude other less common causes of muscle pathology, such as congenital dystrophies, metabolic myopathies, etc. An MR scan of his proximal muscles may reveal areas of focal inflammation, which can be useful when directing the site for a muscle biopsy, etc.

b. Further pulmonary investigations are required including pulmonary function tests to assess lung volume and carbon monoxide transfer factor. A high-resolution CT scan will help distinguish active inflammatory disease in the lung from chronic interstitial fibrosis. With regard to serological testing the ANA is frequently positive, but is a non-specific finding. In the context of myositis with associated alveolitis, antibodies to Jo-1 are also positive.

c. There is an increased risk of malignancy associated with dermatomyositis and a careful history and examination is warranted to look for potential associated signs. In a young male, testicular tumours and lymphoproliferative disorders should be particularly considered and, therefore, a genital examination, as well as a CT scan of his chest and abdomen, is appropriate to exclude these possibilities.

3. This patient has both myositis and interstitial pneumonitis, so initial treatment is with high-dose corticosteroid (prednisolone 60–80 mg daily). This should be continued for 4–6 weeks until clinical improvement has occurred and the CK has begun to normalize. Intravenous immunoglobulin (2 g/kg body weight) is a useful additional therapy to help gain rapid control of his muscle weakness. Interstitial pneumonitis will also frequently respond to this treatment regimen; however, some authorities would recommend the addition of an immunosuppressive agent (azathioprine or cyclophosphamide) in order to gain control of the inflammatory lung disease. These agents also have steroid-sparing effects and will reduce the overall exposure to steroids in the medium to long term.

CASE 100 ANSWERS

13, 16, 18, 21

1. The patient is unable to extend her 5th finger.

2. Extensor tendon rupture of the 5th extensor tendon. The 5th extensor tendon slip runs in its own sheath, but the synovitis that eroded the tendon may also be present in the common extensor tendon sheath and lead to subsequent rupture of the other tendons sequentially.

3. Surgical repair of the tendon is usually not possible. However, the tendon may be attached to its neighbour. If the ulnar styloid is very prominent and eroded, it may be contributing to the rupture of future tendons and may need excision at the same operation.

▍Index

Note: Page numbers in *italics* refer to figures.